# THE
# BEAUTY
# BIBLE

## THE ULTIMATE GUIDE
## TO SMART BEAUTY

## PAULA BEGOUN

# ALSO BY PAULA BEGOUN...

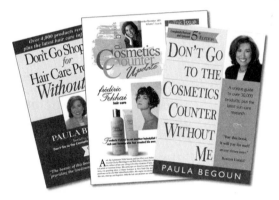

### *Don't Go to the Cosmetics Counter Without Me*, 5th Edition
Item # DG5        $24.95

Candid reviews of over 30,000 products and almost 250 lines!  Guaranteed to save you money and help you find the best skin-care and cosmetic products available.

### *Don't Go Shopping for Hair Care Products Without Me*, 2nd Edition
Item #  HAIR2      $19.95

Are salon products better than drugstore brands? Is it possible to repair, nourish, or reconstruct hair? Find answers to all your hair-care questions in this informative book, containing more than 5,000 hair-care product reviews.

### *Cosmetics Counter Update* Newsletter
Item # SUB, 1-year subscription (6 issues)
$18.75 in U.S., $26.25 in Canada, $33.75 all other countries
Online subscription $12.50 (all countries)

Keep up with the constantly changing cosmetics industry with Paula's bi-monthly newsletter. In every issue, she evaluates new cosmetics and hair-care lines, reviews new products, and provides valuable insights in response to readers' questions.

---

**800.831.4088 • www.CosmeticsCop.com**

Beginning Press   •   13075 Gateway Drive, Suite 160   •   Seattle, WA 98168

# STAY UPDATED WITH PAULA'S WEB SITE
## www.CosmeticsCop.com

### Subscribe to Paula's FREE Beauty Bulletin

Sign up today for Paula's FREE bi-weekly update and stay informed of the latest industry trends, and new products. In each Beauty Bulletin you'll find:

- Product reviews
- "Dear Paula" Q & A
- Myth-busting
- Money-saving tips

### Dear Paula

Beauty Q & A from readers, covering everything from Acne to Wrinkles.

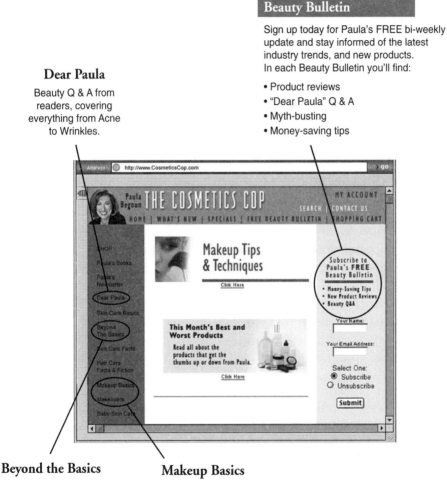

### Beyond the Basics

From Antioxidants and Retin-A to chemical peels and cosmetic surgery...find in-depth, money-saving information.

### Makeup Basics & Makeovers

Learn how to apply makeup simply and beautifully, then see the tips in action with makeovers by Paula.

Contributor: Bryan Barron
Editors: Sigrid Asmus, John Hopper, Jennifer Forbes Provo
Art Direction, Cover Design, and Typography: Erin Smith Bloom
Printing: Publishers Book Services, Inc.
Research Assistants: Bryan Barron, Kate Mee

Copyright June 2002, Paula Begoun
Publisher: Beginning Press
        13075 Gateway Drive, Suite 160
        Seattle, Washington 98168

Second Edition Printing: June 2002

ISBN   1-877988-29-4
       10 9 8 7 6 5 4 3 2 1

This book is distributed to the United States book trade by:
  Publishers Group West
  1700 Fourth Street
  Berkeley, California 94710
  (510) 528-1444

And to the Canadian book trade by:
  Raincoast Books Limited
  9050 Shaughnessy Street
  Vancouver, B.C., CANADA V6P 6E5
  (604) 633-5714

# TABLE OF CONTENTS

## CHAPTER FOUR—SKIN CARE BASICS FOR EVERYONE

## CHAPTER FIVE—SUN SENSE

## CHAPTER SIX—SKIN-CARE PLANNING

## CHAPTER SEVEN—SKIN-CARE BATTLE PLANS

## CHAPTER EIGHT—BATTLE PLANS FOR WRINKLES

## CHAPTER NINE—BATTLE PLANS FOR DRY SKIN

## CHAPTER TEN—BATTLE PLANS FOR BLEMISHES

## CHAPTER FOURTEEN—COSMETIC SURGERY

## CHAPTER FIFTEEN—MEN'S SKIN CARE

## CHAPTER SIXTEEN—BABY SKIN CARE

# CHAPTER SEVENTEEN—BODY AND NAIL CARE

## CHAPTER EIGHTEEN—MAKEUP APPLICATION STEP BY STEP

## CHAPTER NINETEEN—PROBLEMS? SOLUTIONS!

# CHAPTER TWENTY—ANIMAL RIGHTS

# NOTE FROM THE PUBLISHER

The intent of this book is to present the author's research, ideas, and perceptions regarding skin care, makeup, cosmetic surgical procedures, and the marketing, selling, and use of cosmetics and skin-care products. The author's sole purpose is to provide consumers with information and advice regarding skin care, the purchase of beauty products, and cosmetic procedures. The information and recommendations presented are strictly those of the author, reflecting the author's opinions about the subjects and the products described. Some women may find success with a skin-care routine or product that is not mentioned herein. It is everyone's inalienable right to choose and to judge products and procedures on the basis of their own criteria, research, and standards, and to disagree with the author. More important, because everyone's skin can react differently to external stimuli, any product can cause a negative reaction. If you develop sensitivity to a skin-care product or cosmetic, stop using it immediately and consult your physician. If you need medical advice regarding your skin or the various cosmetic procedures available, it is best to consult a dermatologist, board-certified plastic surgeon, or your own medical practitioner.

# CHAPTER 1

## COSMETICS COP

## WHY A NEW EDITION?

Much has changed in the world of cosmetics since I wrote the first edition of this book back in 1995. Serious research has increased exponentially on all fronts—from antioxidants, anti-irritants, and the aging of skin, to why skin wrinkles, how skin heals, what the effects of hormones are on skin function, and how to treat blackheads and acne, not to mention a better understanding of how sun and oxygen destroy skin. Cosmetic dermatology and plastic surgery procedures have greatly improved, though the array of options has become more extensive and the risks more difficult to evaluate. As I compiled the research and began rewriting this book, I was amazed at how far the cosmetics world has advanced in understanding how skin behaves and reacts to environmental factors, to the passing of time, and to the products we put on it. I also am dismayed at how much has remained the same when it comes to misleading claims, poor formulations, products that contain ingredients that can hurt skin, and products that are priced with nothing more in mind than seducing women who are tempted by high prices because they are convinced that expensive means better. It was an amazing process to assemble all this information. At first I thought it was going to be a fairly simple update. It turns out that almost 75% of this book was completely rewritten and reorganized. I hope you find the information as eye opening as I did.

## WHY YOU NEED TO READ THIS BOOK

Here's the answer, in simple terms: Because reading this book will save you money. Lots of money! Depending on how you spend money on skin care, it can add up to savings of thousands of dollars over the years. More important, it can also help you take better care of your skin. It may literally save your skin if you happen to be using products that are poorly formulated or just plain bad for skin. What you don't know about skin care and makeup can waste money and hurt your skin. The bottom line is simple too: Getting ripped off isn't pretty.

For those of you who don't know me, let me introduce myself. I am the author and publisher of several best-selling books on the cosmetics industry. My first was *Blue Eyeshadow Should Be Illegal* (which was revised four times and reprinted dozens more); then came *Don't Go to the Cosmetics Counter Without Me* (the sixth edition will be published in January 2003); and *Don't Go Shopping for Hair Care Products Without Me*. In addition, I am a syndicated columnist with Knight Ridder News Tribune Service, and a consultant to other cosmetics companies, helping them understand the latest research regarding ingredients in relation to skin health.

Over the years my writing has been based strictly on my earnest desire to get beyond the hype and chicanery of the cosmetics industry and to disseminate straightforward information a consumer can really use to look and feel more beautiful.

My expertise, like that of any other consumer reporter who covers such topics as food, cars, or toys, is based on extensive research in the subject area. What makes my situation unique is that I also have over 20 years of personal experience from working as a professional makeup artist and aesthetician and from selling makeup and skin-care products at department stores, salons, and my own stores, and, recently, selling my own product line.

I use my reporting background to continually and extensively research the cosmetics industry. I base all my comments on comprehensive interviews with dermatologists, oncologists, cosmetics chemists, and cosmetic ingredient manufacturers, and on information I've gleaned from both medical journals and cosmetics industry magazines. I am constantly reviewing scientific abstracts and studies. I do not capriciously or abruptly make any conclusions. Everything I report is supported by studies and information from experts in the field, and I document my sources throughout this book. Naturally, there are many who disagree with my assertions, and I do the best I can to present other points of view whenever possible. However, I assure you that a great number of people in the industry agree with my conclusions, even if they can't do so publicly.

In many ways I'm surprised that reviewing, researching, investigating, and questioning the cosmetics industry is what I do for a living. When I started out as a makeup artist back in 1978 it was never my intent to end up writing as a consumer advocate about the cosmetics industry.

At first my quest was personal. I had suffered with acne for many years. I visited over a dozen dermatologists, I tried hundreds of skin-care products from both inexpensive and expensive cosmetics lines, and still I had acne. How could that be? How could all the stuff I diligently applied to my skin—which salesperson after salesperson and doctor after doctor assured me would work—not work? Sometimes one routine worked a little, but not as well as I had hoped and not for very long. And there were always side effects. Most products made my skin so red and irritated I thought it was going to fall off. Slowly but surely I worked my way through the confusion, and after much research and lots more frustration I began to recognize some fundamental problems with the information provided and the products sold by the cosmetics industry. I also found that many of the same difficulties were present in the field of dermatology.

The cosmetics industry's information was little more than marketing mumbo jumbo with exaggerated or misleading claims. In the field of dermatology most doctors don't have time to give their patients the information they need or to explain the limitations and pros and cons of treatment. There is also a great deal of misinformation, not to mention myths that dermatologists generate on their own now that almost 50% of them are selling skin-care products.

In truth, I started out wanting to be an actress, and being a makeup artist was a way to pay the rent. In a very short time it became clear to me that I wasn't going to enjoy much success at acting, or at least I didn't have what it takes to persevere, but I did have what it takes to be a good makeup artist and skin-care consultant. My clientele quickly grew, as did my income. I found I definitely preferred a paycheck to struggling with acting auditions and rejections. Of course, that didn't mean everything was rosy. Along the way, when my freelance makeup business was slow, I supplemented my income with work at department-store makeup counters. But each new job for a different cosmetics line resulted in my being fired.

My first dismissal came after an argument with the line representative of a department-store cosmetics company where I was working. The representative wanted me to say that a toner could close pores and a moisturizer could heal, when I knew it wasn't true. (If a toner could close pores, everyone who used toners would have flawless, poreless skin, and if moisturizers could heal skin, no one would have a pimple or a wrinkle or a scar.) That job lasted about two months.

Several months later, at another department store and for a different cosmetics company, I was involved in a conflict with several of the cosmetics saleswomen working at the other counters. If a customer wanted a particular type of product and I didn't think the product from the line I was selling was right, or if my line didn't offer one, I would walk her over to another counter that I knew had the right product and sell it to her. That caused a nuclear meltdown. I was told to stay behind my counter and not touch another product from any line other than the one I was assigned! (When I recommended that the woman could walk over to the other counter herself, I got in trouble with the sales representatives from my line.) How ludicrous! A great product, five feet away, was out of my reach because it wasn't from the counter I was standing behind.

My final department-store cosmetics counter experience ended when I just couldn't take listening to the distortions and exaggerated claims anymore, and decided to go out on my own. I opened my own makeup stores in 1981. I didn't sell blue eyeshadow, wrinkle creams, or toners that claimed to close pores. Along the way, I hooked up with a business partner who was at first thrilled with my ideas and concept, mainly because of the media attention my rather controversial stores attracted.

My stores were generating a lot of attention from the press, and eventually I was asked to make regular appearances on a local TV station in Seattle, KIRO-TV. I also started receiving national and international TV and print exposure.

Eventually my ideas and concept no longer pleased my partner. The department store counters were crowded with women buying blue eyeshadow, wrinkle creams, and toners, so why shouldn't we sell them too? After all, if you saw women throwing away their money on those sorts of products, at prices ranging from $25 to $250 an ounce for items that cost 75 cents to $4 to produce, you wouldn't want a partner like me either. I sold my shares back to her in 1984 and stayed at KIRO-TV for the next two years. Sadly, the stores went out of business shortly after I sold them—but I learned a lot about investigative reporting and writing during my time at KIRO-TV in Seattle.

I left the TV station in 1986 after finishing my first book, *Blue Eyeshadow Should Be Illegal*. I decided to self-publish after receiving several rejection letters from major publishing companies telling me that, although they liked my manuscript, I wasn't a celebrity or model, and no one would be interested in my point of view. I disagreed. I believed lots of women (OK, not all) were tired of hearing useless, and at times incorrect, information from models and celebrities who were born beautiful and knew which makeup artists, photographers, and managers to hire, but very little about the cosmetics they promoted.

I was right, and I sold several hundred thousand copies of my first book! I believed I had given the consumer the more balanced complete information she needed to tackle the cosmetics industry. I was wrong. After I wrote *Blue Eyeshadow*, I received thousands of letters from women asking me, now that they knew how crazy the cosmetics industry was, what they should buy or what I thought of this product or that. It was one thing to have an overview of the cosmetics industry, but quite another to have specific information about a specific product. How could anyone tell if the formulation was effective? How would a person know whether the information about the research done by the doctor or scientist who formulated it was valid? How could someone find out if a company's claims about their impressive study backing up their miracle skin-care product were true? That's when I wrote *Don't Go to the Cosmetics Counter Without Me*.

Meanwhile, the demand to know what works and what doesn't has grown, mainly because the industry has grown. The number of new product lines emerging every day is sheer madness. Between keeping up with infomercials, multilevel direct marketing lines, home shopping network lines, new lines at the department stores and drugstores, and the endless parade of new product launches from existing cosmetic lines, my job was only beginning.

That brings me to today and the revision of this book. The cosmetics industry has gone through many changes since I wrote *Blue Eyeshadow* and the first edition of *The Beauty Bible*. In many ways the industry has gotten more complicated, yet as the research into skin and skin-care products has increased it has also become more exciting. My goal with this revised edition of *The Beauty Bible* is to compile and clarify the new data and research to help each woman create the best skin-care routine possible for her specific needs. In addition, I want to help women achieve the best makeup look possible in the fewest steps with the easiest and most effective techniques.

As is true in all the books I write, I also want to separate cosmetics fact from cosmetics fiction and reality from myth, because the fiction and myths spread by the cosmetics industry are nothing less than startling and frustrating. Compared to the information provided by the cosmetics industry, Mother Goose stories sound like the *Encyclopedia Britannica*.

Perhaps the most difficult part of my job is keeping a straight face when I hear the crazy things cosmetics salespeople tell consumers. Combating this endless parade of useless and bizarre information can be maddening. But it's my job and, thankfully, it has been far more rewarding than I ever expected.

## EVALUATING PRODUCTS

How I evaluate skin-care formulations deserves some straightforward explanation. Think of the ingredient lists you find on prepared or processed food products, and information on the nutrition content of whole foods. These are the best analogies I can make to ingredient lists on cosmetics products. When it comes to dietary health concerns or awareness, most women start by judging a food on the basis of its ingredient list, or the nutrition content. Information about fat, sodium, preservatives, coloring agents, calories, and many other details, is spelled out there. Then the consumer, using various health resources (books, health professionals, research journals, reliable Web sites) can evaluate the Food and Drug Administration (FDA) mandated ingredient information. Without that information, regardless of how the item tastes (everyone has their own bias), you would never know what you were putting into your body. You could be causing yourself harm by eating more fat than you should, or eating more calories than you should, or skimping on vitamins, antioxidants, fiber, or protein, and on and on, leading to a variety of health problems.

Food labels are incredibly important, and so are the labels on skin-care products. To continue with the food analogy, for example, if one cake mix contains 100 calories per serving but a different cake mix contains 500 calories per serving, that's fundamental information you can use to decide which one you want to buy. Or suppose you are looking for chocolate cake and you find that the mix contains artificial chocolate flavoring—you would probably want to consider another choice. Likewise, if a skin-care product says it is good for sensitive skin but contains ingredients known to cause irritation or breakouts, that is crucial information for making a decision. If a skin-care product sells for $100 but contains the same ingredients as a product that costs $20, that is important information. If a product says it is good for breakouts but contains alcohol and peppermint oil, it would be helpful to know how those ingredients could hurt your face and actually cause more breakouts. That's why the ingredient list is important: It helps you sort through the jungle of choices. Besides, it is a far better starting point for making decisions than are unsubstantiated or one-sided advertising claims.

The fundamental review process for each ingredient or product formulation starts with analyzing the published research about whether or not those ingredients or formulations are capable of providing the asserted benefit.

When it comes to makeup, my team and I actually test a large percentage of the products reviewed. I have purchased over $100,000 worth of cosmetics and I spend a great deal of time at the cosmetics counters. I use, and test, a lot of makeup, relying on my years of experience along with the feedback I receive from thousands of women.

For makeup application, I make it a point to explain tools and techniques that makes sense for everyday use. This isn't the book to use for elaborate or trendy makeup looks. Fashion magazines are replete with those and you don't need another book to help you paint black smudges all around your eyes or apply glitter from head to toe.

## COSMETICS CHEMISTRY–AN ART AND A SCIENCE

I had the opportunity to speak at a meeting of the Society of Cosmetic Chemists, Chicago Chapter, in October 2001. I told this group of accomplished scientists that, despite my anger at the cosmetics industry when it comes to their claims and misleading information, I wanted to affirm that there are wonderful products out there. I know I tend to overemphasize the negative—the crazy claims, prices, and poor quality—but there are also countless extraordinary products to choose from. This boundless parade of superlative makeup and skin-care products is nothing less than exciting for the consumer.

Every step of the way I am in awe of how beautifully most cosmetics work. Where would we be without the brilliant work of the cosmetics chemists who make the exquisite products we use? Because of their astonishing skill, we have moisturizers that take care of dry skin and help skin heal. They create mascaras that can build thick, lush lashes without flaking or smearing, and foundations that smooth out skin tone, making it look flawless. We have sunscreens that protect skin from sunburn as well as from wrinkles and the potential for skin cancer. There is an endless array of sensuous lipsticks that add relatively long-lasting color and definition to the mouth (and keep it there even longer with the advent of Procter & Gamble's PermaTone lip color—but I'll get into that in the makeup section of this book). Not to mention blushes that softly accent cheekbones and eyeshadows that define eyes, and, well, the list is endless.

I want to sincerely thank all the cosmetics companies who have provided so much of their time and information to me for this book, as well as for my newsletter and my other books. We often don't see eye to eye, but despite our differences, more companies than ever have been generous and forthcoming with information and products.

I also want to thank all the cosmetics chemists everywhere who strive to produce the better and better products that continue to make the beauty industry so incredibly beautiful. I also want to ask cosmetics chemists to do the best they can, whenever they can, to combat the insane marketing departments they have to work with! After interviewing and talking to hundreds of cosmetics chemists over the years, I know most of you don't believe even a fraction of what the advertisements, salespeople, infomercial hucksters, or editorials in fashion magazines say about the products you create. Your work is rooted in science, not hyperbole. I also know this is a risky business. After all, creating products that no one buys is not going to get anyone a promotion, and the marketing department knows all too well what women love to hear, no matter how ridiculous. But try anyway, just to bring a bit of fresh air into an otherwise very cloudy business.

## IS BEAUTY EVER NATURAL?

Beauty is definitely in the eye of the beholder, but in our culture, where the cosmetics industry is a $40 billion a year industry, beauty takes effort and money. From celebrities to models, and from homemakers to lawyers, hair care, skin care, and makeup are part of a woman's morning ritual. It is probably important for me to make it clear (as the picture of me on the cover of this books shows) that I am hardly anti-makeup, anti-skin care, or anti-hair care—far from it. I do use several skin-care products, I wear makeup (sometimes a lot of makeup), I dye my hair, I have had corrective cosmetic medical procedures (including BoTox, breast implants, and nonablative laser resurfacing), I get manicures and pedicures, and I am diligent about wearing sunscreen. Some women may be shocked at the fact that I am not writing about "a return to basics" or making your own cosmetics. My entire perspective throughout every book that I've ever written is to be as nonjudgmental as possible about a woman's personal decisions on what she chooses to do around her own appearance. When it comes to almost all aspects of beauty, I am interested in relating the research in regard to what works and what doesn't. The final decision is always up to the consumer. No matter what that decision is, I want every woman to know what is possible (or impossible) to gain by using a product, so she can purchase what works and not waste money on gimmicks or products that can't possibly live up to their claims.

# CHAPTER 2

# UNDERSTANDING THE HYPE

> If you don't understand how the cosmetics industry
> works—the good, the bad, and the ugly—you will
> be a victim of its advertising manipulations,
> exaggerations, and deceptions, and that isn't
> good for your skin or your budget.

## WHY COSMETICS COMPANIES CAN MISLEAD LEGALLY

One of the most beguiling aspects of the cosmetics industry is that the Food and Drug Administration (FDA) doesn't require cosmetics companies to prove their claims. ("Neither cosmetic products nor cosmetic ingredients are reviewed or approved by FDA before they are sold to the public"[Source: FDA *Office of Cosmetics and Colors Fact Sheet*, February 3, 1995]). That means cosmetics companies get to say just about anything they want about their products without any substantiation or proof whatsoever. Pharmaceutical and over-the-counter drug regulations are infinitely stricter than those dealing with cosmetics. If a drug company makes a claim about what an antihistamine can do to prevent sneezing, the product must contain particular ingredients in specified amounts to win approval from the FDA. The same is true for aspirin and other analgesics, antacids, decongestants, anti-inflammatories, and drugs across the board in the world of pharmaceuticals. It is not true for cosmetics. A cosmetics company can say a product provides all sorts of alleged benefits, from firming to closing pores to repairing skin, yet the benefits don't have to be proven.

The only fundamental FDA restriction on cosmetics companies' claims is the legal prohibition of phrases that directly state or promise a permanent change in the skin. Of course, there are a million ways to make something sound permanent to consumers without sounding permanent to the FDA.

What about federal regulations concerning truth in advertising? That issue generally falls under the jurisdiction of the Federal Trade Commission (FTC) and the Federal Communications Commission (FCC), but it doesn't take much to get around these guys either. For example, I can describe at great length how miraculously my product works as long as I throw in phrases such as "appears to," "seems to," "feels as if," "looks like," "you may experience," and lots more variations on these themes. All of these phrases invalidate any promise about a product's performance. A company is not considered to be lying to the consumer when these kinds of terms are used because the purported results are subjective, not actual. It may "seem" like your cellulite has disappeared, or you may "appear" to look younger, or you can "experience" a clear complexion, but nothing has happened except that you may be convinced something has taken place. That's how cosmetics advertising gets around truth-in-advertising restrictions every time.

One of the other ways cosmetics companies deal with claim substantiation is to create "studies" that prove that their product is effective. This isn't difficult to do, because there's an entire industry of labs that can help cosmetics companies support whatever they want to say about a product. A laboratory test can show miraculous results from any product by using nonscientific protocols. This means the tests are not double blind, a placebo isn't used, and the product isn't compared to any other competing formulation. For example, a typical study set up to prove that a moisturizer reduces wrinkles places the company's moisturizer on one side of the face and nothing on the other side. No wonder the side with the moisturizer looks 150% better! Yet any moisturizer would net the same results.

Aside from the lack of regulation and the manipulation of research to create a veneer of scientific authority, advertisements that promise everything from younger skin to smoother thighs give a woman plenty of psychological incentive to see a difference in her skin.

## HYPOALLERGENIC? NONCOMEDOGENIC? DERMATOLOGIST TESTED?

Cosmetics companies give their claims a scientific coating with words like "dermatologist tested," "noncomedogenic," "hypoallergenic," "designed for sensitive skin," "laboratory tested," and "our research shows." But those claims are smoke and mirrors, with nothing behind them but artifice and half-truths. Essentially, none of those terms can hold an ounce of meaning—because there are no regulations setting up standard definitions for them. That's why there are no regulations to make cosmetics companies live up to their claims regarding any of these terms

(Source: *FDA Office of Cosmetics and Colors Fact Sheet*, December 19, 1994, revised October 18, 2000).

"Dermatologist tested" does not tell you which dermatologist did the testing, or what he or she tested. "Noncomedogenic" makes it sound as if the product won't cause blackheads, but where are the data on how that was determined? Assuming a test was conducted, was it done on the skin of someone who never had a blemish in his or her whole life? Surely the results would be radically different from the results of a test performed on someone who suffered from acne.

"Hypoallergenic" and "designed for sensitive skin" are nonsense words that imply a product is unlikely to cause allergic reactions. Here, too, without firm standards every company can make its own determination of what those words mean. I've seen lots of products that claim to be "safer for sensitive skin," yet they contain problematic plants, fragrance, camphor, alcohol, and myriad other ingredients that are known to cause skin reactions.

"Laboratory tested" and "our research shows" might be all well and good, but if the research was conducted by the company's own lab, it's not exactly independent or unbiased information. Furthermore, the test results may just have been the cosmetics chemists saying they like the product a lot. Although a lot of cosmetic testing does go on in the world, there is a stunning lack of it as well. Some endlessly hyped cosmetic ingredients have absolutely no research showing efficacy of any kind. I've searched for abstracts (studies) that evaluate the effectiveness of such heralded cosmetic ingredients as bovine extract, spleen extract, placenta extract, wild yam extract, myriad plant extracts, minerals, emu oil, milk protein, royal jelly, and many, many more in treating aging skin or acne. Other than research commissioned by the companies that sell these ingredients or make products that contain these ingredients, there is nothing proving that these are helpful for skin. The lack of independent research is astounding.

Despite the empty promises made for these wonder ingredients, and the fact that only minuscule amounts show up in absurdly expensive products, consumers desperately hope that this lotion or that cream may finally be the fountain of youth. Of course they aren't. In fact, the emphasis on miracle plant extracts or animal byproducts takes a consumer's attention away from ingredients that do have substantial proof that they can be helpful for skin. For ingredients such as sunscreens, ceramides, glycerin, silicones, glycosaminoglycans, salicylic acid, topical disinfectants, alpha hydroxy acids, various antioxidants, and anti-irritants, the research is real. The same is true for over-the-counter and prescription products whose effectiveness is well substantiated, such as Retin-A, Renova, Differin (adapelene), topical antibiotics, and Accutane.

**The only part of the cosmetics industry that is closely regulated is the ingredient list.** In the United States since 1978, in Australia since 1993, and in the European Union since 1997, ingredient lists have been mandatory on every cosmetic product sold, whether it is makeup, skin care, or hair care. (Come on, Canada, what's taking you so long? You still don't have mandatory ingredient lists and there is still no set date for changing this [Source: Health Canada *Cosmetic Fact Sheet*, July 2001].)

Cosmetics ingredients must be listed in the order of their quantity, beginning with the largest one and going to the smallest, which is why water is almost always the first ingredient listed. The ingredient list is the only place where a consumer can readily find the truth about what she is buying. Ironically, as accurate and truthful as it is, it's also the most difficult part of the label to decipher. There are thousands of cosmetic ingredients available to a chemist to create any of a wide variety of products. It's no easy task for the consumer to differentiate between highly technical ingredient names. Yet even if you had a good basic understanding of cosmetic ingredients, which some consumers do, neither the exact amounts nor the formulation specifications are discernible just from reading the ingredient list.

I absolutely don't want to dissuade anyone from reading ingredient lists, quite the contrary. But the ingredient list provides just an overview. Some very good ingredients work best in very minute amounts, while others are useless if they aren't among the first on the list.

It's my job to help you figure out what doesn't work and what does, and what the most effective quantities are to get results. Over the past 20 years I've continually reviewed and discussed formulary considerations with cosmetics chemists and pored over the available research on a wide range of cosmetic ingredients. Reading this book will help you learn what to pay attention to and what to ignore, so you can take better care of your skin and stop wasting money.

## ARE ALL-NATURAL PRODUCTS BEST?

That's a trick question, because in the world of cosmetics there are truly no such things as "all-natural" cosmetics. They don't exist, and if they did they would not be good for the skin.

Whatever preconceived or media-induced fiction you might believe about natural ingredients being better for the skin has no factual basis or scientific legitimacy. Not only is the definition of "natural" hazy, but the term isn't even regulated, so each cosmetics company can use it to mean something different. "If a company wants to call their products natural, it can, and it doesn't matter what they contain. [The] FDA has tried to establish official definitions for the use of certain terms such as 'natural...' but its regulations were overturned in court. So companies can use them on cosmetic labels to mean anything or nothing at all. Most of the terms have considerable market value in promoting cosmetic products to consumers, but dermatologists say they have very little medical meaning" (Source: FDA *Consumer Magazine*, August 2000).

Further, the 1999 November-December issue of *Consumer Magazine* stated: "Don't be fooled by the term 'natural.' It's often used in health fraud as an attention-grabber; it suggests a product is safer than conventional treatments. But the term doesn't necessarily equate to safety because some plants ... can kill when ingested.... And, any product—synthetic or natural—potent enough to work like a drug is going to be potent enough to cause side effects."

So what is a "natural" cosmetic? Good question. It can mean anything and nothing. For most cosmetics companies it means including plant extracts in their formulations along with an array of synthetic ingredients.

Companies like Aveda that claim to be based on an all-natural concept do list the technical-sounding ingredients along with their natural sources. Although this appears to be helpful information, it still leads consumers in the wrong direction. For example, ammonium lauryl sulfate, a standard detergent cleansing agent, is listed on the Aveda ingredient label as being derived from coconut oil. Doesn't that make it sound pure and pleasant? Ammonium lauryl sulfate is the salt of a sulfuric acid compound, neutralized with an ingredient like triethanolamine. None of that is bad for the skin, and I wouldn't tell anyone to avoid ammonium lauryl sulfate, but that is the more accurate description of that ingredient. Associating it with coconut oil, a far-removed organic source, just makes for better (though misleading) marketing lingo. (It is important to point out that Aveda products also contain a vast array of synthetic ingredients, including synthetic coloring agents, preservatives, film formers, and slip agents.)

Even if an "all-natural" product did exist, you wouldn't want to use it on your skin anyway. Think about a bunch of plants, fruits, or vegetables sitting in your refrigerator (or bathroom for that matter). What would happen if they didn't contain preservatives? In just a few days they would become moldy and disgusting. In contrast, skin-care products contain very "unnatural"-sounding preservatives, and that's great. According to many cosmetics chemists, a reliable preservative system helps avoid the risk of microbial contamination, which could cause problems for the eyes, lips, and skin.

Many natural ingredients can cause allergies, irritation, and skin sensitivities. Just think of how many people have a hay fever response to a wide variety of plants, and that these plants often show up in cosmetics. Citrus often shows up in skin-care products, but most of us have gotten lemon on a slight cut while cooking and know it burns like crazy because it's irritating to skin. "Natural" doesn't tell you anything about the efficacy of the ingredients in a product.

Hanging on to the notion that "natural" equals good skin-care or better makeup products will waste your money and probably hurt your skin. I'm not sure if the majority of women who buy cosmetics are ever going to believe this. For many women, it's hard to resist the pressure to believe the lie about natural products being better for the skin. What makes this natural craze so annoying and undesirable is that it perpetuates myths that can hurt a woman's skin. All of the following natural ingredients can cause skin irritation, allergic reactions, skin sensitivity, and/or sun sensitivity: almond extract, allspice, angelica, arnica, balm mint oil, balsam, basil, bergamot, cinnamon, citrus, clove, clover blossom, cocoa butter, cornstarch, coriander oil, cottonseed oil, fennel, fir needle, geranium oil, grapefruit, horsetail, lavender oil, lemon, lemongrass, lime, marjoram, lemon balm, oak bark, papaya, peppermint, rose, sage, thyme, witch hazel, and wintergreen. The label might say natural, but you could be buying a purely irritating product that might cause an allergic reaction.

Furthermore, the notion that natural ingredients are better than synthetic ingredients is even more distressing, because it just isn't true. **While vegetable or plant oils may sound better for the skin, varying forms of silicones (i.e., siloxanes, dimethicones, cyclomethicones) are just as beneficial and offer impressive benefits for the skin. But it's hard to glamorize and advertise a "synthetic," unnatural-sounding ingredient.** Silicones show up in over 80% of all skin-care, makeup, and hair-care products you buy. Yet you rarely hear about them because the cosmetics companies think consumers won't find them as sexy or alluring as plants, or oxygen therapy, or cellular repair, or a thousand other marketing angles that have nothing to do with what really works for your skin.

I'm not saying there aren't some natural-sounding ingredients that are exceptional for the skin, because there are—lots of them—but the idea that they are the "best option" or are still natural once they have been extracted from their source and mixed into a cosmetic is ludicrous.

The following letter from a reader epitomizes the misconceptions many men and women have regarding natural products:

## Dear Paula,

**I read your newspaper column about the lady who is allergic to hair color. I realize that you are not a fan of natural products, but to not tell this lady to try some of the natural hair colors on the market is terrible. There are many, including Naturtint and Herbatint for full gray hair coverage. These are great**

for sensitive people. Please Paula, look into these. To tell this lady to get allergy testing rather than suggest a natural product is almost a crime. Is your goal to help the consumer or the big companies who likely provide kickbacks? If it is the latter then you should change your name from Cosmetics Cop to Big Company Employee. [I don't understand] your continued disregard for natural products and getting help to consumers (which may not always be with a natural product), [and] I am mad.

**Vicki, via e-mail**

Dear Vicki,

I can't even get many cosmetics companies to return my phone calls much less provide products for reviews (and money would just be a joke—that's reserved for celebrity endorsers, not critics of the industry). While I understand your concern about my recommendations, please understand that I did not overlook the options you mentioned, nor am I opposed to natural ingredients, as long as they are safe and effective. However, the products you mentioned, Naturtint and Herbatint, are not natural in the least. In fact, they are decidedly unnatural, and include as many problematic ingredients as you may find in any other permanent hair-dye product, whether from the drugstore or the salon.

Herbatint is a permanent hair coloring that claims to have "a natural herbal base and no ammonia [and] that gently colors and protects hair structure while giving hair a deep natural gloss and brilliance. It is the only color that has the advantage of coloring without damaging the hair structure." Yet it only takes a quick glance at the ingredient list to notice that this is not gentle or natural and that there are ingredients that can damage hair. Here is the exact ingredient list for Herbatint's hair-color products. [My comments and concerns about specific ingredients are shown in brackets.] "Water, Nonoxynol-6, Nonoxynol-4 [these are forms of phenol], Ethanolamine [releases nitrosamines], Propylene Glycol [popularly referred to as anti-freeze], EDTA, Sodium Metabisulfite [a reducing and bleaching agent; it is extremely alkaline and potentially damaging to hair], Walnut Extract, Rhubarb Extract, Cinchona Extract, P-Phenylenediamine [this is the ingredient suspected of being carcinogenic in hair-dye products; Source: FDA Center for Food Safety and Applied Nutrition], Resorcinol [a form of phenol, which is derived from petroleum and is irritating to skin; there is serious concern about its use in cosmetics], O-Aminophenol, M-Aminophenol [both are derived from phenol]." Naturtint's ingredients are just as problematic, at least from any natural perspective.

Although those ingredients pose concern, there are no alternatives for permanently dyeing hair (changing hair color or covering any amount of gray for an extended length of time) that do not contain an assortment of problematic ingredients. I wish that wasn't the case, but there is no way around it, except for not dyeing your hair.

Many consumers believe in the trustworthiness and reliability of products that are called natural. It is a misplaced conviction. I feel strongly that your anger at me is misdirected; your ire should instead be aimed at the companies who are asserting false information that is potentially dangerous to the consumer.

## ADVERTISING VICTIMS

While the absence of consumer information plays a role in most women's cosmetics buying, it is pervasive and endless advertising that fuels their decisions. Advertising must work or the cosmetics industry wouldn't spend billions of dollars on television, print (particularly fashion magazines), and radio advertising to get you to buy their products. If you don't understand how advertising manipulates your purchases, you will always be a victim of its wiles and contrivances. Lots of consumers make decisions about what they are going to buy based strictly on advertising. Is it any wonder that the advertising industry in the United States is a multibillion-dollar business? Procter & Gamble alone spends $1.3 billion annually to advertise its products to the American public. L'Oreal and Estee Lauder each spend about the same. Companies spend these vast sums on advertising because they want (and get) more sales. Cosmetics companies sign celebrities to multimillion-dollar endorsement contracts because they know certain faces can sell millions of dollars' worth of products.

We may think we recognize the influence advertising can have on us, and even feel we are above this kind of blatant artifice. But whether we like to admit it or not, we are greatly influenced by the power of advertising.

As you flip through fashion magazines or watch television, notice that a typical ad for makeup or skin-care products showcases a beautiful young (and I mean really young) model. The underlying message is that if you buy the right makeup or skin-care products, you will be beautiful, have a good body, win male attention, eliminate wrinkles, reap praise from those you know, enjoy increased fun, and radiate sex appeal just like the model.

Although gorgeous models are an especially obvious advertising tool, the technique of persuading consumers to buy is limited only by the creativity of Madison Avenue (the advertising bastion). One basic tenet of the business is repetition, repetition, repetition. Typically, when a new product is launched by a company, it is promoted via radio, television, newspapers, magazines, counter displays, and promotional literature. With these constant reminders, it soon becomes apparent, either subconsciously or consciously, that you are missing out on something if you don't have whatever it is you've been hearing about. (Repetition as a reinforcer is most evident in the world of infomercials, but more about that later in this chapter.)

Without a pretty face, a cosmetics company ensures its longevity by creating the impression of superiority to other companies. Establishing a solid reputation in the minds of the consumer is a significant goal, although superiority is only a perception. Cosmetics companies spend billions of dollars to promote their logos as symbols of reliability and value. Once a woman has confidence in a company's ability to produce a good product, for example, Estee Lauder's Creme de la Mer moisturizer, she can be easily persuaded that the other ten or so products with the same Creme de la Mer logo (though completely different formulations) are just as good and worth the extremely high price tag. Whether that's true or not is another story, but the perception is all that counts.

Price, another consumer issue, has its own tricky, elusive attraction. It may motivate more decisions to buy than any other appeal. The magic words "sale" or "discount" are directed at consumers with great frequency and in all price categories. Clothes with designer labels such as Donna Karan, Chanel, and Ralph Lauren can be found on sale (eventually) in the most chic department stores. But when it comes to cosmetics, discounts are found only in drugstores, through in-home sales, and on infomercials. There are no discounts at the department-store cosmetics counters because discounts have a "cheap" connotation that high-end cosmetics companies want to avoid like the plague. Instead, these companies maintain the image of exclusivity by offering "gift with purchase" or "purchase with purchase" deals. The "something-for-nothing" appeal of this bizarre marketing style has women waiting in line as if they really were getting something for nothing.

In essence, the more expensive cosmetics companies very quietly, though quite plainly, control prices. Have you ever seen a sale at a high-end department store's cosmetics counters? After all, if Nordstrom had a sale on Estee Lauder products, what would Macy's do? Macy's would have to cut its prices, and so would Lord & Taylor, and then Marshall Fields, and then Bloomingdale's. Can you imagine the competitive cosmetics retailing that would get established at the department stores? The "gift with purchase" would pale as a consumer incentive. Everyone would just wait for sales, and the glamour and status of shopping the counters would evaporate. It would be great for the consumer who shops sales regularly at the department store, but the cosmetics companies, which keep a tight rein on the department stores, think of it as a nightmare that could become reality all over the country. Keep in mind that price fixing (although the cosmetics companies would never call it that, because it brings up antitrust questions) is quite illegal. Yet it is business as usual at the cosmetics counters.

Celebrity endorsements are another powerful advertising tool in the cosmetics industry. Celebrities are visible everywhere in infomercials and fashion editorials (information about which celebrity is using which new product or skin treatment racks up lots of sales) because we as consumers equate acting ability or celebrity status with knowledge and integrity. An endorsement by someone with a well-known face carries weight. But is what a movie star uses on her skin in any way relevant to your skin-care needs? Do a world-famous model's beauty, fame, and money mean she knows something you don't? Enticing as it is to believe that listening to celebrities can help you have better skin and a better look, that's not the way it is. Do we really believe that the celebrities in the ads for Revlon or Estee Lauder are there because they love the company's products? Or is it more realistic to see the truth that these models sign million-dollar contracts to smile brightly, showing their tacit, paid-for approval? A celebrity whose name is attached to a specific line has signed some type of lucrative contract; she's not endorsing the products because she loves them.

Fashion magazines often comment about products celebrities use separate from a signed endorsement. But actresses and models don't all use the same products (or the same makeup artist, plastic surgeon, or dermatologist). They use lots and lots of different products in all price ranges from a vast array of lines, and, like all women, they can be fickle. What they use today may not be what they use tomorrow. Celebrities look for "perfect" products just like the next person and are just as subject to being misled and wasting money as anyone else. Besides, what someone else is using doesn't necessarily have anything to do with your own skin-care or makeup needs.

Perhaps the most insidious and consistent form of cosmetic advertising ploy is showcasing an impossibly perfect, incongruously young woman (or several of them), groomed and photographed at the perfect moment by the best in the fashion world, and seeming to show how well a product works. As if their perfection is a result of any product or product line! In essence, this is fear advertising. Fear that everyone else has the answer, that everyone else is more beautiful and has more perfect skin than you do because they're using products that you aren't. This is a compelling, though completely false, message. The women hired for these ads weren't chosen because they used the product and became beautiful, they were selected from head shot photos provided by modeling agencies. Product use is completely irrelevant, they might even be using and wearing products from other companies.

Be aware of the vast difference between the information provided in advertising and information that is objective. Advertising is one-sided. There are no negatives in ads, except in regard to the competition's products. The truth about almost all products, whether in the cosmetics industry or another industry, is that they all have their pros and cons. It is the task of the company paying for the ad, or the salesperson selling you the product, to portray the product in absolutely glowing, positive terms. **It is, however, your job to search out as much impartial information from independent sources as possible. You might still buy the product, but at least you will have some facts to base your decision on and not just pretty pictures and catchy words.**

As far as cosmetics are concerned, the only objective information is found on the ingredient list. Of course, that's the only part of the package that never gets featured in the magazine or on television, yet it is the only place that legally has to tell you the truth.

## THE BUSINESS OF CLAIM SUBSTANTIATION

How many ads or cosmetic brochures proudly use the phrase "our studies show" and then list astounding results from what appears to be a scientific study? According to an article in *Cosmetics & Toiletries* magazine (December 1999, pages 52–53), "Skin moisturization studies using bioengineering methods are commonplace today. If data generated for a new test product demonstrate a statistically significant difference between the test product and untreated skin in favor of increased hydration, then claims indicating this to the consumer would be substantiated. ... For example, [the claim] 'moisturizes your skin for up to 8 hours' would be substantiated by a study where a statistical difference was observed between the test product and untreated skin for up to 8 hours following application of the test product." In essence, in examples like this, what the words "our studies show" are telling you is that, when compared with plain, unmoisturized, washed skin, the moisturizer made skin moist! That isn't exactly shocking. Using any moisturizer would show the same results.

There is an entire industry of claim substantiation at work in the world of cosmetics. Claim substantiation is also growing in response to new European Union cosmetic legislation regarding animal testing, substantiation of claims, and product safety (Source: 6th Amendment to the European Union Cosmetics Directive). That means the industry is fast and furiously establishing standards that basically meet regulatory standards, yet give you no information that is helpful for your skin. A test that compares dry, unmoisturized skin with dry skin that is moisturized, and then proclaims that "our product works great!" is not much of a test. It would be like doing a test that measures how drunk you can get on a martini versus not drinking a martini—it provides no information at all because the result is already known: of course you don't get drunk when you don't drink. Likewise, of course, moisturized skin looks better than skin that isn't moisturized.

Another public relations ploy used in the world of cosmetics takes advantage of reporters who are trying to be unbiased. Fashion magazines carry lots of reports and articles about the results of some new study by so-and-so, a respected doctor, pharmacist, or chemist. Yet the reporter rarely poses questions about who paid for the study, how the study was conducted (was it peer reviewed, double blind, independent?), whether the study had a broad enough scope to be significant, whether there is any independent corroborating research, and, most important, who benefits from the study. All that information is vitally important and relates directly to the study's validity and credibility.

Very few consumers, or reporters for that matter, are aware of the number of skin-care "research" laboratories whose only clients are cosmetics companies that want to use enticing statistics or validate incredible claims they can use as a marketing strategy. These research labs exist solely to provide pseudoscientific material for the cosmetics industry. That way, if the marketing copy claims that a moisturizer provides an 82% increase in moisturization or a 90% increase in the skin's water content, the company may very well be able to point to a study that says this is true. Whether the study is the least bit valid is another question altogether. Quoting these inconclusive, vague studies in a news story or ad can make them sound significant and meaningful, but in truth they are more often than not just more hype and exaggeration generated to sell products. One of these claim-substantiation companies actually advertises its ability to deliver "creative claim generation/substantiation."

Here's a perfect example of how these feigned studies are performed. Let's take a typical claim about a moisturizer providing a large increase in the skin's moisture content. Without some basic information about how the study was conducted, that percentage is meaningless. You can take almost anyone's skin, rub some alcohol on it or even just wash it with plain soap, then put on any moisturizer in the world, and the skin would reflect anywhere from an 82% to a 200% increase in moisture content. (In fact, you can sit in the bathtub for 30 minutes and come out with your skin well saturated with water and have a 500% increase in its moisture content.) Furthermore, perhaps the test included only five or ten women and compared only two products, one with an unknown formula. It may indicate that for this small group, brand A worked better than brand X—but what about how it worked compared with the 5,000 other moisturizers on the market? Maybe lots of those work just as well as brand A.

Such features are very typical in these types of studies. At first glance, the study sounds impressive, yet it is virtually meaningless. It doesn't tell you anything about the product's effectiveness, or even whether that product is good for the skin (it turns out a high moisture content isn't!), but it gives the cosmetics company statistics it can show off in its press releases.

I've seen this process at work firsthand, and it is disturbing. Whoever is paying the bill hires the research lab. The lab is handed the products and told what to look for and what kind of results are needed—for example, proof of moisturization, exfoliation, smoothness, or some other parameter. Then the lab goes about setting up a study to prove that position. Rarely are these studies done double blind, or do they use a large group of women, or show long-term results, and rarely (actually never) are the results negative. More to the point, these studies are never published. Unpublished research is nothing more than sheer fantasy and illusion. It's completely unscientific and considered invalid by independent researchers. Yet consumers are led to believe this unverified information is fact when they read about it in editorials in fashion magazines and even, on occasion, in newspapers.

This same sleight of hand is used quite effectively in brochures and ads. Many cosmetics counters hand out impressively designed, scientific-looking brochures showing how well a product works on the skin. You might see, for example, a microscopic close-up of a patch of skin paired with an explanation of why it looks bad. Beside it is another close-up of the same patch of skin after the product is applied. See how wonderfully the product worked? The deception here is that you are not given enough "before" information. For example, if the woman had acne, what was she doing before to take care of her skin? Was she using products that clogged pores or aggravated breakouts? Had she never used any effective skin-care products for acne? In that case, any basic skin-care routine for acne could make a difference. And was this the one best result of the lot? Were there perhaps others who still had breakouts despite treatment? Just because information looks scientific doesn't mean it is.

Next time you see stories about test results showing younger-looking skin, new cell growth, or any other claim that sounds too good to be true, regardless of who is making the claim, stop and think. Ask yourself how many times you have heard this "perfect skin in a bottle" message before. Is this "story" about only one study, or are there any corroborating studies? Does it sound too good to be true? You may also want to ask yourself how many more times you are going to swallow another exaggerated claim about a skin-care product, or spend money believing that you've finally found the "best" product available. (Do you really believe that gorgeous, childlike model in the picture looks like that because of the products being advertised?) Think about how many times you've been sucked in by a cosmetics ad, claim, or fashion magazine story, only to be disappointed again and again, until the next advertising campaign for a new product catches your attention. There are many wonderful things that you can do to take care of your skin! But there are also a ton of things that are an embarrassing waste of money.

# HOW COSMETIC ADVERTISING MISLEADS

The huge number of things we are told about skin care and other beauty concerns is nothing less than astounding. That's why, when you begin thinking in terms of reality, facts, and balanced information, it is important to ignore the baseless, unfounded claims that are constantly bandied about in the guise of serious information. You may have run into the following terms and sales pitches for myriad skin-care and makeup products. These come-ons entice purchasers, even though they are vague or illogical.

**"Antiaging."** Ah, if only it were true. As one cosmetic surgeon explained to me, "If any of these antiaging products worked, or even did a little of what they claimed, wouldn't I be out of a job? If anything, younger and younger women are coming in to medically erase wrinkles because that's the only thing that really makes a long-term difference. Women can hardly help themselves when it comes to antiaging products because they'll try anything in the hopes of staying young or looking more beautiful. But they rarely do what it really takes, which is staying out of the sun. Yet even if they do start staying out of the sun, they can't undo what they've been doing to their skin since they were babies, namely going out in the sun without protection. That's why I became a cosmetic surgeon: what I do as a cosmetic surgeon will never become obsolete; never."

Thousands of skin-care products make promises about removing wrinkles or preventing the skin from aging. They contain a hodgepodge of ingredients and formulations. There is no consistent pattern among any of them. Yet they all claim to stop aging, and still no one stops getting wrinkles or sheds a wrinkle. There are great products that can make skin look better, but none of us have lost a wrinkle from any of the skin-care products we purchased.

**"Insulates skin from premature aging factors so it's free to repair itself."** It sounds very impressive, but the only unique aspect of this particular product is that it contains a sunscreen. That can indeed help skin a great deal, but it doesn't erase wrinkling as this claim asserts. Unfortunately, in this case, it's not a very good sunscreen because, while it may block some burning from UVB rays, it doesn't contain UVA-blocking sunscreen agents. And it's the UVA rays that cause skin cancer and wrinkles. If a product doesn't contain avobenzone, titanium dioxide, or zinc oxide, it simply can't protect against the sun's UVA radiation. Sunscreens that do contain UVA protection agents can prevent continuing damage. Sun damage is like any injury, and while the skin has some capacity to repair itself, it can't if you continually reinjure it. As to skin repairing itself, that's an interesting claim. In some ways, all moisturizers allow skin to "repair" itself by protecting the skin's barrier function. But whether or not the repair involves more than that (as in the apparent suggestion that a product can repair your wrinkles) remains to be proven for any product. The only research showing that products can repair wrinkles comes from the companies selling the products.

**"Closest to your skin's own strengthening lipids."** Lipids are fats, and skin is made up of lipids. The sebum your skin secrets as oil is also a lipid, and there are lipids in the layers of skin between the cells. If you put a lipid that resembles skin lipids into a skin-care product, that's nice, but lots and lots of ingredients can do that, including everything from glycerin, cholesterol, and hyaluronic acid to ceramides, and almost every moisturizer made has a varying assortment of these types of ingredients.

**"Soothing botanicals."** Botanicals is simply another name for plants, such as herbs and flowers, or plant extracts in the form of oils or juices. Is any of that soothing? There are definitely some soothing botanicals, such as green tea, kola extract, willowherb, bisabolol, licorice root (glycyrrhetinic acid), and burdock root to name a few. But there are also a great many natural ingredients, from lemons to strawberries, lavender oil, and jojoba, that can be problematic for lots of skin types, either as irritants or because they can clog pores. I can't tell you the number of products I've found that make claims about being good for sensitive skin, even though they contain a host of these irritating ingredients.

**"Independent tests confirm up to 45% reduction in visible lines and wrinkles, as well as significant firming and smoothing."** I called to ask if I could see these independent tests. I was told I couldn't, that they were secret. If that's the case, why quote them at all? If a test was truly independent, it would be open to public review just like all scientific research is.

**"Soon expression lines appear smoother."** What you think "appear smoother" means is one thing; what it literally means is something else. Dry skin can look "superficially" wrinkled; if you put on moisturizer, the dry skin can absolutely look smoother, but the effect is gone the next day. If you have dry skin and you don't reapply the moisturizer, the wrinkles come back. A moisturizer won't get rid of wrinkles—but then, the ad doesn't say the product will eliminate wrinkles, just that it appears to. That boast can easily be made for any and all moisturizers.

**"Superficial lines."** Watch out for the word "superficial"; it is a powerful tool when used in cosmetics advertising. "Superficial lines" really refer to the temporary, transient lines caused by dryness, not sun damage (sun-damaged wrinkles are hardly superficial). Most products could make elaborate claims about smoothing superficial wrinkles and they would not be lying to you. Superficial wrinkles go away when you put on any moisturizer, and that is wonderful. But—and I repeat, *but*—superficial wrinkles are not the ones you are worried about. Permanent wrinkles, like laugh lines, furrows between the eyes and on the forehead, and expression lines, are not eliminated by a moisturizer unless it contains irritants that temporarily swell the skin. The word "superficial" is misleading because it doesn't really refer to the lines and wrinkles women are most concerned about.

**"Start today and see a young tomorrow."** First, this line doesn't say that young has anything to do with you; rather, it has to do with tomorrow being young. So exactly what is a young tomorrow? The implication is that tomorrow you will see a younger you. That's not what it says, but that's the impression you are supposed to get. Even if the phrase did say "see a younger you," how much younger are you supposed to see yourself being tomorrow? Five minutes? An hour? A day? "See a young tomorrow" may suggest something will soon happen to your wrinkles, but that is not actually what the words say; it's only what you hope is being said.

**"Helps neutralize free radicals."** While most of us now know that free radicals are bad for skin, very few have any idea what a free radical is or why it's so bad for skin. I'll explain about free-radical damage, and antioxidants in Chapter Three, but for now understand that when skin-care products are applied topically (on the surface of the skin) there is no way to measure or evaluate whether they can "neutralize" or in any way stop free-radical damage, and definitely not in a way that gets rid of wrinkles. How much of an ingredient is needed to combat free radicals and how long its effect lasts on the skin are unknown. Theoretically, antioxidants are an exciting group of ingredients, but claims about their function and abilities are marketing illusion, not fact (Sources: *Current Problems in Dermatology*, 2001, volume 29, pages 157–164; *Clinical Experimental Dermatology*, October 2001, pages 578–582).

**"Just for your ultra-delicate eye area."** The advertiser may want you to use the eye cream only around your eyes, which means you have to buy a face lotion separately, yet the ingredients of these products are rarely different enough to warrant the extra expense and rarely have any special formulary function specific to the eye area. There is no reason an eye cream can't be used on the face or the face lotion can't be used around the eyes. The only time a special eye cream would be necessary is when the skin around the eyes is different from the skin on the rest of the face, which may require a more or less emollient moisturizer, but that's a different issue from the need for an eye cream.

**"Visible lift with proven results."** The claim is that this product "reduces fine lines in just 30 days, firms skin, pores look smaller, skin tone evens out, and becomes more resilient." First, this foundation product is only an SPF 12, so the notion that it can reduce fine lines when it can't protect skin from what is really causing damage (sun exposure) is not true (the American Academy of Dermatology states that an SPF 15 or greater is minimum for sufficient protection). The study mentioned in this ad doesn't say what the improvement was based on. A comparison to another product? To one side of the face that was stripped bare with alcohol? It also doesn't comment on who made the assessment about the improvement. If it was the company's own appraisal, they clearly had reason to notice that the skin looked better. Claims like these are meaningless, but sound great.

**"Makes dark circles seem to disappear."** There's that word "seem" again—watch out for it! There are no creams that can eliminate puffiness or dark circles. However, dry skin can seem puffier and make naturally dark skin tissue look darker. Any moisturizer applied over an eye area that is dehydrated will make it "seem" to be less dark and puffy. Another cause of dark circles is surface circulation showing through the thin skin around the eyes; that can't be altered by skin-care products either.

**"Dimpling seems to virtually disappear."** Aside from the word "seems," the word "virtually" is also a disclaimer. According to the dictionary, "virtually" means "in effect, but not factually." So this statement doesn't really say if anything is going to happen when you put the product on. "Dimpling" here refers to cellulite, which cannot and should not be altered from the outside in. If these products did work, a woman would never have to diet, and she could use the product to break down fat in every part of her body, and then no one would be overweight or have cellulite. If fat could be eliminated via some external process, it would be seriously dangerous for the body and pose critical health concerns.

**"Nighttime repair."** The suggestion here is that somehow a cream can help increase cell reproduction and undo skin damage. You can do some impressive things with a moisturizer and create smoother, healthier-looking skin, but it is all temporary. Stop using it and things will go back to the way they were. If you could change the way cells reproduce, no one would have wrinkles or sun damage, and no one would get skin cancer.

**"Nourishing hydrobeads release vitamins and minerals."** You can't feed the skin from the outside in. Vitamins and minerals applied on the surface of the skin don't work in the same way as the vitamins and minerals you swallow. For vitamins and minerals to have a "nourishing" effect on skin, they must be digested and combined with a vast array of other nutrients before they are converted to a form the body or skin can use. Some vitamins can function as antioxidants, but that effect isn't unique to this product. "Hydrobeads" sounds like a special delivery system that can somehow transport these vitamins and minerals into the skin. It can't. Literally, hydrobeads means "beads of water." Big deal.

**"So advanced, it's patented."** Patent law just means that the company was able to show a formula or ingredient was in some way unique. It can also establish that an existing ingredient or formula has a unique use. None of that has anything to do with efficacy. A company could patent a terrible formula or a good formula; an erroneous or verifiable claim; as long as it's unique—that's all a patent means. The patent is simply about who can use or sell the formula or ingredient, or who can make a specific public claim about the use of a formula or ingredient. Most major cosmetics companies own thousands of patents, but that doesn't tell you anything about how advanced or mediocre those patents are.

**"Microtargeted skin gel—rebuilding the skin's appearance."** "Microtargeted" is a good word. It sounds like this gel will zap just the area where you need it to work. If you have a wrinkle right next to your eye, no other area will be affected by the gel, right? That is what "microtargeted" seems to mean. But the ad doesn't say that, even though you are supposed to jump to that wrong conclusion. The term could mean anything.

**"Test results reveal the cream beneficially affected the appearance of the skin surface."** Whose test results? In almost every case the cosmetics company is quoting its own results, which are not substantiated by any other source, nor are they published or available for review. That means you just have to take the company's word for it.

**"Natural bonding materials slow down loss of critical moisture."** You know what these bonding materials are? Hairstyling agents, plastic-like ingredients that put a microscopic film layer over the skin that helps keep water from evaporating. Hairspray ingredients show up in lots of skin-care products these days. This is a decent way to keep moisture in the skin, but making it sound impressive is at best stretching the point.

**"Dramatically diminishes wrinkles by penetrating the top layer of skin to create a balloon effect, pushing the skin out from beneath the surface."** I had a tough time deciphering this one. But after reading the ingredient list, it was obvious that all the product could do was irritate the skin, which would make it swell. Swollen skin can look temporarily less wrinkled. Of course, this ad doesn't mention that many dermatologists warn against using products that irritate the skin, because irritation can damage skin, and that eventually makes wrinkles worse. Ironic, isn't it, that many of the very products advertised as diminishing wrinkles can actually make them more pronounced because of chronic irritation?

**"Works with the microcirculation of your skin."** "Works with" is always a good phrase, but exactly what kind of work is being referred to? "Microcirculation" also sounds very impressive. Yet technically, all creams can affect the microcirculation of your skin. If the idea is to stimulate circulation, then rubbing any cream onto the skin will do that. It isn't the cream doing the stimulation, it's the action of your fingers rubbing the cream into your skin. But suggesting in an ad that—product or no product—all you need to do to stimulate circulation is massage your skin wouldn't sell anything.

**"Penetrates deeply into the layers of the skin."** "Penetrates" is another very impressive, though imprecise, word. Almost any cosmetic ingredient, if its molecules are small enough, will penetrate the skin, but the molecules of many cosmetic ingredients are too large to penetrate the skin. When cosmetic ingredients are able to penetrate the skin, the word "layers" is frequently added to confound you.

Layers of skin are so microscopically small they are negligible. A cream can penetrate many layers of skin and still not have traveled anywhere.

**"The skin's ability for self-rejuvenation is helped."** The skin can self-rejuvenate (up to a point) if we don't get in the way of that process with sun damage, smoking, or irritating the skin. You can't rejuvenate the skin if you continually damage it. Yet this product does not have a sunscreen or any warnings about irritation or smoking.

**"Deep cleansing."** This term has always baffled me. How deep is deep? Sounds like a dentist cleaning out a cavity in your teeth. I can vividly hear the sound of a drill trying to get into your pores! If a product could clean deeply—I mean *really* deeply— you would be bleeding, but no one would ever have blackheads because you would eliminate them through "deep cleansing." In this case, "deep cleansing" probably means "thorough cleansing"; well, that's fine. But cosmetics companies encourage the belief that deep-cleansing products can get into a pore and eject a blackhead. There are ways to dissolve the stuff that is inside a blackhead, but "deep cleansing" won't do it.

**"Gentle to the skin"** or **"Good for sensitive skin."** Products described as "gentle to the skin" often contain ingredients that actually can cause irritation—a lot of it. Remember, there is no guideline or specification about what constitutes a gentle product. If you don't read the ingredient list, you could be buying something that's neither gentle nor good for sensitive skin, and you won't know until you put it on your face (and even then you may not know because irritation is not always evident on the surface of the skin).

**"Cellular protein nourishes the skin to visibly tighten and tone."** Even if cellular protein could nourish the skin, which it can't, protein molecules are too large to get past the surface of the skin. You can't feed the skin from the outside in. Nourishment is a very complicated process that does not rely only on a single chemical, vitamin, mineral, or food. It requires an intricate digestive process that delivers site-appropriate chemical substances (thousands of them, not just one) precisely where they are needed. Adding protein sounds good, but by itself, and especially when applied to the skin's surface, it does nothing for the human body and skin.

# THE CRAZY THINGS COSMETICS SALESPEOPLE SAY

Apart from the world of advertising mumbo jumbo, there is an entire realm of appallingly inaccurate or just plain wrong information that is disseminated on a daily basis by cosmetics salespeople all over the world. These false sales pitches are tomorrow's new myths, ingrained into the minds of a captive audience. Here are my latest favorites, though I have to admit these only skim the surface.

**"In order for the products to achieve dramatic results you must use all of them; the skin must be properly conditioned to accept all the products in the line in order for any of the products to work."** This is one of my all-time favorites because its purpose is to convince you to buy all the products from one line. It is a classic sales technique. In essence, what you are being told is that the line's wrinkle cream won't work unless all the other products are used first, so don't bother buying the wrinkle cream unless you are going to buy everything. In my years of reviewing skin-care routines, I have never seen a cosmetics line with products so unique that you couldn't substitute a dozen other products for them, if not many that would work better. Further, every cosmetics line has products you should avoid because they contain irritating ingredients, or inadequate amounts of sunscreen, or moisturizers that oversaturate the skin. The term to note here is "dramatic results." What the cosmetics company considers dramatic results may be dramatically different from what you would really like to see the products do—even if you do use all of them.

**"Our ingredients are high quality; that's why they are so expensive."** It would be nice if that were true, but I can't get any cosmetics company to give me proof of it. I've asked for the names of their suppliers to find out what grades of products they are selling and if they have inferior grades that go to some companies but not others. From what I've been able to find out on my own after talking to several cosmetic-ingredient manufacturers, the grades of cosmetic ingredients don't vary that much, and everyone buys cosmetic-grade ingredients, which are all high quality. For example, DuPont is one of the largest suppliers of glycolic acid to the cosmetics industry (they supply over 99% of the industry who use this ingredient), and they supply the same version to everyone.

**"You need to wear makeup because it acts as a barrier between your skin and pollution."** It's just not true. Perhaps the more opaque, solid particles in foundations, powders, and lipsticks can reduce the skin's exposure to the sun's rays, but that's not pollution. Inorganic pollutants such as smog, car exhaust, and other industrial fumes can be absorbed right through makeup and moisturizers (Source: *Cosmetics & Toiletries*, August 2001, "Pollution and Aging: Antioxidants for Skin").

**"See how smooth it makes your skin feel. That's the vitamins and plant extracts working."** Take some vitamins or plants like chamomile, lemon, or peppermint; rub them on your skin; and then tell me how that makes your skin feel. You wouldn't feel any difference (unless you have an allergic reaction) because it would have no effect at all. Often the amount of vitamins and plant extracts used in cosmetics is so minute as to be undetectable by your skin. When significant amounts are used, many vitamins and plant extacts can have an impact on skin, but not as emollients. The ingredients that make the skin feel smooth are usually the standard oils, waxes, emollients, and slip agents (glycerin-like ingredients that slip over the skin and help give it a smooth feeling) that show up in product after product.

**"We only use natural ingredients; synthetic ingredients are bad for your skin because they are fake and made from gasoline, such as mineral oil and petrolatum."** I have yet to see any cosmetic that is "all" natural. Some synthetic ingredients are awesome for your skin, and regardless of the protestations of cosmetics companies to the contrary, every cosmetics product in the world contains its share of synthetic ingredients.

Synthetic ingredients are derived from many sources, but they all start as natural because everything comes from our environment; nothing is created via alchemy. Petrolatum and mineral oil are indeed by-products of the gasoline industry, but what is unnatural about that? Ironically, gasoline, which is derived from crude oil, is decidedly natural in and of itself as it comes from organic material, such as tiny aquatic plants and animals, that has been buried in the earth for millions of years. Petrolatum and mineral oil are remarkably good skin-care ingredients; they are also recognized by cosmetics chemists the world over for being superior emollients and completely harmless (Source: *Dermatologic Surgery*, June 1998, pages 661–664). Even the claim that these ingredients are occlusive (blocking) and, therefore, bad for skin is also without proof (Source: *Contact Dermatitis,* September 1996, pages 163–168).

Why mineral oil and petrolatum continue to get a bad rap from the so-called natural skin-care world is a mystery. For dry skin, you'd be far better off having petrolatum or mineral oil in your moisturizer than most plant extracts any day.

**"You need to use facial masks and give yourself regular spa treatments that include steaming to pull toxins out of the skin and remove debris from the pores."** Or

**"Facials can stimulate blood circulation and the flow of oxygen to purge skin of toxins embedded in pores."**

It's actually the liver, kidneys, and lymph system that purge toxins from the body, not the skin or sweat glands. Sweat glands are a cooling system for the body, they do not harbor toxins. Interestingly, oxygen itself acts as a toxin because it generates free-radical damage—but I'll get to more of that later, in Chapter Three.

However, there is nothing lurking around in one's skin and pores that can be pulled, sucked, or squeezed out of the skin. If "toxins" are to be found in skin, exactly which toxins are we talking about? I have yet to find anyone who can name these toxins that we need to get rid of.

What does need to be removed is cellular debris (dead skin cells) that fills the pore, along with wax and tiny hairs that have built up in there. These take more than an occasional mask to remove; it takes daily effort and salicylic acid or alpha hydroxy acids (which exfoliate skin), and sometimes prescription drugs such as Retin-A and Differin (which improve and alter cell production to reduce or eliminate cell debris).

**"A famous scientist [doctor, chemist, pharmacist, dermatologist, or whatever—I've heard it all] created this formula and it is only now available to the public."** Lots of doctors and chemists are involved in creating all kinds of products in the world of cosmetics, but all cosmetics contain standard cosmetic ingredients. They can't contain anything else, as drugs do, or they would be regulated quite differently.

My favorite example of this type of claim is Estee Lauder Creme de la Mer. Quite a story accompanies this very costly little cream *($165 for 2 ounces)*! It was created by Max Huber, a NASA aerospace physicist, supposedly to take care of burns he received in an accident. He sold and marketed this product himself. After his death, his daughter continued selling the cream until recently, when Estee Lauder purchased the rights to manufacture and distribute it.

As enticing as this dramatic story sounds, the reality is that this very basic, and I mean *really* basic, cream doesn't contain anything particularly extraordinary or unique, unless you want to believe that seaweed extract (sort of like seaweed tea) can somehow be worth this much money, or that it can in some way heal burns and scars. Even if it could heal burns, heat and sunburns don't have much to do with wrinkling. UVA radiation is what causes most wrinkling, even though those aren't the burning rays. According to Susan Brawley, professor of plant biology at the University of Maine, "seaweed extract isn't a rare, exotic, or expensive ingredient. Seaweed extract is readily available and used in everything from cosmetics to food products and medical applications." Creme de la Mer contains mostly seaweed extract, mineral oil, petrolatum (similar to Vaseline), glycerin, waxlike thickening agents, plant oils, plant seeds, minerals, vitamins, more thickeners, and preservatives. How expensive can it be to stick some seaweed and vitamins in a cosmetic? According to the cosmetics chemists I've interviewed, it costs pennies, not hundreds of dollars.

Moreover, several additional products with formulas that are unrelated to the first now accompany Creme de la Mer's original miracle product. If the first one was so spectacular why did it need company, and why did the subsequent products have completely different formulations? I guess the original wasn't quite the miracle formula they thought it was.

**"The reason you have oily skin is because you don't have enough moisture in your skin. Your skin produces excess oil to protect it from moisture loss. If you had enough moisture in your skin it would stop producing oil. That's why it is so important for someone with oily skin to wear a moisturizer."** Oil production has nothing to do with the state of dryness in your skin. If that were true, wouldn't someone with dry skin have her oil production turned on and thereby not have dry skin? Women with dry skin do not find their oil production increases when they don't wear a moisturizer. Oily skin appears to be primarily the result of genetic inheritance and hormonal influences, but no one knows exactly why some people have oily skin and others have dry skin.

**"Just because the surface of your skin is oily doesn't mean the underlying layer of skin isn't dry and in need of moisture."** I could help a large number of women eliminate their complaints of oily, combination, or acne-prone skin if I could just get them to stop using moisturizer. Moisturizer is actually the most abused skin-care product because unless you have dry skin you absolutely don't need it. There is nothing protective about moisturizers: They don't stop stress, they can't feed the skin, they can't thwart sun damage (unless they contain sunscreen), and they can't permanently alter the skin's structure. If your skin has a dry layer it can be the result of using drying soaps, cleansers, and toners that contain alcohol or other drying ingredients (like lemon or grapefruit). Even using too much moisturizer can be a problem when it prevents skin from sloughing off naturally created, built-up layers of dry skin. There are lots of ways to obtain benefits from water-binding agents, antioxidants, and anti-irritants, but they don't have to come in the form of a lotion or cream.

**"This moisturizer is perfect for someone with oily or combination skin because it is oil-free."** I can't tell you the number of products touting this claim when they indeed do contain oils, or waxes that feel oily, or other ingredients that can clog pores. They may not be oils you recognize, like plant oils or mineral oils, but they are nonetheless in there, with names you may not have heard. Regardless, hearing that a product is oil-free still gives you no information about what it may or may not do to the skin. What is most confusing is that ingredients known for causing breakouts may not leave a greasy feel on the skin. Surprisingly, one of the greasiest ingredients, mineral oil, has been shown in study after study to not cause breakouts, although it can still feel greasy. Go figure. The fewer skin-care products a woman with oily or blemish-prone skin uses, the better off her skin will be.

**"The sage, lemon, and grapefruit in this product help normalize skin oils."** Lemon and grapefruit can irritate skin, but that's about it. Plus, oil in the skin is regulated primarily by hormone production, and there are no plants you can rub on your face to alter that. Finally, irritation itself can trigger a breakout response and that definitely isn't good for skin.

**"By using this product at night you can prepare the skin to offset the visible effects of daytime aggression."** There is nothing you can do for your skin at night to change or reduce the effects of sun damage, and sun damage is the only daytime aggression you should worry about, skin-wise.

# BRAND-NAME LOYALTY

Estee Lauder owns Stila, Aramis, Aveda, Clinique, Jane, Tommy Hilfiger, Bobbi Brown, Prescriptives, M.A.C., Origins, and Creme de la Mer.

L'Oreal owns Maybelline, Lancome, Helena Rubinstein, BioMedic, Vichy, Biotherm, and La Roche Posay.

Procter & Gamble owns Cover Girl, Max Factor, and Olay.

Johnson & Johnson owns Neutrogena, Aveeno, Clean & Clear, and RoC.

So ask yourself: Why should you be loyal to a cosmetics company if the cosmetics company isn't even loyal to itself?

Ever since I began evaluating cosmetics, the question I am asked most frequently is, "Which product line do you like the best? What do you think of Lancome, Estee Lauder, Mary Kay, or hundreds of other lines?" That was the major reason I wrote *Don't Go to the Cosmetics Counter Without Me*. By actually reviewing each line, I could point out specifically what we already know is true: That every line, regardless of price, has good and bad products. Brand-name loyalty does not make any sense. Clinique makes great mascaras and some great foundations, but several of its toners contain alcohol, which is too irritating and drying for all skin types. Lancome has some excellent blushes and mascaras but their foundations with sunscreen typically don't contain UVA protecting ingredients and their moisturizers are overly fragranced. Neutrogena offers some wonderful makeup products and sunscreens but most of their cleansers are extremely drying and irritating and some of their sunscreens don't contain UVA protecting ingredients. Revlon has some great foundations, good mascaras, and terrific lip pencils, but its original ColorStay foundation goes on way too thick (their revamped ColorStay Lite is far better) and some of their foundation colors are too pink, peach, or rose.

Even our own experience tells us that all the products within one product line aren't great because we've all purchased expensive products that didn't work or that we didn't like. Yet the success of the major product lines in establishing brand-name loyalty is astonishing. It is particularly apparent in the way a woman responds to questions about what brand of makeup she is currently using. The answer usually reflects the amount of money she has spent on the product. A customer usually whispers or acts embarrassed when she admits to using a drugstore brand, but if she's using an expensive brand you can hear her across the room. The reality is that the cost of a cosmetic has nothing to do with whether it will work for you. I have used both inexpensive and expensive makeup that looked wonderful and was good for the skin, as well as inexpensive and expensive makeup that looked awful and was bad for the skin.

We've already heard about the claim that you need to buy all your skin-care products from one line because the products are designed to work together. That may be the company's sales concept, but it doesn't hold up. Lots of skin-care products contain ingredients that could be problematic, some by containing irritating ingredients or ingredients that may clog pores; others because of what they don't contain—effective sun protection.

Why is it, then, that a particular brand of cosmetics is so expensive compared with a less-expensive brand made by the same manufacturing company? In the final analysis, price is determined by what the market will bear. If you're willing to pay $25 for a foundation because you believe you'll look twenty-five dollars' worth better, they'll sell it to you for just that. Hopefully, by now, your ideas of brand-name loyalties have changed. Go to any library and check out a copy of *Global Cosmetic Industry* or *Cosmetics & Toiletries* magazines and read about the manufacturing of cosmetics and cosmetic ingredients. These industry periodicals reveal how the cosmetics industry really works.

## WHY WE BELIEVE

I'm often asked why we believe all of this foolishness, given the copious amounts of information to the contrary. I sometimes wonder, too. But our willingness to believe has little to do with being foolish. It is much more complicated than that, both from the emotional and sociological perspectives. There are extremely compelling reasons why we get taken in by empty, meaningless ads and claims time after time.

**Reason No. 1.** For the most part, skin-care products and, more specifically, wrinkle creams feel good and take very good care of skin. We all need to clean our faces, and many of us have to fight dry, oily, or combination skin. One way or another, without skin-care products we would be left with more problems than we started with. Soap all by itself, for the majority of women, leaves the face dry and irritated. Even though many toners contain irritants, they at least take off that last layer of makeup, which can clog pores. Moisturizers (wrinkle creams are, after all, just moisturizers) can be an essential part of taking care of dry skin. So the reason we buy the stuff in the first place is because a lot of these products take great care of our skin. They don't perform the miracles they suggest; they aren't worth the big bucks they frequently cost; but, in general, they do help. The fact that lots of skin-care products perform well can lead one to believe that another brand or price range may perform better yet.

**Reason No. 2.** Even though many skin-care products do their job, many also fail miserably. Women frequently buy the wrong products for their skin type. Sometimes the formulations are so irritating and poorly conceived they cause complications, making matters worse, or they simply do not eliminate the skin problems they were bought for. That's why women are in a constant search for the right products. They believe the right ones for their skin type are out there somewhere, if they could only find them. Skin problems are a recurrent headache. It is the rare individual who doesn't have to be concerned about acne, wrinkles, dry skin, oily skin, irritation, or a combination of these. Anything but perfect skin seems to be what we all have, but perfect skin is what we are all after.

Most women think the major questions to ask about skin care are "Which products will be best for my skin?" and "Which products work and which ones don't, and where do I find them?" The questions themselves show where the problem lies. The search should not be so much for the right product, but for the right (and wrong) ingredients. If you just look for products, but don't know what's inside them, you could buy the same formulation over and over again without really changing what you are doing for your skin. You will be way ahead of the game once you understand that even with the most expensive products you can overmoisturize the skin while trying to eliminate dryness, irritate the skin in the name of drying up acne, or make oily skin worse by using so-called oil-free moisturizers.

**Reason No. 3.** Beauty myths die a long, hard death. Once we believe something about our skin, it is very hard to change our minds. I discuss many myths throughout this book, but they are almost countless, and letting go of them isn't easy. It takes information, and some of that information is boring, technical, and hard to grasp. But once you've mastered some of the basics, none of the bogus facts you hear or see will catch you off guard again.

**Reason No. 4.** Everything the ads, brochures, and cosmetics salespeople tell us sounds very convincing. Given the amount of money cosmetics companies spend on packaging, promotions, and advertising, it should! Just remember that all that glitters is not gold. The glitter and shine at the cosmetics counters sure looks like gold, but it rarely (if ever) is. Do not be convinced again and again that because something "sounds" good, it is, or that expensive means better—because it isn't.

**Reason No. 5.** It is very difficult to believe that cosmetics companies want to take advantage of us when what they are selling seems so beautiful and attractive and comes in such stunning containers. This desire to trust in a company's higher purpose is part of what we all want to presume. It is tiresome to be cautious about everything. And the spokesmodels for these companies look so convincing and sweet; surely they wouldn't lie to us.

The truth is, cosmetics companies have one purpose, and that is to sell their products. That is their bottom line. Anything else is less important than that one objective. Many companies do make good products, and there is nothing wrong with selling them. But to assume that a company is in business for the good of the consumer and that, as a result, they really do sell miraculous formulas or that everything in their line is automatically good, is unwise and potentially costly.

**Reason No. 6.** We want to believe that what they tell us is true. It is reassuring to assume that the $10 or $50 or $150 you just spent is somehow going to take care of your skin-care or makeup problems. Surely all those scientists and dermatologists must have invented something by now!

We also want to believe that there are wrinkle creams that get rid of wrinkles and astringents that close pores and lipsticks that last all day, but be skeptical. If wrinkle creams can work, why do any of us have wrinkles? If astringents or toners can close pores, why do any of us have open pores? If lipstick really can last all day, why must we constantly reapply it? It is OK to accept reality, because being realistic will not make you any less beautiful or prevent you from taking good care of your skin.

**Reason No. 7.** Most cosmetics companies aren't really lying to us. They aren't telling the truth, but even the most extreme ads hedge their promises and claims with vague language that doesn't really say anything specific. When you see an ad for a wrinkle cream that reduces fine lines, restores suppleness, and rejuvenates the skin, you must remember that any moisturizer can make that claim and not be lying. The company may really have a study showing that their skin-care product performed well, even though the study is often poorly controlled, doesn't compare the product against a placebo or a competing brand, and, more substantially, isn't published.

**Reason No. 8.** Salespeople are well trained to sell you their products. They can be very skilled in subtle, but effective, sales techniques. Their best sales tactic is to reinforce a woman's insecurity. This emotional battleground is the salesperson's best weapon and one that the consumer is least equipped to avoid or resist. See if these routines sound familiar:

(1) The salesperson reminds the consumer that she is not as beautiful as she could be because she isn't yet using the salesperson's products. The salesperson offers a lipstick and says, "This color would look much better on you."

(2) The salesperson helps the consumer notice all the problems her skin is having

(after all, she's the expert—she's supposed to notice these problems). She may ask, "Aren't you concerned about how dry your skin is, particularly around your eyes?" or "You aren't using a moisturizer [shocked reaction]? Everyone needs a moisturizer to protect their skin from the environment, stress, hormones, or makeup."

(3) The salesperson suggests that if a woman continues to make the same skin-care mistakes over and over, she will pay for it down the road: "You can't start too soon using this product because it can only get worse if you wait, and then it may be too late to do anything about it."

It is essential to know that cosmetics salespeople are not necessarily trained in skin care or makeup; they are trained to sell products. To assume these people have a scientific or even a basic knowledge about skin is a serious mistake. A 1992 study by the city of New York's Department of Consumer Affairs assessed the statements and claims made by cosmetics salespeople and stated that "more than one in three [cosmetics salespeople] stretched the truth beyond recognition, making claims the company attorneys would never allow." Another one-third gave ambiguous or cryptic responses to skin-care questions, and the rest just recommended products.

The only way to defend yourself against sales techniques like these is with a strong sense of self-esteem. Security in who you are is important in life—and at the cosmetics counters. If you are willing to accept the idea of being rescued by the products being sold to you, you are at the mercy of a good sales pitch. You must recognize right now that there are no answers inside these glittering, slick boxes and jars and that what you need is information from independent sources (not from fashion magazines or salespeople) that can help you understand your skin and recognize what cosmetics can and can't do.

I admit that I repeatedly come down hard on cosmetics salespeople. It isn't that I haven't met some wonderful cosmetics salespeople, because I have. Many times these remarkable women and men have given me insight into the cosmetics industry that otherwise would have been impossible for me to obtain. I would also like to acknowledge from experience that, for the most part, particularly at department stores, selling cosmetics is not an easy or lucrative way to earn a living. Unfortunately, I have also had some difficult encounters with cosmetics salespeople. I have listened to and overheard hundreds of crazy conversations about skin care and makeup application that are nothing more than sales pressure and incorrect information. It is generally hard to distinguish sales technique from valid information, but it is safe to assume that when you are buying skin-care or makeup products you are far more likely to encounter salesmanship than factual information.

**Reason No. 9.** It's hard to question advice you receive from a cosmetics representative. For one thing, it isn't customary for women to refute what they hear, either directly or indirectly. Asserting your doubts and scrutinizing what you are told when dealing with cosmetics salespeople (or any salesperson) is difficult, but once you do, you will start noticing that the information being doled out is baseless and mostly unbelievable. As you start questioning what you hear, the salesperson inevitably gets caught in the pretense and fumbles about, trying to find a plausible explanation. I wish this were as easy as it sounds, but it can be tricky. I can't promise you'll receive a pleasant reaction when you imply you don't believe what you are being told. My suggestion is to take it one step at a time. The next time you're at a cosmetics counter, try a few probing questions, or ask to see the ingredient list when they start explaining the wondrous potion inside. Once you do, you will be less likely to leave feeling oversold. The more information you have, the less susceptible you will be to the hype and fantasy the cosmetics industry confronts us with everywhere we turn. Once you've finished reading this book, you will know more than most of the women and men selling makeup and skin-care products.

**Reason No. 10.** Fashion magazines make everything the cosmetics industry sells look and sound amazing. Ninety percent of the time their editorial comments glorify cosmetics, with only occasional, buried hints of objectivity. Cosmetics companies have a stranglehold on the way fashion magazines present information on skin care and makeup. What makes this so pathetic is that reading fashion magazines is the primary way women get advice, news, and reports on their beauty needs. Gloria Steinem, in an article in *Ms.* magazine, once explained why she would no longer accept advertisements for cosmetics. She said her advertisers demanded that their ads be placed near compatible and positive editorial stories, that they must not be near material that challenged the nature of the product, and that stories in the entire magazine must not contain anything the advertiser found objectionable or displeasing. That concisely explains why you never see a negative article about the cosmetics or fashion industry in the pages of fashion magazines.

# IF IT SOUNDS TOO GOOD TO BE TRUE ...

The great consumer words of wisdom for this millennium, or any millennium for that matter, are these: If it sounds too good to be true, then it probably isn't true. Not everything being sold can be a miracle. In essence, any sales technique that tries to convince you that a product can live up to most, if not all, of your wildest dreams for clear, smooth, wrinkle-free, acne-free skin, and without any negative side effects, is the essence of snake-oil salesmanship. Scams like this are abundant in the world of cosmetics, from every angle—from antiwrinkle products to acne cures, from hair-growth miracles to stopping hair growth, or to the one perfect foundation, and on and on and on. How can you stop getting taken? That's more difficult to change.

Consumers have heard for years that if it sounds too good to be true, it is, but we just don't want to believe it *isn't* true. Whatever the emotional or psychological reasons are that make us weak in the presence of such otherwise repetitive and blatant deceptions, the net result is that it costs us a lot of money and wasted time, not to mention problems when we buy things that can potentially hurt us. Perhaps what we need are a few reminders of how to identify a potential scam when we see one. If you can recognize these fraudulent marketing contrivances, you are well on your way to helping your hair, your skin, and your budget.

**If a company claims their products (or their research) are being suppressed by the government or by big pharmaceutical companies, it's guaranteed that you have encountered a hoax.** This is a pathetic attempt to cash in on the fear that "Big Brother" or a major corporation is keeping you from finding out about something that is truly spectacular for your health. Yet legitimate, verifiable research can be carried out by any company, of any size, and publication of those results can come from any sector. It does take money, but any business involved in selling products must make capital outlays. How dare a company attempt to make money (and some companies are making millions) without doing the work to prove its claims are possible and that the products present no risk to the consumer?

**A corollary to the Big-Brother-is-out-to-get-us ploy is the one that states "We are releasing our products without FDA approval because it would take too long for us to wait for their endorsement."** Of course it takes a long time to prove something is safe and effective, and if a product really can do something significant, like play around with your hormones in the case of hair-growth products or hormone creams, don't you want to know if there is a risk of cancer or other biochemical and systemic side effects? The FDA asks for serious proof, and we should demand no less if someone is asking us to spend our hard-earned money.

**Another sure sign you and your skin or hair are being taken for a ride is if the company claims the secret ingredient is from some faraway, exotic land.** As nice as it would be if there were such miracles hiding in the rain forest of some remote region of the world, there just aren't. Regardless of locale, whether it comes from New Jersey or the Amazon, if an ingredient can perform, then the research and resulting patent wouldn't be a secret, it would be shared with the world just like all legitimate research.

**One of the most frustrating fraudulent schemes taking place in the world of cosmetics is the use of pseudoscience.** Studies are quoted, scientific-sounding publications or journals are cited, well-known universities are mentioned, doctors in good standing are referred to, and serious-sounding awards are attributed to whatever product is being sold. Sadly, more often than not, the studies are taken out of context or misquoted, the study is done on a small population (80% of five people is not proof of anything), the journal mentioned doesn't exist or is published by the company that makes the product, or the study or the results are meaningless given the methodology used—all of which is very difficult for the average person who isn't familiar with scientific protocol to understand. Even more ludicrous, though it happens often, is that the doctor or university mentioned has never heard of the ingredient or product or there is no such award given anywhere in the world.

How do you know when the "scientific results" referred to aren't true when you don't have time to do the research? The clearest sign you're being scammed is when the results are overwhelmingly positive and there are no downsides or disadvantages. When the conclusions point only to the product being sold as being the absolute best, most wondrous thing ever created and there are no negative reactions, you can be assured you're about to be taken in by a great marketing ruse.

**An addendum to the scientific, proof-positive approach to snake-oil selling tactics is the all-embracing, absolutely-everyone-loves-our-products approach.** Infomercials do this form of selling the best. Glowing enthusiasm, stunning before-and-afters, and no downside or risks are all extolled by seemingly impartial users. Yet the reason why hundreds of new lines are being sold is that the previous ones weren't really the "best" after all (and that women are amazingly fickle about the products they like). Plus, do you think these companies are ever going to air the voices of women who aren't happy?

**Medical expertise is the most seductive selling tactic of all.** A neat white coat and stethoscope draped around the spokesperson or owner of a product line are all it takes to establish instant credibility with most consumers. Physicians are believed almost instinctively, and whether the product is related to their field or not, if they are doctors, they must know. But doctors and medical experts exaggerate their positions and lie about products to make sales just like the worst salespeople. Expensive products and overly hyped, ordinary formulations abound in physicians' offices. Again, if it is all positive and wonderful and miraculous, it just isn't true.

**It's ironic that American medical know-how can sell a horde of nonmedical products, while at the same time the notion that a product is anything but American-made or developed from Western science is a strong come-on for a large range of susceptible consumers.** Companies love taking advantage of the belief that anything foreign-made is better. The selling points are distinctive: Either the research has taken place in a far corner of the world or the ingredient has been hidden away in a remote forest or jungle somewhere. Hair-care or skin-care revelations from outside the purview of Western medicine are impossible to confirm or refute because there are rarely any hard data to analyze. A bigger mystery is why people are so quick to believe that American technology is not up to speed with that from these distant locales when most other parts of the world envy our technological proficiency.

**While I love money-back guarantees and consider them a primary, major motivation when finalizing a purchase, they can also be problematic if you don't read the fine print.** First, most money-back policies are good only for a 30-day period and that 30-day period can be deceiving. I've found that most 30-day money-back guarantees include the time it takes for the products to be shipped back—so you would have to pack up the products you don't like and get them in the mail in about three weeks to get your return. By the time you receive the product you've ordered and given it a good test run to discover if you like it or not or if it can even vaguely live up to its claims, it could be far more than four weeks. Skin irritations and allergic reactions can also take weeks to show up. With regard to hair-growth products, or for products that make claims to stop hair from growing, a 30-day guarantee is pointless. It can take months and many repurchases to discover if a hair-related product is working because hair growth takes months to develop. Hair growth is also cyclical, so a product may seem to work and then a few months later the hair you thought grew back may actually fall out.

I've never said it was easy being an informed consumer, but it is well worth the trouble! For the sake of our beauty, health, and budget, say the following phrase the next time you see an ad for a miracle product of any kind: "If it sounds too good to be true, then it probably isn't true." Now those are words you can live by, year after year after year.

## THOU SHALT ...

Feeling and looking beautiful is a wonderful, satisfying, joyous process as well as a state of mind women can revel in with much pleasure and reward. Yet all the delightful and beautiful possibilities can get zapped by frustration caused by poor information and broken promises. Is there anything quite as irksome as spending $70 on a lavishly hyped wrinkle cream or $200 on a whole new skin-care routine, only to end up with more problems than you started with and none of the changes you were hoping for?

The truth is, beauty isn't easy (I wish it were effortless, but we all know better) because human skin and contemporary definitions of beauty are complicated realities. Skin-care problems are complex, arising from both external and internal sources, and related research can be exceedingly technical and difficult to understand. Skin is the body's largest organ, and exists primarily on the outside of the body. That's a lot of area to take care of. Also, skin isn't static: It can change from day to day, month to month, season to season, and year to year. And then there's the skin's intricate, complex structure and its dependence on hundreds of elaborate, integral chemical processes. All this makes it an understatement to say that skin care is complicated. Yet skin is one of the first things people notice about us. Our skin tells the world where we stand in terms of beauty and age. Skin displays the ravages of time, via sun damage, gravity, and genetically determined signs of aging, well before any of us want to see it. In our culture, flawless and wrinkle-free skin on the face is considered an obligatory component of beauty. And let's not forget that whole region from the neck down.

There are ways to take beautiful care of your skin, but the first step is to acquire a clear understanding of how the so-called "beauty" industry works so you don't repeatedly get waylaid by bad or ineffective products. Let's start at the beginning with some basic guidelines that can help you get through most of this information. I call them "The Ten (Plus Five) Commandments of Beauty." Get to know them before you go shopping at another cosmetics counter, see another infomercial, have a friend introduce you to a new multilevel cosmetics line, or read another fashion magazine. Once you've taken them to heart, you will have a better perspective on what you are really buying at the cosmetics counters, what these products can and can't do, whether what you are using is worth the money, and, most important, whether any of this can hurt your skin.

## The Ten (Plus Five) Commandments of Beauty

Actually, there are a lot more "thou shalts" and "thou shalt nots," and I go through each and every one of these throughout this book, presenting the information you need to make an educated decision about your skin care, body care, and makeup.

1. THOU SHALT NOT believe expensive cosmetics are better than inexpensive cosmetics. Women who spend more money on cosmetics do not necessarily have better skin than those on a tighter budget. Many expensive lines own inexpensive lines, ingredient lists don't differ between inexpensive and expensive lines, and cosmetics chemists are not chained to one company.

2. THOU SHALT NOT believe there is any such thing as a natural cosmetic (or that natural means better).

3. THOU SHALT NOT believe in miracle ingredients that can cure skin-care woes.

4. THOU SHALT NOT covet thy neighbor's perfect skin (or believe her perfect skin came from a particular product or cosmetics line; skin is more complicated than that).

5. THOU SHALT NOT believe everything a cosmetics salesperson tells you. (Cosmetics salespeople are not there to tell you their products are useless.) Read the ingredient list, try the product on, and be willing to return what doesn't work or fails to live up to the claim on the label, while also being very, very skeptical.

6. THOU SHALT NOT use the tiny applicators that come packaged with eyeshadows and blushes. Professional makeup artists never use these so why should you?

7. THOU SHALT NOT believe in the existence of antiwrinkle, firming, toning, lifting, or filling-in creams, lotions, or masks that can permanently erase wrinkles. (I wish it were so, but nothing on the horizon other than surgery can do that. I'm praying that this changes, and I'll let you know the second it does so we can all have truly wrinkle-free visages without the help of a surgeon.)

8. THOU SHALT NOT be seduced by every new promotion, new product, or new product line that the cosmetics industry creates.

9. THOU SHALT NOT get a tan. Sun is your enemy, not your friend; it is the primary reason that skin wrinkles and develops skin cancer.

10. THOU SHALT NOT buy a cellulite cream, nor shalt thou assume it's possible to dissolve fat from the outside in, because you absolutely cannot. Any product that could do that would be regulated as a drug and extremely dangerous and risky to use. Where would the fat go? Into the bloodstream? The lymph system? The liver? The heart? Certainly not where it goes when it is naturally metabolized. Anyway, if these products did work, who would be fat?

11. THOU SHALT NOT see pictures of pubescent, anorexic models (who spend two hours getting their hair and makeup done and another two hours posing while the photographer and a corps of assistants determine the most flattering lighting, after which the resulting picture goes through a battery of digitally enhanced touch-ups and adjustments) and believe you will get the same (or even similar) results from using the products being advertised (unless you happen to be pubescent, anorexic, and a model and that can somehow stay in the right lighting all the time).

12. THOU SHALT NOT buy products from an infomercial or a home shopping network, especially when the praise goes on and on with no opposing information. You are receiving an extremely one-sided point of view. It isn't natural for anyone to ever applaud a skin-care product.

13. THOU SHALT NOT believe words and phrases such as "hypoallergenic", "noncomedogenic", "for sensitive skin", "dermatologist tested", "exclusive formula", "increases moisture content" (by some astronomical percentage), or any other gross, unsupported generalization about a product.

14. THOU SHALT NOT buy cosmetic hormone creams assuming you can replace dietary sources of plant hormone or medically prescribed hormone therapy.

15. The ultimate commandment is: THOU SHALT be an informed consumer, because what you don't know can cost you dearly in terms of your skin, appearance, and money.

# INFOMERCIALS

I may be the only person in the world who has a recurrent dream that all women change channels every time an infomercial comes on the air. Of course, that is sheer fantasy on my part. The charisma of the salesperson/celebrity/doctor, the stunning before-and-afters, and the heartfelt testimonials always drive viewers to buy. Objective information is never part of the sales pitch in the cosmetics industry, and this is painfully obvious in the field of infomercials.

For as long as I have been researching and monitoring the cosmetics industry, I have been most amazed by the overly enthusiastic rantings and the ardent, rapturous claims espoused in infomercial after infomercial and on shopping channel after shopping channel. They are all, with their slick settings, attractive celebrity hosts, authoritative-looking doctors, and breathtaking before-and-after shots, shockingly redundant. It is little more than snake oil, but it all sounds so good women can hardly help themselves. Infomercials and shopping channel pitches are no worse than other kinds of advertising, but they are phenomena that take the meaning of hype to an entirely different level.

I wish I could divulge everything I've heard via the people I've met and interviewed in the infomercial business about what goes on behind the scenes, but none of it is substantiated. (I got the information from what I consider to be a reliable source, but I couldn't get corroboration. Without a second reliable source repeating the exact same story, I feel it would be unethical to share what I've learned. I use this standard rule about substantiation in all my books and newsletters.) For example, I would love to let you know about two very popular skin-care infomercials in which the celebrity spokeswomen both carried on at length about the quality of the products, yet neither had even seen them before they walked on the set the day of the shoot. Or about another very popular skin-care infomercial that cost about $5 million to produce, but lost a huge amount of money when more than 40% of the products were returned by disappointed consumers.

I've also personally seen how in-home shopping channels choose the skin-care products they put on the air. One person responsible for getting these products on the air admitted to me that they couldn't do anything about how useless or poor quality the cosmetics were or about the exaggerated claims made by the people selling the products. I was told that if the spokesperson is entertaining enough and appears to have a good pitch or angle, that is enough to get the product some air time.

I've often wondered how many more infomercials women will swallow about miracle skin-care products, skin-care regimes, and makeup products before they start to yawn (or laugh) and keep their money in their pocket. On the other hand, it is sadly true that women have an insatiable appetite for being misled by every slickly positioned sales pitch they hear. I'm not saying there aren't some truly good products in lines sold via infomercials, but the vast majority of the claims and adulation for all of these are manufactured and fabricated and based on hype and false promises.

## DOCTORS SELLING SKIN-CARE PRODUCTS

In the world of cosmetics, a growing number of dermatologists and plastic surgeons have crossed the line from physician to cosmetics salesperson. It is completely reasonable to expect your doctor to be an objective and impartial source of information based on the most current, documented, and peer-reviewed published research. However, that objectivity is at best questionable when the only options presented to you are the doctor's own products or the products the doctor is selling. Crossing the line from physician to cosmetics salesperson sidesteps the issue of medical ethics and the use of scientific modalities when treating or providing recommendations to patients.

From a scientific perspective this is at best problematic territory, though from a profit viewpoint it's good business and looking better all the time. Highlighting how prevalent and serious an issue this is, an article in the August 1999 issue of the *Tufts University Health & Nutrition Letter* stated that the "American Medical Association has issued guidelines advising physicians not to sell health-related products for profit. When a doctor stands to gain from something a patient buys, it creates a conflict of interest." The American College of Physicians–American Society of Internal Medicine issued ethical guidelines for physicians selling products reported on in the *Annals of Internal Medicine* (December 7, 1999). The paper stated that sales of cosmetics and vitamins by physicians are "ethically suspect."

When it comes to skin-care products being endorsed and sold by physicians, the most notable of this group of physicians are Dr. Sheldon Pinnell of Cellex-C and SkinCeuticals fame, Dr. Murad of Murad Skin Care (sold for years via infomercial), Dr. Zein Obagi, a dermatologist with a product line named after himself, and Dr. N.V. Perricone. What all of these doctors have in common is that they sell expensive skin-care products while making exaggerated claims about what their products can do, based almost exclusively on animal or in vitro testing, no testing at all, or conjecture.

For lots of women, the conflicting research and lack of proof among these dueling doctors doesn't matter in the least or pose any concern whatsoever. When it comes to getting rid of wrinkles, high prices rarely faze most women. If it sounds like magic and comes in the guise of medical authenticity, their pockets are now hundreds of dollars lighter and their vanity tables are lined with products that can't possibly live up to their claims.

Dr. N.V. Perricone, with his book *The Wrinkle Cure*, is now at the head of this group. His résumé is more than impressive. He is certified by the American Board of Dermatology and is a member of the Society of Investigative Dermatology, as well as Volunteer Clinical Attending Staff at the Dermatology Department at the Yale School of Medicine. What does Perricone want you to believe? His Web site states that his products are "The only clinical line of skin care treatments that is researched, created and patented by a Board-Certified Dermatologist and Research Scientist," referring to himself, of course. But Perricone's promise to "Defy aging and look ten years younger in days without chemical peels, cosmetic surgery or lasers with N.V. Perricone M.D. all-natural cosmeceutical skin treatments" is where he leaves his medical standing far behind and joins the overhyped world of those selling empty promises and unsubstantiated antiwrinkle products. Where he really gets off track is when his Web site states that these "are not cosmetics" because, according to the FDA, that is exactly what they are.

The entire arena of so-called professional or dermatologic products is nothing more than one of marketing distortion and aggrandizement. There isn't a single aspect of any "physician"-sold or -endorsed line that is specially formulated in any way or has any research showing that it's superior to anyone else's.

# CHAPTER 3
# MIRACLES, FRAUDS, & FACTS

Whether it's royal bee jelly, yeast extract, vitamins, amino acids, minerals, gems, special water, volcanic mud, DNA, placenta extract, a variety of animal organ extracts, or plants from every corner of the planet, the cosmetics industry wants you to believe that they have a miracle ingredient that can take care of your skin-care woes. To put it simply, every ingredient can't be a miracle. Before you can decide how to take care of your skin, you need to understand what ingredients can and can't do. This chapter focuses on the ingredients that get showcased on a label along with a product's promises of delivering wrinkle-free, acne-free, or just generally flawless skin, as well as the ingredients that have been questioned as being dangerous or a risk to skin. I've included all of the significant ones I am asked about most often. Among the ones listed there are definitely some genuine, incredibly effective ingredients that can have a positive effect on skin. But there are also many with overblown reputations, or with scant evidence that they are worthwhile for skin when it comes to daily skin care. And, of course, there are those that are just downright silly.

## ANTIOXIDANTS AND FREE-RADICAL DAMAGE

An "antioxidant" isn't a type of ingredient. Instead, the name describes the function or action a specific ingredient can have on the skin. Free-radical damage is what antioxidants are supposed to take care of, either by stopping new damage or by reversing earlier damage caused by free radicals. Antioxidants and free-radical damage are considered so vital to our understanding of the origins of cancer, aging, illness, and disease that they have become a profound area of research. Many major universities have an antioxidant or free-radical research department. Dozens of scientific journals are dedicated to these topics alone, including *Free Radical Research, Free Radical Biology and Medicine, Antioxidants and Redox Signaling, Oxidative Stress and Aging, Journal of Anti-Aging Medicine, Mechanisms of Ageing and Development, Photochemical & Photobiological Sciences, Photodermatology, Photoimmunology, Photomedicine,* and *Photochemical & Photobiological Sciences.*

Before you can understand the claims being made about many of the skin-care ingredients listed in this section, it is important to have an awareness of what free-radical damage is and what antioxidants can and can't do.

Let's begin by saying that free-radical damage is bad for the skin. It is well known that oxygen, sunshine (UV rays), and pollution are the main catalysts of free-radical damage. Theoretically, free-radical damage can cause deterioration of the skin's support structures, decreasing elasticity and resilience. What plays a part in slowing down free-radical damage is the presence of antioxidants in the diet, and, possibly, the topical application of antioxidants in skin-care products. Antioxidants are ingredients such as vitamins A, C, and E; superoxide dismutase; flavonoids; beta carotene; glutathione; selenium; and zinc. Technically there are thousands (yes, thousands) of viable antioxidant compounds in the plant world, of which we have so far discovered a mere handful.

Despite the proliferation of skin-care products containing antioxidants, according to many researchers, including Dr. Jeffrey Blumberg, chief of antioxidants research at Tufts University, "there is no conclusive scientific evidence that antioxidants really prevent wrinkles, nor is there any information about how much antioxidant(s) or exactly which one(s) has to be present in a product to have an effect" or if any noticeable effect is even possible.

Even if antioxidants did work on the skin to prevent free-radical damage, the results would hardly be immediate. Free-radical damage in the human body can continue for years and years before any noticeable deterioration can be detected. By the same token, you can't slap the stuff on and expect to immediately notice your wrinkles disappearing.

Despite this lack of hard evidence, fashion magazines and cosmetics companies have heralded the elimination of free-radical damage as the fountain of youth. The excitement about antioxidants is understandable. According to many skin experts (both legitimate experts and those who endorse specific products), all aspects of aging, including wrinkling, are caused by free-radical damage. Vitamin companies and cosmetics companies alike want you to believe their antioxidant products can eliminate it. The evidence is fairly convincing that free-radical damage is an insidious "natural" process that causes the body to break down. What isn't known is whether you can really stop free-radical damage that is taking place on the skin.

## FREE-RADICAL DAMAGE

Explaining free-radical damage is like trying to explain how television works. No matter how many times you're told how transmission and reception happen, unless you have a grasp of technology it all sounds like a foreign language. Nevertheless, here's a simplified explanation of free-radical damage.

Free-radical damage takes place on an atomic level. That's really small. To get a sense of an atom's size, imagine that 1 tablespoonful of water is made up of about 120 billion trillion molecules. Molecules are made of atoms, and a single atom is made up of protons, neutrons, and electrons. Electrons are always found in pairs. However, when oxygen molecules are involved in a chemical reaction, they can lose one of their electrons. This oxygen molecule that now has only one electron is called a free radical. With only one electron the oxygen molecule must quickly find another electron, and it does this by taking the electron from another molecule. When that molecule in turn loses one of its electrons, it too must seek out another, in a continuing reaction. Molecules attempting to repair themselves in this way trigger a cascading event called "free-radical damage." The action of free-radical damage takes place in a fraction of a second.

How does this affect our skin? Skin cells are formed of numerous parts, including the nucleus, where genetic material in the form of DNA resides; mitochondria, which are responsible for cell respiration and energy production; ribosomes, which are involved in protein synthesis and are composed of RNA which communicate genetic information; and lysosomes, which are responsible for a cell's enzymatic activity (its chemical actions). These elements are all encased in a plasma membrane (the cell wall). Any of these basic cellular elements—RNA, DNA, mitochondria, and lysosomes—can be broken or impaired by free radicals going about their business of looking for spare electrons.

While we can't see free-radical damage taking place in our skin (at least not without the aid of a skin biopsy and a powerful microscope), we can see it quite clearly in food or even paint. When paint is kept away from air (oxygen) and sunlight in a sealed container, it remains liquid. When it is exposed to air, however, it hardens. What makes this take place? The hardening occurs when an oxygen molecule interacts with the paint and becomes unstable, losing one of its electrons. In searching for another electron, it takes it from the molecule in the paint. This single event happens trillions of times until the paint dries and there are no more electrons available.

What triggers a molecule to let go of one of its electrons, generating free-radical damage? The answer is the presence of oxygen or any compound that contains an oxygen molecule (such as carbon mon**oxide**, hydrogen per**oxide,** and super**oxide**), sunlight, and pollution. Please note that super**oxide** dismutase is an antioxidant enzyme catalase to disarm and destroy the superoxide free radical.

In the human body, free-radical damage is taking place all the time. If you smoke, live in a city, or drive on the highway, that can accelerate the free-radical events taking place in your body at any given moment.

However, to refer to free-radical damage as "damaging" can be misleading. What we call free-radical damage is actually a common life function, in plants and animals as well as in the human body. Immune systems, metabolism, cells communicating with each other, and collagen production (as well as destruction) are all affected both positively *and* negatively by the presence of free-radical damage. This is referred to as the oxygen paradox. We need oxygen for life, but oxygen is also killing us. If you were to breathe pure oxygen for longer than one hour you would die! For all intents and purposes, and in basic terms, oxygen is probably one of the major reasons why, as we grow older, our body's systems start to shut down.

The question that you may be asking at this very moment is this: With all that free-radical damage taking place, and all this oxygen all around us (the air we breathe contains about 20% oxygen), how is it that we are still walking around? Why are we still living? The answer is antioxidants.

## ANTIOXIDANTS

Any substance that impedes or slows down free-radical damage by preventing the oxidative action of molecules is referred to as an "antioxidant". Antioxidants prevent unstable oxygen molecules (made unstable by loss of one electron) from interacting with other molecules (taking one of their electrons) and in turn causing them to become unstable, a process that starts the free-radical chain reaction. Fortunately, a vast assortment of antioxidants are found in both the human body and in the plant world. The full list is beyond the scope of this book. Some of the major categories in the plant world are the carotenoids and flavonoids. Many vitamins have antioxidant properties, including vitamins A, E, and C, as do amino acids such as methionine, L-cysteine, and L-carnitine; enzymes such as superoxide dismutase and ecatalase; and coenzymes such as lipoic acid and coenzyme Q10. Other antioxidant compounds include glutathione and methylsufonylsulfate.

So what does that have to do with wrinkles? No one is exactly sure, but theoretically when free-radical damage originates from natural environmental factors and fails to be cancelled out by antioxidant protection, then wrinkles appear. If we don't get enough antioxidant protection, either from our own body's production, from dietary sources, or from other sources, including antioxidants we put on our skin, free-radical damage continues unrestrained, causing cells to break down and impairing or destroying their ability to function normally. Instead of helping build collagen or other skin components, free-radical damage destroys them.

There's just one problem with the hope that stopping free-radical damage with antioxidants can protect your skin, and that's the fact that free-radical damage is constant and extensive. How could you ever use enough antioxidants to stop it?

How much oxygen, sunlight, or pollution can you really keep away from all skin cells, or even some skin cells? How fast do the antioxidants get used up? Do they last 20 minutes, one hour, two hours, or more on the skin? At this time, no one knows for sure.

Major investigations are now under way in this fascinating area of human aging (intrinsic aging) and sun damage (extrinsic aging), factors that most unquestionably influence wrinkling. However, even though many respected researchers are working on this issue, the research is still in its infancy, and suggesting anything beyond that is sheer fantasy.

Almost every company makes moisturizers that contain antioxidants, so they aren't hard to find. You won't see any difference in your skin, but if free-radical damage, and thus the destruction of the skin's structure, can be slowed or if sun damage can be reduced, then antioxidants should help. Many scientists think that if there is a fountain of youth, antioxidants could be in it. For now, that's only theoretical, and no one can give you any definitive amounts or specific ingredients to look for, despite the cosmetics industry's attempts to do so.

## ACETYL GLUCOSAMINE

Acetyl glucosamine is an amino acid sugar, the primary constituent of substances called mucopolysaccharides and hyaluronic acid that are found in all parts of the skin. It has value as a natural moisturizing factor (a natural component of the skin's composition) and is effective (in large concentrations) for wound healing. There is also research showing that chitins (also known as chitosan—which is composed of acetyl glucosamine) can help in the complex process of wound healing (Source: *Cellular-Molecular-Life-Science*, February 1997, pages 131–140). As impressive as that sounds, the tiny amount of acetyl glucosamine found in some skin-care products is several orders of magnitude less than the amount of acetyl glucosamine used to heal wounds. Further, it is important to understand that none of this relates to wrinkles. Wrinkles are not wounds. Injuries that cause a breach or tear in the surface of the skin, like those caused by a cut, stab, puncture, or scrape, are unrelated to what causes wrinkles. Something that may help heal a tear in skin is not going to change a wrinkle.

## ALGAE

For all intents and purposes algae is little more than pond scum or seaweed (seaweeds are large algae that grow in a saltwater or marine environment). Algae are very simple, chlorophyll-containing organisms, in a family of more than 20,000 different known species. That's a lot of scum and seaweed! A number of these have been used for drugs, where they can work as anticoagulants, antibiotics, antihypertensive agents, blood cholesterol reducers, dilatory agents, and insecticides. In cosmetics, algae are used in thickening agents, water-binding agents, and antioxidants. But algae are also potential skin irritants. For example, the phycocyanin found in blue-green algae has been suspected of allergenicity or causing dermatitis on the basis of patch tests (Source: *Current Issues in Molecular Biology*, January 2002, pages 1–11). Other forms of algae, such as Irish moss and carrageenan, contain proteins, vitamin A, sugar, starch, vitamin B1, iron, sodium, phosphorus, magnesium, copper, and calcium. For the most part, algae, in their many forms, are probably less of a risk and more of a help to skin when used as antioxidants. But the claims that algae can stop or get rid of wrinkling are completely unsubstantiated.

Names of the algae typically found in cosmetics include *Ulva lactuca, Ascophyllum, Laminaria longicruris, Laminaria saccharine, Laminaria digitata, Alaria esculenta,* various *Porphyra* species, *Chondrus crispus,* and *Mastocarpus stellatus.*

## ALPHA LIPOIC ACID

A large quantity of information shows that alpha lipoic acid, when taken *orally* as a dietary supplement, has many potential health benefits. Nevertheless, when it comes to research on what it can do to get rid of wrinkles and make a woman look younger, the information is at best theoretical and (more realistically) inconclusive. While studies of alpha lipoic acid do exist, none have been carried out on people and none have been double blind or placebo-controlled to evaluate wrinkling (Source: *Clinical & Experimental Dermatology*, October 2001, pages 578–582). All of the research has been done on human dermal fibroblasts "in vitro" in cell culture systems. In vitro (test tube) results are always interesting, but it's not known if they translate to human skin. These models do mimic human skin, but something that mimics human skin is still not the same as living skin. It is clear from the research that alpha lipoic acid is a potent antioxidant, but there are many potent antioxidants. Alpha lipoic acid is not the be all and end all when it comes to your skin's health.

## AYURVEDA

Ayurveda is an alternative health practice developed in India. The term "Ayurveda" is based on two Sanskrit words: *ayu,* meaning life, and *veda,* meaning science. Ayurveda is said to be 5,000 years old. That may impress a lot of people, but given that the average human life span prior to the 1900s was less than 50 years, and that the antibiotics developed in the mid 1940s provided health cures previously unknown, the benefits of this ancient science are not necessarily the panacea its adherents would have you believe. Regardless of your belief system, what is absolutely true is that the claims of Ayurveda's effectiveness or lack thereof are primarily anecdotal. That has been changing, however, with some plants proving to be beneficial and others not.

According to an article in the *Indian Journal of Experimental Biology* (May 2000, pages 409–414), the Ayurvedic system of treatments believes that the "living system is made of panch-mahabuta, in the form of vata, pitta and kapha at the physical level and satwa, raja and tama at the mental level. This covers the psychosomatic constitution and [is] commonly known as the Tridosh theory. The imbalance in these body humours [mechanisms] is the basic cause of any type of disease manifestation."

Another interpretation of Ayurvedic theory, in *Alternative Therapies Health Medicine* (March 7, 2001), noted that "The body is composed of 3 body doshas, 3 mental doshas, 7 dhatus, and malas. The harmony among the body doshas of vata (nervous system), pitta (enzymes), and kapha (mucus) and the gunas, or mental doshas (which are human attributes: satogun [godly], rajas [kingly], and tamas [evil]), constitutes health, and their disharmony constitutes disease. The management of illness requires balancing the doshas back into a harmonious state through lifestyle interventions, spiritual nurturing, and treatment with herbo-mineral formulas based on one's mental and bodily constitution."

As you can tell, this is not an easily understood subject. I am not capable of commenting on how or if Ayurvedic principles of any kind can affect skin (though I assure you they do not prevent sun damage—that, at least, is certain). A more complete discussion of Ayurveda would be too complex for the scope of this book and, to say the least, there isn't a shred of research documentation to examine in regard to skin. What I can say is that none of the so-called Ayurveda-based lines I've reviewed have any unique or unusual ingredients. All of the ones I've seen contain the same ingredients that show up in skin-care product after skin-care product, whether they are sold at drugstores, department stores, or health food stores.

## BOTANICALS

Is it worthwhile to look for natural ingredients in skin-care products? Leaving aside the fact that the process of removing a plant extract and then stabilizing and preserving it in a cosmetic renders it fairly unnatural, the answer is yes and no. There are bountiful numbers of wonderful plants and plant extracts that have beneficial effects on skin—and there are plenty of plant extracts that present problems for skin, too. Even so, let's say a natural or botanical ingredient is effective as a disinfectant; that doesn't make it better than a synthetically derived disinfectant, it just makes it an alternative. One shortcoming of natural ingredients in skin-care products that the cosmetics industry hasn't addressed is that each natural ingredient has a large range of limitations. These include what happens as a result of the purification process it goes through to get into a product, which part of the plant is effective, bad crops, possible contamination with herbicides, and maintaining consistent concentrations. In many ways synthetic ingredients are often more reliable for the skin.

It is also important to reiterate that just because an ingredient is found growing in nature doesn't mean it's good for the skin. Lots of plants are poisonous if ingested and lots of plants can irritate the skin.

Among the reasons to be wary of natural ingredients (aside from the lack of a regulated definition of the word "natural," as I mentioned in Chapter One) is that their manufacturers do not make their research available to the Cosmetic Ingredient Review (CIR) panel of the Cosmetic, Toiletry, and Fragrance Association (CTFA). This association is the cosmetics industry's attempt at self-regulation. The efforts of this group are interesting, even though the cosmetics industry doesn't always cooperate. According to an article in *Drug & Cosmetics Industry* magazine (June 1997, page 89), CIR panel members were "frustrated by a lack of specific information to allow them to characterize [natural] ingredients in a manner specific enough to determine safety [or benefit]." The panel further noted "botanicals are frequently poorly defined, subject to seasonal variations or variations due to different species sources, and varying extraction procedures." Specifically, what is lacking is sufficient information regarding composition, usage concentrations, and possible contaminants, which raises serious doubts about the safety of botanicals and their use.

While plants sound great, pure and natural and all that, and while sesame oil and licorice extract sound far better than capric/caprylic triglyceride and glycyrrhetinic acid, they aren't better *or* worse. Each has its pros and cons, and it would be a delusion to assume otherwise.

## COENZYME Q10—UBIQUINONE

It turns out that despite all the research available on coenzyme Q10 (CoQ10), there are only a handful of studies showing it to have any effect on wrinkles (Sources: *Biofactors*, September 1999, pages 371–378; *Zeitschrift für Gerontologie und Geriatrie*, April 1999, pages 83–88). However, neither of these studies was double blind or placebo-controlled, so there is no way to tell whether or not other formulations could net the same results. What is truly fascinating about CoQ10 has nothing to do with wrinkles. Rather, it is a well-researched nutrient with many studies demonstrating what it can do to improve health. CoQ10 has received particular attention in the prevention and treatment of various forms of cardiovascular disease, strokes, and hypertension. It also has been shown in a small number of studies to increase the metabolism of fat and to increase brain activity. It turns out CoQ10 resides primarily in organs, particularly the heart, with its presence peaking at around age 20 and declining after that. I've seen articles in *Health News* and *International Health News* suggesting CoQ10 should be taken with vitamin E, with a meal containing some fat, or in combination with soy or vegetable oil, which enhances its absorption substantially. "CoQ10 supplements are readily absorbed by the body and no toxic effects have been reported for daily dosages as high as 300 mg though the safety of CoQ10 has not been established in pregnancy and lactation, so caution is advised here until more data becomes available." (Source: *International Journal of Alternative and Complementary Medicine*, February 1998, pages 11-12).

Aside from those benefits, there is research showing that sun exposure depletes the presence of CoQ10 in the skin (Source: *Journal of Dermatological Science Supplement*, August 2001, pages 1–4). This isn't surprising because lots of the skin's components become diminished upon exposure to the sun. But whether or not taking CoQ10 supplements or applying them to skin stops or alters sun damage is not known.

## COLLAGEN AND ELASTIN

Collagen and elastin are best described as the skin's scaffolding. These two proteins create a cross-linked mesh that comprises more than 75% of the skin's structure and shape. They are also responsible for the skin's strength, smoothness, and elasticity. Clearly, collagen and elastin are fundamental to the health and appearance of our skin. One of the more amazing capabilities of collagen and elastin is that they can easily regenerate, which is why our skin is usually able to heal so quickly when wounded. As we age, from both intrinsic factors (chronological aging, health problems) and extrinsic factors (sun damage, pollution, smoking, free-radical damage), collagen and elastin get damaged and depleted. If collagen and elastin are so important and so capable of regeneration, then surely there must be a way to facilitate that process. From the cosmetics industry's perspective, it seems logical to manufacture moisturizers that contain collagen and elastin, and to attempt to convince women that if you apply these substances topically on the skin they will be absorbed and become part of your skin, shoring up and reinforcing your own collagen and elastin. However, the forms of collagen and elastin originally used in moisturizers were good only as water-binding agents because their molecular structure was too large to penetrate skin.

Using newer forms of collagen and elastin ingredients in skin-care products, however, manufacturers were able to break down the collagen and elastin structure, making them soluble and therefore able to penetrate skin. These new substances were referred to as pro-collagen and pro-elastin. Yet even though these newer substances were capable of penetrating skin, there is no research demonstrating that they had any effect on adding to the collagen or elastin content of skin. On the surface, collagen and elastin are nothing more than good water-binding agents (natural moisturizing factors of skin). That's good, but it won't change the shape or resiliency of skin.

Research indicates that it is possible to stimulate your skin to produce more collagen and elastin, but not by putting collagen and elastin on the skin. Rather, tretinoin, AHAs, BHA, and treatments such as laser resurfacing, chemical peels, and microdermabrasion can all provide that benefit. Antioxidants, anti-irritants, and natural moisturizing factors (water-binding agents) contribute to helping skin heal and may possibly help stimulate the production and growth of new collagen and elastin. Growth factors, discussed in this section, also play a role.

## COPPER

Copper is an important trace element for human nutrition. The body needs copper to absorb and utilize iron, and copper is also a component of the powerful antioxidant enzyme superoxide dismutase. Copper supplements have been shown to increase superoxide dismutase levels in humans (Source: *Healthnotes*— www.healthnotes.com). The synthesis of collagen and elastin is in part related to the presence of copper in the body, and it's important for many other reasons and processes. But is copper important for skin? Some skin-care companies definitely want you to believe this is the answer for your skin. It isn't. However, there is research showing that copper is effective for wound healing (Sources: *Journal of Clinical Investigation*, November 1993, pages 2368–2376; *Federation of European Biochemical Sciences Letter*, October 1988, pages 343–346).

As I've mentioned before, wound healing can't be compared to what happens with wrinkles. Wound healing is related to many biophysical processes that have nothing to do with wrinkling. Further, there are lots of substances that repair wounds. Far more research exists on transforming growth factor and epidermal growth factor for wound healing than on copper. And there is also research on the effectiveness of silver sulfadiazine for wound healing (Source: *Journal of Vascular Surgery*, August 1992, pages 251–257), tretinoin (Source: *Journal of the American Academy of Dermatology*, September 2001, pages 382–386), and curcumin (Source: *Journal of Trauma*, November 2001, pages 927–931) to name just a few. Actually there is far more research about tretinoin and the growth factors than there is concerning copper. Copper is still an option, but what, if anything, it may have to do with combating wrinkles is nothing more than conjecture, not fact.

# DEAD SEA MINERALS

The Dead Sea in Israel is considered dead because nothing can live in it. Many environmental factors have contributed to making the Dead Sea one of the saltiest lakes in the world. Seawater from the Atlantic and Pacific Oceans has a 3% to 4% salt content; the Dead Sea has a 32% salt content, as well as a large concentration of minerals such as sulfur, magnesium, calcium, bromide, and potassium. If you haven't been to the Dead Sea, I can tell you that the aroma from the sulfur water is overwhelming. It is hard to imagine that anything so noxious would be considered a beauty treatment.

It probably won't come as a shock to you when I tell you that there is no research showing that Dead Sea minerals have any effect on wrinkles. There are, however, several studies demonstrating that these minerals can have a positive effect on psoriatic skin (Sources: *Israel Journal of Medical Sciences*, November 2001, pages 828–832; *British Journal of Dermatology*, June 2001, pages 1154–1160; *International Journal of Dermatology*, February 2001, pages 158–159; *Journal of the American Academy of Dermatology*, August 2000, pages 325–326). Psoriasis is a skin condition characterized by rapidly dividing, overactive skin cells. No one is quite sure how the Dead Sea minerals and salts affect psoriasis. One of the more popular theories regarding its benefit is that the mineral content of the water slows down the out-of-control cell division. Some of the research indicates that the benefit is cumulative and the results can last for up to five months.

# DEA—DIETHANOLAMINE

In 1999 the National Toxicology Program (NTP) completed a study that found an association between cancer in laboratory animals and the application of diethanolamine (DEA) and certain DEA-related ingredients to their skin (Source: Study #TR-478, Toxicology and Carcinogenesis Studies of Diethanolamine (CAS No. 111-42-2) in F344/N Rats and B6C3F1 Mice (Dermal Studies), July 1999—http://ntp-server.niehs.nih.gov/). For the DEA-related ingredients, the NTP study suggested that the carcinogenic response is linked to possible residual levels of DEA. However, the NTP study did not establish a link between DEA and the risk of cancer in humans.

This study "found that repeated skin application to mouse skin of the cosmetic ingredient diethanolamine (DEA), or its fatty acid derivative cocamide-DEA, induced liver and kidney cancer." Besides this "clear evidence of carcinogenicity [only to mouse skin in high concentrations]," the NTP also emphasized that DEA is readily absorbed through the skin and accumulates in organs, such as the brain, where it induces chronic toxic effects. The report went on to explain that high concentrations of DEA-based detergents are commonly used in a wide range of cosmetics and toiletries, including shampoos, hair dyes, hair conditioners, lotions, creams, and bubble baths, plus liquid dishwashing and laundry soaps. "Lifelong use of these products thus clearly poses major avoidable cancer risks to the great majority of U.S. consumers, particularly infants and young children," the report stated.

It is important to note that this conclusion was a stretch. Taking results from high concentrations used on mice and extending them to long-term topical use by humans is not exactly scientific.

According to the FDA (Source: *Office of Cosmetics and Colors Fact Sheet*, December 9, 1999), "Although DEA itself is used in very few cosmetics, DEA-related ingredients (e.g., oleamide DEA, lauramide DEA, cocamide DEA) are widely used in a variety of cosmetic products. These ingredients function as emulsifiers or foaming agents and are generally used at levels of 1% to 5%. The FDA takes these NTP findings very seriously and is in the process of carefully evaluating the studies and test data to determine the real risk, if any, to consumers. The Agency believes that at the present time there is no reason for consumers to be alarmed based on the usage of these ingredients in cosmetics. Consumers wishing to avoid cosmetics containing DEA or its conjugates may do so by reviewing the ingredient statement required to appear on the outer container label of cosmetics offered for retail sale to consumers.

"If FDA's evaluation of the NTP data indicates that a health hazard exists, FDA will advise the industry and the public and will consider its legal options under the authority of the Food, Drug and Cosmetic Act in protecting the health and welfare of consumers."

I can see why some people may want to avoid DEA in cosmetics, and it is easy enough to do so, but given the specific research data, the entire issue of risk seems rather alarmist. In essence, there is as yet no real evidence demonstrating that people using cosmetics with DEA are anymore prone to cancers than those not using them.

# DHEA—Dehydroepiandrosterone

DHEA (dehydroepiandrosterone) is a male hormone produced in the adrenal glands that contributes to bone density, muscle mass, and skin tone. DHEA production peaks when we are in our 20s and, like all male and female hormones, declines shortly thereafter. Its popularity as an oral supplement comes from its reputation for increasing strength, boosting the immune system, enhancing memory and concentration, reducing depression, preventing weight gain, and heightening libido function. Talk about seductive! A quick search on the Internet for dehydroepiandrosterone brings up over 46,000 Web sites, a good many of which are linked to companies selling DHEA supplements.

The research on DHEA is interesting, albeit controversial. Libido function improvement was shown in research published in the *New England Journal of Medicine* (September 30, 1999) and brain function improvement was discussed in *Brain Research Reviews* (November 2001, pages 287–293). But according to an article in the *Harvard Men's Health Watch* (September 2001), DHEA is not ready for prime time. "In one small trial, 67% of subjects who took DHEA reported an increase in 'well-being,' but objective measurements found no change in body fat or sugar metabolism. In another study, DHEA treatment was associated with an increase in muscle strength and mass at the knee—but only eight men participated in the trial. More recently, doctors in New York administered DHEA in a dose of at least 50 mg a day to 10 men with an average age of 60; after 18 months, there was no change in blood testosterone or prostate specific antigen (PSA) levels...." This same article also mentioned a new study from the University of Missouri Medical School that "found no evidence DHEA had any benefits. The [39 men in the study] who took the hormone did not exhibit either a decrease in body fat or an increase in muscle mass; body weight did not change appreciably. Insulin and blood sugar levels were also unchanged. DHEA failed to produce an improvement in sexual function; similarly, there were no changes in overall subjective well-being." Further, Dr. Andrew Weil (at www.drweil.com) warns that DHEA "can increase the risk of breast and prostate cancer, and may elevate the risk of a heart attack."

What does any of this have to do with skin? Aside from the suggested association between DHEA and male hormone levels, and hormone levels having an effect on skin, there is no research showing DHEA has any impact on skin in regard to wrinkling or aging (Source: *Clinics in Geriatric Medicine*, November 2001, pages 661–672). Besides, it isn't the male hormones that improve the texture and appearance of female skin. The feel and suppleness of a woman's skin are affected by the levels of her estrogen and progesterone production.

# DMAE—DIMETHYLAMINOETHANOL

In regard to dimethylaminoethanol (DMAE), there is no research associating it with the skin in any way. What little research there is about DMAE relates to its effect as an oral supplement, and the findings are mixed. The claims about it being an instant face-lift or an ingredient that can repair skin come primarily, if not exclusively, from Dr. N.V. Perricone's book *The Wrinkle Cure,* but his assertions are not substantiated in any published study or research paper.

DMAE, known chemically as 2-dimethyl-amino-ethanol, has been available in Europe under the product name Deanol for over 30 years. As an oral supplement it is popularly known for improving mental alertness, much like *Gingko biloba* and coenzyme Q10. However, the research about DMAE does not show the same positive results found with the other two supplements. Because DMAE is chemically similar to choline, DMAE is thought to stimulate production of acetylcholine. And because acetylcholine is a brain neurotransmitter, it's easy to see how it could be associated with brain function. However, only a handful of studies have looked at DMAE for that purpose and they have not been conclusive in the least, and some have shown that DMAE may be problematic or not very effective (Sources: *Mechanisms of Aging and Development*, February 1988, pages 129–138; *Neuropharmacology*, June 1989, pages, 557–561; *European Neurology*, 1991, pages 423–425).

Aside from what it may do as an oral supplement, the question about DMAE and skin is whether or not a topical application can prevent cell deterioration. Perricone's assertion is that it can, though he doesn't cite a single source that backs up his finding (other than himself and a study where a cream containing DMAE that he sells was applied by 17 of his own patients).

Despite the lack of evidence supporting DMAE as having any effect on skin, there are hundreds of Web sites claiming that it can. It is possible that DMAE can help protect the cell membrane, and keeping cells intact can have benefit, but so far that appears to be only conjecture and not fact.

## EMOLLIENTS

Standard to almost *all* cosmetics, both the so-called natural ones and the not so natural ones, are soft, supple, waxlike, emollient, and thickening agents with names that read like a science journal—long and almost indecipherable. These pliable skin-softening agents have many functions. Not only do they have an affinity for skin, effortlessly smoothing over the surface and readily merging with the natural structures of the skin, they also provide the very feel and texture of the cosmetics we use. If a cosmetic has an elegant, smooth feel; or looks like a light, gel-like lotion; or has a soft, translucent appearance; or has a thick, creamy-white texture, it's the mix of these thickening, emollient ingredients that produces those finishes.

The assortment of names these technical-sounding ingredients come in is nothing less than astounding. There are more of them than you can imagine. They range from cetearyl alcohol, to isopropyl myristate, triglycerides, myristic acid, palmitic acid, PEG-60 hydrogenated castor oil, glyceryl linoleate, cyclomethicone, dimethicone, hexyl laurate, isohexadecane, methyl glucose sesquioleate, decyl oleate, stearic acid, octyldodecanol, and thousands more. There are also more understandable or at least familiar "natural" versions such as lanolin, hydrogenated plant oils, shea butter, and cocoa butter.

Together, these unsung heroes of moisturizers, sunscreens, cleansers, foundations, eyeshadows, and blushes are the mainstay of cosmetic formulations the world over. What they all have in common is their molecular resemblance to the natural lipids (sebum or oil) and intercellular substances found in skin. A big issue for dry skin is the very lack of these lipids and intercellular substances. Cosmetics with innumerable formulary recipes are invaluable resources to fill in what the skin lacks. These ingredients are what prevent dry skin, make rough skin feel smooth, soothe irritated skin, and replenish what skin loses from irritation, cleansing products, and sun damage. Although these indispensable substances are relatively indecipherable in the ingredient list, to a cosmetic formulation they are as important as, or even more important than, any natural-sounding ingredient could ever be.

On the other hand, while these thickening and emollient ingredients work great for a wide range of skin types, they may cause problems for someone with oily, combination, or acne-prone skin. Because all of these ingredients to one degree or another mimic the skin's own oil production, they add more to your own naturally abundant oil supply, and that will only make things worse. This is also true for natural-sounding ingredients like jojoba oil, shea butter, cocoa butter, safflower oil, lanolin, olive oil, and so on. This is one of the primary reasons why someone with oily, combination, or acne-prone skin should avoid almost all emollient moisturizers. When you have your own built-in lubrication (the oil produced by the oil glands) flowing freely onto your skin, it makes no sense to apply someone else's fabricated version, too.

# EMU OIL

The emu is a large, flightless bird indigenous to Australia, and emu oil has become an important component of the Australian economy. As a result there is research from that part of the world showing it to be a good emollient that can help heal skin. But along with the evidence that emu oil is a good emollient and the companies promoting it for that, there are also companies promoting products containing emu oil for its antiaging, antiwrinkling, and wound-healing properties. So does emu oil live up to these acclaimed properties? Regrettably, none of these promises are supported by research. A study published in the *Australasian Journal of Dermatology* (August 1996, pages 159–161), looked at the "Cosmetic and moisturizing properties of Emu oil … assessed in a double-blind clinical study. Emu oil in comparison to mineral oil was found overall to be more cosmetically acceptable and had better skin penetration/permeability. Furthermore it appears that Emu oil in comparison to mineral oil has better moisturizing properties, superior texture, and lower incidence of comedogenicity, but probably because of the small sample size these differences were not found to be statistically significant. Neither of the oils were found to be irritating to the skin." That's good, but it's hardly a reason to run out and by a product containing emu oil. Further, another study published in *Plastic and Reconstructive Surgery* (December 1998, pages 2404–2407), concluded that applying emu oil on a fresh wound actually delayed wound healing. Emu oil's reputation is driven mostly by cosmetics company claims and not by any real proof that emu oil is an essential requirement for skin.

## ENZYMES

Whether in the form of papaya fruit or in a substance such as papain (a proteinase derived from unripe papaya), enzymes have been used for quite some time as exfoliants. They're not as good as AHAs, but they're exfoliants nonetheless. The other new enzymes being put in skin-care potions are supposed to stimulate your skin's own biological processes that have slowed down because of age or sun damage.

Enzymes are proteins that function as biological catalysts. They accelerate chemical reactions in a cell, reactions that would proceed minimally or not at all if enzymes weren't there. Most enzymes—and a lot of different enzymes affect skin cells—are finicky about how they interact. Sometimes it takes several enzymes to produce one chemical reaction. Some enzymes depend on the presence of smaller enzymes, called coenzymes, in order to function. What this boils down to is that it is pretty complicated to stimulate enzyme activity in the skin. One little enzyme in a skin-care product won't turn on your skin's ability to create, say, collagen or elastin. It's a nice idea, but the theory is much more impressive than the effect, if any, on the skin.

Furthermore, even if enzymes were effective in skin-care products, they are an exceedingly unstable ingredient. Enzymes deteriorate quickly, depending on the pH of the product, the presence of other enzymes, and changes in temperature. Most likely, in any enzyme product you buy, the enzyme has deteriorated long before you have a chance to open the product.

## GINKGO BILOBA

Research establishing *Ginkgo biloba* as an effective systemic vasodilator (meaning it can increase blood flow and be effective for improving memory and concentration) has increased over the past several years (Sources: *Neuropsychobiology*, January 2002, pages 19–26; *International Journal of Neuropsychopharmacology*, June 2001, pages 131–134). When taken internally, there are other benefits (though there is still conflicting evidence) ranging from improvement in overall body circulation to reduced ringing in the ears in the elderly. However, the effects ginkgo may have on brain function and blood flow when taken as a supplement seem to be unrelated to its effects when applied topically on the skin. For skin, ginkgo has components that make it effective as an anti-inflammatory and an aid in collagen production, and it also has antioxidant properties (Sources: *Skin Pharmacology and Applied Skin Physiology*, July-August 1997, pages 200–205; *Journal of Pharmacy and Pharmacology*, December 1999, pages 1435–1440).

## GLYCERIN

While many cosmetics lines boast all sorts of exotic ingredients, from plant extracts to vitamins, proteins, essential oils, and other exotic and scientific creations, it turns out that plain old glycerin, long known as a humectant, may be a best friend for someone with dry skin. Glycerin is present in all natural lipids, whether animal or vegetable. It can be manufactured by the hydrolysis of fats and by the fermentation of sugars. It can also be synthetically manufactured. For some time it was thought that too much glycerin in a moisturizer could pull water out of the skin instead of drawing it into the skin. That theory now seems to be completely unfounded. What appears to be true is that glycerin shores up the skin's natural protection by filling in the area known as the intercellular matrix and by attracting just the right amount of water to maintain the skin's homeostasis. The intercellular matrix is the mortar that holds layers of skin cells together, creating an intact natural barrier. Keeping the intercellular layer intact keeps bacteria out, moisture in, and the skin's surface smooth. There is also research indicating that the presence of glycerin in the intercellular layer helps other skin lipids do their jobs better (Sources: *American Journal of Contact Dermatitis*, September 2000, pages 165–169; *Acta Dermato-Venereologica*, November, 1999, pages 418–421).

## GRAPE AND GRAPE SEED EXTRACT

A lot of the buzz surrounding grape extracts started with a story in *Consumer Reports* in November 1999 that ranked grape juice just above green tea and blueberries as having strong antioxidant properties. However the benefits reported both in *Consumer Reports* and in a lead story in *USA Today* (February 2, 2000) had to do with drinking the stuff, not putting it on the skin. There are no published studies indicating that grapes in any form, applied topically, can affect the wrinkling process (and vineyard workers are hardly wrinkle-free). But when it comes to skin care, there are lots of unpublished studies that "prove" all kinds of things. For example, one cosmetics line points to research by Dr. Stephen Herber of the St. Helena Institute for Plastic Surgery, who conducted a study on the benefits of grape seed, as proof of the efficacy of their products. Not surprisingly, St. Helena is in the heart of California's wine country. This "study," and I use the word loosely, had 16 volunteers who used pure milled grape seed extract as a topical application to their facial skin twice each day for six weeks. The results? Herber found that most of the volunteers reported improved texture to their facial skin. Others reported effects including an evening-out of complexion pigmentation and excessive oil, a decrease in breakouts, and a decrease in dryness. It only takes a cursory look to notice that this study wasn't done double-blind, that a placebo wasn't used (so we don't know if the results would be the same with a similar or dissimilar type of extract), and that we have no idea of the status of the participants' skin before they started, or what their relation to the product line or researcher was. Even if you buy the results of this study, the study itself used a pure concentration of the substance on the skin, not a product that contained just a small amount of the extract.

Still, none of that would diminish the potential benefit grape extract may have for skin because, aside from the hype, grape seed does contain proanthocyanidin, considered to be a very potent antioxidant (Source: *Current Pharmaceutical Biotechnology*, June 2001, pages 187–200). However, there is no research establishing its efficacy on skin.

As I've stated several times throughout this book, and will several times more, antioxidants are a big issue, and there is every reason to believe that there will be great strides in this area. For now, though, it's too early to suggest that we know which antioxidant is the best, how much of it is needed, or whether or not any of them work on the surface of skin to affect wrinkling in a positive way.

## HERBAL BREAST ENHANCEMENT?

Most women will do or pay anything to be beautiful, right? That's what a good portion of the cosmetics industry counts on, along with much of the herbal supplement business. While antiaging products are big business, there is also money to be made by convincing women they can take a pill, with all-natural ingredients of course, that will safely enhance the size of their bust. Perhaps images of celebrities with their expansive and overflowing breasts leap to mind along with the hope these products will create the same without surgery. Supplements with names like GroBust, Bust Plus, MiracleBust, Erdic, or Natural Contours abound on the Internet, in vitamin shops, and in mail-order catalogs.

What makes all this unnerving is that by overdosing the body with plant estrogens, these pills can, theoretically, have some effect, although there is no published research indicating that this is the case. Since the female breasts are composed primarily of fat tissue, the only reliable way to increase their size is to gain weight—not something most women want to do. Yet excess estrogen seems to pose that risk, and not only for the breast area. It can also cause bloating and acne. Even more to the point, although plant estrogens (also referred to as phytoestrogens) can have overt health benefits for perimenopausal and menopausal women, there is no research establishing what happens when too much of them are taken, or if there is a negative reaction for younger women who already have sufficient estrogen. But, of course, there are never any downsides to herbal supplements of this kind, at least not any we are likely to hear about from the companies busily selling these products.

The entire issue of breast-enhancement pills is a murky one, saturated with unethical companies doing their best to bilk you out of your money and potentially put your health at risk. For more detailed information about this issue, far more than I can address here, see one of my favorite Web sites, www.dietfraud.com. They have done extensive research on some of the companies selling breast-enhancement pills, including those promoted by some physicians with questionable credentials, and who already have numerous charges of fraud and malpractice lodged against them.

# HORMONE CREAMS

The multifaceted and controversial changes a woman experiences, both physiologically and emotionally, during perimenopause and menopause are too complex to cover in this book. However, I would like to provide a bit of insight on the area where perimenopause, menopause, and skin care cross paths, and offer some suggestions and resources so you will be better equipped to make informed decisions.

Thankfully, most cosmetic ingredients are completely benign. I do worry about irritating skin-care products, the lack of sun protection, and how marketing hype about plants and vitamins draws attention away from products that can really help. This last issue has me very concerned about a controversial barrage of skin-care products hitting the market that purportedly contain plant estrogen and/or plant progesterone. Tofu extract is reputedly the source of the plant estrogen, and wild yam extract is the source of the plant progesterone. Skin-care products that contain estrogen and progesterone are aimed directly at female baby boomers who are seeking solutions to the side effects of menopause. When the subject of perimenopause and menopause is on the table, the subsequent discussion usually centers on hormones.

For years, women have relied on oral or vaginally applied hormone replacement therapy (HRT—either estrogen alone or estrogen with progesterone) as their major remedy to ward off perimenopausal and menopausal symptoms such as hot flashes, vaginal dryness, osteoporosis, and changes in skin texture. For many women HRT was nothing short of a blessing. It eliminated hot flashes and vaginal dryness, reduced changes in skin texture, kept osteoporosis at bay, and kept women feeling and looking younger than those women who didn't take HRT. There is compelling research showing that estrogen loss has a significant impact on skin. The *American Journal of Clinical Dermatology* (2001, volume 2, number 3, pages 143–150) states that "Estrogen appears to aid in the prevention of skin aging in several ways. This reproductive hormone prevents a decrease in skin collagen in postmenopausal women; topical and systemic estrogen therapy can increase the skin collagen content and therefore maintain skin thickness. In addition, estrogen maintains skin moisture by increasing acid mucopolysaccharides and hyaluronic acid in the skin and possibly maintaining stratum corneum barrier function. Sebum levels are higher in postmenopausal women receiving hormone replacement therapy. Skin wrinkling also may benefit from estrogen as a result of the effects of the hormone on the elastic fibers and collagen. Outside of its influence on skin aging, it has been suggested that estrogen increases cutaneous wound healing by regulating the levels of a cytokine. In fact, topical estrogen has been found to accelerate and improve wound healing in elderly men and women…."

As beneficial as taking estrogen for skin can be, recent studies have brought to light the serious risks associated with HRT in regard to an increased risk of breast cancer. According to a study conducted by the Fred Hutchinson Cancer Research Center in Seattle, Washington, and a study published in the *Journal of the American Medical Association* (January 26, 2000), and reiterated in another article, August 2001 (page 907), there is a correlation between use of ERT [estrogen replacement therapy] and increased risk of heart attack. This is completely opposite from what ERT was originally thought to do, namely, preventing an increase in heart-attack risk that resulted from declining hormone levels. The recent Fred Hutchinson Cancer Research Center study also reported an association between endometrial cancer and ERT, though this is not conclusive due to conflicting research results. (The National Cancer Institute Information Resources, November 1999, released the following statement: "Because reports have shown that estrogen increases the risk of developing endometrial cancer … the National Cancer Institute is sponsoring a clinical trial to determine the effects of estrogen in women treated for early stage endometrial cancer.")

A recent follow-up study from Fred Hutchinson Cancer Research Center, Group Health Cooperative, and the University of Washington reported that long-term use of HRT increases the overall risk of breast cancer by about 70%. For one specific type of breast cancer, the risk increases by as much as four times (Source: *Seattle Times*, February 13, 2002).

## PLANT ESTROGEN

It isn't surprising that alternative, nonprescription sources of estrogen and progesterone would appeal to a wide audience of women enamored with "natural" products, especially given the risks of the medical options available. Plus, there is enticing anecdotal information suggesting that Asian women, who have diets high in soy (an estrogen-laden food), experience low rates of estrogen-positive cancers (particularly breast cancer) and that their menopausal symptoms are reduced (but not eliminated).

According to the research I've seen and the experts I've interviewed, there is indeed reason to believe that a diet consisting of foods high in estrogen, such as tofu, kudzu (a root from Japan but also grown in the United States), dates, pomegranates, and flax seed can prevent some of the side effects of menopause and potentially reduce some risks of estrogen-related cancers. But this is all strictly theory—encouraging, but with simply not enough research to make a definitive statement one way or the other.

The current understanding regarding plant estrogen is that it may work by interfering with the body's own estrogen, preventing it from being out of balance. Plant estrogen may fool the body into thinking it has the right balance of this hormone. If the body has too much estrogen, the plant estrogen may prevent the body from utilizing it (thereby preventing estrogen-related cancers); if the body has too little estrogen (as during the stages of menopause), plant estrogen might make the body think it has more, reducing some of the more uncomfortable side effects. In essence, a woman's estrogen level needs to be in balance for things to go right internally and externally. Too little or too much and you can have problems. It's like any other physical issue. Insulin is a hormone secreted by the pancreas. If too little insulin is present you have diabetes; too much, and you go into insulin shock. The same is true for estrogen: too much or too little can cause havoc with the body (and the emotions).

As many researchers and gynecologists have pointed out to me, diet may play a significant part in menopausal symptoms. But whether the American diet can duplicate the traditional Asian diet is a good question. There is little information about how many estrogen-laden foods a woman must consume (and for how long) to reduce or eliminate the effects of menopause. In other words, adding estrogen-rich foods or supplements to your diet won't necessarily prevent breast cancer, heart attack, or osteoporosis. (Keep in mind that, unlike the Asian diet, the typical American diet is high in animal protein, which, combined with a low rate of physical activity and exercise, can have an adverse or aggravating effect on menopausal symptoms.)

There are also studies that have shown no improvement or benefit from dietary estrogens (Sources: *Journal of Clinical Endocrinology & Metabolism*, January 2002, pages 118–121; *Toxicological Science*, February 2002, pages 228–238), although these were hardly sweeping or conclusive reviews. Clearly this is a health issue that needs to be examined more closely.

But what about estrogen creams? There is no research about plant estrogens showing they provide any benefit when applied topically to skin. But even if there were benefits, how much do you need to rub on your skin to obtain it? When it comes to cosmetics, there is no way to know how much of a plant estrogen extract is being used, or how much may be in a moisturizer. More to the point, because the cosmetics and natural-supplement industries are not regulated, there is no way to really know what you are getting. Until there is, leaving your health up to guesswork and marketing schemes is not a wise choice.

## PROGESTERONE IN SKIN-CARE PRODUCTS

At the forefront of the female hormone battle is a Dr. John Lee, with his books *What Your Doctor May Not Tell You About Menopause: The Breakthrough Book on Natural Progesterone* (Warner Books, 1996) and *What Your Doctor May Not Tell You About Premenopause* [perimenopause]*: Balance Your Hormones and Your Life from Thirty to Fifty* (Warner Books, 1999). Lee's primary thesis is that ERT and HRT were flawed for many reasons. On one level, Lee feels ERT is problematic because it utilizes synthetic estrogen and/or synthetic progesterone. But a matter of more concern to Lee is that ERT (without progesterone, as it was typically prescribed for years) puts the emphasis on the wrong hormone, namely estrogen, instead of progesterone. Lee's research suggests that too much estrogen, or "estrogen dominance" as he calls it, is the problem, and that natural progesterone is the only option to combat a woman's hormonal changes.

So what is the difference between progesterone and estrogen? Progesterone is manufactured in the body from the steroid hormone pregnenolone, and is the source or precursor of other steroid hormones, including cortisol, androstenedione, estrogens, and testosterone. For women, progesterone and estrogen work together in a subtle symphonic harmony. This hormonal balance creates the rhythm of the menstrual cycle, and when that harmony gets out of tune, particularly during perimenopausal and menopausal years, the problems for women are significant. Estrogen levels drop by 40% to 60% at menopause, which is just enough to stop the menstrual cycle. But progesterone levels drop, too, and for some women, they may drop to almost nonexistent. According to Lee, "Because progesterone is the precursor to so many other steroid hormones, its use can greatly enhance overall hormone balance after menopause, even for estrogen …" although estrogen itself cannot affect progesterone levels.

Menstruation depends on what is taking place in the ovaries and uterus, including the hormones generated by the hypothalamus and pituitary gland in the brain and the corpus luteum in the ovary. During the first half of the menstrual cycle, as an egg follicle grows in the ovary, estrogen is manufactured and released into the blood. As the egg follicle matures in the lining of the ovary, a hormone called luteinizing hormone (LH) causes the egg to be released directly into the ovary. The ovary then starts producing progesterone while estrogen production declines. Progesterone's role is to help the egg to mature even faster, increasing fertility. As you may know, this hormonal fluctuation in estrogen production versus progesterone takes place at midcycle, when a woman is the most fertile. Not surprisingly, the increased progesterone levels correspond to a surge in a woman's sexual drive (after all you can't get pregnant if your libido—brain—doesn't want to have sex). If fertilization does not occur, ovarian production of progesterone falls dramatically. It is this sudden decline in progesterone levels that triggers the shedding of the uterine lining that results in a menstrual cycle. In essence, estrogen encourages the growth of endometrial tissue in the uterus, and progesterone causes this lining to be shed.

In a recent interview with Dr. John Lee, he told me that he "wants people to understand that natural progesterone brings everything back into balance. Around the time when progesterone is low in women, approximately age 45, there is an estrogen dominance occurring in the body, which causes such things as auto-immune disorders, hair loss because there are more androgens [in the body not counterbalanced with progesterone], risk of breast cancer, and a low libido." Lee went on to explain that "natural" progesterone "is the same identical hormone found in women as opposed to the use of synthetic forms of progesterone (progestins) found in prescription-only drugs that merely mimic the effect progesterone has on the body."

So, if Lee is right, why is the research about natural progesterone so controversial? According to Lee it's because "natural progesterone cannot be patented, it is available to everyone and anyone who wants to [can] put it into any lotion or cream they make. Pharmaceutical companies do not fund research that has no likelihood of netting a profit. Therefore, pharmaceutical companies put a lot of money into researching synthetic hormones that … can be patented and sold exclusively by the patent holder. It follows that there is a lot of research out there to show that synthetic progesterone and synthetic estrogen work and [explains] why there is little research about the use of natural progesterone [there is simply no profit in the latter]. Pharmaceutical companies do not even broach the issue of natural hormonal options versus synthetic ones with physicians because there is no financial motivation to do so."

There is also controversy among physicians as to whether or not progesterone applied topically can provide the body with the same amounts as synthetic forms of progesterone taken orally. Physicians point out that anecdotal information about positive results from natural progesterone is flawed because in double-blind studies the placebo effect for hot flashes or other physical improvements is about 40% when compared to a test vehicle. Further, when actual blood levels of progesterone are measured, physicians found low levels of natural progesterone, confirming their suspicion that not enough of the natural progesterone is absorbed through the skin. Lee is frustrated by this finding because the medical profession will not accept that "natural" progesterone levels are best tested in saliva and not in blood serum, the way synthetic progesterone is measured. Lee's saliva tests indicate that the natural progesterone creams do produce normal levels of progesterone that can be accurately read.

Is there any risk to applying natural progesterone topically? Lee said he has not seen adverse effects since he began studying it over 20 years ago. This is one aspect of Lee's work that requires more research. Although Lee may not have seen any problems, that doesn't mean they don't exist. After all, Lee would not be the doctor to visit; if problems occurred, women would turn to other doctors for uterine or breast difficulties (he was a family physician). Lee does acknowledge that there is a risk of hyperplasia (an abnormal increase in the number of cells in an organ or a tissue with resulting swelling) and a feeling of lightheadedness and lethargy. However, Lee also points out that "during pregnancy, the placenta produces 300 to 400 milligrams of natural progesterone daily during the last few months of pregnancy, so we know that such levels are safe for the developing baby. But [synthetic progesterones—progestins] even at fractions of this dose, can cause birth defects."

Clearly, more research is needed to settle the issue. But without question this is a growing option for treating the symptoms of hormonal changes. Understanding the options and risks, and being able to separate the truth from what is truly intense hype, both by the "believers" in natural progesterone cream and the "believers" in pharmaceutical or synthetic hormonal therapy, is imperative for women facing this change in their bodies.

And there are lots of formidable believers on both sides of the issue. Typing the term "natural progesterone" into a search engine on the Web brings up over 40,000 hits (and most of those are from companies or doctor's offices selling natural progesterone creams), and searching for "estrogen replacement therapy" brings up just about the same number from medical professionals prescribing ERT. When it comes to natural progesterone products, Lee explained that right now there are about 140 companies marketing natural progesterone creams that come from 20 different labs. And with the baby boomers coming full-fledged into their perimenopausal and menopausal years, there will probably be more and more coming to market. Given that natural progesterone creams are not regulated in any way by the FDA, and that they are, in actuality, merely cosmetics, that means anyone can put them into any product they want to.

According to an associate of Lee's, David Zava, PhD, director of research for ZRT Laboratory in Portland, Oregon, "nearly all of the [natural] progesterone cream products are formulated to deliver about 15 to 30 milligrams of USP grade progesterone per 1/4 teaspoon of cream." For perimenopausal women, Lee recommends 15 to 24 milligrams applied daily for 14 days before the menstrual cycle is expected to begin and then stopping the day before the menstrual cycle starts. For menopausal and postmenopausal women, he suggests reducing the application to 15 milligrams per day for 25 days and then not using it for 5 days. Lee states that 15 to 20 milligrams "… is the same amount the ovaries make naturally."

A study published in the *American Journal of Obstetrics and Gynecology* (June 1999, pages 1504-1511) concurs with Lee's position, stating that "In order to obtain the proper (effective) serum levels with use of a progesterone cream, the cream needs to have an adequate amount of progesterone in it [at least 30 milligrams per gram]. Many over the counter creams have little [for example, 5 milligrams per ounce] or none at all. The creams that are made from Mexican yams are not metabolized to progesterone by women. The cream used in the above study (Pro-Gest) contains pure United States Pharmacopoeia [USP] progesterone." Ironically, Pro-Gest was the only cream around at the time Lee started his research.

Lee explains that "The USP progesterone used for hormone replacement comes from plant fats and oils, usually a substance called diosgenin, which is extracted from a very specific type of wild yam that grows in Mexico, or from soybeans. In the laboratory, diosgenin is chemically synthesized into real human progesterone. Some companies are trying to sell … 'wild yam extract' [or other plant extracts] … claiming that the body will then convert it into hormones as needed. While we know this can be done in the laboratory, there is no evidence that this conversion takes place in the human body." Lee is quick to explain that he doesn't sell any of these products and receives no profit from their sale. He also does NOT recommend the use of natural progesterone creams with any other active hormones or herbs.

So what should you use if you want to give natural progesterone creams a try? Lee recommends creams that contain between 400 and 500 milligrams per ounce of cream. That amount would provide about 20 milligrams per day when applying a quarter teaspoon of the cream. But before you venture out shopping for natural progesterone creams, I strongly encourage you to check out Lee's books (available on www.amazon.com and in most bookstores) and to visit his Web site at www.johnleemd.com. Lee lists the companies that sell products that meet his criteria. There is also a list of products that meet the recommended amount of USP progesterone provided by Aeron LifeCycles Laboratory, San Leandro, California, on their Web site at www.aeron.com.

# HUMAN GROWTH FACTOR

It is important to make clear that the topic of human growth factor (HGF) is exceedingly complicated. The physiological intricacies of the varying HGFs and their action challenge a layperson's comprehension. Nonetheless, because the use of HGF seems to be a direction some skin-care companies are taking, and because there is a large body of research showing its efficacy for wound healing (but not for wrinkles), it does deserve comment. Grasping the full depth of this issue, however, is not within the scope of this book.

HGF is a complex family of hormones that are produced by the body to control cell growth and cell division in skin, blood, bone, and nerve tissue. Most significantly they regulate the division and reproduction of cells. They also can influence the growth rate of some cancers. HGFs occur naturally in the body but they are also synthesized and used in medicine for a range of applications, including wound healing and immune system stimulation. The following are the body's primary HGFs:

**Epidermal Growth Factor (EGF):** Stimulates cell division of many different cell types.

**Erythropoietin (Epo):** Stimulates the growth of cells that carry oxygen to the body.

**Fibroblast Growth Factor (FGF):** Stimulates growth of the nervous system and bone formation.

**Hepatocyte Growth Factor (HGF):** Stimulates division in cells lining the liver, skin cells, and cells that produce skin color.

**Insulinlike Growth Factor (IGF):** Stimulates fat cells and connective tissue cells.

**Interleukins (IL):** Stimulate growth of white blood cells.

**Nerve Growth Factor (NGF):** Stimulates growth of nerve tissue.

**Platelet Derived Growth Factor: (PDGF):** Promotes the growth of blood clotting factor.

**Transforming Growth Factor (TGF):** Stimulates wound healing and collagen growth.

**Vascular Endothelial Growth Factor (VEGF):** Stimulates the growth of blood vessels.

All of these HGFs are chemical messages that bind to receptor sites on the cell surface (receptor sites are how cells communicate with any substance to let them know what or what not to do). HGFs need to communicate with cells to instruct them to activate the production of new cells or to tell a cell to create new cells that have different functions. Another way to think of HGFs is that they are messengers designed to be received or "heard" by specific receptor sites or "ears" on the cell.

Many HGFs are quite versatile, with the ability to stimulate cellular division in numerous different cell types, while other HGFs are specific to a particular cell type, say blood cells or bone cells.

We are most familiar with HGFs like TGF, in their role in surgical-wound healing. The main task for HGFs is to cause cell division, which is helpful; however, at certain concentrations and lengths of application they can cause cells to over-proliferate, which can cause cancer or other health problems.

Skin is an elaborate network of growing tissue that continually regenerates and can usually heal after it is cut, punctured, burnt, or scraped. How skin goes about this process is in many ways a physiological miracle directed by an intricate network of HGFs. "In skin, the most actively regulated growth occurs in the epidermis, the visible, outermost layer. A finely regulated growth factor system maintains homeostasis or biological status quo in the epidermis by adjusting the rates of cell growth versus cell death in response to injury, sunburn, or disease. Failures in this system lead to skin disorders such as psoriasis or even skin cancers" (Source: http://www.wound-healing.net/).

But what happens when you put HGFs on skin, particularly TGF and EGF, as some companies claim their products contain? The risk is that they could accelerate the growth of skin cancer by stimulating the overproduction of skin cells. In the case of TGF, which stimulates collagen, that can encourage scarring. Scars are the result of excessive collagen production; if you make too much collagen you get a scar or a knot on the skin such as a keloidal scar. Most of the research on the issue of HGFs for skin has looked primarily at the issue of wound healing, and at short-term use of HGFs. In skin-care products, they would be used repeatedly, possibly over long periods of time.

There is another body of research concerning HGFs, one being touted as the answer for wrinkles. Here is what the research shows: Based on established scientific protocol, you can create "living" skin cells in a petri dish. It is known that normal human skin cells divide a predictable number of times and then die. At first skin cells grow and divide rapidly, and then the division rate slows as we age. Finally the cells cease replicating. In vitro, you can re-create the skin cell's life process and accelerate the effect, so you can watch the growth process of cells in a short period of time (weeks, as opposed to a normal person's life span). If you leave these skin cells alone, they go through a normal life span and eventually stop replicating. However, when you add some forms of HGFs, the skin cells live far longer than they would have on their own. While that sounds like your skin would stay young forever, the other part of the picture is that if you add too much HGF, the skin cells die off sooner than they would have if you hadn't added any! This part of the information is often left out of the impressive data that companies like to publicize in regard to their products.

One other significant shortcoming of HFGs, according to an article by Dr. Donald R. Owen in the March 1999 issue of *Global Cosmetic Industry*, is that "The body produces these [HGFs] in exquisitely small concentrations at just the right location and time.... Actual growth factors such as [EGF and TGF-B] are [large] configurations, which do not penetrate the skin.... They [also] lose their activity within days in water or even as solids at normal temperatures.... [Yet], even after all these complications, the siren's song is too strong. We [the cosmetics chemists] will use them."

The research into HFGs is without question intriguing, but there is much that's not known, especially in terms of long-term risk or stability when they're used in cosmetics and applied to skin. In this arena, if cosmetics companies continue to use HGFs, it's the consumer who will be the guinea pig.

# KINETIN

Kinetin is a plant-growth hormone with the technical name N6-furfuryladenine. Several companies, including The Body Shop, Almay, Osmotics, and Kinerase, sell products containing kinetin. (Kinerase is not in any way special just because it is sold through a doctor's office; it contains the exact same kinetin as the less-expensive versions from The Body Shop and Almay, and the more expensive option from Osmotics.)

The unpublished study that created the excitement around kinetin was conducted in part by Dr. Jerry L. McCullough, Professor, University of California, Irvine (UCI). In a letter to me McCullough stated that in the research done by his team "The UCI study was a double-blind study, which involved subjective assessments of clinical improvement and safety by both the physician and the subject. This is the protocol design used in the pivotal multicenter clinical trials of Renova, which were reviewed by the FDA and led to FDA approval. The above studies focused on the clinical assessment of safety and efficacy as did the kinetin studies. The only objective measures of efficacy in the Renova clinical studies were skin replica analysis and histologic evaluation. The studies at UCI involved over 160 subjects in two studies, each lasting one year.... These studies employed objective assessment of the skin-barrier function using measurements of transepidermal water loss (TEWL) in addition to state of the art clinical photography (Canfield Scientific) to document clinical response. I think that the efforts made by Senetek PLC [the company that licenses kinetin to the cosmetics companies] to document the efficacy and safety of this product far exceed those of the numerous anti-aging skin products [that] flood the cosmetic counters and Web pages making unsubstantiated claims."

While on the surface it does appear that kinetin can perform like Renova, it is important to recognize that the UCI study does not indicate any results about cellular effects or changes. This study looked at surface improvements. As I've reported in the past, the studies the FDA accepted about Renova's performance for wrinkles were hardly definitive. TEWL tells you about moisturization, not about wrinkles, and while visual assessments may be impressive, they don't tell you if other moisturizers with other ingredients would net you the same improvements. The main interest in kinetin for skin care actually has nothing to do with wrinkles. By contrast, the active ingredient in Renova, tretinoin, has a wealth of established literature regarding its effect in improving abnormal skin-cell production caused by sun damage. That makes Renova (or any other drug containing tretinoin) significant. Kinetin has no such effective data.

What does make kinetin far more interesting are the in vitro and animal studies demonstrating its effect as a growth factor, and how that may affect cellular production. Most of the in vitro or animal-model studies about kinetin were conducted by Dr. Suresh I.S. Rattan, PhD, DSc, Associate Professor of Biogerontology at the University of Aarhus, Denmark, who happens to hold the patent for N6-furfuryladenine for use on aging skin. Rattan discovered this plant growth factor in 1988 and obtained the U.S. patent in 1994. That is, Rattan discovered what happens to skin cells in a petri dish when N6-furfuryladenine is added.

Rattan told me, "Normal cells, as they divide and age, go through a progressive accumulation of changes that are irreversible until they reach a stage where they finally die. This in vitro [meaning in a petri dish as opposed to in humans or animals] form of creating cellular aging, which takes place over one year—consider that it takes our cells more than 70 years to age—is a well-known biochemical phenomenon called the Hayflick Phenomenon, named after the researcher who discovered this method of studying cellular aging in a laboratory setting."

All this relates to N6-furfuryladenine and what it does when added to cells that are aging in a petri dish. Rattan continued, "Normally when we grow cells in culture, as they become older, regardless of sun exposure, they go through over 300 varying changes and alterations. A young cell is plump, round, smooth (and the functions and chemical processes orderly and vigorous). As the cells age, they become irregular, flattened, and large, full of debris—debris meaning they fill up with waste products that they can't get rid of. Further, when you grow normal cells in the lab they have a limited number of times they multiply and divide—termed a cell's replicative life span. But when I added N6-furfuryladenine to these cultures the cells did not age as fast, the process slowed down dramatically. In the presence of various concentrations of N6-furfuryladenine, cells act younger, longer."

As exciting as this sounds, and Rattan is indeed excited about his research, he also said, "Topically [applied to the surface of skin] no one knows how or if N6-furfuryladenine is being taken up or used by the cell. There are no studies done on the biochemical action on human skin or animal skin. It has only been observed for in vitro systems. On one level I feel this compound can be a health-preserving molecule. But it would take a lot of money to find out its full potential.

"What will put my mind at rest is knowing what the full up and down side is. We are curious about negative effects; even water is toxic in certain doses. In cell cultures when a concentration of say 250 micromolars [a chemical measure of extremely small sizes] of N6-furfuryladenine was used, we got good results, but when we used 500 micromolars of N6-furfuryladenine the cells started dying."

I suspect that when it's applied topically, kinetin isn't of much use to the skin cell, and even if it could somehow be utilized, there probably isn't enough kinetin in any product to have a negative or positive impact—but that is only a guess, no one knows for sure (Source: *Dermatologic Clinics*, October 2000, pages 609–615).

If kinetin isn't a problem for the skin cell, other research does demonstrate quite clearly that it can be a potent free-radical scavenger (antioxidant), which can hypothetically prevent oxidative damage on the skin (oxidative damage is one theory of why skin wrinkles or eventually looks old). But there are many potent antioxidants found in skin-care products these days, from beta glucan to vitamin C, vitamin A, green tea, grape extract, and on and on, that don't have the possible risks and disturbing unknowns associated with kinetin.

## LANOLIN

Lanolin has long been burdened with the reputation for being an allergen or sensitizing agent. That has always been a disappointment to formulators because lanolin is such an effective moisturizing agent for skin. A recent study in the *British Journal of Dermatology* (July 2001, pages 28–31) may change all that. This study concluded "that lanolin sensitization has remained at a relatively low and constant rate even in a high-risk population (i.e., patients with recent or active eczema)." Based on a review of 24,449 patients who were tested with varying forms of lanolin, it turned out that "The mean annual rate of sensitivity to this allergen was 1.7%"—and it was lower than that for a 50% concentration of lanolin. It looks like it's time to restore lanolin's good reputation, which is a very good thing for someone with dry skin to know.

## MAD COW DISEASE IN COSMETICS?

Mad Cow Disease and the risk it poses for humans (and, of course, animals) has mostly affected countries outside of the United States, primarily England, and does not yet appear to be of concern here. According to the FDA, the USDA (United States Department of Agriculture), and the CDC (Centers for Disease Control and

Prevention), no incidents of Mad Cow Disease have been reported in the United States. There are some sources who disagree with that declaration, but substantiation is hard to come by.

Mad Cow Disease (technically known as bovine spongiform encephalopathy or BSE) is a chronic degenerative disease affecting the central nervous system of cattle. The concern for humans is the risk of eating meat or meat products that contain the BSE pathogen. When the BSE pathogen takes hold in people, it can trigger a variant form of the disease called Creutzfeldt-Jakob disease (after the researchers who identified it). In Europe, over 100 people are now known to have contracted Creutzfeldt-Jakob disease, which leads to dementia and can cause death. The CDC (www.cdc.gov) reports that "… in the United Kingdom, this current risk [of Creutzfeldt-Jakob disease] appears to be extremely small, perhaps about 1 case per 10 billion servings [of beef]." It also states that "Milk and milk products from cows are not believed to pose any risk for transmitting the BSE agent." While the human toll is infinitesimally small when compared with many other known potentially serious diseases, from malaria to AIDS and even the flu, scientists are concerned that we are on the verge of an epidemic that they want to stop before it gets worse.

While it is important to pay attention to the issue of Mad Cow Disease in relation to eating beef or meat, the question is whether or not bovine-derived ingredients used in cosmetics can harbor the disease and cause health risks. The answer is that no one knows for sure, but theoretically a remote possible risk does exist. Some researchers feel that there is no evidence BSE can be contracted through the skin (Source: *Cosmetic Dermatology*, December 2001, pages 43–47); however, neither cooking, preserving, or any of the other processing most cosmetics go through can eliminate BSE pathogens. That means if animal by-products are used in cosmetics (in particular placenta and spleen bovine extracts), they can pose a risk, albeit remote, to the user. The British BSE Committee (http://www.bse.org.uk/) in varying reports has mentioned a concern that people could become infected if the creams were used on broken skin. It is important to realize that very few products use those kinds of ingredients.

If you are thinking of buying any cosmetics that contain animal organ extracts of any kind, you may want to reconsider, or discard them if you have already made a purchase. Other than that, at this point, I feel strongly that it isn't necessary to worry about the other ingredients on your cosmetics labels. Aside from the evidence, which does not point to a single case of BSE associated with cosmetics, checking the ingredient label wouldn't be of much help anyway because there is no way to know whether the collagen or ceramide in your product is sourced from animals or plants. I want to stress that from all the research that is out there, this appears to be a negligible issue for your beauty routine.

## MINERAL OIL

The notion that mineral oil and petrolatum (Vaseline) are bad for skin has been around for some time, with Aveda being the most visible company to mount a crusade deriding these ingredients. According to many companies that produce "natural" cosmetics, mineral oil and petrolatum are terrible ingredients because they come from crude oil (petroleum) and are used in industry as metal-cutting fluid (among other uses) and, therefore, can harm the skin by forming an oil film and suffocating it.

This foolish, recurring misinformation about mineral oil and petrolatum is maddening. After all, crude oil is as natural as any other earth-derived substance. Moreover, lots of ingredients are derived from awful-sounding sources but are nevertheless benign and totally safe. Salt is a perfect example. Common table salt is sodium chloride, composed of sodium and chloride, but salt doesn't have the caustic properties of chloride (a form of chlorine) or the unstable explosiveness of sodium. In fact, it is a completely different compound with the harmful properties of neither of its components.

Cosmetics-grade mineral oil and petrolatum are considered the safest, most non-irritating moisturizing ingredients ever found (Sources: *Cosmetics & Toiletries*, January 2001, page 79; *Cosmetic Dermatology*, September 2000, pages 44–46). Yes, they can keep air off the skin to some extent, but that's what a good antioxidant is supposed to do; they don't suffocate skin! Moreover, petrolatum and mineral oil are known for being efficacious in wound healing, and are also considered to be among the most effective moisturizing ingredients available (Source: *Cosmetics & Toiletries*, February 1998, pages 33–40).

## NATURAL MOISTURIZING FACTORS AND LIPIDS

One of the primary elements in keeping skin healthy is making sure the structure of the epidermis (outer layer of skin) is intact. That structure is defined and created by skin cells that are held together by something called the intercellular matrix. The intercellular matrix is the "glue" within the skin that keeps skin cells together, helps prevent individual skin cells from losing water, and creates the smooth, non-flaky appearance of skin; these components are called natural moisturizing factors (NMFs). Lipids are the oil and fat components of skin that prevent evaporation and provide lubrication to the surface of skin. It is actually the intercellular matrix along with the skin's lipid content that gives skin a good deal of its surface texture and feel.

When the skin's intercellular matrix and lipid content are impaired, the skin is subject to dryness, an increase in the bacteria that cause blemishes, irritation, flaking, redness, roughness, and a tight, uncomfortable feeling on skin. How do you know if your intercellular matrix and lipid content are intact? A wound or cut is easy to understand because you can see that the skin's intercellular matrix has been impaired and is no longer an intact structure. Damage like that is at one extreme end of the type of problems that can make the skin unhealthy. On the less obvious end are sun damage, irritating skin-care products, dry climates, indoor heat, smoking, and intrinsic aging factors, which all injure the skin's intercellular matrix by depleting the skin's lipid content as well as its content of NMFs. When the lipid content and NMFs are intact they form an adequate barrier that keeps foreign substances out and keeps the appropriate amount of water inside the cells. When the lipid and NMF content of skin is reduced, we experience surface roughness, flaking, small facial wrinkles, and a tight, uncomfortable feeling (Source: *Skin Research and Technology*, August 2000, pages 128–134).

It is logical to think that if you replace the components of skin that have been exhausted or destroyed from the varying causes mentioned above, then you can help "repair" skin and keep it intact, allowing it to heal, appear smoother, look healthier, and feel more comfortable. NMFs and lipids make up an expansive group of ingredients that include ceramide, hyaluronic acid, cholesterol, fatty acids, triglycerides, phospholipids, glycosphingolipids, amino acids, linoleic acid, glycosaminoglycans, glycerin, mucopolysaccharide, and sodium PCA (pyrrolidone carboxylic acid). All of these skin-care ingredients are present in the epidermis' intercellular structure between skin cells and in the lipid content on the surface of skin. When any of these ingredients are used in skin-care products, they appear to help stabilize and maintain this complex intercellular-skin matrix. None of these very good NMFs and lipids can permanently affect or change skin, but they are great at temporarily keeping depleted skin from feeling dry and uncomfortable. More important, all of these ingredients, and many more, can help support the intercellular area of the skin by keeping it intact. This support helps prevent surface irritation from penetrating deeper into the skin, helps keep bacteria out, and aids the skin's immune/healing system.

Mimicking the lipid content of skin ingredients are apricot oil, canola oil, coconut oil, corn oil, jojoba oil, jojoba wax, lanolin, lecithin, olive oil, safflower oil, sesame oil, shea butter, soybean oil, squalane, and sweet almond oil which can be extremely helpful for skin.

Are any one of these ingredients the be-all and end-all for your skin? Hardly! All of them perform similarly. That means that limiting yourself to a single ingredient to answer to your skin-care needs, or to a single concept, such as "natural" or "purifying," is the way to do the greatest disservice to your skin.

# OLIVE OIL

In the world of skin care, startling antiaging and antiwrinkling properties can be attributed to almost any plant-sourced ingredient. One of the latest ones is olive oil. The concept of olive oil having antiaging properties stems from some evidence that diets high in olive oil may help prevent heart disease (Sources: *European Journal of Clinical Nutrition*, January 2002, pages 72–81; *Lipids*, November 2001, Supplemental, pages S49–S52; *Lipids*, November 2001, pages 1195–1202). There are also a small number of animal tests showing that topically applied olive oil can protect against UVB damage (Sources: *Carcinogenesis*, November 2000, pages 2085–2090; *Journal of Dermatological Science*, March 2000, Supplemental, pages S45–S50).

It does seem that olive oil is a good antioxidant and assuredly it's a good moisturizing ingredient. But research shows similar results for other oils as well. How olive oil's status got elevated so that it's now a showcased ingredient in expensive skin-care products epitomizes the caprice of the cosmetics industry.

# OXYGEN FOR THE SKIN

Here is the most pathetic but clear-cut demonstration of how insane the world of cosmetics truly is. After selling us products to ward off oxygen's effects on the skin (the word antioxidant means anti-oxygen), the beauty industry then turns around and sells us products that claim to provide oxygen *to* the skin. Doesn't the beauty industry have anything better to do? (No, it doesn't, especially if there is an interested consumer willing to make a purchase.)

Many cosmetic products contain antioxidants, ingredients that keep oxygen off the face, such as vitamin C, superoxide dismutase, selenium, curcumin, plant extracts, and vitamin E, among dozens and dozens of others. At the same time, the cosmetics industry also sells products that contain hydrogen peroxide ($H_2O_2$) or some other oxygen-releasing ingredient, which supposedly delivers an oxygen molecule when it comes into contact with skin. It makes sense to wonder if the extra oxygen would just trigger free-radical damage and cause more problems for the skin. But if you were also using products that contained antioxidants, wouldn't they "scavenge" up that free-radical oxygen? The answer is that if the product could deliver extra oxygen to the skin it would indeed generate free-radical damage and, based on data from almost every imaginable published study on the subject, that's bad for skin.

So why the concern about supplying oxygen to the skin? Oxygen depletion is one of the things that happens to older skin, regardless of whether it's been affected by sun damage or any other health issue. Why or how that happens is a complete unknown, though it is thought to have something to do with blood flow and a reduction in lung capacity as we age. Nevertheless, delivering extra oxygen to the skin doesn't reverse it. After all, there is plenty of oxygen in our environment. The earth's atmosphere is 21% oxygen; the oceans, lakes, and rivers are about 88% oxygen. Oxygen is a constituent of most rocks and minerals, and 46.7% (by weight) of the solid crust of the earth. Oxygen makes up 60% of the human body, and is in every cell and organ. It is a constituent of all living tissues; almost all plants and animals, including humans, require oxygen to maintain life. However, oxygen is utilized by the body almost exclusively through respiration. Oxygen on the surface may affect the very top layer of skin, but so what? How much extra oxygen does skin need? Again, no one knows. Can it be absorbed? No. Plus, none of this addresses the issue about oxygen generating more free-radical damage, which is one of the reasons the veins and capillaries of the body stop working efficiently.

That brings us to the question, How did this caprice of oxygen booths get started? Oxygen booths (hyperbaric chambers) are used medically to repair skin ulcers and wounds that have difficulty healing. According to the American Diabetes Association's *Diabetes Forecast* (June 1993, page 57), "When you have a stubborn [wound] that won't heal, the white blood cells that fight the infection in the [wound] use 20 times more oxygen when they're killing bacteria. Also, the more oxygen your body has to work with, the more efficiently it lays down wound-repairing connective tissue. Yet just when you need more oxygen, you may have less. If you have neuropathy (diabetic nerve damage), that may cause changes in blood flow, resulting in islands of low oxygen levels in your foot. Less oxygen means slower healing, and a [wound] that doesn't heal could eventually lead to an amputation. So it seems that you should try to get extra oxygen in your blood when you have a foot ulcer, to bring the oxygen levels in the tissues around the ulcer up to normal, or even higher. But sitting in your living room and breathing in 100% oxygen won't do the trick. Under normal circumstances, only so much oxygen will dissolve in your blood." Pressure is needed to allow the oxygen to be used by the body; and sitting in a hyperbaric booth serves that purpose. The article continues, "But it is the inhaled oxygen, which is then absorbed by your blood after you breathe it, that speeds wound healing, not the oxygen drifting past the wound. You may have seen advertisements for devices that encase a person's leg and deliver oxygen to the skin. This is not hyperbaric oxygen therapy, and it's not effective—your skin doesn't absorb oxygen that way. These devices may even reduce the amount of oxygen that gets to your leg."

Moreover, leg ulcers and wounds are a temporary condition, but skin aging is ongoing. The notion that oxygen treatments affect aging, wrinkles, or any other skin malady is a joke. Nary a study exists anywhere to support those ideas, though there is a ton of research showing that the oxidative process generated by oxygen is partly responsible for wrinkles and skin aging in general.

## HYDROGEN PEROXIDE

Given what is now known about free-radical damage, I no longer recommend hydrogen peroxide as a topical disinfectant for acne. Oxygen is clearly a problem for skin, and hydrogen peroxide is a significant oxidizing agent. Hydrogen peroxide works by releasing an unstable oxygen molecule onto the skin, and that generates free-radical damage. Hydrogen peroxide is $H_2O_2$ (water is $H_2O$). The extra oxygen molecule in hydrogen peroxide is extremely unstable. That's why hydrogen peroxide is packaged in a dark brown, airtight container. On exposure to air or sunlight, hydrogen peroxide's extra oxygen molecule is released and the product becomes just plain water. For skin prone to acne this extra oxygen molecule is capable of killing the bacteria that cause blemishes. Acne bacteria are anaerobic, meaning they don't like oxygen. By giving the skin an extra dose of direct oxygen in the form of hydrogen peroxide, hydrogen peroxide can reduce the presence of these problematic bacteria. But because of the cumulative problems that stem from impacting the skin with a substance that is known to generate free-radical damage (which can hurt the healing process, cause cellular destruction, and reduce optimal skin functioning), other options need to be sought. In Chapter Ten, *Battle Plans for Blemishes*, in the section "Topical Disinfectants," I discuss the different options for combating the bacteria that cause acne.

# PROPYLENE GLYCOL

Propylene glycol (along with other glycols and glycerol) is a humectant or humidifying and delivery ingredient used in cosmetics. You can find Web sites and spam e-mails stating that propylene glycol is really industrial antifreeze and the major ingredient in brake and hydraulic fluids. These sites also state that tests show it to be a strong skin irritant. They further point out that the Material Safety Data Sheet (MSDS) on propylene glycol warns users to avoid skin contact because systemically (in the body) it can cause liver abnormalities and kidney damage.

As ominous as this sounds, it is so far from the reality of cosmetic formulations that almost none of it holds any water or poses real concern. It is important to realize that the MSDS sheets are talking about 100% concentrations of a substance. Even water and salt have frightening comments regarding their safety according to the MSDS. It is true that propylene glycol in 100% concentration is used as antifreeze, but—and this is a very big *but*—in cosmetics it is used in only the smallest amounts to keep products from melting in high heat or freezing when it is cold. It also helps active ingredients penetrate the skin. In the minute amounts used in cosmetics, propylene glycol is not a concern in the least. Women are not suffering from liver problems because of propylene glycol in cosmetics.

And finally, according to the U.S. Department of Health and Human Services, within the Public Health Services Agency for Toxic Substances and Disease Registry, "studies have not shown these chemicals [propylene or the other glycols as used in cosmetics] to be carcinogens" (Source: http://www.atsdr.cdc.gov).

Polyethylene glycol (PEG) is another ingredient "natural" Web sites have attempted to make notorious. They gain a great deal of attention by attributing horror stories to PEG. For example, several Web sites state the following: "Because of their effectiveness, PEGs are often used in caustic spray-on oven cleaners, yet are also found in many personal care products. Not only are they potentially carcinogenic, but they contribute to stripping the skin's Natural Moisture Factor, leaving the immune system vulnerable." There is no research substantiating any of this. Quite the contrary: PEGs have no known skin toxicity. The only negative research results for this ingredient group indicate that large quantities given orally to rats can cause tumors. How that got related to skin-care products is a mystery to me.

## PROTEINS AND AMINO ACIDS

Proteins are fundamental components of all living cells and include a diverse range of biological substance, such as enzymes, hormones, and antibodies that are necessary for the proper functioning of any organism, plant or animal. There are 20 different amino acids that link together by peptide bonds to form proteins. In skin-care products, proteins and amino acids act as emollients and water-binding agents that help keep the skin's structure intact—they cannot affect, change, or rebuild the structure of skin. Whether the protein in a skin-care product is derived from an animal or a plant, the skin can't tell the difference. There is no research demonstrating that either proteins or amino acids have special properties for skin other than as moisturizing agents.

## PYCNOGENOL

There is a great deal of research on pycnogenol, a plant-derived substance found in everything from pine bark to apples, cocoa beans, unripe strawberries, peanut skin, grape seeds, and red wine. However, most of the research dates back to 1990 and earlier (Source: U.S. Patent No. 4,698,360 entitled "Plant Extract with a Proanthocyanidins Content as Therapeutic Agent Having Radical Scavenging Effect and Use Thereof"). But a recent study supports the notion that pycnogenol is a potent antioxidant with strong free-radical-scavenging properties (Source: *Free Radical Biology and Medicine*, September 1999, pages 704–724). So what about pycnogenol for skin and wrinkles? Like all antioxidants, it can offer benefits for skin, but there isn't a shred of evidence that your wrinkles will melt away or change in any significant manner.

# RETINOL

See the section, "Vitamin A: Retinol vs. Retin-A and Renova" toward the end of this chapter.

# SODIUM LAURYL SULFATE

Are sodium lauryl sulfate (SLS) and sodium laureth sulfate (SLES) serious problems in cosmetics? I have received more e-mails and letters than I care to count about this concern. I believe that this entire mania was generated by several Neways Web sites, and has been carried over as if it were fact into other so-called "all natural" cosmetics lines.

It seems that most of this issue is based on the incorrect reporting about a study at the Medical College of Georgia. As a reminder, here is what is being quoted: "A study from the Medical College of Georgia indicates that SLS is a systemic, and can penetrate and be retained in the eye, brain, heart, liver, etc., with potentially harmful long-term effects. It could retard healing and cause cataracts in adults, and can keep children's eyes from developing properly." This is supposedly quoted from a report given to the Research to Prevent Blindness conference. While the report on animal models extrapolates concerns about the use SLS, it draws no hard conclusions stating that the amount of SLS used was 10% greater then that used in shampoos and done on animals not people. The doctor who conducted the study and delivered the final report is Dr. Keith Green, Regents Professor of Opthalmology at the Medical College of Georgia, who received his doctorate of science from St. Andrews University in Scotland. I had an opportunity to talk with Dr. Green who stated that he was completely embarrassed by all this. He told me in a telephone interview back in 1997 that his "work was completely misquoted. There is no part of my study that indicated any [eye] development or cataract problems from SLS or SLES and the body does not retain those ingredients at all. We did not even look at the issue of children, so that conclusion is completely false because it never existed. The Neways people took my research completely out of context and probably never read the study at all." He continued in a perturbed voice, saying, "The statement like 'SLS is a systemic' has no meaning. No ingredient can be a systemic unless you drink the stuff and that's not what we did with it. Another incredible comment was that my study was 'clinical,' meaning I tested the substance on people, [but] these were strictly animal tests. Furthermore, the eyes showed no irritation with the 10-dilution substance used! If anything, the animal studies indicated no risk of irritation whatsoever!" That lack of outcome is in fact why, as of 1987, Green no longer pursued this research. When I asked if anyone has done any follow-up studies looking at SLS and SLES in this regard, Dr. Green said, "No one has done this because the findings were so insignificant."

Resulting mass e-mails continued for some time, carrying on the SLS and SLES myth with a slightly different bent. Yet, according to Health Canada, in a press release, February 12, 1999 (http://www.hc-sc.gc.ca/), "A letter has been circulating the Internet which claims that there is a link between cancer and sodium laureth (or lauryl) sulphate (SLS), an ingredient used in [cosmetics]. Health Canada has looked into the matter and has found no scientific evidence to suggest that SLS causes cancer. It has a history of safe use in Canada. Upon further investigation, it was discovered that this e-mail warning is a hoax. The letter is signed by a person at the University of Pennsylvania Health System and includes a phone number. Health Canada contacted the University of Pennsylvania Health System and found that it is not the author of the sodium laureth sulphate warning and does not endorse any link between SLS and cancer. Health Canada considers SLS safe for use in cosmetics. Therefore, you can continue to use cosmetics containing SLS without worry."

Further, according to the American Cancer Society's Web site, "Contrary to popular rumors on the Internet, Sodium Lauryl Sulfate (SLS) and Sodium Laureth Sulfate (SLES) do not cause cancer. E-mails have been flying through cyberspace claiming SLS [and SLES] causes cancer … and is proven to cause cancer. … [Yet] A search of recognized medical journals yielded no published articles relating this substance to cancer in humans."

That's not to say that sodium lauryl sulfate isn't a potent skin irritant, because it is, and it's considered a standing comparison substance for measuring skin irritancy of other ingredients. In scientific studies when they want to establish whether or not an ingredient is problematic for skin, they compare its effect to the results of SLS. In amounts of 2% to 5% it can cause allergic or sensitizing reactions in lots of people (Sources: *European Journal of Dermatology*, September-October 2001, pages 416-419; *American Journal of Contact Dermatitis*, March 2001, pages 28–32). But irritancy is not the same as the other dire, erroneous warnings floating around the Web about this ingredient!

# TEA (GREEN, BLACK, AND WHITE)

A significant amount of research has established that tea, including black, green, and white tea, delivers many intriguing health benefits. Dozens of studies point to tea's potent antioxidant as well as anticarcinogenic properties. However, a good deal of this research is on animal models that do not directly relate to human skin (Source: *Skin Pharmacology and Applied Skin Physiology*, 2001, pages 69–76). There is only limited information about its effect on skin. The *Journal of Photochemistry and Photobiology* (December 31, 2001) stated that polyphenols "are the active ingredients in green tea and possess antioxidant, anti-inflammatory and anti-carcinogenic properties. Studies conducted by our group on human skin have demonstrated that green tea polyphenols (GTP) prevent ultraviolet (UV)-B…-induced immune suppression and skin cancer induction."

Green tea and the other teas show a good deal of promise for skin but it is not quite the miracle that cosmetics and health food companies make it out to be. As the *Annual Review of Pharmacology and Toxicology* (January 2002, pages 25–54) put it, "Tea has received a great deal of attention because tea polyphenols are strong antioxidants, and tea preparations have inhibitory activity against tumorigenesis. The bioavailability and biotransformation of tea polyphenols, however, are key factors limiting these activities in vivo [in humans]. Epidemiological studies … have not yielded clear conclusions concerning the protective effects of tea consumption against cancer formation in humans."

What aren't disputed are the anti-inflammatory properties of tea (black, white, and green). They are also definitely potent antioxidants. All of that is very good for skin but whether or not it has any effect on wrinkles or scars is speculation, not fact.

## TEA TREE OIL—MELALEUCA

Tea tree oil has some interesting research demonstrating it to be an effective antimicrobial agent. The *Journal of Applied Microbiology* (January 2000, pages 170–175) stated that "The essential oil of *Melaleuca alternifolia* (tea tree) exhibits broad-spectrum antimicrobial activity. Its mode of action against the Gram-negative bacterium *Escherichia coli* AG100, the Gram-positive bacterium *Staphylococcus aureus* NCTC 8325, and the yeast *Candida albicans* has been investigated using a range of methods…. The ability of tea tree oil to disrupt the permeability barrier of cell membrane structures and the accompanying loss of chemiosmotic control is the most likely source of its lethal action at minimum inhibitory levels." In addition, "In a randomized, placebo-controlled pilot study of tea tree oil in the treatment of herpes cold sores, tea tree oil was found to have similar degree of activity as 5% acyclovir" (Source: *Journal of Antimicrobial Chemotherapy*, May 2001, page 450). For acne there is also some credible published information showing it to be effective as a topical disinfectant for killing the bacteria that can cause pimples (Source: *Letters in Applied Microbiology*, October 1995, pages 242–245). However, the crux of the matter for tea tree oil is: How much is needed to have an effect? *The Medical Journal of Australia* (October 1990, pages 455–458) compared the efficacy of tea tree oil to the efficacy of benzoyl peroxide for the treatment of acne. A study of 119 patients using 5% tea tree oil in a gel base versus 5% benzoyl peroxide lotion was discussed. There were 61 in the benzoyl peroxide group and 58 in the tea tree oil group. The conclusion was that "both treatments were effective in reducing the number of inflamed lesions throughout the trial, with a significantly better result for benzoyl peroxide when compared to the tea tree oil. Skin oiliness was lessened significantly in the benzoyl peroxide group versus the tea tree oil group." However, while the reduction of breakouts was greater for the benzoyl peroxide group, the side effects of dryness, stinging, and burning were also greater—"79% of the benzoyl peroxide group versus 49% of the tea tree oil group."

Given these results, a 2.5% strength benzoyl peroxide solution would be better to start with to see if it is effective, rather than starting with the more potent and somewhat more irritating 5% or 10% concentrations. However, if you were interested in using a 5% strength tea tree oil solution to see if that would be effective, at this time I know of no products stating the amount of tea tree oil they contain. It appears that almost all of the tea tree oil products on the market contain little more than a 1% concentration, if that, which is probably not enough to be of much help for breakouts.

# TOURMALINE

Semiprecious stones and metals have shown up in skin-care products on and off over the years, with silver and gold appearing on the scene periodically. Lately, tourmaline is the gemstone that is showing up in Aveda and Creme de la Mer products (both are owned by the Estee Lauder company), and many women want to know if it has special properties for skin.

Tourmaline is an inert, though complex, mineral. One of its unique properties is that it is piezoelectric, meaning that it generates an electrical charge when under pressure. That's why tourmaline is typically used in pressure gauges. Tourmaline is also pyroelectric, which means that it generates an electrical charge during a temperature change (either increase or decrease). Neither of these actions can take place in a cosmetic, though—and why would you want them to? For example, one of the results of generating an electric charge is that dust particles will become attached to one end of the tourmaline crystal. Who wants that on their skin?

There is a patent for using tourmaline to decrease the need for surfactants, but this patent is for a complicated device and the effect is not generated by the tourmaline itself. Here is a quote from U.S. Patent number 6,308,356, Frederick, et al. October 30, 2001, entitled *Substantially environmental-pollution-free cleaning method and device employing electric energy and surface physical properties*. "The treatment of water by the electrically polar crystalline substance tourmaline requires much longer time to fill up one washing machine tub than the effect lasts. This yields this process of batch treatment before use as impractical as a laundry solution. In the current inventive method the treatment is done simultaneously with the work of cleaning and in the same location as the work of cleaning is being done." In other words, it is a process that uses tourmaline in some way, but the cleaning is not a result of the tourmaline itself (the language is not clear). It doesn't translate to electrifying or illuminating your cosmetics, and especially not in the trace amounts this mineral is found in cosmetics.

After an extensive search, I found no research showing tourmaline has any proven effect on skin whatsoever.

# VITAMIN A: RETINOL VS. RETIN-A AND RENOVA

Retinol is the technical name for vitamin A and, despite its recent popularity in skin-care products that proclaim it as an answer for wrinkles, it is hardly new. In fact, it has been around for some time. Retinol gained immense popularity shortly after Retin-A made headlines as a prescription wrinkle cream back in 1987. The active ingredient in Retin-A (and Renova) is tretinoin, which is also referred to as all-trans retinoic acid, an acid form of vitamin A. It wasn't a big stretch for cosmetics companies to take this information and try to convince the consumer that a product containing retinol could produce the same effects as Retin-A. Both are related to vitamin A and they sound almost identical. Headlines everywhere made most people aware of vitamin A, and in no time there was a flurry of knock-off Retin-A sound-alike products containing retinol or retinyl palmitate (another vitamin A derivative). It is important to discuss what role, if any, retinol plays in skin care.

As I discussed in Chapter Two, there is an abundance of research that shows tretinoin to be effective. Skin does age, whether from sun damage, smoking, or just growing up, and the results are wrinkles, rough skin, sagging, skin discolorations, and thinning of the skin. Changes in the skin are multi-fold, but one of the primary causes is cellular damage and resulting abnormal growth. An article from *Clinics in Geriatric Medicine* (November 2001, pages 643–659) said "Studies that have elucidated photoaging pathophysiology have produced significant evidence that topical tretinoin (all-trans retinoic acid), the only agent approved so far for the treatment of photoaging, also works to prevent it." (Sources: *Cosmetic Dermatology*, December 2001, page 38; *Journal of Investigative Dermatology*, 2001, volume 111, pages 778–784).

But what about retinol's effect on skin? There is limited evidence demonstrating that retinol can exert the same activity as tretinoin on skin. The problem is that, in the skin, tretinoin (all-trans retinoic acid) is the form of vitamin A that can affect actual cell production by binding to the tretinoin receptor sites on the cell. Retinol needs to *become* tretinoin in the skin if it is to do the same thing. Theoretically, retinol can become tretinoin in the skin, but the process isn't direct. Retinol can be absorbed into the skin and if certain enzymes are present it could then be converted to tretinoin. The question is whether or not, after retinol gets into skin, it is converted into tretinoin, and the research results are conflicting (Sources: *Journal of Investigative Dermatology,* 1998, volume 111, pages 478–484; *Journal of Investigative Dermatology,* 1997, volume 109, pages 301–305; *Skin Pharmacology and Applied Skin Physiology,* November-December 2001, pages 363–372).

One more point. Keep in mind that even Retin-A and Renova (the prescription topicals that contain tretinoin) don't produce the kind of results touted by the companies selling retinol products. Ironically, Neutrogena, who sells a retinol product boasting about its antiwrinkle benefits, is owned by Johnson & Johnson, who also happens to own the Retin-A and Renova formulas. If retinol works as well as the label on Neutrogena's product claims, then why would you ever need to use Retin-A or Renova? Perhaps Johnson & Johnson was hoping no one would notice the conflict.

# VITAMIN C

Ever since the distinguished Nobel Prize laureate Linus Pauling wrote his now-legendary book *Vitamin C and the Common Cold* back in 1970, vitamin C has become the darling of the alternative health-care world. The amount of research on vitamin C fills volumes of scientific journals. Vitamin C is essential for collagen formation and helps maintain the viability of the body's lymph system, connective tissue, bone, and cartilage. It is also essential for wound healing and facilitates recovery from burns.

While the information about vitamin C as a dietary supplement abounds, the same cannot be said for what it may do for skin when it comes to wrinkles or aging. In the world of skin care, vitamin C became a cause célèbre after Dr. Sheldon Pinnell from Duke University published a paper in 1992 showing how L-ascorbic acid reduced UVB damage (namely redness and swelling) when applied to the backs of hairless pigs. That was big news and generated product lines based on L-ascorbic acid.

Other doctors, such as N.V. Perricone, M.D. (whose product line bears his name) tout magnesium ascorbyl phosphate as the best form of vitamin C for skin. Still others assert that ascorbic acid is best and can be stabilized. Much of this information is derived from researchers who happen to endorse or are involved in selling products that contain their preferred form of vitamin C. So is there a best form of vitamin C or are any forms of vitamin C the answer for your skin? The answer is a confusing yes and no.

An article in *Plastic and Reconstructive Surgery* (January 2000, pages 464–465) discussed the issue of vitamin C and concluded that the answer is a resounding yes. "Vitamin C is a valuable antioxidant and protectant against photodamage that is created by sunlight in both the UVB and UVA bands.... Although oral supplementation may also be useful, topical preparations are able to deliver a higher dosage to the needed area. Topical vitamin C does not absorb or block harmful ultraviolet radiation like a sunscreen. Instead, it augments the skin's ability to neutralize reactive oxygen singlets [free-radical damage] that are created by the ultraviolet radiation, thereby preventing photodamage to the skin. It becomes an integral part of the skin and remains unaffected by bathing, exercise, clothing, or makeup. Used appropriately, topical vitamin C is an important adjunct to the use of sunscreens, an adjunctive treatment to lessen erythema [redness] in skin resurfacing, a helpful adjunct or an alternative to Retin-A in the treatment of fine wrinkles, and a stimulant to wound healing."

If that answer is yes, the answer to the question about which form of vitamin C to choose is not clear. Conflicting research indicates there is no way to know which type of vitamin C is the best. L-ascorbic acid is a good option in terms of its potential bioavailability on skin, but Pinnell's own research shows it is highly sensitive to formulary concerns, including concentration and the pH needed for it to remain stable (Source: *Dermatologic Surgery*, February 2001, pages 137–142).

On the other hand, magnesium ascorbyl phosphate is considered stable and there is reliable research showing it to be effective as an antioxidant (Sources: *Photochemistry and Photobiology*, June 1998, pages 669–675; *Journal of Pharmaceutical and Biomedical Analysis*, March 1997, pages 795–801). A small number of studies also show that magnesium ascorbyl phosphate can be effective for skin lightening (Source: *Journal of the American Academy of Dermatology*, January 1996, pages 29–33). In terms of stability, ascorbyl palmitate may be reliable for skin as well (Source: *Biochemical and Biophysical Research Communications*, September 1999, pages 661–665).

Adding to the tangle of information about ascorbic acid, the entire vitamin C molecule has also been shown to be effective as an antioxidant (Sources: *Journal of Investigative Dermatology*, February 2002, pages 372–379, and June 2001, pages 853–859). However, you have to balance that with information that ascorbic acid in its pure form is neutralized with water, and given that almost all moisturizing formulations are more than 50% water the chance of ascorbic acid remaining stable (and so available to skin as an antioxidant) is unlikely.

I wish I could point to one clear answer, but there isn't one. Aside from the matter of which form of vitamin C to select, perhaps the fundamental question is whether or not vitamin C is more helpful than any of the other antioxidants described in this chapter? Given the abundance of research on many antioxidants, it is apparent that this vitamin can play a role, but it is hardly the only one to do so, and it is definitely not the "best." What is true for any issue involving skin wrinkling is that aging is more complicated than just the loss or need of vitamin C—or any other vitamin, enzyme, protein, fatty acid, amino acid, or lipid in the skin. We should be concerned about the entire picture, not just one aspect. Besides, there are many other antioxidants that are as good as or even more impressive than vitamin C, including beta-glucan, vitamin E, vitamin A, green tea, grape extract, selenium, curcumin, and superoxide dismutase to name a few; and, according to many researchers dedicated to the study of antioxidants, there are probably thousands of undiscovered antioxidants out there that may be even more significant.

## VITAMIN E AND TOCOTRIENOLS

Vitamin E is without question one of the most well-researched vitamins for skin health. It is also, for all intents and purposes, the most well-known antioxidant, both when taken orally as a health supplement and when used in skin-care products. Simply put, vitamin E is an antioxidant superstar. It is a lipid-soluble vitamin (meaning it likes fat better then water) that has eight different forms, of which some are known for being potent antioxidants when applied topically to skin, particularly alpha tocopherol and tocotrienols (Sources: *Free Radical Biology and Medicine*, May 1997, pages 761–769; *Journal of Nutrition*, February 2001, pages 369S–373S; *International Journal of Radiation Biology*, June, 1999, pages 747–755). However, other studies have indicated the acetate form is also bioavailable and protective for skin (Source: *Journal of Cosmetic Science*, January-February 2001, pages 35–50).

Pointing to the significance of vitamin E for skin is an article in the *Journal of Molecular Medicine* (January 1995, pages 7–17), which states: "More than other tissues, the skin is exposed to numerous environmental chemical and physical agents such as ultraviolet light causing oxidative stress [free-radical damage]. In the skin this results in several short- and long-term adverse effects such as erythema [redness], edema [swelling], skin thickening, wrinkling, and an increased incidence of skin cancer.... Vitamin E is the major naturally occurring lipid-soluble ... antioxidant protecting skin from the adverse effects of oxidative stress including photoaging [sun damage]. Many studies document that vitamin E occupies a central position as a highly efficient antioxidant, thereby providing possibilities to decrease the frequency and severity of pathological events in the skin."

In essence, vitamin E functions in the body and on the skin to protect cells against free-radical damage, and an abundant assortment of researchers from diversified medical fields have theorized that this can slow the aging process (Sources: *Skin Pharmacology and Applied Skin Physiology*, November-December 2001, pages

363–372; *Free Radical Biology and Medicine*, October 1999, pages 729–737). Theory is not fact, yet the research is definitely compelling for this ingredient. Right now, though, we simply don't know how much is needed or how long it lasts and whether or not any of the benefit shows up as a reduction of wrinkles.

If you thought vitamin E was fascinating, wait until you start hearing about tocotrienols! Tocotrienols are one of vitamin E's eight components and they are fast becoming a popular word in the world of skin care. There is some research showing tocotrienols to be more potent than other forms of vitamin E for antioxidant activity (Source: *Journal of Nutrition*, February 2001, pages 369S–373S), but the studies cited in this review were all done on animal models or in vitro. According to the University of California at Berkeley's *Wellness Guide to Dietary Supplements* (October 1999) "[Tocotrienol] research in humans is very limited, and the results conflicting." The research that has been done has centered on large doses of oral tocotrienols, animal studies, or test tubes. Companies that want you to believe tocotrienols are now the answer for your skin are guessing whether or not the laboratory evidence translates to human skin as it exists in the real world (Source: *Healthnotes*, http://www.healthnotes.com).

As I have written before about antioxidants, the jury is still out on how much of any topically applied antioxidant is needed to be effective. Full-scale clinical studies on humans to assess the benefits of topical tocotrienols have not yet been performed, so for now (as is true for all antioxidants) choosing it as the "best" one is a leap of faith.

## VITAMIN K AND SPIDER VEINS

You may have seen advertisements or heard cosmetics salespeople discussing the effectiveness of vitamin K creams and lotions for reducing or eliminating surfaced spider veins (technically referred to as telangiectasias). These creams can't change spider veins, but let me explain why some people erroneously think they can. Vitamin K in skin-care products is considered a cosmetic ingredient, not a pharmaceutical or drug. As a cosmetic, it is not necessary for companies to prove their claims about what it can do. The only research concerning vitamin K's effectiveness on skin or surfaced spider veins comes from the companies selling these products. One medical source in particular, Dr. Melvin Elson, who sells creams that contain vitamin K, makes a lot of claims about treatment of spider veins. His company, Cosmeceutical Research Institute, is the only source of information suggesting this stuff works. There are no published or peer-reviewed studies that add up to results you can even remotely count on.

According to Dr. Craig Feied, MD, director of the American Vein Institute and Associate Clinical Professor of Emergency Medicine at George Washington University, vitamin K is associated with veins and blood because it is a prominent factor in the blood's ability to clot. If you take too much vitamin K orally, it can cause blood clots (which can lead to death). Blood clots can choke off the blood flow through a vein or capillary and make it atrophy. However, shutting down a vein or a surfaced capillary (spider vein) this way can be risky. Applying vitamin K to the surface of the skin does nothing, and that's good. If vitamin K could penetrate the surface of the skin to affect the blood flow in spider veins, it could also affect the blood flow in healthy veins. If you're already using a vitamin K product, don't worry; for vitamin K to form blood clots to shut down a vein or capillary, you would need to take large doses that would then need to be digested and metabolized in the liver, where proteins are formed. These special proteins are what cause the blood to clot. It isn't the vitamin K that shuts down veins, but a by-product that is created after digestion.

If you are interested in doing something that truly eliminates tiny surfaced spider veins from the face, the Photoderm laser is an option. Photoderm zaps the tiny spider vein and literally makes the blood boil for a moment, which closes down the vein and the surrounding surfaced spider veins. The sensation is about the same as being poked by a tiny needle. It is best for tiny spider veins because it treats only the surface of the skin, where the problem exists. Photoderm can't get deep enough to cause damage or problems for veins you don't want it to affect. Scleratherapy, or salt injections into the surface veins, is another option. (This procedure is discussed further in Chapter Thirteen, *Cosmetic Surgery*.)

Getting rid of spider veins is one issue, but preventing them is even more important. Sunburn, heat (prolonged exposure to saunas, Jacuzzis, or just cooking for long periods over a hot stove), pressure on the face (from severely blowing your nose, facial exercises, or rough massages), injury, smoking, and repeated local irritation and inflammation from irritating skin-care ingredients can all increase the occurrence of spider veins. Avoid these things and you can reduce the appearance of these veins, as well as their formation.

# YEAST

It is a bit odd to think of yeast as a skin-care ingredient worth looking into, yet in many respects it is one of the most paradoxical organisms occasionally found in cosmetics. A simple computer search for brewer's yeast's Latin name, **Saccharomyces cerevisiae**, brings up over 85,000 references. That's amazing! Yeasts are basically fungi that grow as single cells, producing new cells either by budding or fission [splitting]. Because it reproduces well, *Saccharomyces cerevisiae* is the most widely used organism in biotechnology. Nevertheless, some forms of yeast are human pathogens, such as **Cryptococcus** and **Candida albicans**.

In relation to skin there is limited information about how **Saccharomyces cerevisiae** may provide a benefit. Live yeast-cell derivatives have been shown to stimulate wound healing (Source: *Archives of Surgery*, May 1990, pages 641–646), but research like this is scant. Most of what is known about yeast is theoretical, and is about yeast's tissue-repair and protective properties (Source: *Global Cosmetic Industry*, November 2001, pages 12–13) or yeast's antioxidant properties (Source: *Nature Genetics*, December 2001, pages 426–434). As a skin-care ingredient yeast has potential, but what its function may be or how it would affect skin is not understood.

# CHAPTER 4

## SKIN CARE BASICS FOR EVERYONE

### SUNSCREEN

Sunscreen, without question, is the most basic and essential part of any skin-care routine—it plays a pivotal role from birth into our old age. No other skin-care product can so greatly and unquestionably influence the health of skin. It may sound simple, but it's a complicated product to understand, thanks to federal Food and Drug Administration (FDA) regulations, formulary considerations, application issues, reapplication concerns, risk of breakouts or irritant reactions, interpreting the SPF number, waterproof claims, and controversial research about ingredients. Because of that complexity, along with the seriousness of sun damage and the vital protection effective sunscreen offers, it deserves a chapter all its own. See Chapter Five, *Sun Sense*, where it will deservedly receive the attention it merits.

### FORGET SKIN TYPE

Some women are quite aware of their skin type; for other women it's a complete mystery, an elusive conundrum of changes that never settles down in one specific direction. What you should know is that regardless of how sophisticated some cosmetics companies are in approaching the issue—whether with computers and questionnaires to help you discover what is going on with your skin, or seemingly knowledgeable salespeople looking at your face and evaluating what you need—their final determination of your skin type is often inaccurate. **That's not to say understanding skin type isn't important, because it is, but not in the way the cosmetics industry approaches it or the way we've been indoctrinated to think about it.**

What I'm really saying is to forget about skin type as the cosmetics industry defines it. The rigid categories you find at cosmetics counters and the information about what your skin needs as analyzed by a salesperson are often wrong or at best incomplete. The concept of skin type, in terms of the standard normal, oily, combination, or dry types, is one of the most misused beauty concepts around. Yet it is usually where making decisions about our skin-care routines begin.

The primary difficulty in understanding your skin type is that, in addition to your skin's condition, you must recognize that outside factors can and do influence what you see and feel on your face. You can't know what skin type you have or what to do about it until you know why skin behaves the way it does. There can be no rational discussion of your skin-care needs until you evaluate what you may be doing that affects your skin's health, such as smoking, subjecting your skin to unprotected sun exposure, or using irritating and drying skin-care products.

What kind of environment you live in absolutely has an impact on skin. Someone living in cool, moist Seattle has radically different skin-care concerns from someone coping with the hot, dry air of Phoenix or Los Angeles. Your skin-care routine also plays a significant factor. Too many of the wrong skin-care products can wreak havoc on your face. For example, over-using moisturizers, scrubs, AHAs, BHA, and masks can all adversely affect skin. Further, health problems such as rosacea or psoriasis or internal health conditions such as a thyroid disorder can affect skin, too.

Those complex, integrated circumstances, combined with your skin's genetic predisposition for certain traits (oily versus dry, prone to breakouts, or sensitive skin), contribute to what takes place on and under your skin. To complicate matters further, skin type is not static. **What you see today may not be what you see tomorrow, next week, month to month, or season to season.** Judging skin type from one moment in time (like when you are shopping at a cosmetics counter and the salesperson says you have dry, oily, or combination skin) doesn't give you enough information to create an effective skin-care routine.

While cosmetics salespeople may ask what skin type you have, their ability to factor in any or even part of this intricate list is at best limited, and may be nonexistent. Nevertheless, aside from genetic traits, environmental factors, hormones, or skin disorders, your present skin-care routine is the pivotal element in the appearance of your skin. The products you use can affect the skin's oiliness, dryness, and sensitivity. The wrong skin-care products can trigger allergies, redness, surfaced capillaries, or changes in skin texture, and can aggravate breakouts. The way your face feels right now can largely (though not solely) be a result of the way you clean your face. Your skin-care routine could be creating the very problems you're trying to eliminate.

For example, if you wash every day with a bar soap (which is drying), followed by a toner (which may also be drying), and several moisturizers (which can be greasy and potentially can block pores), you can create a severe combination skin condition and cause breakouts. Or if you wipe off your makeup with a cold cream (even expensive ones can be greasy) and then follow up with a toner (which might also be greasy or contain irritants), you should not be surprised if you develop breakouts and dull-looking skin. If you have fairly normal skin but you use an alcohol-based AHA toner, plus a scrub, an AHA moisturizer, and a clay mask, your skin may end up looking very dry and irritated, along with showing rashlike pimples.

Typing skin without taking into consideration the products you use relies on the assumption that the skin is the way it is all by itself, regardless of what you do to it, but that is rarely the case. **Before you can know what your skin type really is, you have to start at square one to discover what your skin type is not and find out what is causing the conditions you see on the surface.**

Another problem with what's called skin typing is the assumption that once you've been told your skin type, your skin will be the same forever, or at least until you age. That, too, is rarely the case. Emotions, weather conditions, hormonal levels, menstrual cycles, stress, physical changes, weight fluctuations, and whatever else life brings can directly affect your skin. If your skin-care routine focuses on skin type alone, it can become obsolete the moment the season changes, your work life becomes stressful, or hormonal influences fluctuate (as hormones often do).

To complicate things even more, in any given period of time a woman may have many skin types! Over the years, even when using gentle, irritant-free products, I've experienced irritated skin patches at the same time I had oily skin, or acne flare-ups along with dry skin around my eyes. **It is not unusual for women to have a little bit of each skin type simultaneously or at different times of the month or week. An overview of how your skin behaves and changes is necessary to assess what your skin needs.**

Once skin type is identified, the biggest problem is how the cosmetics industry handles that information. As far as the cosmetics industry is concerned, every woman can and should have normal skin. Yet the very idea of acquiring normal skin is like trying to scale a peak with a slippery, precarious slope. Like the rest of our bodies, skin is in a constant state of change. Even women with perfect complexions go through phases of having oily, dry, or blemish-prone skin. Almost every woman after the age of 40 will have some amount of sun-damaged skin. In reality, no one is likely to have normal skin for very long, no matter what she does. Those of us who struggle with oily skin, breakouts, dry skin, sensitive skin, or sun damage know that normal skin is at best fleeting. **Chasing after normal skin can set you up on an endless skin-care buying spree, running around in circles trying everything and finding nothing that works for very long.**

In any case, identifying skin type is highly subjective. Many women have really wonderful skin but refuse to accept it. The smallest blemish or wrinkle or the slightest sensation of dry skin distresses them. I can't tell you how many women I've met who get one blemish and run to the dermatologist complaining about acne. Or the women who see a line or two around their eyes and immediately buy the most expensive antiwrinkle creams they can find in the hope of warding off their worst imagined nightmare. Overreacting to what you see in the mirror makes for more mistakes in cosmetics purchases than almost any aspect of skin type. **This is one of those times where being realistic is the most important part of your skin-care routine.**

Identifying your skin type is made even more difficult by the omnipresent combination-skin complaint. Almost everyone at some time or another, if not all the time, has combination skin. This is not out of line—it just happens to be the way the skin functions. The nose, chin, center of the forehead, and the center of the cheek all have more oil glands than other parts of the face. It is not surprising that those areas tend to be oilier and break out more frequently than the other areas. Problems occur when you buy extra products for combination skin because many ingredients that are appropriate for the T-zone (the area along the center of the forehead and down the nose where most of the oil glands on the face are located) won't help the cheek or jaw areas. Some products claim they can regulate themselves over each area of your face, but that's a complete impossibility. The ingredients that can absorb oil can promote dryness and the ingredients that moisturize dry skin can cause breakouts. Mixed together they don't self-regulate, they cancel each other out. **You may need separate products to deal with the different skin types on the face because you should treat different skin types, even on the same face, differently.**

The most frustrating aspect of the skin type idea is the fact that it's often used (by cosmetics salespeople and by the cosmetics industry in its ads) to instill a sense of immediate need. Once your skin is classified as a "type" that isn't normal, or if it stops being normal, then panic can set in. Cosmetics salespeople aim this ploy at the 30-something crowd, with the pitch sounding something like "You had better do what you can do now to make sure your skin doesn't get worse." I've seen it happen a thousand times as I've listened to or been personally subjected to a salesperson's scolding about skin-care mistakes that are destroying my skin. **What destroys skin is unprotected sun exposure, smoking, and using irritating skin-care products. Not using the right skin-care products (other than a good sunscreen) may cause problems, but it does not damage skin in the long run, and that includes not using a moisturizer.**

Determining skin type is not the answer to other skin care needs that may not be apparent on the skin's surface. For example, sun damage is not evident when you are young, but sun protection is imperative for all skin types. Dry and oily skin that are present at the same time, along with some redness, may be an early sign of rosacea, a condition that cannot be treated with cosmetics and may not be easily diagnosed. Your skin may be breaking out now, but those blemishes on the surface took a few weeks to get there. Breakouts begin in the pores, and may involve sebum (oil), cellular debris (dead skin cells), dead hair shafts, and/or bacteria. It takes consistent, long-term planning to handle each aspect of the blemish problem, and treating only what you see (as in "zapping zits" or "spot treatment") can make matters worse. Large patches of flaky, dry, red skin may be caused by psoriasis, and cosmetics can make this condition worse. Dry patches of rough, abraded skin can be caused by an allergic reaction or by eczema. What you see on the surface of the skin does not always indicate the type of skin-care products you should buy, or even that you need a skin-care product at all.

# SKIN TYPE HAS NOTHING TO DO WITH YOUR AGE

**Older skin is different from younger skin. That is indisputable. Yet it is a mistake to buy skin-care products based on a nebulous age category.** Treating older or younger skin with products supposedly aimed at dealing with specific age ranges is inappropriate because not everyone with "older" or "younger" skin has the same needs. An older person may have acne, blackheads, eczema, rosacea, sensitive skin, or oily skin, while a younger person may have dry, freckled, or obviously sun-damaged skin. Products designed for older skin are almost always too emollient and occlusive, and those designed for younger skin are almost always too drying. Both extremes can cause problems when the key issue becomes your age as opposed to the actual condition of your skin.

Treating older or younger skin with an age-related, unified skin-care routine is a trap lots of women fall into, particularly older women. I understand the anxiety a woman feels when she passes the age of 40 and notices her skin is changing. And when a skin-care routine claims it is best for your age group it is hard not to believe that isn't true. Yet an effective skin-care routine should be based on the current condition of your skin, along with protection from sun damage, regardless of your age. Age is not a skin-care condition! In fact, many of the skin-care concerns associated with age are more often than not shared by women of all ages.

All women, regardless of age, need sun and antioxidant protection, and possibly treatment of skin discolorations (either potential or existing), dry or oily skin, or breakouts. Wrinkles may tend to separate younger from older skin, but the care you give the skin doesn't necessarily differ. Not everyone in their 40s and older has the same skin care needs. In a way it's simple: You need to pay attention to what is taking place on your skin, and that varies from person to person.

# DOES SKIN COLOR OR ETHNICITY AFFECT SKIN CARE?

Regardless of skin color or ethnic background, all skin is subject to a range of problems. These skin problems almost always have less to do with color or ethnic background differences than with what they have in common with skin problems in general. Whether it is dry or oily skin, blemishes, scarring, wrinkles, skin discolorations, skin disorders, skin sensitivity, and even risk of sun damage, all men and women share similar struggles. So, while there are some distinctions between varying ethnic groups when it comes to skin problems and skin-care options, overall these differences are minor in comparison to the number of similarities.

According to an article in the *Journal of the American Academy of Dermatology* (February 2002, pages 41–62) "People with skin of color constitute a wide range of racial and ethnic groups—including Africans, African Americans, African Caribbeans, Chinese and Japanese, Native American Navajo [and other] Indians, and certain groups of fair-skinned persons (e.g., Indians, Pakistanis, Arabs), and Hispanics.... There is not a wealth of data on racial and ethnic differences in skin and hair structure, physiology, and function. What studies do exist involve small patient populations and often have methodological flaws. Consequently, few definitive conclusions can be made. The literature does support a racial differential in epidermal melanin [pigment] content and melanosome dispersion in people of color compared with fair-skinned persons. Other studies have demonstrated differences in hair structure and fibroblast size and structure between black and fair-skinned persons. These differences could at least in part account for the lower incidence of skin cancer in certain people of color compared with fair-skinned persons; a lower incidence and different presentation of photo aging; pigmentation disorders in people with skin of color; and a higher incidence of certain types of alopecia [loss of hair] in Africans and African Americans compared with those of other ancestry."

One arena where differences do exist was explained in *Contact Dermatitis* (December 2001, pages 346–349). It noted that "There is a widespread, but largely unsubstantiated, view that certain skin types may be more susceptible to the effect of skin irritants than others. One expression of this would be that certain ethnic groups may also be more likely to experience skin irritation.... In this study, we have investigated 2 carefully matched panels of Caucasian and Japanese women volunteers to determine their topical irritant reaction, both acute and cumulative, to a range of materials. The results indicated that the acute irritant response tended to be greater in the Japanese panel and this reached statistical significance with the stronger irritants. Cumulative irritation was investigated only with the weaker irritants and, although again the trend was to a higher response in Japanese compared to Caucasian panelists, this rarely reached significance."

Throughout this book I will point out the special needs, concerns, and treatment options that affect men and women of color when they differ from those of Caucasian skin types. Specifically, I will describe what takes place in keloidal scarring and hyperpigmentation (darkening of the skin).

## AVOID IRRITATING YOUR SKIN

I started my career as a cosmetics consumer advocate by warning women about the damage being done to their skin by irritating skin-care ingredients. Over the years my fears about irritation have been confirmed and reinforced by many dermatologists and cosmetics chemists. Indeed, irritation is a bigger problem for the skin than even I had suspected. Irritation can cause an immediate breakout response, it can cause redness, flaky skin (which can clog pores), or rashes, and it can even cause capillaries to surface on the face. More significantly, irritation can destroy the skin's integrity by breaking down the skin's protective barrier, which, over time, damages the skin's structure. Inside the skin, irritation impairs the skin's immune and healing response (Source: *Skin Pharmacology and Applied Skin Physiology*, November-December 2000, pages 358–371). Additionally, breaking down the skin's protective barrier can allow the introduction of bacteria, thus raising the risk of more breakouts.

What causes skin irritation? Many elements are responsible for hurting skin including hot water, cold water, sun exposure, pollution, irritating skin-care ingredients, soaps, and drying cleansers, plus just scrubbing the skin. You may think that none of those things bothers your skin. However, it is startling to learn that even if your skin doesn't feel or appear irritated after exposure to those things, it is still being irritated and the skin breakdown is nonetheless taking place. That means if you are out in the sun, sitting in a sauna, or using a skin-care product that contains potentially irritating or sensitizing ingredients, the irritation damage is still taking place even though the skin doesn't show it (Source: *Skin Research and Technology*, November 2001, pages 227–237). We can get a clearer idea of how this secret damage takes place by likening it to what happens to skin in response to unprotected sun exposure. Getting tan or sunburned when we are young and throughout our teens seems to be a lot like using a cosmetic coloring because the cumulative damage takes place beneath the skin's outer surface and doesn't show until after many years of exposure.

Avoiding the obvious substances and elements that irritate skin is crucial for healthy skin. This includes not smoking, avoiding unprotected sun exposure at all costs, and not using irritating or harsh skin-care products. Not paying attention to the irritation potential of certain ingredients in skin-care products can be damaging to the health of your skin. What skin-care ingredients irritate skin? That list is presented in the next section. Keep in mind that throughout this book when I indicate something is a possible skin irritant, it means it can be irritating to everyone's skin, even if your skin doesn't appear to have a reaction. Some ingredients always create irritation beneath the skin's surface and cause damage, and that is not good for anyone's skin.

(**Note:** Some irritating ingredients can also have positive results for skin, such as AHAs, BHA, Retin-A, Renova, sunscreen ingredients, some antioxidants, and some preservatives [which keep products stabilized]. All of those can be considered essential for many skin types and product formulations, yet they do pose a risk of irritation. In this case, it is simply a tradeoff in which the benefits outweigh the potential negatives. On the other hand, some ingredients are not only irritating but also have no positive impact on skin, meaning they don't help it in any way and are best avoided. Those are the ones I consistently warn about.)

## LEARNING TO BE GENTLE

Irritation takes a toll on all skin types. Although many things can cause irritation, the skin can respond the same way regardless of the source. While the skin's reaction to irritation is not always visually apparent, when it does react it isn't pretty! Irritation can cause an assortment of problems, from redness to dry patches, blemishes, rashes, cracks along the side of the nose and corners of the mouth and eyes, flakiness, increased skin sensitivity, other skin disorders, and a reduction in the skin's immune/healing response.

Here it's important to say that it is generally believed that irritation is *not* responsible for wrinkles and premature aging of the skin. Some dermatologists suggest, however, that repeatedly using irritating ingredients on the skin can suppress the skin's immune/healing response, making the wrinkling process worse. Many products that are advertised as making skin look instantly younger when placed over the lines on the face contain irritating ingredients (such as alcohol) that swell the skin temporarily. With repeated use, they could actually make the skin more wrinkled.

Take this rule at face value: Thou shalt always treat thy skin gently or it will complain loudly that something is wrong. The skin might react to topical irritation immediately, or it may take some time before signs of irritation show up. Possibly the most ominous aspect of irritation is that your skin doesn't have to exhibit a reaction at all. Your skin can become irritated and you won't necessarily feel or see anything different. If you use irritating skin-care products, your skin may suffer the negative effects whether or not you can see it taking place on your skin (Source: *Contact Dermatitis*, November 1998, volume 39, issue 5, pages 231–239).

It logically follows that learning how to be gentle to your face is one of the most important parts of any skin-care routine. There is no way you can ever hope for soft, smooth skin when your face is being irritated every time you take care of it. Irritation-free skin is the goal.

# HOW TO BE GENTLE

We do many things to our skin and buy an assortment of skin-care products that can cause serious irritation. Yet it is far easier than you may think to eliminate these skin-"care" culprits. With that in mind, here is a list of typical skin-care and makeup ingredients and specific cosmetics products and tools to avoid or use cautiously. The skin can react negatively to all of the following products, procedures, and ingredients.

**Irritating Skin-Care Steps and Products**

- Abrasive scrubs
- Astringents containing irritating ingredients
- Toners containing irritating ingredients
- Scrub mitts
- Cold or hot water
- Steaming or icing the skin
- Facial masks containing irritating ingredients
- Loofahs
- Bar soaps and bar cleansers (Source: *Dermatology*, March 1997, pages 258–262)

**Irritating Ingredients**

(These are of greater concern when they appear in the beginning of an ingredient list.)

- Acetone
- Alcohol or SD alcohol followed by a number (Exceptions: Ingredients like cetyl alcohol or stearyl alcohol are standard, benign, waxlike cosmetic thickening agents and are completely nonirritating and safe to use.)
- Ammonia
- Arnica
- Balm mint
- Balsam
- Bentonite
- Benzalkonium chloride
- Bergamot
- Camphor
- Cinnamon
- Citrus juices and oils
- Clove
- Clover blossom
- Coriander
- Cornstarch
- Eucalyptus
- Eugenol
- Fennel
- Fennel oil
- Fir needle
- Geranium

- Grapefruit
- Horsetail
- Lavender
- Lemon
- Lemongrass
- Lime
- Linalool
- Marjoram
- Melissa (lemon balm)
- Menthol
- Mint
- Oak bark
- Orange
- Papaya
- Peppermint
- Phenol
- Sandalwood oil
- SD alcohol
- Sodium C14-16 olefin sulfate
- Sodium lauryl sulfate
- TEA-lauryl sulfate
- Thyme
- Wintergreen
- Witch hazel
- Ylang-ylang

These ingredients are extremely common; you would be surprised how often they show up in skin-care products for all skin types. Ingredients like camphor, menthol, mint, alcohol, and phenol are sometimes recommended because they are considered anti-itch ingredients. The theory works like this: When your skin itches, the nerve endings are sending messages begging you to scratch. If you place these irritating ingredients over the area that itches, the nerve hears the irritation message louder than it hears the itch message and interprets this as a reason to stop itching. That reasoning is fine if minor, sporadic, occasional itching is your problem. If it is not and those ingredients are present in skin-care products meant for everyday use, they introduce a constantly irritating insult to the skin and causing dryness, rashes, increased oil production, redness, and breakouts. None of those side effects are attractive.

**Skin doesn't have to hurt, tingle, or be stimulated even a little to be clean. (If the skin tingles, it is being irritated, not cleaned.) The major rule for all skin types is, if a product or procedure irritates the skin, don't use it again.**

Exceptions to the rule: When you initially begin to use an AHA or BHA product or Retin-A, Renova, azelaic acid, or Differin, stinging or tingling can occur. You may need to cut back if it is more than a little tingling, or stop altogether if these symptoms persist for more than a few weeks or worsen with repeated use.

## ANTI-IRRITANTS AND ANTI-INFLAMMATORIES

Avoiding irritating ingredients is important for the health of your skin, but it is also helpful to use skin-care products containing ingredients that mitigate or counter the effects of irritation on skin. Anti-irritants and anti-inflammatories are a group of ingredients known for reducing or relieving skin irritation and inflammation. Because irritation and inflammation are well known to be problematic for skin, anti-irritants as well as anti-inflammatories have become popular and necessary terms and components in the cosmetics world and in most medical fields, particularly in dermatology. Many ingredients perform the function of anti-irritants or anti-inflammatories and better ones are being discovered all the time. Interestingly enough, most antioxidants function as anti-irritants, and one of the skin's responses to free-radical damage is irritation and inflammation. Some of the more popular anti-irritants used in cosmetics are willowherb, willow bark, allantoin, oat extracts, bisabolol, borage, chamomile, comfrey, dogwood, fireweed, *Gingko biloba*, green tea, black tea, grape seed, licorice, coenzyme Q10, and vitamin C to name a few. These ingredients go a long way toward helping the skin deal with its daily struggle against sun exposure, pollution, skin-care routines (topical disinfectants, sunscreens, and exfoliants can be irritating to skin), makeup, and seasonal environmental extremes.

## HEAT IS A PROBLEM

Because irritation is a problem for skin, anything that irritates the skin should be avoided as much as possible. Heat is one of those things that should be avoided. As good as hot water, direct steam, or dry saunas feel on the skin, they end up causing more problems for the health of the skin. For years, I have recommended washing the face with tepid water. This is because hot water burns the skin and cold water shocks it, and both leave it irritated and dry. These two temperature extremes can also injure skin cells, dehydrate the skin, and cause capillaries to surface. Extreme temperatures in any form cause problems for the skin, but heat is the more attractive alternative (most people avoid a cold shower or bath).

Dry heat is clearly dehydrating. Whether the dry heat comes from a dry sauna or an arid desert climate, it pulls water right out of the skin cell. That's bad for any skin type, but especially for someone with dry skin.

Wet heat is a bit more deceptive. We all know how great the skin feels initially when we exit a hot shower, Jacuzzi, or sauna. It feels plump and saturated with water because the skin absolutely loves drinking up all the water it can. After even a short soak in a tub, your skin can swell and become engorged with water. When you leave a bathtub and your fingers are all thick and wrinkly, it isn't because they are dry, but because they are distorted and swollen with water-saturated skin cells. Because the surface layer of skin likes water so much, hot water can enter the skin, stay there, and cause a burn-like reaction. As a general rule, if water feels hot to the touch, it's too hot for the skin, especially the face. Be very skeptical about facial treatments that involve the use of heat or washing your face with hot (or cold) water; down the line, they could cause more trouble for your skin than you want.

# DON'T SMOKE

Smoking is, at the very least, equal to the sun in the direct damage it causes to the skin's surface. In actuality, smoking is probably even more insidious than sun exposure when it comes to damaging healthy skin. Not only does smoking cause serious free-radical damage and block the body's ability to utilize oxygen, it also creates necrotic (dead) skin tissue that cannot be repaired. Even more unattractive is the breakdown of the elastic fibers of the skin (elastosis), which gives rise to yellow, irregularly thickened skin (Sources: *Journal of the American Academy of Dermatology*, July 1999, "Cigarette Smoking-Associated Elastotic Changes in the Skin", and May 1996, "Cutaneous Manifestations and Consequences of Smoking").

Moreover, smoking causes a progressive cascade of damage inside the body (restricted blood flow, reduced capacity of the blood to take in oxygen, impairment to the body's immune system) that eventually shows up on the surface of skin, making it look haggard and dull. It also creates serious deep wrinkling around the lips and lip area.

While smoking can make skin look prematurely wrinkled and aged, it's unattractive for many other reasons as well, including the permeating smell of smoke on clothing, breath that smells like smoke, and yellow stains on hands, nails, and teeth. Smoking isn't pretty and it can be deadly. Quitting smoking is one of the most healthful things you can do for your skin and body.

# EVERYONE HAS SENSITIVE SKIN

Most of us have sensitive and/or irritated skin. Regardless of your primary skin type, ethnic background, or age, minor or major irritating skin conditions can be present, even those you can't feel. The skin can burn, chafe, or crack, and you may have patchy areas of dry, flaky skin related to weather conditions, hormonal changes, the skin-care products you use, or sun exposure. Skin can also break out in small bumps that look like a diaper rash. Skin can itch, swell, blotch, redden, and develop allergic reactions to cosmetics, animals, dust, or pollen.

If that isn't enough to make you itch just a little, then think about the number of cosmetics most women use daily. The average woman uses at least 12 different skin-care, makeup, and hair-care products a day, with each one, on average, containing about twenty different ingredients. That means her skin is exposed to about 240 different cosmetic ingredients on any given day. The fact that any of us have skin left is a testimony to the skin's resiliency and the talent of cosmetics chemists. Whether we like it or not, most of us will react to something along the way, perhaps even daily.

Your skin is the protective armor that keeps the elements and other invaders from entering the body. We protect most of our anatomy with clothing, but our faces are left painfully exposed to everything. It's no wonder the skin on our faces acts up now and then. Sensitive skin is probably the most "normal" type of skin around.

Everyone has the potential to develop sensitive skin, so women of every skin type should heed the precautions for sensitive skin. What are the precautions? There is really only one and it goes for all skin types: **Treat your skin as gently as you possibly can. Whether you think of your face as oily, dry, or mature, you still need to be gentle with your skin and avoid things that cause irritation.**

The operative word is gentle. Preventing skin irritation, regardless of your skin type, is the course of action I recommend throughout this book. Of course, some skin types can and should try to tolerate certain potentially irritating ingredients. A topical disinfectant (like 2.5% benzoyl peroxide, for instance) is helpful for someone with acne, while a BHA solution (a salicylic acid exfoliant) is good for someone with blackheads. Likewise, an AHA (an alpha hydroxy acid product used to exfoliate) or Retin-A or Renova (to improve cell formation) are beneficial for someone with sun-damaged skin. But aside from those exceptions to the gentleness rule, if something is irritating it can be detrimental for all skin types. If it is bad for sensitive skin, it is probably bad for oily skin, acne-prone skin, combination skin, dry skin, or menopausal skin. As you integrate this gentleness philosophy into your skin-care routine, you will slowly solve many of the skin problems you have been experiencing.

# FRAGRANCE IN SKIN-CARE PRODUCTS

Hopefully by now you are sensitive (pun intended) to the fact that the cosmetics industry doesn't always tell you the truth about how its products can affect your skin. They are particularly silent on the issue of allergic reactions and unfavorable skin flare-ups that result from ingredients in lots and lots of skin-care products. Allergic reactions and skin sensitivities are not technically the same thing, but they can feel the same on your skin. Regardless of the physiologically precise definition, we have all used some type of cosmetic that causes part of our face or body to burn, tingle, swell, flake, redden, itch, blister, break out, or just feel bad. How could this happen? Given how many products we use and the diversity of ingredients, I'm shocked it doesn't happen more frequently. Interestingly enough, two ingredients almost universally added to cosmetics, fragrance and preservatives, are often thought to be the major culprits when our skin goes a little crazy from a cosmetic (Source: *Contact Dermatitis*, June 1999, pages 310–315).

An article in the January 24, 2000, issue of *The Rose Sheet* discussed an advisory report issued by the Scientific Committee on Cosmetic Products and Non-Food Products, a European Commission agency. The report stated that "Information regarding fragrance chemicals used in cosmetic products that have the potential to cause allergic reactions should be provided to consumers." According to the article, "It is seen that a significant increase in fragrance allergy has occurred and that fragrance allergy is the most common cause of contact allergy…." Concurring with this conclusion is an editorial by Pamela Scheinmann, MD, entitled "The Foul Side of Fragrance-Free Products" (Source: *Journal of the American Academy of Dermatology*, December 1999, page 1020). She states that "Products designated as fragrance-free should contain no fragrance chemicals, not even those that have dual functions." She continues by saying that "hypoallergenic, dermatologist tested, sensitive skin, or dermatologist recommended are nothing more than meaningless marketing slogans." Further research presented in the *American Journal of Contact Dermatitis* (June 1999, pages 310–315; September 1998, pages 170–175) poses this same concern.

Preservatives are impossible to avoid because without them our skin-care products would become contaminated with mold, fungus, and bacteria and pose a serious problem for our skin in just a short period of time. However, you can and should stay away from cosmetics, particularly skin-care products, that contain fragrance. It smells nice, but fragrance serves no purpose for skin. Even fragrant ingredients that may also offer a positive benefit are easily replaced with ingredients that can perform the same function without the irritation aspect of the fragrant component. It sounds simple enough to avoid products with fragrance, perfume, or parfum by just reading the ingredient list and then not buying those products. But ingredient lists aren't always that easy to decipher.

The cosmetics industry knows that most women emotionally and psychologically prefer cosmetics that smell nice, even if they say they want to avoid fragrance. But if a cosmetics company produces products without fragrance, you will instead get the scent of the ingredients, which are not in the least as appealing as an added sweet, floral, or citrusy fragrance. This is why, in order to kill two marketing birds with one cosmetic stone, companies often list the fragrance components as essential oils or plant extracts rather than listing fragrance or perfume on the label. As lovely as essential oils sound, they are still nothing more than fragrance. **So while you don't see the word "fragrance" on the list, and you may approvingly think wintergreen oil, lemon oil, cardamom oil, ylang-ylang oil, or other oils sound pleasant and healthy, your skin may still respond disapprovingly.**

The next time you admire the fragrant quality of a skin-care product you're about to apply to any part of your body or face, think twice. Similarly, aromatherapy shouldn't be a skin-care treatment, however therapeutic it is for the sense of smell and emotions. Fragrance might be nice for your spirits, but it is a health risk for skin. And it doesn't matter if the source of the fragrance is essential oils or plant extracts; as far as the health of your skin is concerned, they are all the same.

## ALLERGIC REACTIONS

An allergic reaction to a substance can look like an irritation or sensitizing reaction but when it comes to what is going on beneath the surface of your skin it is a completely different reaction. Simply put, an allergic reaction happens when our immune system reacts to a familiar or an unfamiliar substance in a unique way. When our system or skin encounters a particular ingredient or combination of ingredients, the immune system decides whether or not it should accept, reject, or ignore the substance. If the body determines that the substance is unwanted, even when no allergic response existed before, it all of a sudden produces histamines to get rid of it. Allergies can develop immediately or build over time with each additional exposure to the ingredient. That is why many women develop an allergic reaction to a cosmetic that they were able to use for years. What makes identifying the source of the reaction even more difficult is that you can develop an allergic reaction at any time, or even find that you are no longer allergic to a substance you had problems with for years.

In addition to the multiple problems associated with irritation and that cause skin to react negatively, it can be both disconcerting and aggravating to have an allergic reaction to the cosmetics you use! Reactions can be subtle, such as a little itching, minor redness and swelling, or small rashlike pimples. They can also involve a full-blown flare-up that causes intense, but temporary, discomfort and an unsightly appearance or they can trigger a chronic condition requiring medical attention. If you have a tendency toward allergic reactions, your skin's condition can be greatly affected and you will have to pay close attention to what you use. Someone with allergy-prone skin needs to use fewer products with smaller ingredient lists.

I would love to list ingredients that I could guarantee won't cause your skin to have an allergic reaction, but there is no single ingredient or combination of ingredients that can live up to that sweeping claim. Why not? Because everyone is biochemically different. Each of us has a unique chemical makeup, and the endless paradoxical differences in the way our bodies perform is why we can react so differently when exposed to the same thing.

Because of the almost limitless combinations, in all sorts of cosmetic formulations, it is truly impossible to know if, when, or how anyone's skin will react to any cosmetic. Your only recourse, and this is not the best news, is to keep experimenting until you find what works for you. If you do get a reaction, stop using the product immediately. Consult your physician if the reaction is serious or prolonged, return products that are suspect, and keep track of the ingredients included in products to which you seem to be allergic. Also, keep in mind that just because you've used a cosmetic for a long time doesn't mean you won't develop an allergic reaction to it.

Whenever I mention the risks of plants and other potentially sensitizing or allergy-related ingredients throughout this book, remember that the amount of a suspect ingredient can also determine how a product will affect your skin. The less there is of an ingredient—the farther down in the ingredient list it is—the less likely you are to have a reaction to it. Just because the ingredient is suspect or may have a potential for causing skin sensitivities doesn't mean it will always cause problems. Listen to your skin, err on the side of gentleness and be cautious. **Moreover, be patient. If you do have an allergic reaction, wait until it subsides before you venture out to try something new or different. Pare down to the absolute basics, usually just cleanser and a touch of moisturizer over very dry areas, try a bit of over-the-counter cortisone cream to reduce irritation, and stay out of the sun.**

Reminder: If you have an allergic reaction of any kind to a cosmetic product, stop using it immediately and consult your physician if the problem persists. Also, do not hesitate to return the product to the place where you purchased it and get your money back. It is not your fault that the product caused problems. Also, returning the product gives the cosmetics company essential information about how their formulas are working.

Is there one line of cosmetics that's best for sensitive or allergy-prone skin? It would be great if there were, but it just doesn't exist. Allergic skin reactions are amazingly random and dissimilar. What you're sensitive to often has little to do with what someone else reacts to, and beyond that there's the intricate interaction of ingredients being combined on the face. The culprit may not be the product you think caused the problem. You may think a new moisturizer made your eyes swell, but it could be the resins from that reliable nail polish you were wearing in combination with the new moisturizer that triggered the problem.

## BATTLE PLAN FOR ALLERGY-PRONE OR SENSITIZING SKIN REACTIONS

Whether or not you have sensitive or allergy-prone skin, the chances are that at some point you've had a sensitizing or allergic reaction to a cosmetic you've applied somewhere on your face or body. For some, simply identifying which product caused the problem and stopping its use is enough to improve the appearance of skin almost immediately, or at the very least in a day or two. For others, even after you've stopped using the offending item or items, your skin can remain rashy, reddened, flaky, dry, swollen, and irritated for days—and for some, even months. There is no known medical reason why some skin types can't shake a sensitizing or allergic reaction, but there are a few relatively simple things you can do to wage a successful battle against your skin's response to a product or products it doesn't like.

1. **Be certain you are dealing with an allergy or sensitizing reaction to a product and not with a skin disorder.** Many skin conditions such as psoriasis, rosacea, eczema, folliculitis (an inflammation of the hair follicle), and reactions to food can account for the skin becoming irritated, swollen, red, itchy, flaky, or rashy. A great resource for identifying whether or not what is occurring on your face is a skin disorder, is the *Primary Care Dermatology Atlas* at http://www.medscape.com/mp/dermatlas, where you can search over 2,600 images of skin problems. (You will need to create a user name and password, but otherwise this amazing source is a free online service of Medscape.) This gives you a way to identify whether or not your skin is similar in appearance to the images found for a particular skin disorder.

2. **Find what product(s) or ingredient(s) are causing the problem and stop using them.** Sometimes that is a simple enough procedure. If you started using a new concealer and within a few hours that area became red, itchy, and swollen, it would be clear that the concealer is the problem and you would stop using it. Unfortunately, it isn't always that easy. This discovery process can be very difficult because many skin reactions don't happen all that quickly. It may be several weeks or even months or years of using a product before your skin has a negative reaction to it. For some unknown reason your skin can develop allergic or sensitizing reactions over time. Further, given the number of cosmetic products women use daily, each one containing a disparate range of ingredients, it is no wonder that pinning down exactly which one caused the problem can be a challenge. To make matters even more complicated, it may not be a single product but the combination of products worn one over the other that caused the problem (maybe the concealer isn't the problem, but the mix of concealer, foundation, and moisturizer together that sparked the reaction). The key is to be patient and diligent, experimenting with the item or items you suspect and then watching how your skin responds when you discontinue using them.

3. **Whether or not you've been able to identify the problem product, an over-the-counter cortisone cream can be your skin's best friend.** Lanacort or Cortaid are excellent over-the-counter cortisone creams that function as anti-inflammatories. When either of these are applied to irritated, inflamed skin they can turn off the reaction that is causing the problem. It is essential to be conscientious about using these on a regular, methodical, though short-term, basis while your skin is having problems. For example, once the skin irritation shows up, keep applying the cortisone cream over the affected area for several days, even a day or two after everything seems back to normal. Remember that the skin can hold on to a sensitizing or allergic reaction for a long period of time, even after you've stopped using the offending product. And don't be afraid about the short-term use of an over-the-counter cortisone cream. It is the long-term, consistent use (for more than two or three months) of cortisone creams that can damage collagen and elastin in the skin, not short-term use.

4. **While you are combating the allergic or sensitizing reaction, do not use any other skin irritants of any kind over the affected area.** Fragrances, scrubs, washcloths, AHAs, Retin-A, Renova, benzoyl peroxide, skin lighteners, or other skin-care products with active or abrasive ingredients can trigger skin irritation and will only add to the problem.

5. **Avoid saunas, steam, sweating (if possible), or rubbing the affected area, all of which can help re-trigger the reaction.**

6. **Finally, if matters don't improve after four to six weeks, or if the reaction is severe from the beginning, you should see your dermatologist for an evaluation.**

7. **If you suspect that you are having a serious allergic reaction (in the form of hives, extremely swollen skin and eyes, or red patches over the skin that feel warm or tingle), consult your physician to discuss varying options. Prescription-strength topical cortisone, oral cortisone or oral antihistamines may be necessary.**

## WHAT ABOUT MOISTURIZER?

Not everyone needs or should use a moisturizer, especially women with oily, combination, or acne-prone skin! That sums it up. I can't think of any other skin-care product that is more misunderstood, misused, and abused than moisturizer.

How did things get so out of hand? The only answer is that things tend to get out of hand in the world of cosmetics!

Ironically, from a formulary point of view, I like more moisturizers than I dislike (putting aside the nasty debates over cost versus performance or exaggerated claims). Yet I've found that because most women overuse moisturizers, these products can cause some surprising skin problems. A lot of women (maybe most) still cling to the erroneous belief that moisturizers somehow prevent wrinkles. Not just moisturizers with a high SPF, which do stop further skin damage if they contain titanium dioxide, zinc oxide, or avobenzone, but all moisturizers. The mistaken notion that dry skin is more prone to wrinkles than oily skin remains firmly implanted in the mind of the consumer, and that's on top of all those claims about firming, toning, repairing, and lifting the skin made by companies that sell all sorts of other creams, gels, and lotions.

The only reason to use a moisturizer is if you have dry skin or wrinkled skin and you want it to look smoother (moisturizers can smooth over, not change, wrinkles). If you don't have dry skin, there is no reason to use a moisturizer. If you have oily skin or skin that breaks out, the worst thing you can do is use a moisturizer of any kind. It really is that simple. What happens when you overuse a moisturizer? Pores get clogged and blackheads can develop; dead skin cells get trapped and have a harder time naturally sloughing off, which can leave the skin looking dull; and you run a higher risk of getting patches of dermatitis, increasing the number of breakouts, and creating your own combination-skin predicament. Additionally, oversaturating the skin can turn off the skin's own immune/healing response. Overdoing it with moisturizers can actually prevent the skin from repairing itself.

Recognizing that a moisturizer isn't for everyone doesn't mean that your skin doesn't need the benefit of sunscreen ingredients, anti-irritants, antioxidants, or water-binding agents. It just means you need to reconsider the type of products you use that contain these kinds of ingredients. Many toners use no thickening agents that can clog pores or occlude skin but do contain antioxidants, anti-irritants, and water-binding agents. Further, many foundations now contain effective sunscreens, so that you don't have to load up your skin with layers of unnecessary products.

## DO YOU NEED A MOISTURIZER?

Dry skin is technically a condition caused by a lack of moisture in the skin's top layers, combined with a breakdown of the skin's intercellular matrix (the components that fill the area between skin cells) and an inadequate supply of lipids and oils from the oil gland. If the oil glands aren't doing their job of forming a protective barrier composed of lipids and other substances that prevent evaporation, you can have dry skin. In addition, anything that depletes or damages the skin's intercellular matrix, such as sun damage, environmental factors, or drying skin-care products, can create the need for a moisturizer.

Generally, you can assume that if you are using a gentle skin cleanser and no other irritating skin-care products and your skin still feels dry several minutes after you wash your face, you should use a moisturizer. **(This assumes you are not using a drying or irritating cleanser. It is critical to make sure the dryness of your skin isn't caused by your cleansing products.)** If your skin feels tight, dehydrated, taut, or uncomfortable from dryness by midday or at the end of the day, it is essential to use a moisturizer. Fine lines that improve with the application of a moisturizer, especially around the eyes, are a great reason to use a moisturizer. Just keep in mind that it is best to use the most lightweight moisturizer possible that makes a difference. If none of these problems are present, you don't have dry skin, so don't use a moisturizer. (Obviously, sunscreen is another story, but I'll delve into that in the next section.)

I know giving up a traditional moisturizer may be hard to do, but think about it the next time you reach for one. Ask yourself if your skin really needs this or if it would be better off with an AHA product or a lightweight moisturizer for just around the eyes instead. Or perhaps a well-formulated toner with antioxidants, anti-irritants, and natural moisturizing factors (also called water-binding agents) may be all your skin needs. You can even try a simple experiment to see if your skin does better by using moisturizer only on the dry spots or wrinkled areas rather than applying it all over. (Again, this presumes your skin-care routine is not drying out your skin.)

It's important to note that several skin conditions can look like dry skin but are not, and that they may be exacerbated by the use of moisturizers. Eczema, seborrhea, rosacea, early signs of skin cancer (called actinic keratosis), psoriasis, sun-damaged skin, and even overuse of heavy moisturizers can all resemble dryness but are not helped by using moisturizer. Eczema requires a cortisone cream; seborrhea, rosacea, and psoriasis require topical prescription medications to control the condition; skin cancer or actinic keratosis demands immediate medical attention; and sun-damaged skin is better off with an alpha hydroxy acid product to help exfoliate skin. Overusing moisturizers can not only mask these problems, but also can cause breakouts, make the skin appear dull and thick (by holding down skin cells and preventing exfoliation), and inhibit the skin's natural immune/healing response.

## WHAT MAKES A GREAT MOISTURIZER?

As any cosmetics chemist will tell you, there are countless formulary possibilities for moisturizers, far too many to narrow them down to any one ingredient or even to a handful of ingredients. There are truly myriad possible ingredient combinations that can be used to create a great moisturizer. There simply isn't a single best one, which explains why a company like Estee Lauder can sell over 300 antiaging products when you count the varying cosmetics companies under their banner. The cosmetics-industry-induced hype that one ingredient holds the answer for skin is a complete fabrication. Whether it is vitamin C, green tea, grape extract, seaweed, beta glucan, alpha hydroxy acid, or some rare mushroom extract, to name just a few, none of them can deliver on the promise for wrinkle-free skin. Instead, each one has a specific benefit to consider, and there is no research establishing any one of them as being preferred over the other (Source: *Cosmetic Dermatology*, December 2001, pages 37–39).

So what does constitute a great moisturizer? For daytime, the crucial aspect of any moisturizer is that it must be a well-formulated sunscreen. Besides protecting your skin from the sun, an excellent moisturizer will contain emollients, water-binding agents (ingredients that attract water to the skin and help keep it there), anti-irritants, and antioxidants.

## EMOLLIENTS

Emollients are lubricating ingredients that are critical for making dry skin not feel dry. These provide dry skin with the one thing it's missing—lubrication—in the form of substances that resemble those the skin produces for itself. Emollients are ingredients like plant oils, mineral oil, shea butter, cocoa butter, petrolatum, cholesterol, and animal oils (including emu, mink, and lanolin, the latter probably the one ingredient that is most like our own skin's oil). All of these are exceptionally beneficial for skin and are easily recognizable on an ingredient list. Far less easy to comprehend on the label are a wide range of ingredients like triglycerides, palmitates, myristates, and stearates. These substances are generally waxy in texture and appearance but are what give most moisturizers their elegant texture and feel. Overall, emollients create the fundamental base and texture of a moisturizer and impart a creamy, smooth feel on the skin. Silicones are another interesting group of lubricants for skin. These have the most exquisite silky texture and an incredible ability to prevent dehydration without suffocating skin. All of these ingredients, in endless variations, spread over the skin to create a thin, imperceptible layer, re-creating the benefits of our own oil production, preventing evaporation, and giving the skin the lubrication it is missing.

## NATURAL MOISTURIZING FACTORS (NMFS) OR WATER-BINDING AGENTS

Natural moisturizing factors (NMFs) or water-binding agents work great for dry skin, and most are suitable for all skin types. "Water-binding agent" and NMF are general terms that refer to ingredients that can keep water in the skin or repair the skin's intercellular matrix (fundamental external structure). There are many ingredients that have these functions. Humectants, for example, attract water to skin and are one vital component of a moisturizer. But what good is getting water to the skin if the structure isn't there to keep the water from leaving? It turns out skin cells usually have plenty of water if they don't become degraded or damaged. Once skin is irritated, overcleansed, exposed to the sun, dehydrated from air conditioning or heaters, and so on and so on, the integrity of the skin is compromised. That means the substances that keep the skin cells bound together to create the surface structure we see as skin (the intercellular matrix) are depleted. This intercellular structure is made up of many different components, ranging from ceramides to lecithin, glycerin, polysaccharides, hyaluronic acid, sodium hyaluronate, sodium PCA, collagen, elastin, proteins, amino acids (of which there are dozens), cholesterol, glucose, sucrose, fructose, glycogen, phospholipids, glycosphingolipids, and glycosaminoglycans to name just a few. All of these give the skin what it needs to keep skin cells intact. Just adding water is meaningless if the skin doesn't have the wherewithal to keep the water inside, or if the intercellular matrix is damaged. When a moisturizer does contain a combination of these NMFs and water-binding ingredients, it reinforces the skin's natural ability to function normally and that temporarily reduces the presence of dry skin.

## ANTI-IRRITANTS

Anti-irritants are another vital component of any skin-care formulation. Regardless of the source, irritation is a problem for all skin types, and is ubiquitous and almost impossible to avoid. Whether it is from the sun, the environment, or from the skin-care products a person uses, irritation is a constant assault on the skin. Ironically, for skin-care products, even such necessary ingredients as sunscreen agents, preservatives, exfoliants, and cleansing agents can cause irritation. And other ingredients are irritating or have no real benefit for skin care, such as fragrance and sensitizing plant extracts. Further, oxidative damage from pollution, sun exposure, and air can cause irritation and damage to skin. Anti-irritants thus are a growing addition to many skin-care products to help skin handle the impact or to reduce the irritation skin is subjected to on a daily basis. Anti-irritants are incredibly helpful because they allow skin healing time and can reduce the problems oxidative damage causes. Anti-irritants include substances with names like bisabolol, allantoin, burdock root, aloe, licorice root, grape extract, glycyrrhetinic acid, green tea, vitamin C, chamomile extract, willowherb, white willow, willow bark, and many many more.

## ANTIOXIDANTS

Antioxidants are a fascinating part of a moisturizing formula. There's now a growing body of research that shows antioxidants to be a potential panacea for skin's ills and it's nothing less than impressive. What makes antioxidants so intriguing is that they seem to have the ability to reduce or prevent some of the oxidative damage that destroys and depletes the skin's function and structure, while also preventing some solar degeneration of skin (Source: *Cosmetic Dermatology*, December 2001, pages 37–40; *Current Problems in Dermatology*, 2001, volume 29, pages 26–42, "The Antioxidant Network of the Stratum Corneum"). All of that is incredibly beneficial for cell turnover, healing, and reducing dehydration. I suspect that antioxidant research for skin will become even more fascinating over the years. Meanwhile, lots of antioxidants are showing up in skin care these days, such as selenium, superoxide dismutase, vitamin A (retinyl palmitate and retinol), vitamin C (ascorbyl palmitate and magnesium ascorbyl palmitate), beta glucan, vitamin E (a-tocopherol, tocotrienol), curcumin, coenzyme Q10, alpha lipoic acid, green tea, grape extract, and forms of rosemary and lemon bioflavonoids to name a few.

All of these, combined in more permutations than you can imagine, create the moisturizers I consider "best" for skin. There is no one mixture or "best" ingredient though, just like there isn't just one "best" chocolate cake. I wish there were, but the brilliance of cosmetics chemists lies in their ability to put these ingredients together in many ways to create wonderful products. There are just too many options to sum it up in any one formula. (Find out more about antioxidants in the discussion in Chapter Three, *Miracles, Frauds, & Facts*.)

# ARE SERUMS NECESSARY?

Hearing the word "serum" evokes a sense of a medical fluid of some kind, something more technically advanced for your skin. It may make you think of blood serum, the fluid, colorless part of the blood. It may even trigger memories of being given a shot of specially prepared serum to protect you from an illness. But in cosmetics serums are not an authentic or distinctive formulation. Cosmetic products labeled as serums are using a term with no real meaning or specific definition of any kind. Rather it is just a clever marketing ploy used to make a standard product sound like something impressive and different from a moisturizer. This way the cosmetics industry can lead women to believe that they are purchasing a unique product that is worth the extra money and a necessary addition to their skin-care routine.

Technically, serum is defined as any watery animal fluid, and surely that doesn't sound appealing! Yes, the name "serum" may give you the sense that they are something medical or therapeutic, but that is nothing more than a psychological impression, not a tested formulary attribution. In the cosmetics world a serum is just a lightweight, gel-like moisturizer with a consistency that is less viscous or emollient than the average lotion or creamy moisturizer. These serums also tend to contain more silicone than other moisturizers, as opposed to thickening agents, so it's very likely that the silky feel you experience is from the silicone they contain. Serums may moisturize, but the name is nothing more than a marketing term. They are not a uniquely formulated product that provides an uncommon benefit for skin.

## EXFOLIATING SKIN

The issues around skin exfoliation are complicated, but exfoliation itself is essential for skin health, and most skin types can benefit from exfoliation. Despite the risks of irritation, removing the damaged outer layer of skin is an essential skin-care need of many different skin types. If you have dry skin, oily skin, blackheads, acne, sun-damaged skin, flaky skin (not caused by a skin disease or a skin disorder), or a rough surface texture, those problems are best handled by products that exfoliate and help dead skin cells slough off from the surface of the skin. (Disinfectants, which can also be irritating, are essential for treating acne; see Chapter Ten, *Battle Plans for Blemishes*, for more information about the pros and cons of disinfectants.) The goal is to use the most effective, least irritating products for exfoliating skin. The only skin types that need to be very cautious about using exfoliating products are those with extremely sensitive skin or older skin, and those with skin diseases or disorders such as rosacea, eczema, dermatitis, or seborrhea.

## EXFOLIATING OILY SKIN

Let's start with oily skin or skin with clogged pores. Blackheads or blemishes can occur if the oil gland produces too much sebum. Sebum is a soft wax that should liquefy when it reaches the surface of the pore, spreading a thin, imperceptible protective layer over the skin. But when too much sebum is produced, the liquefying process can get backed up. Add to that problem a tendency for skin cells that should be naturally sloughing off to instead fall inside the pore and get stuck. The more skin cells that build up in the oil gland, the more oil will be held back from flowing easily out of the pore (the pore is the exit path for oil), and the result can be a blackhead or a blemish.

Often with oily skin, cells that should be shedding on a regular, daily basis are being held back. One thing that keeps cells from sloughing off is that self-same oil (sebum). The oil works as an adhesive, preventing the shedding skin cells from going where they are supposed to go—off the face. One way to keep pores from getting clogged is to help skin cells shed as freely as possible so they don't get trapped inside the pore. The more you keep skin cells exfoliating in a normal manner, the less cell debris can fill up the pore.

Another issue for oily skin with clogged pores is that the oil gland itself has a skin lining (epithelial lining). For some reason, this lining inside the pore can become thickened or misshapen and choke off and block the flow of oil out of the pore. Using exfoliants that can exfoliate the lining of the pore, thus restoring a more natural shape, can encourage a normal flow of oil and eliminate clogged pores.

# EXFOLIATING DRY SKIN

The reasons for exfoliating dry skin are different from the ones for treating oily, blemish-prone skin, though the objective is the same: removing dead skin cells that are not shedding normally. Skin can be dry for many reasons, including lack of moisture, a buildup of dead skin cells that don't easily shed, and abnormal skin cells that adhere together in a way that prevents normal exfoliation and normal moisture retention. (Dry-looking skin can also be caused by moisturizers that are too emollient and hold dead skin cells in place, preventing healthy shedding. When this happens, the surface of the skin feels "greasy" or moist, and the underlying layer feels dry.) When you help dry skin shed dried-up, dead skin cells, it can make room for plumper (moisture-filled), less-dry skin cells to come to the surface, which can lend a fresher look to the skin. This also allows moisturizers (the least amount and lighter texture, the better) to more easily penetrate the skin because there are fewer dried-up skin cells in the way to block absorption. Exfoliating helps the dead surface-skin cells shed at a more normal rate, making room for the lower layers of newer skin cells. And for dry skin it is also helpful to efficiently remove dead skin cells to reduce the chance of pores becoming clogged and creating blackheads and whiteheads.

# EXFOLIATING SUN-DAMAGED SKIN

One of the primary manifestations of sun-damaged skin is that the outer layer of skin becomes thickened, similar to a callous. This thickened layer is your skin's response to the damage caused by unprotected exposure to ultraviolet (UV) radiation from the sun. While this thickened layer provides a minimal amount of sun protection (it is thought to protect with the equivalent of an SPF of 2), it ends up creating far more problems than advantages. As you will learn in Chapter Five, *Sun Sense*, on sun protection, an SPF of 2 is truly meaningless and useless for skin. This thickened outer layer of the skin produced by sun damage causes skin to look dull and more wrinkled than it really is; it also adds a yellowish or gray tint to skin and reduces the ability of good skin-care ingredients to penetrate. Using effective topical exfoliants to remove this thickened, unattractive outer layer of skin can help skin feel smoother, look less wrinkled, have a healthier, more normal skin color, and reduce the chance of clogged pores. (Removing this layer of unhealthy skin does make the skin more sun sensitive, the way it was before it became sun damaged. Though it is always imperative to use a sunscreen, it is even more so if you are regularly using an exfoliant of any kind.)

## WHICH EXFOLIANTS TO USE?

For many skin types, the issue is not whether to exfoliate, but which type you should use and how often. There are a lot of exfoliating products out there waiting to peel the money from your pocketbook as well as skin cells from your face. Scrubs, soaps with exfoliating ingredients, toners, facial masks, facial peels, abrasive sponges, washcloths, and facial brushes are all designed to exfoliate. Overkill (as in doing too much to the skin) becomes an issue when your skin-care routine includes more than one exfoliating product or if the one you are using is too strong. In the world of consumerism, if a little is good, a lot must be better, and the cosmetics industry is right there with a host of products. Ignore them; it only takes one product to do the job, and your task is to choose the best product for your skin type.

I do not recommend exfoliating facial masks because often, in addition to the exfoliating ingredient, they also contain a number of other irritating ingredients. Also, exfoliation works best when done consistently, while facial masks tend to be used irregularly and infrequently.

Facial brushes and washcloths are options, but I find they are both almost impossible to keep clean, they tend to exfoliate unevenly, they exfoliate only on the very surface of the skin, and they are not as effective or as gentle as other alternatives. Abrasive sponges, such as loofahs, are way too irritating from the neck up, and are also very difficult to keep clean, meaning they could cause problems by harboring bacteria that can cause infection.

Cosmetic scrubs can be a good way to remove the dead surface layer of skin, but there are difficulties with these types of exfoliants, too. Many of them contain gritty abrasives that can be unnecessarily irritating. These abrasive fragments are not uniform in shape and can literally cut the skin. In addition, cosmetic scrubs often contain thick waxes and creams so you can smooth them more easily over your skin, yet these waxes can clog pores and leave a film over the face, which reduces exfoliation. Some scrub products also contain harsh ingredients such as peppermint, menthol, eucalyptus, alcohol, and roughly ground scrub particles that are simply unnecessary and overly irritating. The problems with all mechanical scrubs—even the one I recommend, namely plain baking soda or baking soda mixed with Cetaphil Cleanser—are that the scrubbing action is mostly on the surface, and the mechanical action against the skin can cause too much irritation. You need to exfoliate, but how to do that gently is the question.

# AHAS AND BHA

There are two primary topical ways to exfoliate skin, either with a product containing alpha hydroxy acids (AHAs) or one with beta hydroxy acid (BHA). AHAs have lost much of the popularity they enjoyed since they were first introduced when Avon launched its Anew line with AHAs in 1992, but nevertheless their effectiveness for skin remains a convincing option.

There is only one BHA (beta hydroxy acid, or salicylic acid), but there are a variety of AHAs. The five major types of AHAs that show up in skin-care products are glycolic, lactic, malic, citric, and tartaric acids. Of these, the most commonly used AHAs are glycolic and lactic acids because of their special ability to penetrate the skin, plus they have the most accumulated research on their functionality for skin. A search of the published literature for glycolic and lactic acids lists over 200 varying studies, while there are only a handful for the other three AHAs put together. A similar search for salicylic acid (BHA) reveals over 450 different published studies evaluating its effectiveness.

What glycolic, lactic, and salicylic acids can do is "unglue" the outer layer of dead skin cells, helping increase cell turnover by removing the built-up top layers of skin, allowing healthier cells to come to the surface. Removing this dead layer can improve skin texture and color, unclog pores, and allow moisturizers to be better absorbed by the skin. Both AHAs and BHA affect the top layers of skin, and they help to improve the appearance of sun-damaged skin, dry skin, and thickened skin caused by a variety of factors, including abnormal cell growth, smoking, and heavy moisturizers. Reminder: Sun damage in particular causes the top layer of skin to thicken, creating a dull, rough texture and appearance on the surface of skin; AHAs nicely remove this thickened layer, revealing the more normal-appearing skin cells underneath (Sources: *Archives of Dermatologic Research*, June 1997, pages 404–409; *Dermatologic Surgery*, May 1998, pages 573–577).

There is even a good deal of research showing that the use of glycolic acid can improve the appearance of skin discolorations, increase collagen production, and reinforce the barrier function of skin (Source: *Dermatologic Surgery*, May 2001, pages 429–433).

Because AHAs and BHA work through a chemical rather than a mechanical process, they can produce better results than cosmetic scrubs, which work only on the exposed surface of the skin. And because AHAs and BHA work just on the surface of skin (or, in the case of BHA, inside the pore), there is no risk that you will lose too much skin. That is, they don't keep on exfoliating away layers of skin without stopping, as can happen with a scrub. Technically, there is a drop-off rate, meaning the AHA and BHA will exfoliate just the dead or damaged skin and leave the healthy skin alone.

**The fundamental difference between AHAs and BHA is that AHAs are water-soluble, while BHA is lipid-soluble (oil-soluble). This unique property of BHA allows it to penetrate the oil in the pores and exfoliate the built-up skin cells inside the oil gland. AHAs are much less able to do this because they can't get through the fat content of the oil (sebum). Therefore, BHA is indicated for use where blackheads and blemishes are the issue, and AHAs are more suitable for sun-damaged, thickened, dry skin where breakouts are not a problem** (Source: *Global Cosmetic Industry*, November 2000, pages 56–57).

I wish the discussion of AHAs and BHA could end here. I wish you could find a good AHA product by looking for glycolic or lactic acid on the ingredient list if you have sun-damaged, thickened, dry skin. Or that if you tend to have blackheads or blemishes and wanted to find a good BHA product, you would only need to look for a product that contains salicylic acid. But, alas, it isn't that simple. AHAs and BHA are effective as exfoliants only at certain concentrations (the quantity of the ingredient present in the product) and at very specific pHs (referring to the acidity or alkalinity of a product).

## PH-SENSITIVE AHA AND BHA

When it comes to AHAs and BHA, the crucial information comes in two parts: One is the type of ingredient and its concentration in the product, and the other is the pH of the product. AHAs work best at concentrations of 5% to 8% and at a pH of 3 to 4 (this is more acid than alkaline or neutral), and their effectiveness diminishes as you go past a pH of 4.5. BHA works best at concentrations of between 1% and 2%, and at an optimal pH of 3, diminishing in effectiveness as you go past a pH of 4. Both AHAs and BHA lose their effectiveness as a product's pH goes up and the concentration of the ingredient goes down. This is so central to the whole subject of exfoliation and cell turnover that it bears repeating: **AHAs work best in a 5% to 8% concentration, in a product with a pH of 3 to 4; BHA works best in a 1% to 2% concentration, in a product with a pH of 3 to 4** (Source: *Cosmetic Dermatology*, October 2001, pages 15–18).

If the cosmetics industry isn't forthcoming about the necessary percentages and pH for a BHA or AHA product (and most companies aren't), how can you tell if it provides decent or effective exfoliation? Consumers can't, not unless they are shopping with pH measuring paper in hand, which is exactly how I went about rating exfoliant products for my book *Don't Go to the Cosmetics Counter Without Me*. As a general rule, it is best if the AHA ingredient is either second or third on the ingredient list, making it likely that the product contains a 5% or higher concentration of AHAs. For salicylic acid, because such a small amount is required, it is fine if the ingredient is located toward the middle or end of the ingredient list. (To establish the pH of a product you can always do what I do, test each product with a pH strip, but that is hardly practical for most women.)

Aside from the way they can exfoliate the skin when the concentration and pH level are right, AHAs can also have water-binding properties. They can provide an added benefit by helping to keep water in the skin at the same time that exfoliation is taking place. They also have water-binding properties at any pH, so even if the product can't exfoliate skin it still can aid in moisturizing the skin.

BHA, though it provides more penetrating exfoliation into the pore, ends up being less irritating than AHAs. This is due to BHA's relation to aspirin. BHA, as salicylic acid, is derived from acetylsalicylic acid, which is the technical name for aspirin, and aspirin has anti-inflammatory properties. On the skin, BHA retains many of these anti-inflammatory effects.

Keep in mind that none of these AHA or BHA products, regardless of concentration, pH, or type, can prevent aging or change a wrinkle. Researchers theorize that AHAs, and possibly BHA, can increase collagen and elastin, much as Retin-A and Renova can. But this is only theory, and there is no research to prove it. Meanwhile, AHA and BHA products can definitely smooth the skin, improve texture, unclog pores, and give the appearance of plumper, firmer skin (because more healthy skin cells are now on the surface). And when you stop using them the skin goes back to the condition it was in before you started.

## AHA CONFUSION

Estee Lauder was one of the first department-store lines to launch an AHA product, Fruition. It was an overnight success, but not because of its AHA content: Fruition contained less than 2% AHA. At that percentage, AHAs are little more than good water-binding agents. That isn't bad; it just isn't what makes AHAs and BHA such fascinating ingredients. Consumers must have complained, because shortly thereafter Lauder launched Fruition Extra, which contains a decent amount of AHA and has a good pH. It's absurdly expensive for what you get, and of course the company never bothered to explain why you now needed Fruition Extra if the original Fruition was supposed to be so amazing and wondrous for the skin.

Another example: Clinique's TurnAround and Total Turnaround products, all of which contain about a 1% concentration of BHA, and have a pH of around 5. That high pH makes them ineffective as exfoliants. In reality, TurnAround can't turn around even one skin cell.

Then there are AHA sound-alikes, including sugarcane extract, mixed fruit acids, fruit extracts, milk extract, and citrus extract, and BHA sound-alikes such as wintergreen extract. You may think these are better, more natural AHAs or BHA products when you see these less technical, more familiar names, but that absolutely isn't the case. Without knowing exactly what type of AHA or BHA ingredient you are buying, there is no way to know for sure what you are putting on your skin or how effective it really is. Although glycolic acid is derived from sugarcane and lactic acid is derived from milk, that doesn't mean sugarcane extract or milk extract are the same as glycolic or lactic acid. Just because a product contains sugarcane extract doesn't mean that the acid has been extracted from the sugarcane. And even if the acid has been extracted, you can't tell how concentrated it is, and what about the pH? It's all too vague and meaningless, making it impossible to determine what you are really buying. My advice is to be very suspicious of any product that claims an association with AHAs or BHA but contains a variety of sound-alike ingredients.

## BHA CONFUSION

Products boasting that they contain a natural source of salicylic acid (BHA) usually add willow bark. Willow bark contains salicin, a substance that when taken orally is converted by the digestive process into salicylic acid. That means the process of converting willow bark to salicylic acid requires the presence of certain enzymes to turn the salicin into salicylic acid. The digestive conversion processes can turn salicin into saligenin, and then into salicylic acid, but they are complicated. Further, salicin, much like salicylic acid, is stable only under acidic conditions. The likelihood that willow bark in the tiny amount used in cosmetics can mimic the effectiveness of salicylic acid is at best problematic, and in all likelihood impossible. However, willow bark may indeed have some anti-inflammatory benefits for skin because, in this form, it appears to retain more of its aspirin-like composition.

## WHAT ABOUT HIGHER CONCENTRATIONS OF AHAS?

I am very concerned about the introduction of products with higher percentages of AHAs, as is the FDA (Source: FDA *Consumer Magazine*, March-April 1998, revised May 1999). Various cosmetics lines have introduced products like this, including one called M.D. Formulations, sold by doctors and salons. M.D. Formulations sells AHA products at 10%, 15%, and 20% concentrations in appropriate pHs of 3 to 4.

Removing the outer layer of skin can be taken too far, however, and many cosmetic dermatologists and researchers worry that increased irritation and exfoliation caused by such high concentrations of AHAs can actually hurt skin. Without more evidence showing a genuine benefit from higher concentrations (none exists at this time), I am not willing to recommend that anyone put their skin at risk in that way. Most likely the positive results women and men may perceive with higher concentrations of AHAs come from the swelling and edema they cause. That may diminish the appearance of wrinkles and make the skin feel smoother, but it is most likely not best for the long-term health of the skin due to the increased amount of constant irritation.

If you use a well-formulated AHA product (5% to 8% concentration, with a pH of 3 to 4) or BHA product (1% to 2% concentration with a pH of 3 to 4) but you don't "feel" it working on your skin, that doesn't mean it isn't working. Quite the contrary, it is indeed working—without causing your skin any discomfort or irritation.

## POLYHYDROXY ACIDS

It's no secret that alpha hydroxy acids (AHAs) may be irritating. In fact, for them to be effective they need to produce a little bit of irritation. Yet for some skin types that little bit can be too much. The search for an effective form of AHA (as mentioned above, glycolic acid and lactic acid are considered the most functional forms) or an extra ingredient that can enhance performance and reduce irritation has been a popular topic of discussion among cosmetics formulators. Gluconolactone and lactobionic acid are types of polyhydroxy acid that NeoStrata believes serves both ends: They are supposed to be just as effective as AHAs but also less irritating. (NeoStrata is the company that holds the patent on glycolic acid as an antiwrinkle agent, as well as a patent for gluconolactone for reducing the appearance of wrinkles.)

Gluconolactone and lactobionic acid are chemically and functionally similar to AHAs. The significant difference between them is that gluconolactone and lactobionic acid have a larger molecular structure, which limits their penetration into the skin, resulting in a reduction of irritating side-effects. This more controlled release into the skin supposedly doesn't hamper effectiveness. So are gluconolactone and lactobionic acid better for your skin than AHAs in the form of glycolic acid or lactic acid? Probably not, or at least not significantly enough for most skin types to notice a difference. According to an Internet-published class lecture by Dr. Mark G.

Rubin (Source: http://128.11.40.183/lasernews/rubin_lecture/21.html), a board-certified dermatologist who is also an Assistant Clinical Professor of Dermatology at the University of California, San Diego, research on gluconolactone demonstrated only a "6% decrease in dermal penetration" in comparison to glycolic acid, which "isn't a dramatic improvement." Gluconolactone may be slightly less irritating for some skin types but this isn't quite the magic bullet for exfoliation that beauty magazines and some cosmetics companies have been extolling. There is no independent information available about lactobionic acid.

## HOW DO YOU USE AHAS OR BHA?

Strictly based on your skin type and skin-care needs, you can apply an AHA or BHA product once or twice a day. Also, depending on your skin's sensitivity you can apply either of these around the eye area, making sure to keep them off the eyelid and away from the eye itself. Apply the AHA or BHA product after the face is cleansed and after your toner has dried (if you are using one). Once the AHA or BHA has been absorbed, you can apply any other product, such as additional moisturizer, eye cream, sunscreen, and/or foundation. It is not essential to wear moisturizer over an AHA or BHA product. That totally depends on what type of skin you have, how it reacts to the AHA or BHA product, and what kind of base the AHA or BHA is in. Some AHAs and BHA come in moisturizing bases, and most skin types do not require another moisturizer.

I generally recommend using an AHA or BHA in a gel or liquid form so you don't have to apply a moisturizing base where you don't need it. That way the AHA or BHA goes on first and the moisturizer goes over it only where the skin is dry or taut. Never purchase an AHA or BHA product that includes other irritating ingredients such as alcohol, menthol, camphor, eucalyptus, mint, or citrus. AHAs and BHA can be irritating enough by themselves (removing dead, damaged skin cells is not a gentle process), and there is never a reason to add more irritation, especially when it provides no benefit for the skin. The only reason possible irritation from AHAs and BHA is allowable is because their ability to exfoliate is useful for solving many skin-care problems.

I never recommend cleansers that contain AHAs or BHA, for several reasons. First, if they are in a water-soluble cleanser, you run the risk of possible contact with the eyes, which can cause irritation. Second, AHAs and BHA work on the skin or the pores when they have been absorbed. When they are in a cleanser, they get rinsed down the drain before they can work. (Some companies shockingly recommend leaving the cleanser on the face for several minutes so the AHAs or BHA can be absorbed into the skin, but that means the detergent cleansing agents would be left on the skin for longer than necessary, and that absolutely can cause unwanted irritation.) Finally, the skin needs only one good exfoliant, and that's it. Overexfoliating will further irritate the skin, and the long-term effects of that are unknown.

In terms of sunscreens, it would be great if an AHA or BHA product had a good SPF rating (at least SPF 15, with FDA-approved UVA protection). That way, if you wanted to use an AHA or BHA product during the day along with a sunscreen, you would only have to apply one product instead of two. **There are no sunscreens currently on the market that contain an effective concentration of AHAs or BHA with a proper pH level as well as an effective SPF formulation (effective meaning an SPF 15 with one or more of these active ingredients: avobenzone, titanium dioxide, or zinc oxide). Why? Because to be stable, sunscreen formulations require a pH higher than what is acceptable for an effective AHA or BHA product. As a result, sunscreen needs to be a separate step from the application of AHAs or BHA (or Retin-A and Renova, for that matter).**

As you search for an AHA or BHA product, cosmetics salespeople will tell you to use theirs along with their complete program, including two or three other moisturizers, toners, cleansers, eye creams, throat creams, and anything else they can sell you. Be prepared for the hard sell when it comes to AHA or BHA products! Many cosmetics companies treat them like the fountain of youth, and they are not. They do not stop wrinkling, they merely smooth the surface skin for as long as you continue to use them. Some companies deal in specialty AHA products that contain higher percentages (from 8% to 15%). However, higher percentages may guarantee higher irritation, and there is little research indicating what kind of risk or harm that might pose over time. Be aware that many, many AHA and BHA products are poorly formulated, with ineffective concentrations and pH levels. The purpose of AHAs and BHA is to exfoliate the skin. They can do that only at the appropriate concentration and pH. An AHA or BHA product that has a low concentration and a high pH may feel good on the skin, but it is good only as a moisturizer. That isn't bad, but it won't exfoliate the skin.

By the way, many AHA or BHA products designed for oily skin contain alcohol. I do not recommend these because of the risk of increased irritation and sensitization they pose. Likewise, someone with oily skin or breakouts will have problems with an AHA or BHA that comes in a moisturizing base because the ingredients may make the skin feel slick and can clog pores. Those with oily skin types need to look for AHA or BHA products in a gel or liquid form that are irritant-free (meaning no alcohol, plants, fruit extracts, or witch hazel) and as lightweight as possible. More of these are becoming available, but the pickings are still relatively slim if you're looking for a good, reasonably priced AHA or BHA product that won't adversely affect oily skin types.

As a general rule (though there are definitely exceptions and personal preferences that alter this rule), if you are using one good AHA or BHA product, you should not use additional exfoliating products such as cosmetic scrubs, washcloths, and facial masks (clay or drying masks). Also, stay away from overdoing exfoliation. Lots of cosmetics companies put AHAs and BHA in everything they make. Remember, the skin can handle only so much irritation; one effective exfoliant is all that is necessary for anyone's skin.

Most people experience a tingling or slight stinging sensation when they use AHA or BHA products with appropriate concentrations and pH. Some people have had minor to severe flaking and redness. Minor reactions are to be expected, given the nature of AHAs and BHA. However, long-term irritation, redness, flaking, or patches of dermatitis are not healthy for the skin, and if any of these symptoms occur, you should reduce the frequency of application or consider a gentler (less concentrated) product. Listen to your skin. If it gets very dry and flaky, use an additional moisturizer for a period of time until the skin calms down and gets used to the new level of exfoliation. If it gets red and irritated, use the product less frequently, though still regularly (perhaps once a day, or two or three times a week). If it still gets very dry and irritated, consider stopping altogether. Severe irritation is not the goal or the desired result.

One more key point. As you probably already know, it is imperative that you wear a sunscreen every day, one with an SPF of at least 15 that includes avobenzone (trade name Parsol 1789), titanium dioxide, or zinc oxide to protect skin from UVA damage. Exfoliating the skin leaves it more vulnerable to sun damage and that means you need mandatory, maximum sunscreen protection every day.

**The FDA has confirmed that there is a risk of UVB sun sensitivity (sunburn) following the use of AHAs. That makes sense, given that AHAs work to remove sun-damaged skin, and that leaves the skin somewhat more vulnerable. Of course this sensitivity is easily preventable with the diligent use of lower concentrations of AHA (10% or less) and a sunscreen.** Research does show AHAs to be safe in 4% to 8% concentrations with a pH of 3 to 4 (Source: *Journal of Cosmetic Science*, November/December 2000, pages 343–349).

# TRETINOIN (RETIN-A, RENOVA, ETC.)

Even after discussing AHAs and BHA at length, I do not want to play down the considerable importance of tretinoins for skin because they are major players when it comes to changing the way skin behaves. If you have sun-damaged, dry, wrinkled, or acne-prone skin, you should become familiar with the names Retin-A and Renova and their active ingredient tretinoin.

Let me make it perfectly clear from the beginning that **Retin-A and Renova are not exfoliants**, though many people think that's what they do. It is also vital to clarify how important it is to consider these products (or any topical prescription medication containing tretinoin) as elements of basic skin-care treatment. This is because tretinoin affects and improves actual cell production deep in the dermis, far away from the surface of skin (Sources: *Clinical and Experimental Dermatology*, October 2001, pages 613–618; *Clinical Geriatric Medicine*, November 2001, pages 643–659; *Photochemistry and Photobiology*, February 1999, pages 154–157).

Tretinoin can help skin look and feel smoother and function more normally, but the process is subtle and very different from the action of removing surface layers of skin to create a smoother texture and appearance. AHAs and BHA affect the *surface* of the skin (epidermis) or the lining of the pore by actually ungluing or dissolving layers of skin cells. In contrast, tretinoin affects the *dermis*, where new skin cells are produced. Why the confusion about the effect tretinoin can have on the skin? Primarily it's due to the fact that using products containing the drug tretinoin can cause irritation and inflammation, resulting in the skin becoming flaky and dry. This flaking and dryness is not exfoliation, nor is it a desirable or advantageous result. If tretinoin causes your skin to be consistently dry and flaky it is a problem, and you should probably avoid the products that contain it.

For a bit of history, the original patent for the use of tretinoin to treat acne and sun-damaged skin was held by a division of Johnson & Johnson. The only prescription products that contained tretinoin were varying forms of Retin-A and Renova. Johnson & Johnson's patent for tretinoin expired in the mid-1990s. Now there are a handful of other topical prescription drugs containing tretinoin that are also an option for skin, including Tazorac, Avita, and generic tretinoin.

The FDA approved Renova for use as a wrinkle cream in December 1995. That makes Renova the only medication ever approved by the FDA for the treatment of sun-damaged skin and wrinkles. Yet the research concerning Renova in regard to "wrinkles" was not exactly exciting. According to the FDA, "Studies on Renova showed that after 24 weeks approximately 30 percent of people who used the product for fine wrinkles or spotty discoloration had moderate improvement, 35 percent had minimal improvement and 35 percent had no improvement. Among individuals who used the product, about 16 percent had moderate improvement in skin roughness, 35 percent saw minimal improvement and 49 percent had no improvement. Renova does not eliminate wrinkles or repair the sun-damaged skin that leads to cancer. Nor is there evidence that Renova treats coarse skin, deep wrinkles, skin yellowing or other skin problems" (Source: *FDA Talk Paper*, January 2, 1996).

**While Renova and other tretinoin products won't erase wrinkles, they can do remarkable things for the health of the skin.** Tretinoin has the ability to locate receptor sites on the skin cell that accept certain specific components of vitamin A. The tretinoin attaches to this receptor site, which provides information to the cell, telling it to behave in a healthier manner. In this way, tretinoin can play a vital role in changing the way skin cells are formed and shaped. This is different from exfoliating. If a skin cell has a healthier form and shape, it can do its job of natural exfoliation and look the way it did (to some extent) before it was sun damaged.

Regardless of these positive effects, tretinoin products will be useless if you do not wear a sunscreen as well. Not a wrinkle cream in the world, even one approved by the FDA, can have positive results if you don't use an effective sunscreen; without that, you are just putting back more of the damage you don't want.

Tretinoin products aren't cheap. Renova costs about $60 for a 40-gram tube (a one- to two-month supply), and that doesn't include the cost of a visit to your doctor. But Tazorac and Avita or generic tretinoins are half that price and just as effective.

Many physicians recommend applying both tretinoin and AHAs, using AHA in the morning and tretinoin at night or one over the other. How BHA figures into use for different skin types is not clear. Because people react differently to skin-care products, I would suggest experimenting to see which item or items work best for you. There is no reason in the world not to judiciously try out such a combination, always remembering sunscreen, to see what has the most benefit for your skin.

Again, what tretinoin, AHA, and BHA products have in common is that once you stop using them, your skin will revert to the way it was before. These products will not produce permanent change. The smooth exterior lasts only as long as you use them. This is one of the major reasons that researchers don't believe AHAs, BHA, Retin-A, or Renova really change the deeper layers of the skin.

## TRETINOIN CARE

If you do choose to get a topical prescription tretinoin product, it is important to be careful when using it and/or AHA and BHA products. Review and remember the following list of cautions:

- It is always dangerous to tan, but it is especially problematic after you start using topical tretinoins (because they can be irritating and cause peeling) or an AHA or BHA product. As the surface skin peels and the callous of damaged skin is removed to reveal healthier skin, the skin becomes more sensitive to sunlight and is, therefore, even more subject to serious sunburn and sun damage. Also, tanning will negate any positive effects you hope to gain from using these products. You should already be using an effective sunscreen every day, but if you are using any of the above-mentioned products, it is vital to wear a sunscreen rated at least SPF 15, with the UVA-protecting ingredients of avobenzone (Parsol 1789), titanium dioxide, or zinc oxide, whenever you venture outside. The idea is to keep your sun exposure to a minimum.

- Tretinoin, as well as AHA and BHA products, can irritate the skin. If you use any other irritant on the skin at the same time you will exacerbate the initial negative side effects of the product. You must eliminate all of the following from your skin-care routine during your first months of using these products: all astringents, toners, fresheners, clarifying lotions, refining lotions, and the like that contain irritating ingredients. Also avoid scrubs, clay and peel-off facial masks, bar soaps, and skin-care products that contain fragrances. Finally, it is best to avoid saunas and steam rooms (used on a regular basis, saunas and steam rooms can surface tiny capillaries, causing a spider web of tiny red lines on the face).

- If you want products with tretinoin, AHAs, or BHA to work, you must use them regularly. To sustain the results, you must continue using them on a regular, patterned cycle for the rest of your life. The changes they allow to take place on the skin are not permanent. Once you stop using the product, the skin slowly reverts to its original condition. Using something forever is a tremendous commitment. But according to the majority of women I've interviewed and who have written to me, the difference is positive enough to warrant a long-term relationship.

## EXFOLIATING TREATMENTS

While we are on the subject of exfoliation, you should know there are deeper forms of exfoliating than products that contain a 5% to 8% concentration of AHAs or 1% to 2% concentration of BHA. The deeper options are treatments you can receive from a salon or spa or at a doctor's office. These include AHA or BHA peels, microdermabrasion, non-ablative laser resurfacing, and ablative laser resurfacing. All of these are valid options for dealing with wrinkles and some kinds of scarring. You may also be pleased to hear that in many ways the decision to go with one of these is less baffling than you think. That's because it isn't about which method is effective (they are all effective in their own way for removing surface layers of skin); rather, it is a question of money, tolerance, how comfortable you are about the risks (if any), and, finally, what results you hope to achieve. When considering any of these skin-resurfacing methods, the questions you need to answer are how much risk you can tolerate, what your budget is, how long you want the results to last, what the condition of your skin is, and what your skin color is. Once you understand how the answers to those questions affect your choice you can start shopping for what you want as opposed to being sold a service by a convincing doctor or aesthetician.

**Note:** I discuss each of the following procedures further in Chapter Thirteen, *Cosmetic Surgery*.

## SUPERFICIAL MICRODERMABRASION

Facialists typically perform this type of procedure but it is also available from some dermatologists and plastic surgeons. It is little more than a deep surface scrub done with a machine that shoots finely ground mineral crystals onto the skin and then vacuums them back up. This involves superficial abrasion of the skin's surface (removing the nonliving skin cells that occupy the top three to five layers of skin only). This surface layer has no capillaries and is nonpigmented, which is why its removal causes no bleeding, crusting, or skin discoloration. Left on its own, sun-damaged skin takes on a dull or thick appearance and fine lines seem more apparent because the surface skin cells slough off unevenly. Regular superficial microdermabrasion treatments with an appropriate system can temporarily improve the appearance of skin, but that's about it.

Microdermabrasion presents minimal to moderate risk, but that has little to do with your skin type or color and more to do with your reaction to the procedure and the skill of the technician. For some skin types, the irritation is too much; also, some aestheticians get carried away and go over and over an area, causing wounds and oozing. To obtain lasting or noticeable results, microdermabrasion needs to be constantly repeated because once (and even three or four times) is not enough.

The most typical result is a noticeable reduction in the appearance of some wrinkling and red skin discolorations (superficial scarring). However, this takes repeated sessions, and it is believed that the outcome is most likely a reaction to the skin being irritated and not from a change in the lower layers of skin. But that conclusion is open to debate, with most studies substantiating the concern (Source: *Dermatologic Surgery*, November 2001).

There is no downtime associated with superficial microdermabrasion, although the skin of some women does get red, dry, and flaky. The price varies widely, but generally the procedure can be pricey—and to get the smooth skin you are looking for, the repeated treatments can go on forever. The results also vary depending on the skill of the technician.

**Risk: Minimal.** Some women can experience redness, flaking, dryness, and irritation, but this usually diminishes within a few days. If you are prone to cold sores *(Herpes simplex)* around your mouth or on your face, this can trigger an outbreak.

**Cost: Moderate to Expensive.** A series of microdermabrasion treatments can range from $300 to $600 for three treatments. That's pricey, considering the short-term nature of the results, and over a few years the amount can add up.

**Results:** After two to three treatments a noticeably smoother surface, with wrinkles and redness from surface acne scars reduced but not eliminated. Has no effect on ice-pick or dented scars from acne or chicken pox.

**Duration:** Improved appearance can last for one to three months, but treatments must be repeated for improvements to stick around.

## DEEP MICRODERMABRASION

Deep microdermabrasion is (or should be) performed only by physicians and involves disruption of part of or the entire epidermis. The skin cells of the epidermis have capillaries and varying degrees of melanin; therefore, their disruption can cause bleeding, crusting, and skin discolorations, particularly in darker-skinned individuals. It was believed, when microdermabrasion technology was new, that this deeper disruption of the skin would cause dermal remodeling of collagen and should, therefore, reduce the appearance of acne scars, pits, and deeper wrinkles. Histologic confirmation of this has yet to be established and clinical correlation remains controversial (Source: *Cosmetic Dermatology*, March 2001).

Deeper microdermabrasion shares risks that are similar to AHA peels, which are reviewed in the following section. Last, it should be mentioned that both superficial and deep microdermabrasion may in fact be safer than some glycolic or salicylic acid chemical peels in darker-skinned individuals because acid peels may alter pigmented cells in the epidermis.

## AHA PEELS RANGING BETWEEN 20% AND 40% CONCENTRATIONS IN A pH OF 2 TO 3

AHA peels using concentrations of over 50% are done strictly by physicians. There are no BHA peels in any concentration available as a nonmedical treatment. AHA peels in concentrations of 40% or less are done by both physicians and facialists. There is a vast difference between results and risks at these varying concentrations (see the next section). At lower concentrations, AHA peels are similar in efficacy and results to microdermabrasion, with AHAs having a slight to moderate edge in creating a smoother appearance and less noticeable wrinkles and scars with only one to three applications. However, to obtain more significant, lasting results, takes subsequent treatments—up to three or six over the period of a year. Both microdermabrasion and low-concentration AHA peels require repeated treatments.

While microdermabrasion may not produce the same quality of noticeable results, there are far fewer risks associated with it. Even low-concentration AHAs can result in extreme redness, flaking, a burning sensation on the skin, and even some oozing and scabs.

Several cosmetics companies sell products claiming to be at-home peels. Thankfully, none of these are effective. These types of products may have a high AHA content, but none of them have a pH low enough to exfoliate skin. That's good news. The risk to skin of using a truly effective at-home peel include possible burns from leaving it on too long or not treating the skin appropriately afterward.

**Risk: Minimal to moderate.** Some women can experience extreme redness, flaking skin that can last for a week, irritation, and dryness, although this usually diminishes in a week or two. If you are prone to cold sores *(Herpes simplex)* around your mouth or on your face, this process can trigger an outbreak.

**Cost: Moderate to expensive.** A series of AHA treatments can range from $300 to $600 for three treatments, and the treatments need to be repeated to maintain the effect.

**Results:** After two to three treatments a noticeably smoother surface, with less-noticeable wrinkles and less obvious redness from surface acne scars. Has no effect on ice-pick or dented scars from acne or chicken pox.

**Duration:** Improved appearance can last from two to three months.

## AHA PEELS RANGING BETWEEN 50% AND 70% CONCENTRATIONS IN A pH OF 2 TO 3, OR BHA PEELS AT 8% TO 13% CONCENTRATIONS IN A pH OF 3

These high-concentration peels are performed strictly by physicians—and with good reason: The risk to skin is far higher, with many concerns about hypo- or hyperpigmentation, severe irritation, and risk of infection. As you may suspect, the higher risk goes hand-in-hand with more impressive, longer-lasting results. These kinds of medical peels can make a significant difference in the appearance of skin. They can fundamentally change the appearance of wrinkles and surface scarring; however, they still won't have an effect on ice-pick or dented scars from acne or chicken pox. Peels like this also have a far longer duration, with the effects lasting between two and three, and up to five years.

**Risk: Moderate.** Most women will experience severe redness, flaking, and oozing skin, and that can last for one to four weeks. The risk for these effects is reportedly somewhat less with a BHA peel because BHA's relation to aspirin may provide an anti-inflammatory effect along with the peeling action. There is also the possibility of a minimal risk of skin discoloration (either darkened areas of skin or lighter areas of skin). However, when this does occur it more often than not doesn't last, and fades with minimal treatment of prescribed skin lighteners. This risk of discoloration is more significant for those with darker skin tones. If you are prone to cold sores *(Herpes simplex)* around your mouth or on your face, this can trigger an outbreak.

**Cost: Expensive.** A high-concentration AHA or BHA peel can range from $1,000 to $2,500.

**Results:** After healing is completed the skin will have a markedly smoother appearance, with facial lines and surface scarring greatly reduced. High-concentration AHA and BHA peels have no effect on ice-pick or dented scars from acne or chicken pox.

**Duration:** Improved appearance can last from two to five years.

## NON-ABLATIVE LASER RESURFACING

In the world of making skin look younger there are many paths to take, and a number of non-ablative laser treatments ("non-ablative" meaning noninjurious or without damaging or burning skin tissue) are available options. Non-ablative lasers include the N-lite laser, Nd:YAG laser, Flashlamp laser, Pulsed Light laser, and Cool-Touch laser. All of these are options for minimizing the appearance of wrinkles and skin discolorations. But what are non-ablative laser treatments, and how do they compare to other forms of laser resurfacing?

Non-ablative (or coblative) laser resurfacing is very different from ablative laser resurfacing treatments, which became popular over the past several years and involved a machine that would "ablate" skin tissue with extreme heat generated by laser pulses. (The most well-known types of ablative lasers are the $CO_2$ Pulse Laser and the Er:YAG laser.) Ablative laser resurfacing procedures absolutely made a remarkable difference in the appearance of skin, particularly in terms of long-lasting improvement in the appearance of deep wrinkles, surface wrinkles, and skin discolorations. But as wonderful as that sounds, there are risks with ablative laser resurfacing, which include swelling, scabbing, oozing, bleeding, flaking, redness, and irritation that could last for an extended period of time. There is also a definite risk in terms of even longer-term skin discoloration and scarring.

The laser procedure being performed by plastic surgeons and dermatologists alike is termed non-ablative laser resurfacing or dermal remodeling because it does not injure skin tissue. That means little downtime and few to none of the risks associated with ablative laser resurfacing. However, non-ablative resurfacing doesn't produce the same dramatic results as ablative resurfacing can. According to an article by Dr. David Goldberg in *LaserNews* (July 2000) "Non-ablative dermal remodeling leads to improvement in photodamaged skin and rhytids (wrinkles) without any obvious wound.... However, at the present time, the clinical improvement seen with such techniques is less than that following the inelegant ablative laser resurfacing techniques."

**Risk: Minimal.** Some women can experience redness, flaking, dryness, and irritation, but this usually diminishes within a few days. If you are prone to cold sores *(Herpes simplex)* around your mouth or on your face, this can trigger an outbreak.

**Cost: Moderate to expensive.** $300 to $1,000 per treatment. Typically, two to five treatments are needed.

**Results:** After a series of treatments, noticeable improvement is visible on areas of skin discoloration, rough surface texture (sun damage), and reduction of post-inflammatory hyperpigmentation. The impact on wrinkles is not as impressive as with ablative laser treatments but an improved appearance is still possible.

**Duration:** Improved appearance can last from two to four years, but varies depending on how many treatments you have had.

Non-ablative laser resurfacing does require multiple treatments to maintain or achieve better results, but the smaller risk and minimal to no downtime to let the skin heal (relative to that of ablative techniques) is a huge benefit. This method is indeed a consideration, but it is not a panacea for getting rid of wrinkles and skin discolorations—it's just one of the many options to consider.

## ABLATIVE LASER RESURFACING

This is the prince of all peels. Other than a face-lift, this is the last of the effective surface treatments to help reduce the appearance of wrinkles. Because the process is so involved, including a discussion of the different laser options, I provide a more in-depth analysis in Chapter Thirteen, *Cosmetic Surgery*, examining the options for this complicated, though highly effective and long-lasting, resurfacing cosmetic-surgery procedure. Put simply, and aside from questions about the types of machines available, this procedure is both extremely effective and most risky. The results can be astounding, but when it's overdone or done with poor pre- and postoperative procedures, it can give the skin a plastic look. When done right, it can smooth out a good deal of wrinkling, uneven skin texture, skin discoloration, and acne scarring. It can't undo deep folds or heavily sagging skin, but it can retract some sagging. It cannot eliminate dented or ice-pick scars.

Preoperative care, including the use of skin lightener (to reduce the risk of skin discoloration), Renova or Retin-A to improve the skin's healing ability and the general health of the skin, and the use of effective sunscreens is important, and it can help achieve positive results. It is also essential that the patient stop smoking, if not permanently, for at least as long as possible before treatment (smoking not only causes wrinkles but it can also weaken the skin's immune system enough to put the patient in a higher risk category). Postoperative care varies, but silicone bandages are considered one of the best options, along with antibiotic creams and oral antibiotics. There should be minimal exposure to sun and irritating skin-care products of any kind.

**Risk: Moderate to Severe.** Most women will experience severe redness, flaking, and oozing skin that can last for two to five weeks. There is also a possible risk of skin discoloration (either darkened areas of skin or lighter areas of skin). This risk of discoloration is more significant for those with darker skin tones. If you are prone to cold sores *(Herpes simplex)* around your mouth or on your face, this can trigger an outbreak.

**Cost: Expensive.** Prices range from $2,500 to $5,000.

**Results:** After healing is completed the skin will have a markedly smoother appearance, with facial lines and surface scarring greatly reduced and some eliminated altogether. Deep, furrowed lines will not be affected much. Laser resurfacing can greatly improve and eliminate some acne scarring. It cannot eliminate sagging skin but some retraction will be visible.

**Duration:** Improved appearance can last from three to seven years.

# CHAPTER 5

## SUN SENSE

## UNDERSTANDING UV

Before you can understand how to protect skin from the sun it is helpful to know what exactly you need protection from. Sun feels great, especially when you're outdoors and it's shining. But even on a cloudy day, when you can't see the sun, the sun's rays are ever present and ever attacking the skin. Basically, the sun's infrared rays (IR) keep us warm and the visible rays provide daylight. But while the sun's ultraviolet radiation (UVR) is also important, its effects are serious for skin and eyes.

UVR is divided into three different bands: UVA, UVB, and UVC. Virtually all UVC radiation is filtered out by the atmosphere so that none actually reaches the earth's surface (although ozone depletion has some researchers worried about this one, too). In direct contrast to UVC, UVB and UVA rays both reach the earth in significant amounts.

UVB radiation, the rays of the sun that burn, is much stronger in some ways than UVA radiation, and it has a considerable capacity to cause instant skin damage in the form of blistering sunburns. However, the earth is bombarded with about 100 times as much UVA as UVB, so while it may be weaker, UVA radiation still has a potent impact on the skin.

All UVR is strongest between 10 A.M. and 2 P.M. Clouds filter some, but not most, of the UVR, which is why you are still likely to get burned on an overcast day. Different surfaces, such as water, cement, sand, snow, and even grass, can reflect UVR, causing a double whammy for the skin. Altitude is also a sun enhancer because for every 1,000-foot increase in altitude the UVR potency increases by 4%.

Pollution's effect on the ozone layer, located many miles above the earth's surface, is serious business for many reasons, but this discussion is about what that means for skin. When intact, the ozone layer filters out much of the sun's UVB radiation, but it has relatively little effect on UVA. It is the sunburning UVB rays that increase when the ozone layer is eroded, which means more serious burns for those who dare to go outside without protection.

By the way, UVB rays can't get through glass, so there's no risk of sunburn when you sit in a car or next to a window, but that's the good news. The bad news is that UVA rays *can* get through windows. Normal glass doesn't protect skin from UVA damage, so sitting in a car or next to a window that lets daylight through offers no UVA protection whatsoever. (Sunglasses are very important, but I discuss that later in this chapter.)

# TO TAN OR NOT TO TAN? NOT!

**FACT: There is no such thing as a safe tan. ALL tanning is a problem.** Actually, any and all unprotected sun exposure is damaging to skin. Most of us think sun damage occurs from baking in the sun and getting a deep, dark tan. That is only part of the picture. Sun damage begins the moment you walk out of the house, anytime during the day, whether it is sunny or cloudy (at least 40% to 50% of the sun's rays penetrate cloud cover). It may take 20 minutes for some of us to get burned, an hour or two for some of us to start tanning, but the damage associated with wrinkling and skin cancer begins the moment your skin is exposed to sunshine. It is the repeated sun exposure, just several minutes a day, 365 days a year, *even when sitting near a sunny window* (UVA radiation comes through windows), that adds up to a great deal of damage, both aesthetically and physically.

But back to tanning. Turning any shade that is darker than your own natural skin color, whether you have very light or very dark skin, is the skin's defensive response to sun damage. It may look nice, but it isn't nice for the skin. Melanocytes are skin cells that contain the brown-colored protein called melanin. These brown skin cells determine a person's natural skin tone. Surprisingly, the difference between the lightest skin color and the darkest is only a very small amount of melanin. With exposure to sun, the melanocytes produce more melanin, and tanned skin is the result. But here's another shock: Despite the fact that tanning is a protective response, it isn't all that helpful. By some estimates, a tan provides an SPF of only about 2. Sorry, there just isn't any way a tan of any kind can be considered healthy. As one dermatologist described it, a tan is the same as a callus on your foot. Yes, it protects the foot, but who wants that kind of protection and why continue doing what caused the callus in the first place?

Because melanin isn't a very reliable sunscreen, dark-skinned people still suffer negative effects from sun exposure. Ashen skin color, mottled skin, wrinkles, and even skin cancer can happen to those with dark skin. Skin cancer is less likely, but the risk of skin damage and wrinkling is certain.

The most damning result of sun exposure is that it does serious damage to the entire system, beyond the problems that eventually take place on the skin's surface.

The skin contains components that are central to the body's immune system. The Langerhans cells in the epidermis prevent bacteria from attacking the system and prevent cell mutation, making these cells indispensable to good health (Source: *Journal of Investigative Dermatology*, January 2002, pages 117–125). Yet a few minutes of unprotected sun exposure can damage the Langerhans cells in ways that can last for weeks.

In addition to damaging the immune system, the sun also directly attacks the collagen structure of the skin, changing it from a cohesive network of support into a disorderly, weakened mass. While the sun is busy destroying collagen underneath the surface of the skin and the Langerhans cells throughout, it also thickens the exterior of the skin, chokes off the skin's blood supply, and reduces the skin's elasticity (Sources: *Clinical Experimental Dermatology*, October 2001, pages 573–577; *Journal of the American Academy of Dermatology*, July 2001, pages 610–618). Sun tanning is not pretty.

## Dear Paula,

**With summertime just around the corner, I thought that I might share the knowledge I have learned over the years about self-tanning products. I have used self-tanning products since they were first introduced on the market. I am a 49-year-old female and enjoy being "tan." My best advice is to get just a little bit of a real tan. I live in the Houston/Galveston area and usually in late spring (late April, early May) I will lay out in the early part of the day (10 A.M. to 12:30 P.M.) and then apply the self-tanner. This helps achieve a real bronze colored tan. If you like being tanned it's worth your time and effort, because it sure beats the alternative, namely skin cancer.**

**Wanda, Houston, TX**

Dear Wanda,

I am sharing your letter because I am afraid that there are women who may share your belief that a little bit of tanning is safe, but that is absolutely not the case! The skin turning color is a danger sign of damage and abnormal cell production. It is not safe or healthy. Any amount of tanning puts the skin at high risk for cancer, not to mention wrinkles. I cannot advocate your routine and would suggest you reconsider what you are doing. Your belief that you are preventing problems for yourself by tanning in the morning and getting just a "little" color is dangerous thinking and you are putting your health and skin in jeopardy. One more point: In reality you are exposing your skin to sun at the worst time—right in the middle of the day (given that the sun is strongest between 11 A.M. and 2 P.M.) when UVA and UVB rays are at their most potent.

## SUN STRATEGY

If you take to heart only one section of this book, make it this one. What makes the following information so vital is not only the prevention of wrinkles, but also the prevention of many forms of skin damage. We're talking serious skin care.

Perhaps the most important fact about sun protection is that the Food and Drug Administration (FDA) stringently regulates sunscreens as over-the-counter drugs, not as cosmetics. While cosmetics don't have to prove their claims, or their efficacy for that matter, over-the-counter drugs have to prove both efficacy and safety and their formulations are tightly controlled. The FDA also allows only specific claims to be made for specific ingredients. That means if a product is labeled SPF 15, whether it's Chanel or Coppertone, it must utilize one or more of the limited number of approved sunscreen ingredients, in very specific concentrations, that are allowed to receive such a rating (Source: FDA *Cosmetics and Colors Fact Sheet,* June 27, 2000).

SPF stands for "sun protection factor." But the SPF number tells you only about how long a product will protect you from getting a sunburn, protecting your skin from the sun's UVB rays. Surprisingly, it doesn't provide any information about the sun's UVA rays. The sun's UVA rays have no apparent, immediate impact on skin, but they are thought to be the cause of wrinkles, hyperpigmentation, and skin cancer (Source: *Photodermatology, Photoimmunology & Photomedicine,* February 2001, pages 2–10). So, while SPF is important it does not tell you everything you need to know in order to purchase an effective sunscreen.

It turns out that the difference in UVA versus UVB protection is incredibly significant for the health of the skin. Until as recently as 1997, in the United States, the typical SPF 15 formulation provided protection only from UVB radiation, which unquestionably prevented sunburn and deep tanning. Anyone who applied a sunscreen correctly knew they wouldn't get burned and could stay in the sun with no painful side effects. Yet despite this remarkable protection, as well as the notably increased use of sunscreens, skin-cancer rates did not decline. If anything, they increased. So why weren't sunscreens doing their part to reduce the problem?

To the dismay of dermatologists, oncologists, and researchers, it eventually became clear that UVB radiation is not the culprit in many types of skin cancers. Rather, UVA radiation is the primary cause of skin cancer. **In addition, because sunscreens were so successful at preventing sunburn (protecting against UVB radiation), they allowed people to stay out in the sun for even longer periods of time, absorbing more cancer-causing UVA radiation.** It was found that while the typical SPF 15 sunscreen formulation protected against about 97% of UVB radiation, it kept out only a limited amount of UVA radiation. Keeping a large percentage of the UVB rays off the skin felt great, but evidently that wasn't enough for the long-term health of the skin. It is easy to see why cancer rates were going up, not down (Source: *Journal of Investigative Dermatology*, November 2001, pages 1186–1192).

So how do you know if your sunscreen is protecting your skin from the sun's UVA rays? There is only one way to tell. You must look at the *active* ingredient list on the sunscreen you own or are thinking of buying, and then look for one of the following ingredients: avobenzone, titanium dioxide, zinc oxide, and (outside of the United States) Mexoryl SX (Source: *Photodermatology, Photoimmunology & Photomedicine*, December 2000, pages 250–255). If one of these three ingredients isn't present it is a product you should throw out and absolutely should not purchase.

If you are looking for a sunscreen—and everyone must wear a sunscreen 365 days a year—you now need to pay attention to more than just the SPF. The SPF is still important, but it's only part of the story. What counts, and regardless of what sunscreen products you buy—whether tints, foundations, oil-free sunscreens, sprays, or lotions—they must be rated at least SPF 15 or greater and they must have the UVA-protecting ingredients avobenzone (Parsol 1789), titanium dioxide, zinc oxide, or Mexoryl SX on the active ingredient list. It is acceptable to have titanium dioxide and zinc oxide as the only sunscreen ingredients present, while Mexoryl SX and avobenzone can be used in conjunction with other sunscreen ingredients. (Avobenzone may also be listed as butyl methoxydibenzoylmethane.)

## WHAT ABOUT SPF?

A sunscreen's SPF rating is incredibly important, but it is no longer the only guide when buying sunscreens. All the SPF number lets you know is how long you can stay in the sun without burning while wearing that product. For example, let's say you're like me and you can stay in the sun for about 15 minutes before your skin starts to turn pink. Applying a sunscreen rated SPF 15 (both the new formulations with avobenzone, titanium dioxide, or zinc oxide or without) will allow you to stay in the sun 15 times longer (three and three-quarters hours: 15 times 15 minutes) without getting pink. In other words, the SPF number, 15 in this case, multiplied by the amount of time you can normally stay in the sun without getting pink, is how long you can stay in the sun after you've applied the sunscreen. If you normally can stay in the sun 25 minutes without getting pink, applying an SPF 15 sunscreen would let you stay in the sun six and one-quarter hours (15 times 25 equals 375 minutes) without burning.

However, as we now know, the SPF rating refers only to protection from UVB radiation. It gives you no information about protection from UVA radiation, which can cause skin cancer and wrinkles. If that SPF 15 or SPF 30 doesn't contain avobenzone, titanium dioxide, or zinc oxide you are receiving minimal protection from UVA radiation and it is a dangerous product to consider using.

## APPLYING SUNSCREEN

Now that so many products contain sunscreen (foundation, concealers, moisturizers, and even face powders), the next question is, What about application? That's a great question! The major issue for the use of any well-formulated sunscreen (SPF 15 or greater with UVA protecting ingredients) is liberal application. Protection is determined not only by the SPF number and the UVA ingredients the product contains but also by how thick and evenly it is applied, and when, where, and how often the sunscreen is re-applied. There is a mismatch between the expectation versus the reality of actual use (Source: *Journal of Photochemistry and Photobiology*, November 2001, pages 105–108).

Keep in mind that everyday liberal application, applied 20 minutes before you step outside (not once you get to the car, or get to the beach, or do anything—but before you leave the house) is the key element of getting the best protection possible. But within your skin-care routine, exactly when does sunscreen get applied? If you are applying several skin-care products, ranging from toners to acne medications to moisturizers, **the rule is that the last item you apply during the day is your sunscreen.** If you apply sunscreen and then apply, say, your moisturizer or an acne product, you could inadvertently be diluting or breaking down the effectiveness of the sunscreen you've just applied.

Any skin-care product, or even just water (and almost all moisturizers are more than 50% water), applied over a sunscreen reduces its effectiveness. This is why you have to reapply sunscreen after swimming or perspiring. If you use moisturizers, which are always lipid soluble, over your sunscreen you are breaking the sunscreen down via dilution or removal, and that is a serious problem. I have seen information in some fashion magazines suggesting that you should apply sunscreen first because putting it on over other skin-care products would block its absorption and that absorption is necessary for a sunscreen to be effective. This is dangerous information. If anything, research indicates that sunscreen can readily be absorbed through other cosmetic ingredients. An article in the *Journal of Investigative Dermatology* (2001, volume 117, pages 147–150) stated that "In contrast, when applied [in light amounts], thickening agents promote penetration, most likely through greater stratum corneum diffusivity arising from an enhanced hydration by the thicker formulations …" and suggests people "… recognize that thicker formulations may sometimes enhance the penetration of other topical agents when applied 'in use.' "

What about applying foundation (one that doesn't contain sunscreen) over the sunscreen you've just applied? If the foundation is a thin, watery-type foundation or you're using a tinted, lotion-type moisturizer (which doesn't contain sunscreen) you would in all likelihood reduce the potency of the sunscreen underneath. However, if you are applying a standard liquid foundation, a cream-to-powder or stick foundation, a cream foundation, or a pressed-powder foundation, and as long as you are smoothing it over the skin and not wiping it off or rubbing it too heavily into the skin, there is minimal risk that you are affecting the sunscreen underneath. However, if there is even a small risk that you are diluting the effectiveness of your sunscreen with foundation, you should consider wearing a foundation that contains sunscreen, too.

If you are using more than one product containing sunscreen, such as an SPF 15 moisturizer and an SPF 8 foundation, it is important to understand that does not add up to an SPF of 23. You would get some increased SPF value for protection, but there is no way to know what amount of increased protection that would be. If you want to get the protection of SPF 30, then that is the SPF number you should look for. If you are mixing SPF products, both must contain the UVA-protecting ingredients of avobenzone, titanium dioxide, zinc oxide, or Mexoryl SX.

What if your foundation is the product you've chosen for sun protection? **Then the trick is to be sure you've applied it evenly and liberally.** If you apply it too thinly or blend most of it off instead of using it full-depth, you would not get the amount of protection listed on the label.

I am concerned about the new pressed powders with SPF ratings. While I don't doubt the validity of the SPF number, I worry that most women do not apply pressed-powder foundations liberally enough to get the amount of protection indicated on the label. **If you lightly dust the powder over the skin there is no way you will get the SPF protection indicated on the label.** You must be sure you apply the pressed powder in a manner that completely and evenly covers the face. I believe that pressed powders are an iffy way to get sun protection for the face, but they *are* a great way to touch up your makeup during the day and reapply sunscreen at the same time. Several cosmetics companies have their versions; I list the ones with the best sunscreen ingredients and color selection in my book *Don't Go to the Cosmetics Counter Without Me.*

## SUN-BELIEVABLE—AN OVERVIEW

While the world of skin care is definitely providing better and better sunscreen products, and although most of my readers already know the basics and even a lot of the more detailed sunscreen information, it never hurts to go over the salient points one more time. It will also help you handle the new myths that companies generate as they try to defend their products as being the best when they aren't.

- **There is no such thing as a safe tan**, at least not from the sun or tanning beds. Even if you tan slowly without burning, the damage to skin is still hazardous to the health of your skin.

- **UVB** rays are the sun's burning rays, which have an immediate harmful impact on skin.

- **UVA** rays are the sun's silent killers. You don't feel them, but they are the primary cause of skin cancer and wrinkles! (UVA rays also penetrate through clear glass windows.)

- Skin damage from the sun begins within the first minutes your skin is exposed to sunlight.

- Even on a cloudy day the sun's rays are ever-present and ever attacking the skin.

- Sitting in the shade or wearing a hat protects only from a small portion of the sun's rays. Plus, other surrounding surfaces such as water, cement, and grass reflect the rays from the ground to your skin, giving you a double whammy of damage.

- Altitude is a sun enhancer; for every 1,000-foot increase in altitude, the sun's potency increases by 4%.

- According to the FDA, a product's SPF (sun protection factor) number tells you how long you can stay in the sun while wearing it without getting burned. Here's how it works: If it normally takes you 20 minutes in the sun before you start turning pink, an SPF 15 product will let you stay in the sun for five hours without burning. The formula is 20 (minutes) x (SPF number) 15 = 300 (minutes), or five hours. But that five hours applies only if you aren't swimming or perspiring. If you are active or if you get wet, you need to reapply the sunscreen after 60 to 90 minutes.

- SPF numbers are crucial, but they are a measurement that only pertains to sunburn (UVB rays). **There are no numbers to tell you about protection from UVA radiation.** For that protection you have to check the active ingredient list. Make sure that either **avobenzone, titanium dioxide,** or **zinc oxide** (which may also be listed as Parsol 1789 or butyl methoxydibenzoylmethane) or, outside of the United States, **Mexoryl SX** is one of the active ingredients. If one of these doesn't appear in the **active ingredient** list (it doesn't count if it is just part of the regular ingredients) you will not get adequate UVA protection.

- Several sunscreen ingredients are approved for use in the United States for sunburn protection, and they have a wide variety of technical names. Two of these are benzophone and oxybenzone, and while they sound like avobenzone and they do offer some UVA protection, they are not as effective in protecting from the entire range of UVA radiation as are avobenzone, titanium dioxide, zinc oxide, or Mexoryl SX (Source: *Photodermatology, Photoimmunology & Photomedicine*, December 2000, pages 250–255).

- For more technical specifics about the issue of UVA versus UVB protection, refer to the *Skin Therapy Letter* published by the Division of Dermatology at the University of British Columbia (1997, volume 2, number 5, "Update on Sunscreens"). This informative article states that the "UVA [range is] 315 [through] 400 nanometers" [according to the FDA the UVB range is from 280 to 315]. The range of protection for the following sunscreen ingredients is listed as "Padimate O, 290-315 nanometers; Benzophenones, 250-350 nanometers; Octyl methoxycinnamate, 290-320 nanometers; Avobenzone, 320-400 nanometers; Titanium dioxide, 290-700 nanometers; and Zinc oxide, 290-700 nanometers." Skin receives the best protection when a sunscreen uses ingredients that screen the entire range of UVA and UVB.

- **Waterproof sunscreens are actually not waterproof**, and the FDA is ordering manufacturers to eliminate such a claim from sunscreen labels. Sunscreens can be water resistant, but they are never waterproof. Water-resistant sunscreens must be reapplied every 90 minutes if you are sweating or swimming.

- A product with an SPF 2 blocks only about 50% of the UVB rays; an SPF 10 filters out about 85% of the UVB rays; an SPF 15 stops about 95%, and an SPF 30 through SPF 50 stops about 97%. So even if the SPF number on the label of your sunscreens is an ultra-high SPF 50, it still has limitations. (Note that new FDA regulations state that no sunscreens will be allowed to have ratings over an SPF 30+.) These percentages explain why you still might get some color after prolonged exposure to the sun despite slathering sunscreen on your skin.

Another reason you may get color despite using generous amounts of a good sunscreen is because of the following. Along with the change that eliminates SPF ratings over 30, the FDA is going to crack down on all "unsupported, absolute, and/or misleading and confusing terms such as 'sunblock,' 'all-day protection,' and 'visible and/

or infrared light protection.' " Why the concern about "sunblock" as a term? Because all sunscreen agents, even zinc oxide and titanium dioxide (which are often thought of as "blocking" UV rays), work the same way. All sunscreen agents work because they disperse and break up UV radiation, not because they "block" the sun's rays.

- **Always apply sunscreen at least 15 to 20 minutes before going outside.** This gives the sunscreen time to be absorbed and to spread over and into the skin.

- **You must apply sunscreen liberally.** According to a press release from the American Academy of Dermatology (May 21, 1999), "sunscreen users are only applying 50 percent of the recommended amount, so they are only receiving 50 percent of the SPF protection." Is anyone out there really applying the right amount? This is an important issue because liberal application is essential, and skimping on it just because your sunscreen is expensive can be dangerous to your skin's health. After all, how likely are you to liberally apply an expensive sunscreen that would be gone in a few days if you were using it correctly? Not applying sunscreen liberally can negate any benefit you may assume you are getting from the SPF number on the label.

- If you are using AHAs, BHA, Retin-A, Renova, Differin, or any other topical, pharmaceutical tretinoin (Tazorac, Avita, generic tretinoin), they can make your skin more vulnerable to sun damage. This information isn't news for those of you who are already diligent about using sunscreen, but if you are not being diligent then remember that these ingredients expose healthy layers of skin and make it even more at risk for sun damage and sunburn with even minimal sun exposure.

- Getting sunburned is bad enough, but what you may not know is that **sunburn continues to develop for 12 to 24 hours after the initial burn takes place!** For detailed information on how to handle a sunburn, please see the "Sunburn" section in this chapter.

- If you have **babies or small children**, the sunscreen protection issue should absolutely be of primary concern. Their delicate skin is even more sensitive to the sun's damaging rays. Here, you need to know that all sunscreen formulations that have an SPF are regulated closely by the FDA; and the formulations don't differ in any way because of the age of the intended user. Although kids' products often come in very cute packaging, the formulation you choose should be of greater concern and must contain one of the UVA-protecting ingredients mentioned above, either avobenzone, titanium dioxide, or zinc oxide.

- If you are looking for a less-irritating sunscreen for your kids or yourself, choose one that contains only pure titanium dioxide or zinc oxide as the active ingredient; these are definitely less irritating than products made with other types of sunscreen agents.

- If you're determined to tan, the only safe way to do it is with the self-tanning products sold by countless cosmetics lines.

## Is Sunscreen in Foundation Reliable?

An article published in the *Journal of the American Academy of Dermatology* (October 2001, entitled "Degradation and Migration of Facial Foundations") concluded that foundations with sunscreen are not reliable for sun protection. Dr. Zoe Diana Draeolos, the author, is a dermatologist who really and truly does test products, and her work is impressive and considered dependable. However, I wouldn't conclude from her study that foundations with sunscreen are completely unreliable and therefore unusable for sun protection.

The summary of this study was that you would need to reapply a foundation with sunscreen at least every two hours (or apply a sunscreen over it) for continued protection. However, looked at more closely, this conclusion was not based on any sunscreen testing as such. Rather the results were based on examining 12 participants who applied the following foundations: Clinique Pore Minimizer (no longer made), Neutrogena Healthy Skin SPF 20, Revlon ColorStay SPF 6, L'Oreal Visuelle (no longer made), Cover Girl Ultimate Finish, and Estee Lauder Impeccable SPF 20. Over an eight-hour period "the migration of the iron oxide pigment [the coloring agent] over the skin surface was monitored in 12 white female subjects with dry (4 subjects), normal (4 subjects), and oily (4 subjects) skin." Following application, each participant was photographed with a specialized video that magnified the skin. The pictures revealed that after two hours the foundation began to travel into facial lines and eventually, by the end of the day, it also had moved into the hair follicles. About the movement, the study commented that "This was particularly true for those participants who had oily skin and for those who used the cream-to-powder foundations." Cream-to-powder foundations are often the greasiest types of formulations (especially in the case of Lauder's Impeccable).

I agree that this study poses concerns that require further investigation, but please realize that the study did *not* test whether or not sun protection was still present, it just noted that the pigment colors of the foundation migrated into lines and hair follicles. There was no UV skin testing done at any point, which would be the only way to know how much sun protection (if any) was still present. In other words, did the sunscreen protection degrade because of the migration with the foundation's color? Yet sunscreen testing would have been pointless for this study because three of the foundations didn't even have sun protection (and one only had an SPF 6). More precisely, the conclusions were based on the *assumption* that the sunscreen efficacy dissipated in relation to the pigment movement of a foundation. That means the conclusions about what happens to sunscreen protection when foundations with sunscreen are used were not based on actual testing or proof. Instead, an educated guess was offered, based on the opinion that if the iron oxide pigments in the foundation migrate, the migration must take the active sunscreen agents away with it. A guess is not scientific nor a final determination of any kind.

Another issue here was the unrealistic expectation that you're going to reapply your foundation with SPF (or apply a sunscreen over your previously applied foundation) every two hours! That is impractical in every respect because for most women it would mean redoing almost every other part of your makeup, from concealer to blush, eyeshadow, and eyebrows as well. Instead, it would be far more helpful to touch up your foundation during the day with a pressed powder that has an SPF 15 or higher and that also has UVA protection.

On an anecdotal, personal note, as someone who is diligent about wearing foundation with sunscreen and a moisturizer with sunscreen on my body (both containing titanium dioxide), I found that after two months in Florida last year the only part of my body to *not* get a drop of color was my face. There was a decidedly noticeable change of color on my arms and hands.

More important, application and wear are issues for *all* sunscreens. Another study went so far as to suggest that reapplying your sunscreen "liberally to exposed sites 15 to 30 minutes before going out into the sun, followed by reapplication of sunscreen to exposed sites 15 to 30 minutes after sun exposure begins" is the optimal way to ensure the best protection (Source: *Journal of the American Academy of Dermatology*, December 2001, pages 882–885). Liberal application as well as even, smooth application is critical. From there, you should monitor how your sunscreen wears so you know you're not sweating it off, rubbing it off, washing it off (particularly for the hands), or degrading it by virtue of your own oil production. I know this is a lot to pay attention to, but it is our first line of defense against photodamage, which is truly what causes the skin to wrinkle.

## WATER RESISTANT NOT WATERPROOF

The FDA's 2002 regulations regarding sunscreen require companies to eliminate the use of the word "waterproof" as a valid claim. In truth, no sunscreen can be waterproof because it must be reapplied if you have been sweating or immersed in water for a period of time. The only approved terms for use on sunscreens, reflecting studies that prove they have limited ability to stay in place when people are in water or sweating, are "water-resistant" or "very water-resistant." A product that is water-resistant means the label's SPF value has been measured after application and 40 minutes of water immersion; it must keep the same SPF value to use the term water-resistant. A very water-resistant product means the SPF value on the label must remain intact after 80 minutes of water immersion.

If you are swimming or sweating, you absolutely should use a sunscreen that's labeled water resistant or very water-resistant. Water-resistant sunscreens are formulated quite differently from regular sunscreens. Water-resistant sunscreens use acrylate technology in their formulations, which helps them hold up remarkably well under water. Acrylate-type ingredients are, like hairspray, holding agents. These plasticizing ingredients form a film over the skin and can take a great deal of wear and tear in contact with water before the sunscreen protection is rinsed away.

For normal wear, I do not recommend daily application of water-resistant sunscreens. The acrylate-type ingredients that help keep sunscreens on when swimming or sweating also make them somewhat tacky or sticky under makeup. For regular application, when you aren't exercising outside or taking a dip, a regular sunscreen with SPF and good UVA protection is the best choice.

## TITANIUM DIOXIDE AND ZINC OXIDE

Titanium dioxide and zinc oxide are often referred to as "nonchemical" sunscreen ingredients, but this is misleading at best. In every aspect and by every definition titanium dioxide and zinc oxide are chemicals. What these two substances do have in common is that they are inert minerals used as sunscreen ingredients. They also have minimal to no risk of causing an allergic reaction and are considered benign and safe for skin. Along with their safety they have a superior ability to protect skin from the sun's UVA radiation (Sources: *British Journal of Dermatology*, November 2001, pages 789–794; *Lasers in Surgery and Medicine*, September 2001, pages 252–259). One drawback that these two ingredients also share is that, when they are present in large enough concentrations to impart optimal UVA protection, they tend to leave a white cast on the skin. Ingredient manufacturers are working to make better, microfine versions of titanium dioxide and zinc oxide to help reduce or eliminate this problem. In the meantime it is a shortcoming of two otherwise outstanding options for sun protection.

Some media attention has been given to research that indicates microfine zinc oxide is a superior sunscreen ingredient when compared to microfine titanium dioxide (Source: *Dermatologic Surgery*, April 2000, pages 309–314). This study concluded "microfine zinc oxide is superior to microfine titanium dioxide as a sunscreen ingredient." However, this study was about a commercially available form of zinc oxide and no other study has supported the results. Nonetheless, if you feel that zinc oxide is a preferred sunscreen ingredient it only takes a quick review of the active ingredient label to see if the product you are using contains it.

One misconception that often comes up about titanium dioxide and zinc oxide is the notion that they are "sunblocks" and, therefore, better than traditional sunscreens. However, titanium dioxide and zinc oxide function fine as sunscreens. In fact, the FDA is disallowing the term "sunblock" on all products that have an SPF. The *Federal Register* (May 21, 1999, volume 64, number 98) Final Sunscreen Monograph states: "While micronized titanium dioxide does not meet the proposed definition of a sunscreen opaque sunblock, the agency has not included the use of this term in the final monograph (see section II.L, comment 52 of this document).... In addition, the proposed definition of 'sunscreen opaque sunblock' in Sec. 352.3(d) applied only to titanium dioxide and is inconsistent with how micronized titanium dioxide functions as [a] sunscreen active ingredient (Ref. 44)"; and "... micronized titanium dioxide absorbs short wavelength UV radiation and reflects and scatters long wavelengths, thereby functioning similarly to chemical UVB radiation sunscreens." This is a very technical way of saying that titanium dioxide and zinc oxide need to be applied in the same manner as any sunscreen: liberally, and 20 minutes before going outside.

## AVOBENZONE UNDER FIRE

A story that appeared in the May/June 1998 issue of *Health* magazine raised concerns about the stability of avobenzone in sunscreen formulations. According to the article, recent research conducted by Robert Sayre, a physicist in photobiology at the University of Memphis, suggests that avobenzone may break down in as little as 30 minutes when exposed to sunlight.

That published study has created quite a stir in the cosmetics industry and among dermatologists, oncologists, and scientists in the biomedical arena. *Stir* is actually an understatement; shock and confusion may be more accurate. If Sayre is right, a lot of sunscreen products should be thrown in the garbage. But so far the primary response is confusion because no one understands how Sayre came up with his findings, given how incredibly well researched and scrutinized avobenzone is as a sunscreen ingredient. There are no other studies substantiating Sayre's results anyplace in the cosmetics or medical world.

Avobenzone is not some untested or untried sunscreen agent. It has been around since 1981 and is the most-used sunscreen ingredient in the world. It is the number-one sunscreen agent used in Canadian, Australian, and European sunscreen formulations. In the United States, the FDA approved avobenzone's use as a sunscreen agent only after more than seven years of study. Avobenzone had to meet scrupulous performance standards when Hoffman LaRoche applied for it to receive new drug status from the FDA. New drug status is the most stringent FDA classification possible and requires more safety studies and efficacy substantiation than you can imagine. Avobenzone held up under all of the FDA's safety and potency protocols, or it wouldn't have been approved.

Even more significant, the June 1996 issue of *Journal of Chromatography BioMedical Applications* (pages 137–145) contained a study that examined the issue of sunscreens degrading when exposed to sunlight. The conclusion for avobenzone was as follows: "After 72 hours Parsol 1789 [avobenzone] in the sample exposed to the sun was decreased by up to 25% of the initial concentration." That 25% decrease was after 72 hours (far longer than anyone is supposed to rely on a sunscreen) and is a far cry from the 50% decrease reported by Sayre after only 30 minutes.

In particular, one must ask the author of a study like this whether his research has been peer reviewed, published in a scientific publication, and whether the results have been validated. To the best of our knowledge, none of the above has taken place. (There have also been no other studies supporting Sayre's work.) In vitro (meaning in a petri dish) photostability measurements cannot be substituted for in vivo (meaning on a live person) determinations of UVB and UVA photoprotective efficacy.

For many reasons I find Sayre's research and conclusions incredibly suspect. Sayre looked at the issue of stability in vitro only, he did no studies in vivo. Plus, he did not use the required application amount and smaller amounts mean less protection, something the American Academy of Dermatology and I have been warning about for some time. Avobenzone is extremely reliable and a safe source for UVA sun protection.

# SUNBURN

Most of us know about sunburn. Spending even a short time in the sun can be all it takes to get a serious, painful burn. As I stated earlier, sunburn continues to develop for 12 to 24 hours after the initial burn takes place. It goes without saying that it would be best if we all knew enough to take care of our skin and never get a sunburn, or tan for that matter, but that isn't realistic. So knowing how to take care of sunburn is essential, both to keep from making the problem worse and to help skin heal.

Essentially, treating sunburn is the same as treating any other burn. Do not cover it with thick salves (butter is the worst). That will trap the heat and cause more damage. Get the skin in contact with cool compresses immediately (do not put ice directly on the skin—that's too cold and can cause a different kind of burn on the skin). Then keep applying cool compresses on and off for several hours. Do not soak the skin with water; too much water in the skin can inhibit the skin's healing response (Source: *Contact Dermatitis*, December 1999, pages 311–314).

## SUN RISK FROM USING AHAS, BHA, OR TRETINOIN?

As I've already described in the previous chapter one of the major signs of sun-damaged skin is that the outer layer of skin becomes browned, thickened, and wrinkled. To some extent that does serve as protection, but it isn't very good protection (it barely rates an SPF 2), nor is it very attractive! AHAs and BHA (because they exfoliate the built-up damaged surface layer of skin) and tretinoin or products containing it (because they change abnormal cell production back to some level of normalcy) can help remove some of that thickened exterior. That change to the exterior of the skin does leave it more vulnerable to the effects of sun exposure. Yet it is far better to improve the appearance of damaged skin by removing that layer than it is to leave it in place for inadequate, coarse, and defective sun protection. After all, it isn't the AHAs or the tretinoin that cause the skin to be more sensitive to sunlight. All they do is remove the old, sun-damaged skin. Sunscreen is always important, *always*, but it becomes even more essential to protect the fresh skin cells you get if you are using AHAs or tretinoin on a regular basis.

## CAN SUNSCREEN CAUSE CANCER?

Media headlines sometimes have a way of creating news sensations where none exist, or making something sound new and eye-popping when the information is really well established and even dated. You may have seen stories in the media regarding a study claiming that sunscreens do not help protect a person from skin cancer. According to an epidemiological review of ten previously published studies, presented at an American Association for the Advancement of Science meeting in Philadelphia, February 1998, by Dr. Marianne Berwick, an epidemiologist at Memorial Sloan-Kettering Cancer Center in New York, "based on the evidence, we conclude that sunburn itself probably does not cause melanoma, but that it is an important sign of excessive sun exposure, particularly among those who are genetically susceptible because of their skin type." Well, of course!

Dermatologists have debated for some time whether or not sun exposure is related to skin melanomas, so there is conflicting information for this deadly form of skin cancer. However, basal cell and squamous cell carcinoma is directly linked to sun exposure. Further, the fact that sunburn has *not* been implicated in the occurrence of some skin cancers has long been concluded in Europe and Australia, and recently here in the United States (due to the research about the effect of UVAs on skin). But that's about UVA protection versus UVB protection. The importance of protecting skin from UVA rays (skin-cancer and wrinkle-causing rays) as well as UVB rays (sunburning rays) has now been demonstrated. I'm not sure how Berwick missed this one, but she did. Her study did look at sunscreen use over the past ten years. However, she should have checked into the formulations that were used during that period. It is only recently that cosmetics chemists have started formulating sunscreens with ingredients that can protect equally from both UVB and UVA damage. People who used traditional sunscreens over that ten-year period were putting their skin at risk because they were getting sunburn protection only, while still being exposed to harmful UVA rays. At the time, UVB sunburn-preventing products were so effective that people stayed out longer than they might ever have before, thus exposing their skin to the sun's more damaging UVA rays for longer periods of time.

Others have raised questions about how Berwick's study was conducted and the conclusions her team reached. Dr. Roger Ceilley, former president of the American Academy of Dermatology, refuted the suggestion that long-term sunscreen users derived no benefit from sunscreen. "The study looked at patients who were using sunscreens before 1980, well before broad-spectrum, Sun Protection Factor (SPF) 15 became widely available in 1984. There is a period of at least 10 to 20 years from sun exposure to the clinical appearance of skin cancer. Sunscreens would have had little impact on the patients studied. Many well-documented studies from notable organizations such as the U.S. Department of Health and Human Services (Food and Drug Administration), the American Academy of Pediatrics, the American Cancer Society, and the American Society of Plastic and Reconstructive Surgeons join the American Academy of Dermatology in saying that the use of sunscreen products is an important tool in the prevention of skin cancer" (Source: *American Society for Photobiology Online Newsletter*, Summer 1998, volume 27, issue 2).

Studies also abound regarding the appearance of thickened, yellowed, mottled, sun-damaged skin versus the smooth, even, wrinkle-free appearance of someone who has stayed out of the sun; the contrast is a classic in dermatological annals. Staying completely out of the sun isn't possible (nor would it be healthy). However, good sun protection is, at the very least essential for reducing or stopping the damage that causes most of the wrinkles we see on our skin, basal cell carcinoma, squamous cell carcinoma, and very likely melanoma (Source: *American Journal of Clinical Dermatology*, 2001, volume 2, issue 3, pages 131–134).

# CAN SUNSCREEN AFFECT SKIN NEGATIVELY?

A paper presented at the March 2001 meeting of the American Physical Society by Johannes Norrell et al., Department of Physics at the University of Alabama at Birmingham, created quite a stir regarding the safety of sunscreen ingredients. Because his paper is titled "The Sunscreen Octyl Methoxycinnamate Binds to DNA," it is easy to see why someone might be concerned. The abstract from this presentation stated the following: "Sunscreens are designed to prevent skin cancer by absorbing ultraviolet radiation from the sun before it gets to the DNA in skin cells. The purpose of this work is to determine whether or not octyl methoxycinnamate, an active ingredient in many sunscreens, will bind to DNA. If so, the sunscreen could transfer the energy it absorbed from the sun to the DNA and cause damage. To determine this, we prepared samples with varying concentrations of cinnamate added to herring sperm DNA, sonicating the mixture to disperse the hydrophobic sunscreen into solution. We conclude that the octyl methoxycinnamate can indeed bind to DNA in aqueous solution."

Before you go checking your bottles of sunscreen for this very popular sunscreen ingredient, let me add a bit of fuel to the fire and inform you that many sunscreen ingredients, from oxybenzone to titanium dioxide, zinc oxide, padimate-O, homosalate, benzophenone-3, phenylbenzimidazole sulphonic acid, and 2-phenylbenzimidazole, just to name a few, all have some intimidating negative research about their potential effects on skin. These aren't junk science articles either—they are all from very notable publications, including such well-respected journals as *The Lancet, Journal of Investigative Dermatology,* and *Mutation Research.* Rather than elaborate on each specific paper (which would take pages and pages), let me sum up the major issues.

Despite the limited amount of research being conducted on the harmful effects of sunscreen ingredients, the majority of the research on these ingredients has been done in vitro (in test tubes) and not in vivo (on human skin). In other words, how does octyl methoxycinnamate's effect on herring sperm relate to its effect when used on human skin? None of the papers described research conducted on humans and, therefore, the results are not conclusive in the least. Plus, there is much debate between researchers themselves about what any of this research means. For example, an article in *The Lancet* (February 14, 1998) stated that the concerns in regard to using oxybenzone "for large surface area application for extended and repeated periods ... are not warranted." Further, an article in *Science News* (June 6, 1998), which compared the handful of research papers on this issue, concluded that hundreds "of experiments have shown that sunscreen-protected skin seems to suffer less DNA damage than unscreened skin."

Going beyond possible DNA damage, the whole arena of sun protection becomes even murkier, given the way sunscreens interact with the very light they are meant to direct away from skin cells. Several published studies show oxidative damage in vitro from varying sunscreen ingredients. *Science News* (in the same article) mentioned that " 'The sunscreen [ingredient] actually forms oxygen radicals that we would like to protect the skin against, but sunscreen also reacts with and traps them,' mitigating harmful effects…. Some scientists argue that it is by trapping radicals that sunscreen blends offer their protection…"

Some in vitro studies have indicated that there is a possibility that certain sunscreen ingredients can be absorbed into skin. However, there are still many researchers who believe that most sunscreen ingredients stay on the surface of skin (where skin cells are dead) and do not penetrate into lower layers of skin, where the real damage occurs. If that's the case, it means the negative effects seen for surface skin in test tubes may be irrelevant.

Another concern about sunscreen is whether the ingredients may possibly exert estrogenic effects. This was examined in a study published in *Environmental Health Perspective* (March 2001). The research was done on rats that were *fed* sunscreen ingredients, not on topical application to rat skin or anyone else's skin. Eating pure sunscreen ingredients is not the same thing as applying them to the skin, anymore than applying chocolate to the skin is the same as eating it! There is concern that sunscreen ingredients found in lakes, particularly 4-methyl-benzylidene camphor (4-MBC), may be associated with estrogenic effects on fish, but again this is about consumption, not application, and unless you are living in lake water, the issue appears to be unrelated to humans.

All these issues are significant and deserve more research, but none of the findings indicate that anyone should give up using sunscreen. Besides, it is important to realize that no one sunscreen ingredient stands out as more of a problem than any other in these studies. Also, none of the research demonstrates that there are actual, in vivo human risks related to the topical application of the sunscreen ingredients currently being used in products. Finally, it is imperative to note what a massive amount of research does show: That *not* wearing sunscreen is related to lots of serious skin problems.

# WHY YOU MAY STILL GET TAN WHEN USING SUNSCREEN

There are many reasons why you may still be getting some tan despite diligent use of sunscreen. One likely cause is the fact that even the best of sunscreens still let some sun rays through. A high SPF number is not about better or deeper protection, but just longer protection—an SPF 30 means you can stay in the sun 30 times longer than it would normally take you to get a slight burn. For most skin types that would provide over eighteen hours of sun exposure without getting sunburned. It's impressive, but it is also only about the length of time the protection lasts.

High SPF numbers give the false impression of providing enhanced protection when that is not the case (that's why the FDA no longer allows products to be labeled as having SPFs over 30). A well-formulated sunscreen with an SPF 30 still only protects your skin from about 97% to 98% of the sun's rays. That means 2% to 3% of the sun's rays are still getting through, and that can trigger melanin production (the skin's tanning response). This is especially true for those with darker skin tones or for those who have a lot of previous sun damage, because for them hypermelanin production is more likely to take place.

Further, most people misunderstand or have poor information about how to get the best sun protection. Please review the "Applying Sunscreen" and "Sun Strategy" sections in this chapter. It is essential to apply sunscreen liberally and to be sure that the active ingredients include the UVA-protecting ingredients of avobenzone, titanium dioxide, zinc oxide.

Keep in mind that you must:

- Apply sunscreen every day of your life, not just when you think you will be spending extended time in the sun.

- Apply sunscreen liberally.

- Apply sunscreen 20 minutes before going outside.

- Reapply water-resistant or very water-resistant sunscreen every 40 to 80 minutes if you are spending extensive time in the sun and are swimming, exercising, or perspiring heavily.

- Reapply sunscreen on your hands every time after you wash them.

- It always helps to wear a broad-brimmed hat, sunglasses, and long sleeves when you're outside or at the beach, and to avoid direct sun exposure as much as possible.

- Try to avoid spending more than a few minutes out in the sun when it's most intense (between 11 A.M. and 2 P.M.).

- Seek shade whenever possible for "sun breaks" on long days outdoors.

# SPF-RATED CLOTHING

After you've dressed in the morning and because you take great care of your skin, you apply a well-formulated sunscreen to the areas of your body that will be exposed to the sun. You are confident that the parts of your body covered by clothing are protected from the sun and therefore don't need sunscreen. Think again. Just because some of your body is under wraps doesn't mean it is protected from sun damage. While clothing can be an excellent form of sun protection, if the fabric is sheer, lightweight, or has any transparency (meaning it lets daylight through) it also lets the sun's damaging rays through. "The most important determinant is tightness of the weave. Fabric type is less important. Thickness is also less important than regular weave. Protection drops significantly when the fabric becomes wet. Color plays a minor role with dark colors protecting [slightly] better than light colors. A crude test of clothing is to hold it up to visible light and observing penetration. The FDA defines clothing with an SPF rating as a medical device. One approved line of clothing with a SPF 30 or greater rating is Solumbra" (1-800-882-7860) (Source: *eMedicine Journal*, July 31 2001, volume 2, number 7, and http://www.fda.gov).

Sun damage is not to be taken lightly, and lightweight clothing can be a problem. When in doubt, apply sunscreen all over and then get dressed.

# HOW LONG DO SUNSCREENS LAST?

How long does sunscreen last in the container? Should you throw it away after a year or two if you haven't used it up? Sunscreens don't last forever, on your skin or in the bottle. The FDA considers sunscreens over-the-counter (OTC) drugs, meaning they are subject to much more stringent guidelines and regulations than cosmetics. According to the FDA's OTC regulations, sunscreens should be stamped with an expiration date if they have less than three years of acceptable stability testing. If they do have three years' worth of acceptable stability testing they do not need to be stamped with an expiration date. That confusing bit of legislation is almost impossible for the consumer to understand. In the long run you are best off looking for a sunscreen product that is stamped with an expiration date so you know how long it has been on the shelf, but those without expiration dates are not a problem in terms of meeting FDA guidelines.

# SHOPPING FOR SUNSCREENS

To recap, it is no longer good enough (or safe enough) to buy a sunscreen based only on its SPF rating. It is now essential to buy sunscreens that are not only at least

SPF 15 but also contain avobenzone, titanium dioxide, zinc oxide or as one of the active ingredients. When those ingredients are present, either alone or with other sunscreen agents, you are guaranteed of getting equal protection from UVA and UVB radiation. UVB radiation causes sunburn, but UVA radiation is far more insidious and causes skin cancer and skin damage.

Please understand that labeling on sunscreens can be misleading. If the label says "protects from UVA and UVB radiation" but you don't see avobenzone, titanium dioxide, or zinc oxide listed in the active ingredients, the sunscreen will not provide adequate protection from skin cancer and wrinkle-causing rays, despite the claim. The reason products can say this even when they don't contain the pertinent ingredients I've mentioned is because of a technicality. Sunscreen formulations without UVA-protecting ingredients do block a small portion of the sun's UVA rays, it's just insufficient. Yes, you do get some UVA protection with most sunscreen formulations, but not enough to really protect you from skin damage, cancer, and wrinkles. So when the product states you'll be "protected from UVA and UVB rays," it isn't exactly lying even though it doesn't contain avobenzone, titanium dioxide, or zinc oxide. But it isn't telling the whole truth, either. The FDA has not established any guideline or measurement when it comes to UVA protection; the only way the consumer can obtain any information is to check the active ingredients for the UVA-protecting ingredients of avobenzone, titanium dioxide, and zinc oxide.

## SUN PROTECTION FOR DIFFERENT SKIN TYPES

Perhaps one of the most irresponsible, reckless, and unethical marketing positions the cosmetics industry takes is selling skin-care routines that don't include sunscreen. Many cosmetic lines sell an endless array of cleansers, toners, anti-wrinkle treatments, eye creams, throat creams, face creams, and facial masks yet never mention the indispensable need for regular, consistent use of a sunscreen. Almost every line does have "sun-care" products, but they are often promoted separately from the "daily care" routines. I've personally spoken to hundreds and hundreds of cosmetics salespeople about their products and repeatedly found a gross lack of information about sun protection. I'm always told how important moisturizers, eye creams, serums, toners, cleansers, and eye-makeup removers are, but almost never do I hear about the value of daily sunscreen use.

There are indeed many ways to get good sun protection, regardless of your other skin-care needs. This is so important that I consider it unconscionable to discuss any skin-care routines, skin-care problems, or skin-care concerns without also including a discussion of sun protection. If you've been intrigued by a new miracle skin-care line, but a sunscreen is not mentioned, that company clearly does not take skin care seriously or ethically. You should not be wasting your money and hurting your skin by considering a company that would ignore such a vital component of healthy skin care.

Now that you understand the importance of using sunscreen on a daily basis, finding the right product is not easy. Perhaps the trickiest part of sunscreen use is finding one that doesn't cause problems, particularly if you have normal to oily skin, acne-prone skin, or sensitive skin. Active sunscreen agents including avobenzone, benzophone, octyl methoxycinnamate, oxybenzone, padimate O, and many others can cause irritation on the skin, creating patches of dryness, itching, rashlike breakouts, redness, and swelling. Because these particular sunscreen agents can be potentially irritating, many dermatologists feel that titanium dioxide and zinc oxide are the best sunscreen ingredients, since they are almost benign on the skin and are excellent screens for both UVA and UVB radiation. I wish the subject could end here and I could unequivocally recommend titanium dioxide and zinc oxide as the only sunscreen ingredients to look for, but that isn't the case. As safe and effective as titanium dioxide and zinc oxide are they can be occlusive, meaning they can block and clog pores.

The issue for any ingredient that can cause breakouts is threefold: how occlusive it is (meaning blocking oil flow out of the pores), how irritating it is on the skin (perhaps causing rashlike breakouts), and how much the ingredient duplicates what the pore already produces, adding more fuel to the fire. Titanium dioxide and zinc oxide pose the first problem for skin. Are you guaranteed to break out if you use a sunscreen with titanium dioxide? Absolutely not, but it is a possibility. Everyone's skin reacts differently to any and all cosmetic ingredients. One other issue with a sunscreen that uses only titanium dioxide and/or zinc oxide as the active ingredient is a cosmetic one, as these products tend to leave a white appearance and can feel somewhat heavy on the skin. That can be a problem for all skin types. In response to that shortcoming, many sunscreen products combine titanium dioxide with other sunscreen agents, which reduce the amount of potentially irritating ingredients while also decreasing some of titanium dioxide's occlusive tendency.

## SUNSCREENS FOR OILY SKIN

The search for a sunscreen that is appropriate for oily skin can be a frustrating, lifelong pursuit. Even those I've created for my line can have problems for some people. There are difficulties of several kinds. First, the types of ingredients that can be used to suspend sunscreen agents are not exactly the best for oily skin. Regardless of the claim on the label, there are risks that the base formulation can clog pores or feel slippery or greasy on the skin. There's also the problem that the sunscreen ingredients themselves can cause an irritated breakout reaction, a response to the synthetically derived sunscreen agents. (Regrettably, that is the nature of almost all active ingredients used in cosmetics—"active" meaning they actually do something on the skin. Whether they are AHAs, Renova, benzoyl peroxide, hydroquinone, or sunscreen ingredients, if they work, they can be irritating.) In the case of titanium dioxide and zinc oxide, even though they are relatively innocuous and have minimal to no risk of irritation on skin, they can still clog pores, being the thick creamy ingredients that they are. Finally, given the wide variety in formulations, there is no way to quantify which ingredients are more problematic than others for causing problems. What's my advice? The only true answer is to experiment. I wish there was a slam-dunk solution I could offer, but there are no product lines that can legitimately make the claim that their sunscreen won't cause breakouts (and those of you with this problem already know that).

For oily skin, or any skin type for that matter, wearing a foundation with a high SPF is an excellent idea, particularly for women with oily skin who don't want to wear layers of skin-care products. This is also an option for women who are just tired of wearing layers and layers of skin-care products and makeup. Luckily, there are now many well-formulated foundations and tinted moisturizers with good SPF numbers containing avobenzone, titanium dioxide, or zinc oxide. **The one negative about using a foundation with sunscreen is that you need to apply it generously; thin, sheer applications don't work. Plus, as the foundation shifts during the day it is essential to touch it up with a pressed powder containing an SPF 15 and including UVA-protecting ingredients of avobenzone, titanium dioxide, or zinc oxide.**

If you wear a foundation with a good SPF you might forget to use a sunscreen on your hands, neck, throat, chest, or any other area of your body that is exposed to the sun on a daily basis. Those brown "age spots" and crepy skin textures are related to sun damage. Like wrinkling on the face, wrinkling on the rest of the body can't be mitigated without daily use of sunscreen, and that means reapplying your sunscreen every time you wash your hands and taking care to put sunscreen on any exposed parts of your body day in and day out.

## FOR THE LITTLE ONES

If you have babies or small children, the issue of sunscreen protection should absolutely be of primary concern. Their delicate skin is even more sensitive to the sun's damaging energy. Whether or not you are diligent about staying out of the sun or using sunscreen for yourself, you must be diligent when it comes to the health of your children.

An article in the *Archives of Pediatrics & Adolescent Medicine* (August 2001, pages 891–896) stated that "the regular practice of sun protection for children rarely takes place and primarily consists of applying sunscreen rather than methods that reduce sun exposure. This flies in the face of definitive knowledge that skin cancer, both melanoma and nonmelanoma, has reached epidemic proportions, that excessive sun exposure is associated with the subsequent development of most types of skin cancer, and that as much as 80% of lifetime sun exposure takes place during childhood.... [S]un protection should take its place among topics like car seats, smoke alarms, safe water temperature, and bicycle helmets...."

When should you start using sunscreen for children? It's generally thought to be safe when they are six months old or older. But according to an August 1999 press release from the American Academy of Pediatrics, "The issue of whether sunscreen is safe for infants under the age of 6 months remains controversial. Concerns have been raised that human skin under 6 months may have different absorptive characteristics; biologic systems that metabolize and excrete drugs may not be fully developed in children [younger than] 6 months." Despite these concerns, the Australian Cancer Society in a Position Paper entitled, "Sun Protection and Babies," August 2000, supported by the Australasian College of Dermatologists, concluded "There is no evidence that using sunscreen on infants is harmful. Although premature babies may have increased skin permeability consistent with incomplete development of the skin, the structure of the stratum corneum (the skin layer principally determining permeability) in full term babies is indistinguishable from that of adults [thus] providing an effective barrier. If infants are kept out of the sun or well protected from UVR by clothing, hats and shade, then sunscreen need only be used occasionally on very small areas of a baby's skin. When used according to these guidelines, it is unlikely that the small amount of organic sunscreen components absorbed would exceed the metabolic capacities of the liver. In this position statement, the term 'infant' refers to babies from birth to 12 months of age."

Before you make a decision for your child, check with your physician for his or her recommendation.

When choosing a sunscreen for your child it's easy to be attracted to the sunscreen products with pictures of cute babies on the label. However, despite these marketing tactics, formulations of products aimed at children are no different from the formulations of products for adults. All sunscreen formulations that have an SPF are regulated closely by the FDA; the formulations do not differ in any way because of the age of the intended user. The only difference I've ever noted in baby products is the use of fragrance. Certain fragrances may make you think of little ones, but fragrance can be irritating for all skin types, and baby formulas tend to contain more than many adult products do.

Of greater concern is that many sunscreens claiming to be for children do not contain the UVA-protecting ingredients of avobenzone, titanium dioxide, or zinc oxide. If one of these ingredients is not present in the active ingredient list on the label, do not buy it, or if you already own one, now that you know better, do not use it again and throw it out immediately.

If you are looking for a less irritating sunscreen for your kids, choose one that contains only pure titanium dioxide or zinc oxide as the active ingredient, which are definitely less irritating than products with other inorganic sunscreen agents.

## VITAMIN D AND SUN

Sunlight is the primary source of vitamin D, and vitamin D deficiencies can be a serious health problem. Some people worry that if they use sunscreen it will cancel out their body's ability to absorb vitamin D from the sun. Regarding this issue, a June 1999 article in *Cosmetic Dermatology* (page 43) discussed a presentation given by Mark Naylor, MD, assistant professor in the Department of Dermatology at the University of Oklahoma, which described some of "the latest studies proving that ultraviolet exposure is neither required for vitamin D sufficiency nor [that vitamin D is] a scientifically proven cancer fighter. Prospective sunscreen trials examining whether sunscreen contributes to vitamin D deficiency found that regular sunscreen users were not vitamin D deficient."

## THE ART OF SELF-TANNING

Self-tanners are the only way to get a tan that is safe for the skin. All self-tanners are virtually equal in that they use the same ingredient, dihydroxyacetone (DHA), to chemically turn the skin brown. Some products contain a greater concentration of DHA than others, and the higher the concentration the faster the skin will turn color. The key to a good result is the application, which is always tricky. It takes experimentation to figure out how much to use, how dark to go, what areas to go over lightly (like knees and elbows), what areas to avoid (like palms of hands and armpits), and where to start and stop the application (do you stop at your ankles or continue down to your toes?). All of these are questions you need to answer for yourself, depending on your own personal preferences and blending techniques.

**Note:** If you choose to buy a self-tanner, whether it contains a sunscreen or not, please be aware that self-tanned brown skin does not offer any protection from the sun. All of the rules for wearing sunscreens still apply when you are using these products.

During the summer months, fashion magazines are replete with advertisements and stories about the best self-tanners and the optimal application for obtaining the best results. Varying products proclaim they are streak-free, won't turn orange, dry in five minutes, tan in under an hour, or have special color indicators. Those claims are often unreliable or misleading. Essentially, any self-tanner can be streak-free if *you* apply it evenly. A product that has "color indicators" simply refers to one with a temporary color that helps you see where you've applied it. That is helpful, but still not foolproof, because the tint can dissipate quickly in some areas, leaving you wondering where you've applied it. (However, products that aren't transparent are definitely a great place to start, helping improve your odds of putting it on right.)

As far as the color of the tan you get, there are basically no color differences between products. As stated earlier, this is because all self-tanners contain the same ingredient, dihydroxyacetone, which turns skin brown. DHA is a simple sugar involved in plant and animal carbohydrate metabolism, so you can even think of it as being all natural. How fast your skin turns color also has to do with how much DHA the product contains. The true color differences correlate with how much DHA the product contains and how your skin reacts to this ingredient. DHA browns the skin through its interaction with the amino acid arginine, which is found in surface skin cells. (Source: *Chemical Engineering News,* June 2000). Drying time is irrelevant because the tanning effect really depends on the chemical changes taking place in your skin cells. That's why, if you aren't patient and your skin rubs against your clothes (whether the self-tanner is completely dry or not), it will cause smudging or an uneven appearance.

Products that claim to turn your skin tan in less than an hour may actually be a problem because if you make a mistake in application (which is almost inevitable at first) it will also be almost instantaneously noticeable. A self-tanner that takes a few applications to achieve the color you want may be a better option as you learn how your skin reacts and hone your technique.

Regardless of the claims made about any self-tanner, it turns out that which product you choose isn't anywhere near as important as your technique and diligence. The following list will help you get the absolute best results with minimum problems. Just let me warn you, trying to do this fast will make your skin look more strange than tan.

1.  It takes time, so apply self-tanner in the evening, allowing yourself at least a half hour, although an hour would be best. (For those who think the time it takes to apply self-tanner is inconvenient, remember how many hours it used to take in the sun to get the same amount of color? And with self-tanners there's no risk of wrinkles or skin cancer.)

2. Self-tanners grab on to surface skin cells, and you may have more in some areas than others. To help achieve a uniform appearance, take a shower or bath and exfoliate your skin, either with a washcloth or some baking soda, or both. Don't overscrub, but do pay extra attention to your knees, ankles, feet, elbows, and neck.

3. After showering and completely drying off, apply a minimal thin layer of moisturizer over the areas where you will be applying self-tanner. This will help the self-tanner glide on more easily and not stick over dry patches. A little extra moisturizer over ankles, knees, and elbows can prevent those areas from looking patchy. I have seen some recommendations that suggest mixing self-tanner with your moisturizer, but don't do it because that will encourage streaking (unless you can precisely mix the two together), and it will take longer for the self-tanner to absorb and dry.

   **Body Sense:** *Perspiration can make self-tanners streak, so take a cool shower or bath to keep yourself from sweating. Your skin must be completely dry to get the best results. Do not apply self-tanner in a steamy, hot bathroom.*

4. It is best to apply the self-tanner while naked, but wearing an old bathing suit (one you don't plan to wear outside) can help you determine where you want your tan to be. Either way, have a game plan of where you want to stop and start the color. (Do you want tan armpits, the entire arm tan? What about the heels of your feet, your ears, or the palms of your hands?) Remember that self-tanners will stain clothing until they completely absorb into the skin and take effect in the skin cell.

   **Body Sense:** *Applying self-tanner on your back requires a friend with a helping hand, although you can use a long-handled paintbrush. I vote for the friend (or significant other) as the paintbrush poses some issues of dripping and uneven application.*

5. Apply self-tanner to one section of your body at a time. Be more concerned about even application than rubbing it all the way in. Avoid areas of your body where you do not want to have color.

6. To prevent tan palms you can try using surgical or plastic gloves to apply the self-tanner. This can work well, but can also make application trickier. Another option is to wash your hands after you've applied the self-tanner to a section of your body, or just to wash them every few minutes. If you wait too long you will have strange-looking palms. It helps to have a nail brush handy to be sure you get the self tanner off of your cuticles and the area between your fingers.

7. Different parts of your body "pick up" self-tanner more easily than others. For example, some people find that their legs turn brown more easily than their arms or torso, while others find that their faces and necks change color fastest. Experience will help you determine which is true for you. Be careful around your nose, eyes, ears, hairline, and lips. A cotton swab can help blend a thin, even amount smoothly over those areas. To keep your hair from turn ing color, apply a layer of conditioner or Vaseline over the hairline.

8. Wait at least 15 minutes before getting dressed. Do not exercise or swim for at least three hours.

9. If you make a mistake and end up with streaky or dark areas of skin, consider using my 2% Beta Hydroxy Acid Solution or Neutrogena's Clear Pore Clarifying Gel (with 2% BHA) over those spots. Then, in the morning, manually exfoliate those areas with a wet washcloth, and Voila! Bye-bye streaks!

10. Problem Areas. As an option for your hands (which can be particularly tricky to get looking natural) apply self-tanner as you would a moisturizer, but then quickly wipe your palms off on a slightly soapy washcloth. Then take a Q-tip dipped in cleanser, eye-makeup remover (one that is not greasy so it doesn't spread or smear), or nail polish remover and carefully use it to wipe around the nails and cuticle area and between your fingers. Another option is to use a makeup sponge to apply self-tanner to the back of your hands, tops of your feet, temples, and hairline. By holding the sponge deftly be tween two fingers, you only need to worry about preventing this small area from becoming the wrong color.

    **Body Sense:** *Skin-care products such as AHAs, BHA, topical scrubs, Retin-A, and topical disinfectants can affect the self-tanner's action on your skin or even eliminate the color by exfoliating the surface skin cells (self-tanners only interact on the surface of skin). It is best not to apply these products the evening you apply a self-tanner. However, if you must do so, wait at least two to three hours before you do.*

11. Reapply self-tanner as you feel the need. Generally it will start wearing away in about three to four days as the surface layers of skin shed.

All of these are valid application techniques, but none offers a guarantee, which is why it takes experimenting and going slow to get the best results.

# SUN-TANNING MACHINES

According to the FDA, the FCC (Federal Communications Commission), the American Academy of Dermatology, and the Skin Cancer Foundation, sun-tanning machines are nothing more than skin cancer machines and should be made illegal. The research for this is startling. Sun-tanning machines radiate the most damaging effects of the sun only inches away from your body, and, worse, they are available day after day, month after month, in areas of the country where you would not normally see the sun on a daily basis. In addition, they allow exposure of body parts that are usually covered. They pose the same serious risk of skin cancer that unprotected exposure to the sun allows (Source: *Journal of the American Academy of Dermatology*, May 2001, pages 775–780).

Shockingly, I have received pamphlets and brochures from tanning-machine companies and from salon managers who own these machines explaining how safe these machines really are because of the type of radiation they emit. It makes me want to scream, or cry, or both. None of it is true or substantiated by anyone other than those who market the use of tanning machines. Please, if you heed no other information this book provides, protect your skin from sun damage, both artificial and natural. There are lots of ways to look and feel beautiful, but this isn't one of them.

# TANNING PILLS?

Tanning pills come in two forms: those that contain tyrosine and those that contain concentrated does of beta-carotene. Let's start with tyrosine. The FDA has debunked tyrosine as a tanning accelerator. The marketing pitch is that tyrosine is needed by your body to produce melanin, which is a true statement. Ergo, the logic (albeit flawed) follows: taking pills with tyrosine will increase melanin production. It just isn't true—only exposure to UVA or UVB sun rays can activate tyrosine and other elements in skin to initiate (or trigger) melanin production, the pigment we see as a tan.

Here's what the FDA says about tyrosine in the *Office of Cosmetics and Colors Fact Sheet* (June 27, 2000), "Lotions and pills marketed as "tanning accelerators" generally contain tyrosine (an amino acid), often in combination with other substances. Tanning accelerators are marketed with the claim that they enhance tanning by stimulating and increasing melanin formation. FDA has concluded that these 'tanning accelerators' are actually unapproved drugs, and the agency has issued warning letters to several manufacturers of these products. There are no scientific data showing that they work; in fact, at least one study has found them ineffective." Companies that sell these types of tyrosine pills or lotions play on the fact that tyrosine is an amino acid that is a precursor for the production of melanin. Yet, no research supports the oral consumption of tyrosine as having any effect on the color of skin. In another report the FDA stated "In fact, an animal study reported a few years ago demonstrated that ingestion or topical application of tyrosine has no effect on [melanin production]. The [FDA] has … issued warning letters to several major manufacturers of these products (Source: FDA Web site, http://www.fda.gov/ora/inspect_ref/igs/cosmet.html).

A self-tanning pill, called Elusun, shows up on many Internet sites. Elusun's claims are at best misleading and, at worst, potentially dangerous. Elusun claims that it can prevent the skin from aging during sun exposure; that's not only completely false information, but also a truly harmful statement. Without sunscreen that contains UVA-protecting ingredients, *all* sun exposure is damaging, and no oral vitamin or supplement can change that.

Does Elusun color the skin? Yes, by giving the skin high doses of beta-carotene (an FDA-approved vitamin supplement and food-coloring agent). Beta-carotene is the stuff that makes carrots orange and, if you consume enough of it, it can alter the skin's color. However, according to the FDA, megadoses of beta-carotene "enter the blood stream and are partially deposited in skin tissue, giving the skin a tan-like color … [but they are not] approved for [tanning] use, and products containing them are considered adulterated. Some reports of adverse reactions associated with 'tanning pills' have mentioned stomach cramps, hepatitis, nausea, diarrhea, and deposition of the color in the retina of the eye." Megadoses of beta-carotene can be harmful (Source: FDA Web site, http://www.fda.gov/ora/inspect_ref/igs/cosmet.html).

Aside from pills that contain beta-carotene, there are others that contain another food-coloring substance called canthaxanthin. This ingredient works much like beta-carotene, but, according to the FDA "At least one company submitted an application for the approval of canthaxanthin-containing pills as a tanning agent, but withdrew the application when side effects, such as the [formation] of crystals in the eye, were discovered."

The FDA also states on its Web site that "In recent years, 'suntan accelerators' have appeared on the market. They claim to enhance tanning by stimulating and increasing melanin formation.… One type of suntan accelerator is based on bergapten (5-methoxypsoralen) which is found in bergamot oil and is a well-known phototoxic substance (responsible for Berloque dermatitis). Bergapten increases the skin's sensitivity to ultraviolet light, intensifies erythema formation, and stimulates melanocytes to produce melanin. It has also been reported to be photo-carcinogenic in animals" (Source: FDA Web site, http://www.fda.gov/ora/inspect_ref/igs/cosmet.html).

# SKIN CANCER AND SUN DAMAGE

According to the Centers for Disease Control and Prevention (CDC) and the American Academy of Dermatology (AAD), one million new cases of skin cancer are diagnosed each year. That gives skin cancer the unfavorable distinction of being the most common form of cancer in the United States. As reported by Dr. Darrell S. Rigel from the New York University School of Medicine, the chance for an American to develop melanoma in their lifetime is 1 in 84. Those aren't the kinds of odds you want to gamble on, at least not when it comes to losing portions of your skin or your life.

Most skin cancers fall into three categories: basal cell carcinomas, squamous cell carcinomas, and melanomas. Basal cell carcinomas and squamous cell carcinomas are caused by repeated, unprotected sun exposure (Source: *American Journal of Clinical Dermatology*, May-June 2000, pages 167–179).

However, there is some controversy as to whether or not melanomas are caused by unprotected sun exposure. Despite the disagreement, many, if not all, dermatologists feel that the best available evidence suggests counseling patients to lower their exposure to sunlight and advising them that the use of a broad-spectrum sunscreen with a high protection factor decreases the risk of developing melanoma (Sources: *Archives of Dermatology*, December 2000, pages 1447–1449; *Journal of the American Medical Association,* June 2000, pages 2955–2960).

As a general theory, scientists believe that exposure to UVA and some UVB radiation triggers mutations in replicating skin cells, causing their genetic coding to go haywire. The cells forget how to maintain the normal cell turnover process because of the radiation damage. Fortunately, nonmelanoma skin cancers are relatively easy to treat if detected in time, and are rarely fatal. Melanomas are a much more dangerous and life-threatening form of cancer.

An article in the *Journal of Epidemiology* (December 1999, Supplement, pages 7–13) succinctly summed up the issue quite nicely, "Skin cancer is the most commonly occurring cancer in humans…. Descriptive studies show that incidence rates of the main types of skin cancer, basal cell carcinoma, squamous cell carcinoma and melanoma are [highest] in populations in which ambient sun exposure is high and skin transmission of solar radiation is high, suggesting strong associations with sun exposure. Analytic epidemiological studies confirm that exposure to the UV component of sunlight is the major environmental determinant of skin cancers and associated skin conditions and evidence of a causal association between cumulative sun exposure and SCC, solar keratoses and photodamage is relatively straightforward…. Complementary to [population and research] data is the molecular evidence of ultraviolet (UV) mechanisms of carcinogenesis [cancer] such as UV-specific mutations in the DNA of tumor suppressor genes in skin tumors. With increased UV irradiation resulting from thinning of the ozone layer, skin cancer incidence rates have been predicted to increase in the future—unless, as is hoped, human behavior to reduce sun exposure can offset these predicted rises."

Other than sun protection, you should be aware of some early, telltale signs of skin cancer. Early detection of skin cancer can save your skin and your life. If you perceive a change in your skin that you are not sure about, talk to your doctor; even a minor difference in a mole or a freckle, or a blemish that doesn't look "normal," can be an indication of skin cancer.

**The five most typical characteristics of skin cancer are:**

1. An open sore, any size, that bleeds, oozes, or crusts and remains open for three or more weeks. A persistent, nonhealing sore is one of the most com mon signs of early skin cancer.

2. A reddish patch or irritated area that doesn't go away and doesn't respond to cortisone creams or moisturizers. Sometimes these patches crust over or flake off, but they never go away completely.

3. A smooth growth with a distinct rolled border and an indented center. It can look like a small blemish or wound, but tends to grow and doesn't heal.

4. A shiny bump or nodule with a slick, smooth surface that can be pink, red, white, black, brown, or purple in color. It can look like a mole, but the tex ture and shine are what make it different.

5. A white patch of skin that has a smooth, scarlike texture. The area of white skin can have a taut, clear appearance that stands out from the appearance of the surrounding skin.

**The American Academy of Dermatology has a list of the "A, B, C, Ds" of identifying skin cancer, as follows:**

**A.** **A**symmetry: One half of the lesion or suspect area is unlike the other half.

**B.** **B**order: There is an irregular, scalloped, or poorly circumscribed border around a suspected skin lesion or mole.

**C.** **C**olor: Color varies from one area to another, with shades of tan, brown, black, white, red, or blue.

**D.** **D**iameter: The area is generally larger than 6mm (diameter of a pencil eraser).

# ACTINIC KERATOSIS

If you have had any amount of unprotected sun exposure and you are between the ages of 30 and 80 you might have noticed uneven, rough-feeling, slightly raised, occasionally crusty, and generally light brown or light pink patches on your chest, hands, arms, or neck. These discolorations are called actinic keratosis or solar keratosis, and are distinct from other types of brown discolorations that show up on skin. According to the Skin Cancer Foundation, "One in six people will develop an actinic keratosis in the course of a lifetime." The more typical brown spots that appear on skin due to sun exposure are called melasmas. Melasmas look more like brown freckling and are not raised, rough, or crusted, and are considered benign. Actinic keratosis, though not cancerous, are problematic because they are considered indicative of a precancerous skin condition and require evaluation by a dermatologist. If you are in doubt whether or not a brown patch on your skin is a melasma or an actinic keratosis, it is best to ask your doctor.

Prevention is the best method of averting the occurrence of these types of brown patches (meaning daily and liberal use of effective sunscreens). Unfortunately, because most of us were not aware of appropriate sun protection for much of our lives, many of us have a pretty good chance of seeing one of these patches crop up somewhere on our bodies.

There are a number of ways to deal with removing actinic keratosis. The primary techniques are curettage, cryosurgery, and photodynamic therapy, plus topical chemotherapy options (Source: *American Journal of Clinical Dermatology*, May-June 2000, pages 167–179).

Deciding what to do depends primarily on the status of the lesion and how much the appearance bothers you. This requires a discussion with your dermatologist to evaluate your various options.

A typical method of removal is to scrape or cut the lesion off with procedures called **curettage**, **electrodesiccation**, or even simple scraping with a surgical razor. Curettage refers to cutting out the lesion with a curette, a spoon-shaped implement that has a sharp edge. Electrodesiccation uses an electric current to remove the skin tissue while it simultaneously controls bleeding. In both instances a biopsy is done to check on the status of the lesion. Both of these methods can cause scarring, and recurrence of the lesions is a problem.

**Cryosurgery** uses extreme cold, in the form of liquid nitrogen, to get rid of the unwanted tissue. This method doesn't cause bleeding or scarring but it can leave behind a white mark that often doesn't regain normal skin color. There is also a strong likelihood of recurrence.

When there are numerous actinic keratosis lesions present, two topical medications are sometimes used. The first, **5-fluorouracil** (brand name Efudex), a chemotherapy agent for some cancers, is applied to the spots twice a day for three to five weeks. The side effects of this treatment can be significant, though temporary. Inflammation, burning, stinging, crusting, and some discomfort or pain are typical, but healing takes place one to two weeks after treatment is discontinued. It is considered a highly effective treatment.

Another chemotherapy agent used topically, **masoprocol** cream, 10% (brand name Actinex), is similar to 5-fluorouracil in terms of application and results, although there is a far higher risk of contact dermatitis with masoprocol than with 5-fluorouracil.

**Immune response modulators** are capable of selectively destroying abnormal skin cells. In a small study group "six men with actinic keratosis were treated with imiquimod 5% cream (trade name Aldara) three times a week for 6-8 weeks. In the event of a local skin reaction treatment was modified to two times per week. Results: All the AK [actinic keratosis] lesions were successfully cleared…. Histologically [under the skin], no apparent signs of persisting AK could be detected, and no recurrences were reported during follow up" (Source: *British Journal of Dermatology*, May 2001, pages 1050–1053). Aldara is a potential option to discuss with your physician.

**Chemical peeling** uses trichloroacetic acid (TCA), which is applied under light sedation. Much like any other cosmetic chemical peel, this causes the top layers of the skin to slough off, to be replaced within a few weeks by growth of new skin. A TCA peel is used when deeper penetration is needed to remove the lesion. The downsides to this method are the need for sedation, which makes it rather inconvenient, and the prolonged healing time; the upside is that the eventual results are considered quite good.

The newest treatment recently approved by the FDA is called **photodynamic therapy**. This is an interesting procedure that involves the topical application by a physician of a prescription-only cream containing aminolevulinic acid (brand name Levulan Kerastick). About 14 to 18 hours after the cream has been applied the area is exposed to a particular light source, called BLU-U or Blue Light, for approximately 15 to 20 minutes. This is considered a very successful treatment with little risk to skin. However, after the aminolevulinic acid has been applied, the skin becomes abnormally sensitive to daylight or bright indoor lighting until the treatment is completed. It is critical to wear sunlight-protective clothing and to avoid any exposure to the sun because sunscreens will not protect you. It is also important to avoid sitting close to any light source. Side effects during treatment usually include burning, a crawling feeling, itching, numbness, and stinging sensations, darkening or lightening of treated skin, crusting, scabs, and red itchy bumps. However, once treatment is discontinued the reaction and brown spots are gone and tend not to return.

# AFTER-SUN CARE

I worry about the concept of "after-sun care." It sounds as if you can undo all the sun damage you incurred during the day. I admit it's a great marketing concept, but it is risky business for someone to buy into the notion that skin can be repaired following unprotected sun exposure. If you leave your skin defenseless and exposed to the sun's rays, and then slather some lotion, toner, or serum on afterward, you cannot miraculously or even in a minor way heal, eliminate, correct, or cancel the devastating injury to your skin (and all sun exposure over time is devastating). The skin does want to heal on its own, but what we do to it in the name of skin care can get in the way of the skin's own immune/healing response.

Slathering too much moisturizer on after a long day outside, or just in general, can prevent the skin from doing what it does on its own naturally, namely healing. This is because too much moisturizer can turn off the skin's natural ability to heal. Most skin is best left alone or, at most, given a lightweight, thin layer of moisturizer, especially after sun exposure.

What about taking care of sunburn? Well, why are you getting sunburned in the first place? Why would you ever leave your house any time of the day or year without a good sunscreen on (one rated at least SPF 15 that contains either avobenzone, titanium dioxide, or zinc oxide as the active ingredients)? OK, that's enough guilt, just don't do it again, and now take care of your burn wisely.

It is essential to treat sunburns the same way you would treat a burn injury from any heat source. Unquestionably, whenever the skin is burned you first need to cool it off to prevent the skin tissue from either retaining the heat or continuing to react negatively. Trapping the heat in the skin by covering it with a thick, waxy, or heavy lotion or cream will literally let the skin continue to fry, even after the heat source has been removed. Likewise, it promotes swelling, redness, and pain.

Some of you may remember the days when you got burned in the kitchen and your grandmother or mother would slather butter on it. Absolutely nothing could have been worse for the skin. Butter, like any emollient moisturizer, places a relatively occlusive layer over the skin, encapsulating the heat and preventing it from leaving the skin. It does nothing to reduce the swelling or redness.

All burns need to be cooled to dissipate the heat simmering in the lower layers of skin and to reduce the resulting inflammation. If you have sunburn over most of your body, a cool to slightly cold bath (not ice-cold; ice or icy water applied directly on the skin is too severe and can burn the skin in other ways). If you do want to use a moisturizer or soothing agent, I recommend a light layer of aloe vera, but not for the reasons the cosmetics industry tells you to use the stuff. Using aloe vera helps cool the skin and prevents trapping the heat the way creams and emollient moisturizers do.

If your burn is serious or extremely painful, do not hesitate to find the nearest hospital emergency room. Heat trauma from sunburn can be a serious threat to your health.

# WHY ALOE VERA MAY WORK ON SUNBURNS

We are now learning that moisturizers can be overdone and can hamper the skin's healing process. Lots of people attribute miraculous benefits to the aloe plant for helping the skin heal. Yet there is no real evidence that aloe vera helps the skin in any significant way. An article in the *British Journal of General Practice* (October 1999, pages 823–828) stated that "Topical application of aloe vera is not an effective preventative for radiation-induced injuries…. Whether it promotes wound healing is unclear…. Even though there are some promising results, clinical effectiveness of oral or topical aloe vera is not sufficiently defined at present." There is also research that has isolated certain components of aloe vera and demonstrated it has some effectiveness for wound healing and as an anti-irritant (Sources: *Journal of Ethnopharmacology*, December 1999, pages 3–37; *Free-Radical Biology and Medicine*, January 2000, pages 261–265).

Regardless of the disparate information, there is enough anecdotal evidence about aloe vera to make its reputation hard to ignore. It turns out that aloe's reputation may have less to do with what it does for the skin than with the things it helps you keep off the skin. In other words, if you apply pure aloe to sunburn or some other injury site, you won't apply anything else. In essence, you are just cooling off the skin and leaving it alone to do its own thing. Once the aloe juice dries—and because it is mostly water that happens fairly quickly—the skin can heal quite nicely on its own.

# BUYING SUNGLASSES

Wearing sunglasses on a regular basis is critical for the health of your eyes. The lens of the eye turns out to be a pretty good absorber of UVA rays, but, unlike the skin, the lens cannot slough off damaged cells. That means there is no way for the lens to ever repair itself. Protecting the eyes isn't just a cosmetic or a costume, it is about keeping your sight undiminished for as long as possible. Your eyes need protection from ultraviolet radiation, and whether you buy inexpensive or expensive sunglasses, it is a waste of money if they don't supply it.

Eyes exposed to sunlight are at risk for cataracts, sunburn (the eyeball itself can get sunburned), irritation, skin cancer of the eyelid, and dry eyes. Fortunately, most sunglasses do protect us well from the sun, but there is no easy way to know which ones do and which ones don't. Some sunglasses come with labels indicating they offer UV radiation protection, but there are no regulations or standards in this field. It doesn't hurt to buy sunglasses with a UV protection label, but there are some things you need to check out to make sure you purchase a pair that does more than just look good.

I strongly recommend buying sunglasses that hug the face and have wide rims and sidepieces. This way, you shield the eyes from any sunlight coming in from above, below, or around the sides, as well as protect more of the delicate skin around the eyes from sun damage.

The American Academy of Ophthalmology (http://www.aao.org/) offers a few extremely helpful guidelines for finding the best protection:

1. Select sunglasses that block ultraviolet rays. Don't be deceived by color or cost. The ability to block UV light is not dependent on the darkness of the lens or the price tag. You should always buy sunglasses with this feature. Shop for sunglasses that block 99 or 100% of all UV light. Some manufacturers' labels say "UV absorption up to 400nm." This is the same thing as 100% UV absorption.

2. Ideally, your sunglasses should wrap all the way around to your temples, so the sun's rays can't enter from the side.

3. Even if you wear contacts with UV protection, remember your sunglasses.

4. Be sure that the lens tint is uniform, not darker in one area than another.

Another test to be sure the glasses are well made is to hold them out from you at arm's length. Look through them from this distance at a straight line such as the edge of a bookcase or wall. Then slowly move the glasses across the straight line. If the straight edge distorts, sways, curves, or moves, the lenses have imperfections and you should not buy them.

Tinted sunglasses have an impact on what kind of sun exposure you get, aside from their impact on the face. Red- and yellow-tinted lenses can cut haze, but may not adequately protect from sun exposure, though if they had a UV coating they would work to protect against sun damage. Check them in daylight or consult an ophthalmologist. Gray, green, and brown tints are known for providing good viewing as well as good sun protection. Black and blue tints can be too dark, impairing good vision.

# CHAPTER 6
## SKIN-CARE PLANNING

### WHY DOES IT HAVE TO BE SO COMPLICATED?

As I look over the material and research I've accumulated, from magazine articles and books on botanicals and herbs, to medical and scientific journals, as well as from interviews with dermatologists, oncologists, and cosmetics chemists, I am amazed at the depth of information available on skin and skin care. It is also mind-boggling to realize how many thousands of products you can choose from when it comes to everything from cleaning the face, to protecting skin from the sun, moisturizing, fighting blemishes, or treating a large number of skin problems. You wouldn't think that taking care of your skin could be so complicated or shrouded in such controversy, but the truth is, it *is* very complicated.

Despite being such a small part of the whole body, the face has the lion's share of topical problems, far more than what takes place from the neck down. Acne, wrinkles, sagging, sunburn, blackheads, dryness, rosacea, eczema, psoriasis, seborrhea, dry patches, swelling, and allergies, not to mention our concepts of beauty, are most evident on the face. There is a lot of money to be made if a cosmetics company can get a consumer to believe that their product(s) will make her more beautiful and do something to tackle one or more of those facial dilemmas. If a company can make the stuff sound utterly unique for the skin, even when it isn't, the sales figures rise astronomically. No wonder the claims are so hard to decipher!

As complicated and emotional as skin care can be, the actual skin-care routines can really and truly be streamlined and concise. By now you have an overview of what works and what doesn't when it comes to cosmetics claims and various skin-care ingredients. You are also aware of how the cosmetics industry may be damaging your skin and what current research is revealing about optimal skin care. The next step is to arrange all these data in a way that helps you find an effective skin-care routine so you can stop wasting money on useless products that may be hurting your skin.

## CLEANING THE SKIN

No other aspect of skin care is quite as basic as this one. Cleaning the face sets the stage for everything else that will take place on the skin. More so than any other part of your skin-care routine, it is essential that the cleansing products you use be gentle. **Overcleaning or using cleansers that are too drying is a major cause of irritation, dry patches, and redness. Not cleaning the skin well enough can clog pores or leave a residue on the face that can prevent skin cells from sloughing off. Using a cleanser that leaves a greasy film on the face can clog pores and prevent moisturizers from being able to absorb and do their job. It is essential to get this step right, and that means thoroughly, but gently, cleaning the face** (Source: *Cutis*, December 2001, pages 12–19. Note: "cutis" is Latin for skin).

## EYE-MAKEUP REMOVERS

In the past I have been hesitant to recommend wiping off makeup. Repeated pulling at the skin can be problematic because it stretches skin and damages the skin's elastin fibers. Elastin is a stretchable elastic protein found in skin tissue that is responsible for the flexible, resilient nature of healthy skin. When skin is being pulled and yanked, elastin's orderly arrangement can change. Regardless of the direction you pull—up, down, or sideways—if you see the skin move, you are tugging on the skin's elastic fibers and helping the skin to sag sooner than it would otherwise. No matter how gently it's done, this pulling distends the tissue more than enough to stretch it. Watch closely in the mirror the next time you start wiping off your makeup, particularly eye makeup. Notice that even when you are trying to be gentle the skin is shifting around, movement that inevitably causes wrinkles and sagging.

So how do you get your makeup off? If your makeup is water soluble, the process is pretty straightforward. Because so many water-soluble cleansers use mild ingredients that don't affect the eyes any differently than makeup removers do, they can easily remove all of your makeup, including eye makeup. Using water with a water-soluble cleanser that slips over the face and is easily rinsed off decreases friction and minimizes pulling. If you are used to wiping off makeup, it can take a while to get used to washing it off, but it is the most effective and least damaging way to remove eye makeup.

The exception to this rule is when you are using waterproof or water-resistant makeup, waterproof mascara, heavy or thick foundations, or ultra-matte or transfer-resistant foundations such as Revlon's ColorStay foundations. In those instances, it is necessary to use a gentle, wipe-off makeup remover to help get all your makeup off, and to be as delicate as possible in doing that.

If you do use a water-soluble cleanser to remove your makeup, you may find some residual eye makeup gets left behind. In those circumstances, when you are done cleaning your face, dip a cotton swab in the eye-makeup remover to get the last remnants of your eye makeup; you can also use your toner (assuming it is gentle) to gently remove whatever makeup was left behind on your face.

# WASHCLOTHS

Using a washcloth can prove irritating for some skin types and should probably be avoided. However, if you are using ultra-matte foundations, heavy or thick foundations, or layers of makeup, you may find that most gentle, water-soluble cleansers, no matter how effective the cleansing agents are, will have a difficult time cutting through them. To be sure you are cleaning these off thoroughly, especially to help prevent breakouts, it is extremely helpful to use a washcloth in conjunction with a water-soluble cleanser. The goal is to always remove your makeup thoroughly every night (leaving any amount of makeup on all night long can cause irritation, breakouts, or dryness). Be prepared for ultra-matte foundations or heavy makeup to pose a tricky twist to the proceedings.

# THE WATER

It's important to pay attention to the right type of cleanser, but it is also important to pay attention to the temperature of the water you use. For the most part, water is one of the most nonirritating things you can use on your skin (though on rare occasions there are people with serious atopic dermatitis who find water irritating to the skin). Although water is the most gentle part of cleaning the face, it is gentle only when it is tepid. Hot water can burn and irritate the skin, and cold water will shock and irritate it. Because the goal is to always be gentle to reduce irritation, redness, and swelling, and to prevent any negative impact on the skin's immune response, using tepid water is essential (Sources: University of Washington Physicians Web site, http://uwphysicians.org/; *Advances in Skin & Wound Care*, 2000, volume 13, pages 127–128; *Acta Dermato-Venereologica*, July 1996, pages 274–276).

Water is also frictionless, a beneficial quality that is another very important reason to use it. When you splash your face with tepid water, your hands glide over the face, letting you avoid pulling and tugging at the skin. That means you can remove makeup without stretching the skin tissue, making it overall a better way to treat skin.

# HARD VERSUS SOFT WATER

Hard water is a common problem found in many homes. If you live in a hard-water area, the use of a water softener can make a difference in how your hair and skin feel. What is hard water? The term "hardness" simply describes the total concentration of calcium and magnesium ions present in the water. Why is hard water a problem? Hard water is an issue when it comes to any type of washing because with hard water it can take twice as much cleanser, shampoo, or laundry detergent to achieve the same level of cleanliness as it does when using soft water. That's the efficiency side of it. The other issue with hard water is that cleansing agents of any kind combine with the calcium and magnesium ions in the water to form a film that doesn't easily (or even completely) rinse off. That film attaches to all kinds of surfaces, including almost imperceptibly to clothes, and it can be seen on dishes, bathtubs, and, yes, on skin and hair. In fact, the squeaky sound you hear after washing your face or hair is from the presence of calcium, not the effect of having clean skin. That means there really is no such thing as "squeaky clean." And yes, the film remains on your skin even after rinsing, and that clogs pores and coats hair. Moreover, the calcium and magnesium are drying in and of themselves (as are most minerals) when found in high concentrations. According to an article in *Contact Dermatitis* (December 1996, pages 337–343) even "Using the more mild wash procedure, skin sites treated under conditions of hard [water] were significantly drier, had more [redness], and were less hydrated than corresponding sites treated with [soft] water. All [three] surfactant cleansers behaved similarly. We also found the hardness of the rinse water to be the more significant factor versus that of the wash water."

According to several water-softening companies I called, the most economical way for you to soften household water is with an ion-exchange water softener. These units exchange the hard calcium and magnesium minerals for sodium, which has softening properties on skin. This can be a far less costly process than trying to find hair-care products that make your hair feel softer and fuller, when the issue is really the quality of your water supply.

What to expect: If you do choose to try a water softener in your home, you will find, when the "hard" minerals are removed from the water, that cleansers will no longer form a film and you won't get much of a "bathtub ring." You are also likely to experience a slippery feel on the skin and hair, almost too much "softness," and that can take awhile to get used to. Soft water can also tend to make hair more flyaway, which would call for different hair-care products than you would have used when your hair was being rinsed with hard water.

# CHOOSING THE BEST CLEANSER

Using the right cleanser makes all the difference in the world because it determines how your skin is going to react to everything else you put on it. Overcleaning your face and drying it out causes problems a moisturizer can't correct. Greasing up your skin with a wipe-off, cold cream–type cleanser can clog pores and leave a film on the skin, which means all the other products you put on will be sitting on top of that instead of being easily absorbed. Trying to degrease the skin with a drying toner after using this kind of greasy makeup remover can cause irritation and a range of other problems. Using a gentle, water-soluble cleanser is the best option for the entire face, and this is true for all skin types.

Most of us are familiar with the three primary categories of cleansers available: wipe-off cleansers (including cold creams and milky makeup removers), soaps of all kinds (including bar cleansers, which technically are not soap), and water-soluble cleansers (creamy, lotion, or shampoo-type cleansers that rinse off).

A good water-soluble cleanser is a terrific invention. It is a cross between a shampoo and a cold cream, and it is not a soap. What differentiates a good water-soluble cleanser from a poor one? Three basic qualities: (1) it washes off makeup without leaving the face dry (like soaps) or greasy (like cold cream), (2) it contains no fragrance (fragrance is an irritant, though water-soluble cleansers without fragrance are hard to find) or abrasive, scrublike particles (scrubs should be used carefully and judiciously not as part of cleaning skin), and (3) most important of all, it is gentle to the skin. Some cleansers on the market are labeled "water soluble," but in actuality they need to be wiped off with a wet washcloth. If the cleanser must be wiped off with a tissue or washcloth, it is anything but water-soluble. These types of cleansers may still be an option for someone with dry skin but only a very soft, nonabrasive washcloth will be gentle to skin.

Water-soluble cleansers are not only the gentlest way to clean the face, they are also the most efficient. Everything is done at the sink. Using a water-soluble cleanser eliminates the need for a separate eye-makeup remover or for boxes of tissues to wipe the face with. Imagine splashing your face generously with (tepid) water, then massaging a water-soluble cleanser on evenly over your face, including the eyes, and then rinsing it off with more water, preferably with your hands. Once the face is rinsed, it shouldn't feel greasy or dry.

I'm not referring to needing to use a washcloth with water to remove your cleanser when I say a product is water soluble. Water-soluble cleansers should splash off without the aid of a washcloth; if you prefer to use something besides your hands, use the softest washcloth you can find. Many people use smoother cloths on their kitchen counter than they do on their face!

Not all water-soluble cleansers are created equal, and finding a good one can be tricky. Just because a cleanser is labeled water-soluble doesn't mean it comes off with water or is gentle. Plenty of cleansers have names that sound great, with words like "Milky" or "Creamy" or "Foaming" or "Gel". But many of them leave the face feeling greasy and need to be wiped off, or they rinse off too well, leaving the face feeling dry and irritated.

I also recommend that you avoid water-soluble cleansers that contain AHAs, BHA, or disinfectants. These may be well-formulated products but they can all be irritating to the eye area, and because they are rinsed, the active ingredients are washed away before they have a chance to have their intended full, positive impact on the skin.

When I first began recommending water-soluble cleansers years ago, there was really only one available. That was Cetaphil Gentle Skin Cleanser, which is still available and is excellent for someone with dry, sensitive skin. Today, there are more water-soluble cleansers to choose from than I ever thought possible. Not all of them are really water soluble and many are too drying, but many are very gentle on the skin, remove all the makeup without causing irritation or dryness, do not burn the eyes, and leave no greasy residue.

One thing most water-soluble cleansers have in common, regardless of price, is the same basic ingredient list. You'll find they have water and one or more detergent cleansing agents such as sodium laureth sulfate, ammonium laureth sulfate, cocamidopropyl betaine, or sodium cocoamphopropionate, among others. Cleansers designed for dry skin often contain oils and leave a greasy residue. When someone with dry skin uses a cleanser supposedly designed for her skin type, and then follows that with a rich, creamy moisturizer, too many emollients can build up, causing the skin to look dull and preventing cell turnover. On the other hand, cleansers designed for normal to oily skin can contain one or more standard detergent agents that can be overly drying and irritating for skin, such as sodium lauryl sulfate, TEA lauryl sulfate, and sodium olefin sulfate (when listed as one of the first ingredients on the label). Drying out the skin is always a problem and often creates the artificial need for a moisturizer, which just greases things back up. This cycle of greasing up dry skin or drying out oily or combination skin causes more skin problems than almost any other facet of skin care.

The following information from an article in *Cutis* (December 2001, Supplemental, pages 12–19) nicely sums up the need for mild cleansing products: "The choice of a mild cleansing agent is important in the adjunctive management of various skin conditions, such as atopic dermatitis, acne vulgaris, rosacea, photoaging, retinoid-induced irritant dermatitis, and sensitive skin. There are 3 major categories of cleansing agents: soaps, synthetic detergents, and lipid-free cleansing agents. The irritancy potential of cleansing agents is a function of a number of factors, including the pH, type of surfactants, and amount of skin residue. Furthermore, the presence of humectants and emollients also can influence the overall mildness of a cleansing agent. Agents with slightly acidic or neutral pH, nonionic surfactants, and minimal skin residue may be preferable for people who are at increased risk for irritancy reactions."

In my book *Don't Go to the Cosmetics Counter Without Me*, I provide a complete summary of the best water-soluble cleansers for each skin type.

**Summary:** Use only water-soluble cleansers that rinse off completely when water is splashed on the face, leaving the face with a clean, soft feeling that is neither dry nor greasy. Creamy, water-soluble cleansers can be an option for dry skin as long as they are used with an extremely gentle washcloth.

**Basic directions:** Wash your hands first and then splash the face generously, including the eyes, with tepid water (not hot or cold). Once the face is soaking wet, take your cleanser and massage it generously all over the face, including the eyelids. Rinse very well. If traces of makeup are left behind, or if you have very oily skin, you may need to repeat this step. Another option is to first cleanse the eye area and rinse, then do the rest of the face separately and rinse again. Do this step twice a day or whenever you need to clean the face, whether or not you are wearing makeup. Use a gentle washcloth if you are wearing heavy makeup, ultra-matte foundations, or other hard-to-remove makeup.

# What About Bar Soap?

For many reasons it is best to avoid bar soap, especially from the neck up, but it can also be helpful to avoid it from the neck down. This is particularly true if you have problems with dry skin or breakouts. Just be aware that there are issues with using most bar soaps or bar cleansers no matter what type of skin you have.

Many women believe that the tight sensation they feel after washing with soap means that the face is clean. You know the feeling I'm talking about, where if you open your mouth it pulls the skin around your eyes? The thinking is that the more squeaky-clean your face feels, the better off you are. But that feeling you associate with being clean is nothing more than irritated, dried-out skin. The difficulty with asking someone to break a soap habit is that soap really does clean the skin thoroughly. Unfortunately, it cleans too thoroughly, and that can be irritating! If your skin feels tight for more than two minutes after you wash, you have to run to your moisturizer to prevent it from feeling pulled or taut; if you have oily skin, the oil resurfaces in seconds no matter how clean you felt initially; and if you have combination skin, you reinforce that dual condition.

The major issue with bar soap is its high alkaline content (meaning it has a high pH). "The increase of the skin pH irritates the physiological protective 'acid mantle', changes the composition of the cutaneous bacterial flora and the activity of enzymes in the upper epidermis, which have an acid pH optimum" (Source: *Dermatology*, March 1997, pages 258–262). That technical description basically explains that skin's normal pH is about 5.5, while most bar soaps have a pH of around 9 to 10, which negatively impacts the surface of skin by causing irritation and increasing the presence of bacteria in the skin. There is definitely research showing that washing with a cleanser that has a pH of 7 or higher, which is true for many bar soaps and bar cleansers, increases the presence of bacteria significantly when compared to using a cleanser with a pH of 5.5. (Sources: *Clinics in Dermatology*, January-February 1996, pages 23–27; *Dermatology*, 1995, volume 191, issue 4, pages 276–280).

What about specialty soaps that come in clear bars, have nonsoap-sounding names, or contain creams and emollients that appear to have none of the properties of regular soap? Bar cleansers (which are technically not soap) often have a lower pH and are therefore far less irritating to skin. However, the ingredients that keep the bar cleanser in its bar form can theoretically absorb into skin and clog pores. There is also no way for a consumer to test each particular bar to be sure the pH is compatible with skin. Further, many of the so-called gentle bar cleansers I've reviewed contain fairly drying, irritating, and potentially pore-clogging ingredients. So much for specialty soaps being different. Even worse, the soaps designed for oily or acned skin contain even harsher ingredients. Soaps designed for dry and sensitive skin often contain beneficial ingredients such as glycerin, petrolatum (mineral oil), or vegetable oil, and while they might make the face feel somewhat less stiff after you rinse, they won't prevent the irritation caused by the other ingredients.

Here's a rundown of some basic categories of soaps. Remember, just because a product is advertised as gentle doesn't mean it is.

*Castile soaps* use olive oil instead of animal fat, but the cleansing agent, sodium hydroxide, is still fairly irritating to the skin.

*Transparent soaps* look milder or less drying because of their unclouded, clear appearance, but many contain harsh cleansing ingredients, and the ingredients that give the bar its shape can clog pores.

*Deodorant soaps* are always irritating for the face and should be used only on other parts of the body, if at all. The ingredients used to reduce bacteria are too harsh for the delicate skin of the face and they don't stay on the skin long enough to have any real disinfecting effect.

*Acne soaps* often contain very irritating ingredients in addition to harsh cleansers that, especially when combined with other acne treatments, can super-irritate the skin. There is no reason to overclean the skin. Breakouts have nothing to do with how clean your skin is! A study in *Infection* (March-April 1995, pages 89–93) demonstrated that "in the group using soap the mean number of inflammatory [acne] lesions increased…. Symptoms or signs of irritation were seen in 40.4% of individuals…." Furthermore, if the acne cleanser contains antibacterial agents, the benefit would be washed down the drain.

*Cosmetic soaps* or bar cleansers are sold at the cosmetics counters for more money than they are worth. Although these are advertised as being gentle or specially formulated, they are no better than or different from what you can buy at the drugstore. The irritating and pore-clogging ingredients are still included regardless of the price or claim.

*Superfatted soaps* contain extra oils and fats that supposedly make them more gentle for the face. Basis Soap is one of the most popular superfatted specialty soaps. However, the extra glycerin, petrolatum, or beeswax in these soaps won't prevent irritation and can cause breakouts.

*Oatmeal soaps* are supposed to be better at absorbing oil and soothing sensitive skin than other soaps or bar cleansers. There are studies demonstrating that oatmeal can have anti-irritant properties. How that translates into a bar cleanser is unknown, but the benefits are probably nonexistent given the amount of time the oatmeal is actually on the skin and the presence of other irritating ingredients. Plus, the oatmeal particles are fairly large and end up usually being more abrasive on skin and that isn't gentle in the least.

*"Natural" soaps* are those that contain vitamins, fruits, vegetables, plants, flowers, herbs, aloe, and specialty oils; these ingredients are gimmicks and serve no purpose on the face. They don't nourish the skin or provide any other health benefit; that is sheer marketing whimsy and nothing more. Plus, the cleansing agents and the ingredients that keep the soap in bar form are the same as in any other bar cleanser.

*Beauty bars* such as Dove are about 50% sodium cocoyl isethionate (a form of coconut oil) and, although it is not as irritating as other cleansing agents found in soaps, it is still potentially irritating and drying, especially in such a high concentration. Dove claims to be moisturizing, and it does contain emollients to help soften the effect of the cleansing agent. If the manufacturers left out the drying and irritating ingredients altogether, they wouldn't need to add emollients to counteract them. Also, the ingredients that help the bar keep its shape can clog pores.

## WHAT DO TONERS TONE?

In reality, toners—also referred to as astringents, clarifiers, refiners, fresheners, and tonics—don't tone anything. At least not by the dictionary definition of "tone," which refers to the "normal firmness of a tissue or an organ." The term "toner" is a caprice invented by the cosmetics industry and, therefore, it can mean anything they want it to. I have heard that toners do everything from balance the skin and close pores to deep-clean and prepare the skin for other products. They do none of that. In fact, toners of any kind do not close pores; they do not deep-clean pores; and they do not reduce oil production. If toners could do any of that, given the repeated daily use of these items by most women, who would have a pore left?

There are no ingredients in toners that can firm skin and return it to its normal state. What well-formulated toners can do is help reduce inflammation, add water-binding agents and natural moisturizing factors to skin, help remove the last traces of makeup, and impart some lightweight moisturizing ingredients to skin. However, not all toners are created equal, and many are poorly formulated, meaning they have a real capacity to cause irritation, redness, and dryness. No matter what toners may be called (astringent, freshener, pore cleanser, clarifying lotion, witch hazel, and so on) and whether or not they are inexpensive or expensive—if they contain irritants they are bad for skin. The only toners you should ever consider using are those that are as irritant-free as possible.

In the past, the primary ingredient in most toners—even many of those designed for dry skin—was usually SD alcohol with a number following it. This is one of the kinds of alcohol that burn like crazy when you put them on a cut or wound, and it's extremely drying and irritating for all skin types.

Fortunately, the use of alcohol in toners has definitely decreased over the past several years. However, it still shows up in astringents and toners aimed at those with oily or acne-prone skin. If you were under the impression that alcohol is somehow helpful for acne you would be mistaken. For alcohol to be an effective disinfectant, it needs to be 60% to 70% pure alcohol. Most astringents are in the 20% range. Even at a 40% level, you would not get an effective disinfectant, although you would get an effective irritant that kills skin cells and destroys the skin's intercellular layer. Further, irritation and dryness deplete the skin's intercellular matrix and protective outer barrier, and that damages the skin's ability to heal at the same time it increases the presence of bacteria in the skin. All of that can only make breakouts worse in the long run (Source: *Archives of Dermatological Research*, 1995, volume 287, issue 2, pages 214–218).

**Note:** Do not be confused by cosmetics that contain ingredients that sound like alcohol but are not. For example, cetyl alcohol, stearyl, or other alcohol esters are not the type of alcohol I'm warning you about. Remember the ingredient list will say "SD alcohol" followed by a number, or use the term "ethanol" or "isopropyl alcohol" on the label. Those are the kinds to avoid.

Aside from alcohol, other irritating ingredients found in toner-type products include acetone (that's nail polish remover), citrus (lemon, grapefruit, and orange juice are incredibly irritating to the skin because of their high acid content), camphor, mint, peppermint, menthol, volatile plant extracts, fragrance (or essential oils, which are nothing more than fragrance additives), and witch hazel. All of these ingredients can hurt the skin because of irritation or skin sensitivity, and should be avoided.

If a toner does contain irritants, all that irritation does to a pore is temporarily cause it to swell, which can make the pore look smaller for maybe a few minutes. Toners that contain alcohol can remove the surface oil from the skin, but if you've cleansed the skin properly there should be no excess surface oil left. You can't get inside the pore with a toner to deep-clean it without causing damage (if you could, we would all have spotless, empty pores), so toners surely don't work in that capacity. Most of all, toners do not reduce oil production. Oil production is controlled primarily by hormonal activity (Source: *Medical Electron Microscopy*, March 2001, pages 29–40). There is nothing you can put topically on skin to stop the oil production triggered by hormones.

Irritant-free toners are an excellent skin-care option for all skin types. They are fine as an extra cleansing step after removing the cleanser. Toners can also soothe skin, lightly moisturize it, and provide some antioxidant and anti-irritant protection. For some skin types, a toner can be the only moisturizer needed. That makes irritant-free toners a wonderful cleansing, lightweight moisturizing aid. What is in these products that makes them beneficial to the skin? Well-formulated toners usually are a blend of water-binding agents, natural moisturizing factors, anti-irritants, antioxidants, lightweight emollients, and gentle cleansing agents. There are great toners in all price ranges.

It is best if the toner is fragrance-free, but those are hard to find. In my book *Don't Go to the Cosmetics Counter Without Me*, I provide a complete summary of the best toners for each skin type.

**Summary:** Many irritant-free toners are a fine alternative as an extra cleansing step after cleaning the skin with a water-soluble cleanser. Toners won't close pores and they won't deep-clean, but depending on the formulation they can leave the face feeling soft and smooth, remove the last traces of makeup or oil, reduce or eliminate irritation, provide antioxidant protection, soothe the skin, and lightly moisturizer skin. For some skin types, a toner can be the only moisturizer you need to use.

**Basic directions:** After cleansing the face, soak a large cotton ball with the toner and gently stroke it over the face and neck.

# EXFOLIATING THE SKIN

As I explained in Chapter Four, exfoliating skin or removing excess or built-up dead skin cells on the surface of skin or in the pore can be helpful for almost all skin types. During the 1970s the only way to exfoliate the skin was to use toners that contained alcohol, which literally burned skin cells off, leaving dry and irritated skin in their wake. In the 1980s, the main choices were mechanical scrubs with ingredients such as honey and almond pits, cleansers with scrub particles, facial masks, more irritating toners, and loofahs. Most of these worked, but they took a toll on the face and irritation was a typical problem. When it comes to mechanical scrubs, my favorite recommendation was and still is mixing Cetaphil Cleanser with baking soda to create an effective, gentle, and extraordinarily inexpensive scrub. Other mechanical scrubs, with their detergent cleansing agents and wax bases, just can't compare.

However, with the advent of alpha hydroxy acids (AHAs) and beta hydroxy acid (BHA), mechanical scrubs are now a supplement for exfoliation, not the primary choice. AHAs and BHA chemically exfoliate the skin instead of physically abrading it. Chemical exfoliation provides even exfoliation with less physical damage to the skin.

Remember that AHAs exfoliate the surface skin (they do not penetrate into the pore) and, therefore, are the best option for normal to dry skin or sun-damaged skin that doesn't break out. BHA can exfoliate the surface of skin as well as skin within the pore (BHA is lipid soluble) and is, therefore, preferred for those with normal to oily skin that is prone to breakouts or clogged pores.

I provide a complete summary of the best exfoliants for each skin type in my book *Don't Go to the Cosmetics Counter Without Me.*

**Summary:** For oily skin, one of the ways to keep pores from getting clogged is to help skin cells shed as freely as possible so they don't get trapped inside the pore. The more you keep skin cells exfoliating in a normal manner, both on the surface of the skin and inside the pore, the less cell debris can fill up the pore and obstruct oil flow out of the pore (Source: *Journal of the European Academy of Dermatology and Venereology*, 2001, volume 15, Supplement 3, pages 43–49).

When you help dry skin shed excess dried-up skin cells, it can make room for plumper, moisture-filled skin cells to come to the surface, which can lend a fresher look to the skin. It also allows moisturizers (the fewer and lighter, the better) to more easily penetrate the skin because there are fewer dried-up skin cells in the way to block absorption. Exfoliating helps the dead surface-skin cells to slough off evenly and at a more normal rate, making room for the lower layers of newer skin cells to arrive.

If you decide to use a reliable AHA product for dry or sun-damaged skin, or a BHA product for normal to oily skin or skin prone to breakouts, the question is: Do you still need to use a physical scrub? There is no definitive answer, so you will have to judge for yourself. Most women with normal to dry skin that is sensitive, allergic, or mature should use one, and only one, exfoliant and no other. Someone with normal to oily skin with breakouts can use a BHA product and may find benefit from a gentle physical exfoliant as well. Stick with Cetaphil Cleanser and baking soda for the gentlest results and listen closely to your skin; irritation is never the goal.

**Note:** The only skin types that may need to stay away from exfoliating are those with extremely sensitive skin, thin skin, and skin diseases or disorders such as rosacea, eczema, dermatitis, or seborrhea, unless approved by a dermatologist.

**Basic directions:** After cleansing and toning, when the skin is dry, place a small amount of AHA or BHA on your fingertips and smooth it over the entire face, avoiding direct contact with the eyes. First-time users who have sensitive skin should apply it once a day (preferably at night). Depending on your skin's tolerance, you may even want to apply it every other day. If the exfoliant you choose isn't in an emollient base or isn't emollient enough, apply a moisturizer over dry areas. In the morning, apply sunscreen after applying the exfoliant.

If you started out using the chemical exfoliant once a day or every other day, after four weeks you can start increasing usage to twice a day.

If you are using an alkaline cleanser such as bar soap (which you shouldn't be, but just in case you are), wait 15 minutes before applying any chemical exfoliant because the high pH of the cleanser can affect the acidity of the exfoliant. Nearly all other skin-care products are formulated with a pH of 7 or less (pH 7 is neutral, like water), with the majority around a pH of 5.5, and will not affect the efficacy of the AHA or BHA.

## SUNSCREEN

Regardless of the time of year, where you live, the color of your skin, or the amount of time you spend in the sun, sunscreen should be an essential part of your morning skin-care routine. It takes only a few minutes in the sun—the time it takes to walk to your car or to your office—for sun damage to begin. Over time this can cause serious wrinkling, even if you don't tan on a regular basis.

There are several ways to fit this vital skin-care step into your daily routine. Most sunscreens come in a moisturizing base, which means you most likely do not need any additional moisturizer if you have dry skin. As long as one of your daytime products (either a moisturizer or foundation) is an SPF 15 or greater that includes the UVA-protecting ingredients of avobenzone, titanium dioxide, or zinc oxide, it is a fine choice.

**Basic directions:** During the day, sunscreen is the last thing you apply to the skin because applying anything else over it could dilute its effectiveness. Sunscreen is applied after you have finished cleansing, applying toner, disinfectant, chemical exfoliant (AHA or BHA), topical prescription medications such as Retin-A, Renova, Tazorac, generic tretinoin, or Differin), and skin-lightening products. If you have very dry skin and feel the moisturizer in your sunscreen is not enough, you can apply a moisturizer over the drier areas and then apply sunscreen over that.

# MOISTURIZING

If you have dry skin, dry, wrinkled skin, or dry areas (like on the cheeks or around the eyes), you need a moisturizer; otherwise you don't. It's that simple. If you don't have dry skin or you have normal to oily skin, you can obtain many of the benefits moisturizers contain (antioxidants, anti-irritants, water-binding agents, natural moisturizing factors) in a well-formulated toner. Avoiding using a cream-, lotion-, or serum-style moisturizer when you don't have dry skin can help prevent breakouts and feeling greasy and shiny through your makeup by midday, and encourage your skin to do its own natural exfoliation.

Always use the lightest moisturizer capable of making your skin feel soft without feeling greasy or layered. There are more wonderful moisturizers available than bad ones. They contain a vast array of emollients, water-binding ingredients, natural moisturizing factors, soothing agents, anti-irritants, and antioxidants in a dizzying range of permutations with an equally dizzying range of prices. Unfortunately, there is no one formula I can point to as the single best one, so don't let the cosmetics industry convince you such a thing exists. It turns out there are hundreds and hundreds of great moisturizers with great ingredients and very few poor ones.

The worst thing about moisturizers is they are often overpriced and erroneously labeled as wrinkle creams, firming and lifting lotions, and serums to make them seem more exotic and miraculous than they really are. While women the world over search for the best wrinkle creams, you can be ahead of the game, and take better care of your skin, either by leaving this step out altogether (because you now know that overmoisturizing the skin is bad) or by using a great but inexpensive moisturizer that can do the job as well as, if not better than, the expensive stuff. Strangely enough, the expensive stuff almost always has too much fragrance (which can cause allergic reactions or irritation), too many plants (and, therefore, a higher risk of skin reactions), and coloring agents (products sell better if they look pretty, even if the result isn't better for the skin), and all of these can be problematic for skin.

The only thing that distinguishes a daytime moisturizer from a nighttime moisturizer is that the ones for daytime should include sunscreen. All the other claims and descriptions explaining why daytime products are different from nighttime products are bogus. Make sure your daytime moisturizer is rated SPF 15 or greater and contains the UVA-protecting ingredients avobenzone, titanium dioxide, and/ or zinc oxide. There are great, state-of-the-art moisturizers with sunscreen available, and more are being created all the time.

At night almost any moisturizer will do, depending on your skin type. Always use the lightest formula possible and only over dry areas. There is no reason to apply moisturizer where the skin isn't dry. And don't expect any moisturizer you apply at night to work by somehow "banking" or "depositing" the right ingredients in the skin so it would build up interest for the next day's wear and tear.

More than 100 excellent moisturizers are listed in my book *Don't Go to the Cosmetics Counter Without Me.* Refer to that summary to see if the moisturizer you are interested in has an acceptable formulation for your skin type.

**Basic directions:** During the day, follow the guidelines for applying the sunscreen. If you have dry skin that's your daytime moisturizer. At night, over clean, dry, or slightly damp skin, sparingly apply the moisturizer over dry areas. Dab it on and let it be absorbed; don't rub it in (rubbing isn't good for the skin). At night, moisturizer is the last thing you apply. If you are using an AHA or BHA product in an emollient base, or using Renova, which comes in a moisturizing base, azelaic acid in a cream base, or Differin in a cream form, that is the last thing you apply and probably the only moisturizer your skin needs. If you feel some areas of your face need a little more moisturizer, apply that to the drier areas of the face after you've applied the AHA, BHA, Renova, Retin-A, azelaic acid, or Differin.

## WHAT ABOUT EYE CREAMS?

Most women believe that eye creams are specially formulated for the skin around the eye area. Although the eye area does tend to be more prone to allergic or sensitizing reactions and often shows wrinkles before other areas of the face, it turns out that product formulations for eye creams don't differ from those for face products. There is no evidence, research, or documentation validating the claim that eye creams have special formulations setting them apart from other facial moisturizers. It only takes a quick look at the ingredient labels of any moisturizer or eye moisturizer to see that they don't differ except for the price and the tiny containers the eye creams come in. Eye creams are a whim of the cosmetics industry designed to evoke the sale of two products when only one is needed.

The only time you might want to use a different product around the eyes is if the skin there happens to indeed be different from the skin on the rest of the face. For example, if your face is normal to oily and doesn't require a moisturizer except occasionally on the cheeks or around the eyes, then an emollient, well-formulated moisturizer of any kind will work beautifully.

Ironically, one of the drawbacks of many so-called eye creams is that they rarely contain sunscreen. For daytime, that makes most eye creams a serious problem for the health of skin. You could believe that you were doing something special for your eyes, but you would actually be putting them at risk of sun damage and wrinkling by using an eye cream without sunscreen. This is another example of the way cosmetics marketing and misleading information can waste your money and hurt your skin.

## DRY PATCHES OF SKIN

There are many reasons why skin can develop dry patches. Makeup left on overnight can cause irritant or allergic reactions; then there are drying skin-care products, dermatitis, eczema, and heavy moisturizers that can cause a buildup of dead skin cells. Any and all of these can contribute to dry patches of skin. The best advice is to avoid drying skin-care products and use only the lightest-weight moisturizer for dry skin areas.

If the dry patches are chronic or itchy, they are probably a form of topical dermatitis or eczema and may require treatment by a dermatologist. If you've done your best to eliminate the cause of the problem and the problem persists, one of the best ways to calm down the appearance of dry patches is with an over-the-counter cortisone cream. Lanacort and Cortaid are 1% hydrocortisone creams meant for dry patches of skin, for short-term use only. It is amazing how effective they can be. If the problem lingers, consult a dermatologist, but for many people this is all it takes.

## DRY UNDERNEATH AND OILY ON TOP

Several things can cause the combination of a layer of dry, flaky skin combined with oily skin. Often using the wrong combination of skin-care products causes this condition. An emollient, wipe-off cleanser, followed by a toner that is too emollient for your skin type, and then an unnecessarily emollient moisturizer can prevent the lower layer of skin from exfoliating, creating a thick, dry, flaky lower layer and a greasy layer on top. Conversely, if you have oily skin, using a drying face cleanser followed by a toner with irritating or drying ingredients, and then an emollient moisturizer can create the same condition. The drying toner and cleanser can cause the skin to be dry and flaky, while the emollient moisturizer adds to your own excess oil production, aggravating it and making the skin look both oily and dehydrated. The condition of dry skin underneath and oily skin on top rarely requires additional skin-care products. Instead, taking a completely different approach and eliminating overly drying or overly emollient products can help a great deal.

It is also possible that the dry layer covered by an oily layer could be a result of psoriasis, rosacea, seborrhea, or eczema. Chapter Twelve, *Skin Disorders*, deals with these skin problems at length.

# SKIN LIGHTENING

Brown spots on skin are called chloasma or melasma and can happen for several reasons. One repercussion of sun damage is areas of skin discoloration known as solar lentigenes, more popularly called liver spots, sun spots, or age spots. They are definitely not associated with the liver, but they often have everything to do with unprotected sun exposure. On lighter skin types, solar lentigenes emerge as small brown patches of freckling that grow over time. On women with darker skin tones, they appear as small patches of ashen-gray skin that tend to enlarge over time.

Brown or ashen patches of skin can also occur due to birth control pills, pregnancy, or estrogen replacement therapy. In those instances, the discoloration is referred to as pregnancy masking or hormone masking.

Regardless of the source, the issue is the same: site-specific, increased melanin production, or hyperpigmentation. Melanin is the pigment or coloring agent of skin. It is created by melanin synthesis, a complex process controlled partly by an enzyme called tyrosinase.

When it comes to selecting treatment for these areas, one important factor to consider is the depth of the discolored pigment within the skin. In most situations the discoloration is superficial. In a few cases, the discoloration lies deep in the dermis. If the pigment is in the epidermis, it can be helped with skin-lightening products, both over-the-counter and prescription types. If the pigment is deeper, laser treatments are a consideration. For topical treatments, according to an article in the *American Journal of Clinical Dermatology* (September-October 2000, pages 261–268), "[T]opical hydroquinone 2 to 4% alone or in combination with tretinoin 0.05 to 0.1% is an established treatment. Topical azelaic acid 15 to 20% can be as efficacious as hydroquinone…. Tretinoin is especially useful in treating hyperpigmentation of photoaged skin. Kojic acid, alone or in combination with glycolic acid or hydroquinone, has shown good results, due to its inhibitory action on tyrosinase. Chemical peels are [also] useful to treat melasma."

## SUNSCREEN

Diligent use of a sunscreen alone allows some repair as well as protection from further photodamage (Source: *British Journal of Dermatology*, December 1996, pages 867–875). No other aspect of controlling or reducing skin discolorations is as important as the use of sunscreen, SPF 15 or greater with the UVA-protecting ingredients avobenzone, titanium dioxide, or zinc oxide. Using skin-lightening products or laser treatments without also using a sunscreen is a waste of time. Sun exposure is one of the primary, fundamental causes of hypermelanin production. Before you consider any other treatment for skin discolorations, this is unconditionally the first and most practical step.

## LASER TREATMENTS

Pigment deep in the dermis does not respond well to topical agents. Resurfacing procedures such as chemical peels and laser treatments may significantly help some of these problems, but the results are not consistent, problems can occasionally occur, and without strict use of a sunscreen with UVA-protecting ingredients the discolorations almost always come back. Moreover, laser treatments of this kind are often a problem for those with darker skin tones. However, after taking all of the risks into consideration, when laser treatments do work they can make a marked difference in the appearance of the face, arms, hands, and chest, which are the areas of the body most prone to hypermelanin production. The results can be startling, and completely eliminate any appearance of the problem.

## HYDROQUINONE

Over-the-counter skin-lightening products often contain 2% hydroquinone, while 4% concentrations are available only from a physician. Hydroquinone is a strong inhibitor of melanin production (Source: *Journal of Dermatological Science*, August 2001, Supplemental, pages S68–S75), meaning that it lightens skin color. Hydroquinone does not bleach the skin (calling it a bleaching agent is a misnomer); it only disrupts the synthesis of melanin hyperpigmentation.

Hydroquinone in the medical literature is considered the primary topical ingredient for inhibiting melanin production. Using it in combination with other options listed here can make a marked difference in the appearance of skin discolorations (Sources: *Journal of Cosmetic Science*, May-June 1998, pages 208–290; *Dermatological Surgery*, May 1996, pages 443–447).

Some concerns about hydroquinone's safety on skin have been mentioned, but research indicates that reactions are minor or a result of using extremely high concentrations (Source: *Critical Reviews in Toxicology*, May 1999, pages 283–330).

According to Howard I. Maibach, MD, Professor of Dermatology at the University of California School of Medicine, San Francisco, "Overall, adverse events reported with the use of hydroquinone ... have been relatively few and minor in nature.... To date there is no evidence of adverse systemic reactions following the use of hydroquinone"—and it has been around for over 30 years in skin-care products. Maibach also stated that "hydroquinone is undoubtedly the most active and safest skin-depigmenting substance...." Research supporting Maibach's contentions was published in the *Journal of Toxicology and Environmental Health* (1998, pages 301–317).

Hydroquinone can be an unstable ingredient in cosmetic formulations. Upon exposure to air or sunlight it can turn a strange shade of brown. It is thus essential, when you are considering a hydroquinone product, to be sure it is packaged in nontransparent container that doesn't let light in and that minimizes the amount of air exposure. Hydroquinone products packaged in jars are not recommended because once opened they quickly become ineffective.

## TRETINOIN

A great deal of research shows that the use of tretinoin (all-trans retinoic acid) is effective in treating skin discolorations (Sources: *Acta Dermato-Venereologica*, July 1999, pages 305–310; *International Journal of Dermatology*, April 1998, pages 286–292; *Journal of the American Academy of Dermatology*, March 1997, pages S27–S36). However, the response to treatment is less marked than with hydroquinone or azelaic acid. Results can also take far longer with tretinoin than with other treatments, requiring at least six months or more before improvement is seen. As such, tretinoin is generally not recommended as the only treatment option for skin discoloration, but is used in combination with other effective topicals (Source: *eMedicine Journal*, www.emedicine.com, November 15, 2001, volume 2, number 11). Even though tretinoin can be disappointing for skin lightening, that should in no way diminish the critical role it plays in the overall improvement in skin from the standpoint of cell production, collagen production, elasticity, skin texture, and dermal thickness. Tretinoin in combination with more effective skin-lightening treatments is a powerful alliance in the battle against sun-damaged and aged skin.

## ALPHA HYDROXY ACIDS

Alpha hydroxy acid products, in and of themselves, in concentrations of 4% to 10% are not effective for inhibiting melanin production and thereby won't lighten skin discolorations. However, there is evidence that in combination with other treatments such as kojic acid, hydroquinone, azelaic acid, and laser resurfacing they can be very effective for improving the overall appearance of sun-damaged skin and possibly help the other ingredients penetrate the skin better.

Much like laser treatments do, AHA peels (using 50% concentrations) have impressive results for removing skin discolorations (Source: *Dermatological Surgery*, June 1999, pages 450–454). Only a physician should perform these types of facial peels.

## KOJIC ACID

Kojic acid is a by-product in the fermentation process of malting rice for use in the manufacture of sake, the Japanese rice wine. There is definitely convincing research, both in vitro and in vivo, and also in animal studies, showing kojic acid to be effective for inhibiting melanin production (Source: *Archives of Pharmacal Research*, August 2001, pages 307–311). Both glycolic acid and kojic acid or glycolic acid with hydroquinone are highly effective in reducing the pigment in melasma patients (Source: *Dermatological Surgery*, May 1996, pages 443–447). So why aren't there more products available containing kojic acid? Kojic acid is an extremely unstable ingredient in cosmetics formulations. Upon exposure to air or sunlight it can turn a strange shade of brown and lose its efficacy. Many cosmetics companies use kojic dipalmitate as an alternative because it is far more stable in formulations. However, there is no research showing kojic dipalmitate is as effective as kojic acid, though it is a good antioxidant.

## AZELAIC ACID

Azelaic acid is a component of grains such as wheat, rye, and barley. It is effective for a number of skin conditions when applied topically in a cream formulation at a 20% concentration. For the most part, azelaic acid is recommended as an option for acne treatment, but there is also some research showing it to be effective for the treatment of skin discolorations. For example, "The efficacy of 20% azelaic acid cream and 4% hydroquinone cream, both used in conjunction with a broad-spectrum sunscreen, against melasma was investigated in a 24-week, double-blind study with 329 women. Over the treatment period the azelaic acid cream yielded 65% good or excellent results; no significant treatment differences were observed with regard to overall rating, reduction in lesion size, and pigmentary intensity. Severe side effects such as allergic sensitization or exogenous ochronosis were not observed with azelaic acid" (Source: *International Journal of Dermatology*, December 1991, pages 893–895). However, other research suggests that azelaic acid is more irritating than hydroquinone mixed with glycolic acid or kojic acid (Source: *eMedicine Journal*, www.emedicine.com, November 5, 2001, volume 2, number 11). Azelaic acid is a consideration for skin lightening if you have had problems using hydroquinone along with tretinoin.

## ARBUTIN

Plant-derived skin-care ingredients send a definite siren call to consumers. Anyone developing "natural" alternatives to hydroquinone has an eager audience ready and willing to give it a try. To that end, arbutin, a hydroquinone derivative isolated from the leaves of the bearberry shrub, cranberry, blueberry, and most types of pears, serves that purpose.

Because of arbutin's hydroquinone content it can have melanin-inhibiting properties (Source: *Journal of Pharmacology and Experimental Therapeutics*, February 1996, pages 765–769). Although the research describing arbutin's effectiveness is persuasive (even if most of the research has been done on animals or in vitro), concentration protocols have not been established. That means we just don't know how much arbutin it takes to have an effect in lightening the skin. Moreover, most cosmetics companies don't use "arbutin" in their products because there are patents controlling its use in skin-care products for skin lightening. To get around this problem many cosmetics companies use plant extracts that contain arbutin, such as bearberry. No research exists showing that the plant-sourced arbutin has any impact on skin and especially not in the tiny amounts it is used in cosmetics. The only product I've seen with a pure and rather high concentration of arbutin (about 5%) is Shiseido's Whitess Intensive Skin Brightener *($120 for 1.4 ounces)*. I doubt if it's really worth the price just to see if this amount of arbutin can have an effect on skin as an alternative to hydroquinone, given that arbutin doesn't work any better than hydroquinone. Plus this product contains alcohol and menthol, which would make it potentially as irritating to skin as hydroquinone.

## MAGNESIUM ASCORBYL PHOSPHATE

This form of vitamin C is considered stable and an effective antioxidant for skin. For skin lightening there is only a single study showing it to be effective for inhibiting melanin production (Source: *Journal of the American Academy of Dermatology*, January 1996, pages 29–33). The study concluded that a moisturizer with a 10% concentration of magnesium ascorbyl phosphate "suppressed melanin formation.... The lightening effect was significant in 19 of 34 patients with chloasma or senile freckles and in 3 of 25 patients with normal skin." One study is not exactly anything to write home about, not to mention that at present there are no products on the market containing 10% magnesium ascorbyl phosphate. Most skin-care products containing magnesium ascorbyl phosphate have less than a 1% concentration.

## COMBINATION TREATMENTS

Diligent and consistent use of sunscreen with the UVA-protecting ingredients of avobenzone, titanium dioxide, or zinc oxide, is the first line of defense when tackling skin discolorations. Many researchers feel that 2% to 4% hydroquinone lotions can be more effective when combined with Retin-A or Renova and AHAs. Higher strengths of hydroquinone (over 2%) are available only from a physician and can possibly help deeper sources of pigment discoloration, although they can be a problem for darker skin tones. It is also extremely helpful to consider chemical peels or laser treatments to remove or lighten skin discolorations and then use topicals to maintain the improvement (Source: *Cosmetic Dermatology*, August 2001, pages 13–16).

# FACIAL MASKS

If there is one truly optional step in skin care, masks are it. Whatever miraculous properties are attributed to masks, no research supports the assertions of benefit attributed to the special muds, minerals, vitamins, or plant life these products contain. These exotic components range from seaweed to volcanic earth, unusual muds, enzymes, vitamins, and just about anything else you can think of, all associated with a fantastic jumble of characteristics to make the products seem life-altering for your skin. Cellulite is smoothed, wrinkles are eliminated, and acne is cured all with the application of a facial mask! I would offer to sell you a bridge if you believe any of this, but there aren't enough bridges in the world to accommodate the number of women taken in by these claims.

A recent example of the insanity regarding facial masks or mud mask spa treatments are the preposterous claims that revolve around moor mud. Depending on the Web site, the multitude of claims made for this substance range from curing vaginitis to healing arthritis, acne, and wrinkles. Based on the fact that it was used by the Romans in 120 B.C. (at least that was the information proffered by several spas offering moor mud treatments), the association with ancient medicine must have value. (Though I doubt any of the people proposing these claims would want to get sick in ancient Rome.) Here are the qualities another spa attributed to their moor mud: "As biological beings, the atoms in the human body have an intrinsic affinity for like atoms in nature, so whether moor products are taken internally or externally, the body automatically extracts the substance it needs to reestablish order and harmony." First, if that were accurate then there would be no risk of poisonous substances in nature, and that simply is not true. Moor mud refers to wet earth with a limited ability to grow plant life because of the acidic nature of the land.

Other claims for masks say they offer the benefit of detoxifying properties. Again, there is no research showing this to be the case, but the world of cosmetics or spa treatments is all about outlandish claims, not proof. To begin with, what exactly are these toxins that need to be eliminated from our bodies, and that supposedly cause so many skin problems? Where is the information or data indicating exactly what toxins need to be removed from the body and how is this taking place? If it is possible to "detox" by the application of a facial mask, what biological or physiological process is taking place to allow that to happen? Are the toxins being leached through skin? Drained out of the body in some fashion? This all adds up to magic along with some murky smoke and mirrors. It isn't based on a shred of reality.

Despite the litany of bogus claims ascribed to facial masks, they still can have a benefit for some skin types. Someone with dry skin may find an emollient facial mask soothing and relaxing. Someone with oily skin may find a facial mask with oil-absorbing properties beneficial. It is that uncomplicated.

Facial masks, by their very design, are meant to be used occasionally. But they are much like dieting or exercising—when it is done occasionally, little gain can be derived. The skin's need for antioxidants or anti-irritant protection, skin barrier repair, or (for someone with breakouts) the need for disinfecting or oil absorption is a daily one, not solved by a once-a-week fix.

## SHOULD YOU GET A FACIAL?

I suspect there is more pressure lately to spend money on facials than ever before. The rapid proliferation of day spas, which seem to be showing up in every hair salon and mall from Manhattan to Los Angeles, probably brought this form of beauty treatment back into the spotlight. While there are reasons to consider having a facial, it is very important to keep in mind that there is very little a licensed aesthetician can provide that regular use of good skin-care products can't duplicate—and do better.

(Let me emphasize the need to consult only a licensed aesthetician. Although "licensed" doesn't tell you anything about the capability of the aesthetician, it does mean the person has been trained in sanitation and application techniques and, more to the point, has been tested on those procedures and is certified to be able to accomplish those tasks. Of course, while that is just the beginning of what you should expect in the care of your skin, it is essential to know that your skin will be handled in as safe and hygienic a manner as possible.)

Given the popularity and effectiveness of high-concentration alpha hydroxy acid peels and the occasional or regular need to remove stubborn blackheads and deep-rooted blemishes, facials can indeed play an important role in a person's skin-care needs. AHA peels at concentrations of 20% to 35% with a pH of 3.5 are extremely effective at providing a temporarily smooth appearance to the skin. That is within the ability of a good facialist, and the results can be very satisfying. But be extremely cautious. This is, at best, a controversial salon treatment. Many cosmetic surgeons and dermatologists (and the FDA) consider AHA peels unsafe when done by some-one without medical training. That is an extremely rational concern, especially con-sidering the wide disparity in training and licensing, even though there are plenty of doctors who charge exorbitant prices for AHA peels but have an assistant or an aesthetician in their office perform the service instead.

When it comes to acne, a reliable aesthetician can definitely soften the skin and safely remove blackheads and blemishes without scarring. In cases like these, there is every reason in the world to get a facial every six weeks to every other month. But please don't expect any of this to permanently stop breakouts. If anything, facialists can get carried away with applying creams and masks, and rubbing and wiping at the skin, which can cause blemishes and irritation. **Keep in mind that the skin-care products sold by facialists and spas are not any more effective or better formulated than those sold anywhere else.**

Along with the viable and relaxing facial treatments out there, a whole host of facial masks and procedures that pass as premium skin care are really nothing more than a waste of time and money. Lymph drainage treatments are one of the many spa services that are claimed to rid the body of toxins, cellulite, wrinkles, and on and on. Lymph massage does have validity for those with lymphedema, a consequence of diseases such as cancer that require the removal of lymph nodes. However, the massage associated with lymphedema is not about "draining" lymph or removing toxins. Rather it is about preventing the pooling of lymph into the extremities when the lymph system has been compromised in a given area.

The concept of draining lymph glands from the outside in to remove toxins makes as much sense as the idea of draining your hormonal system or blood system from the outside in. The lymph system carries our body's immune defenses. Lymph runs through the body like blood does, in veins and capillaries. You wouldn't want someone draining your blood or hormones (without lots of proof that it was safe and worthwhile), and the same goes for the lymph.

# CHAPTER 7

# SKIN-CARE BATTLE PLANS

## GETTING STARTED

The following list is a fairly comprehensive compilation of the most effective skin-care routines for different skin types. Remember, before you choose a routine for your specific skin type, you must determine if what you are seeing or feeling on your skin is being caused by the skin-care products you are presently using.

Whatever is happening to your skin indicates the direction you should follow, which may indicate treating several different needs at the same time. If your cheeks are dry, your forehead is breaking out, and you have some brown discolorations and patches of rosacea, it will take a combination of products used on different parts of the face to address each issue.

Moreover, your skin-care needs may change depending on the time of year or the climate you find yourself in. **Respond to what you see or feel on your face and change what you are doing based on what your skin is telling you.** (This always assumes that you are using gentle, nonirritating, and nondrying products on your skin.) For example, the cleanser you are using may be fine in a humid, temperate environment, but it may be too drying for an arid, hot climate. It will take some experimentation to find what feels best for your skin in different situations, paying attention to what works and what doesn't. You can always refer to my book *Don't Go to the Cosmetics Counter Without Me* to see if the product you are using could be causing your skin problems.

**Exception to the rule:** Although it is best to only treat what is happening with your skin now, some skin-care problems require consistency even when the problem is not present on the face. If you tend to break out or have psoriasis, rosacea, or seborrhea, a consistent program is essential. For breakouts you must use an exfoliant and disinfectant daily in order to see a continued difference. I explain in Chapter Ten, *Battle Plans for Blemishes*, why you can't spot-treat blemishes. For psoriasis, rosacea, or seborrhea, consistent treatment is also paramount even when the problem isn't present.

The chapters preceding this elaborate on some of the more challenging skin-care dilemmas women face. Here I list some basic skin-care steps for all skin types.

### Normal Skin with no signs of wrinkles or sun damage

A.M.

Water-soluble cleanser

Toner

Sunscreen in a lightweight or matte base (SPF 15 or greater with avobenzone, titanium dioxide, and/or zinc oxide)

P.M.

Water-soluble cleanser

Toner (optional)

Lightweight moisturizer (only over dry patches and around the eyes)

### Normal Skin with signs of wrinkles or sun damage

A.M.

Water-soluble cleanser

Toner (optional)

Sunscreen (SPF 15 or greater with avobenzone, titanium dioxide, and/or zinc oxide in a lightweight moisturizing base)

P.M.

Water-soluble cleanser

Toner (optional)

AHA in a lightweight lotion (can be used in the A.M. as well)

Tretinoin product

Skin-lightening product

Moisturizer for dry areas, including the eyes

### Oily Skin with no signs of wrinkles or sun damage

A.M.

Water-soluble cleanser

Toner (optional)

BHA product in a gel or liquid base

Sunscreen (preferably in a foundation or a very lightweight lotion base with SPF 15 or greater containing avobenzone, titanium dioxide, and/or zinc oxide)

P.M.

Water-soluble cleanser

Toner (optional)

BHA product in a gel base
Moisturizer (for dry areas only, including the eyes)
Absorbent facial mask

## Oily Skin with signs of wrinkles or sun damage

A.M.
Water-soluble cleanser
Toner (optional)
Moisturizer (for dry areas only, including the eyes)
Sunscreen (preferably in a foundation or a very lightweight lotion base with SPF 15 or greater containing avobenzone, titanium dioxide, and/or zinc oxide)

P.M.
Water-soluble cleanser
Toner (optional)
BHA product in a gel base
Skin-lightening product (optional)
Tretinoin product (optional)
Moisturizer (for dry areas only, including the eyes)
AVOID absorbent facial masks

## Combination Skin

A.M.
Water-soluble cleanser
Toner (optional)
BHA product in a gel or liquid base
Moisturizer (for dry areas only, including the eyes)
Sunscreen (preferably in a foundation rated SPF 15 or greater with avobenzone, titanium dioxide, and/or zinc oxide)

P.M.
Water-soluble cleanser
Toner (optional)
BHA product in a gel or liquid base
Tretinoin product
Moisturizer (for dry areas only, including the eyes)
Absorbent facial mask over oily areas only

## Combination Skin prone to breakouts

A.M.
Water-soluble cleanser

Toner (optional)
Topical disinfectant (only over areas with breakouts)
BHA product in a gel or liquid base
Moisturizer (for dry areas only, including the eyes)
Sunscreen (preferably in a foundation rated SPF 15 or greater with avobenzone, titanium dioxide, and/or zinc oxide)

P.M.
Water-soluble cleanser
Toner (optional)
Topical disinfectant (only over areas with breakouts—but not benzoyl peroxide if you are using Retin-A, Differin, Avita, Tazorac, or generic tretinoin)
BHA product in a gel or liquid base
Tretinoin product
Moisturizer (for dry areas only, including the eyes)
Absorbent facial mask over oily areas only

**Combination Skin with signs of wrinkles or sun damage
and prone to breakouts**
A.M.
Water-soluble cleanser
Toner (optional)
Topical disinfectant (only over areas with breakouts—but not benzoyl peroxide if you are using Retin-A, Differin, Avita, Tazorac, or generic tretinoin)
BHA product in a gel or liquid base
Moisturizer (for dry areas only, including the eyes)
Sunscreen (preferably in a foundation rated SPF 15 or greater with avobenzone, titanium dioxide, and/or zinc oxide)

P.M.
Water-soluble cleanser
Toner (optional)
BHA product in a gel or liquid base
Topical disinfectant (only over areas with breakouts—but not benzoyl peroxide if you are using Retin-A, Differin, Avita, Tazorac, or generic tretinoin)
Tretinoin product
Skin-lightening product
Moisturizer (for dry areas only, including the eyes)
Absorbent facial mask over oily areas only

### Dry Skin with no signs of wrinkles or sun damage

A.M.

Water-soluble cleanser

Toner (optional)

Moisturizer

Sunscreen in a moisturizing base (rated SPF 15 with avobenzone, titanium dioxide, and/or zinc oxide)

P.M.

Water-soluble cleanser

Toner (optional)

AHA product in a moisturizing base

Moisturizer (over dry areas)

### Dry skin with signs of wrinkles or sun damage

A.M.

Water-soluble cleanser

Toner (optional)

Moisturize

Sunscreen in a moisturizing base (rated SPF 15 or greater with avobenzone, titanium dioxide, and/or zinc oxide)

P.M.

Water-soluble cleanser

Toner (optional)

AHA product in a moisturizing base

Tretinoin product

Skin-lightening product

Moisturizer (over extremely dry areas)

### Very Dry Skin and Fragile Dry Skin

Follow Dry Skin routine above, only at night the last thing to apply is plain olive oil, or another non-volatile plant oil such as sweet almond or evening primrose, over excessively dry areas

### Sensitive/Allergy-Prone Oily Skin

A.M.

Water-soluble cleanser

Toner (optional)

Over-the-counter cortisone cream (only when irritation or skin reactions occur—if skin reactions are persistent seek medical advice)

Sunscreen (preferably in a foundation rated SPF 15 or greater with titanium dioxide and/or zinc oxide as the only actives, and no other sunscreen agent)

P.M.

Water-soluble cleanser

Toner (optional)

Over-the-counter cortisone cream (only when irritation or skin reactions occur—if skin reactions are persistent seek medical advice)

BHA in a gel or liquid solution

Lightweight moisturizer (over dry patches or around the eyes)

### Sensitive/Allergy-Prone Dry Skin

A.M.

Water-soluble cleanser

Toner (optional)

Over-the-counter cortisone cream (only when irritation or skin reactions occur—if skin reactions are persistent seek medical advice)

Sunscreen in an emollient moisturizing base, SPF 15 or greater, with titanium dioxide and/or zinc oxide as the only actives, and no other sunscreen agent

P.M.

Water-soluble cleanser

Toner (optional)

Over-the-counter cortisone cream (only when irritation or skin reactions occur—if skin reactions are persistent seek medical advice)

BHA in a moisturizing base

Moisturizer

### Rosacea with oily, flaky skin

A.M.

Water-soluble cleanser

MetroGel, MetroLotion, or azelaic acid 20% (prescription-only topical medications)

Sunscreen (preferably in a foundation rated SPF 15 or greater with titanium dioxide and/or zinc oxide as the only actives, and no other sunscreen agent)

P.M.

Water-soluble cleanser

MetroGel, MetroLotion, or azelaic acid 20% (prescription-only topical medications)

BHA product in a gel or lotion base

### Rosacea with dry, flaky skin

A.M.

Water-soluble cleanser

MetroLotion, MetroCream, or azelaic acid 20% (prescription-only topical medications)

Sunscreen in a moisturizing base, SPF 15 or greater with titanium dioxide and/or zinc oxide as the only actives, and no other sunscreen agent

P.M.

Water-soluble cleanser

MetroLotion, MetroCream, or azelaic acid 20% (prescription-only topical medications)

BHA in a moisturizing or lotion base

Emollient moisturizer (for dry areas)

For other prescription options for rosacea refer to Chapter Twelve, *Skin Disorders*.

### Seborrhea

A.M.

Water-soluble cleanser

BHA product and/or prescription steroids and coal-tar lotions

Sunscreen in a moisturizing base, SPF 15 or greater with titanium dioxide and/or zinc oxide as the only actives, and no other sunscreen agent

P.M.

Water-soluble cleanser

BHA product and/or prescription steroids and coal-tar lotions

Emollient moisturizer (for dry areas)

For associated prescription options for seborrhea refer to Chapter Twelve, *Skin Disorders*.

### Psoriasis

A.M.

Water-soluble cleanser

BHA product

Sunscreen in a moisturizing base, SPF 15 or greater with titanium dioxide and/or zinc oxide as the only actives, and no other sunscreen agent

P.M.

Water-soluble cleanser

BHA product

Emollient moisturizer (for dry areas)

For associated prescription options for psoriasis refer to Chapter Twelve, *Skin Disorders.*

### Any skin type with patches of dermatitis, eczema, or rashlike areas

A.M. & PM

Follow the skin-care regime for your skin type. Before applying the appropriate sunscreen, apply an over-the-counter cortisone cream over inflamed areas only and only intermittently. (Lanacort® and Cortaid® are over-the-counter cortisone creams found at the drugstore.) Repeated use of topical cortisones can thin skin. If your skin condition persists seek medical advice.

**All Skin Types prone to blemishes or blackheads:** see Chapter Ten, *Battle Plans for Blemishes.*

# CHAPTER 8

## BATTLE PLANS
## FOR WRINKLES

Note: Cosmetic medical procedures such as BoTox and face-lifts as well as some spa procedures such as microdermabrasion and low-concentration chemical peels are discussed in Chapter Thirteen, *Cosmetic Surgery*.

## HOW SKIN AGES AND WRINKLES

How the skin ages and wrinkles is a very complicated process that involves an almost limitless range of physiological occurrences. There isn't any one cause that can be addressed with a cosmetic to erase or minimize the inevitable, because the "aging" process itself is so complex and intricate. Skin, all by itself, ages in many identifiable ways. Adding one plant extract or a vitamin to the skin won't address what is needed to deal with the myriad issues for slowing down the aging process. A series of extrinsic factors (sun damage, pollution, free-radical damage, smoking) and intrinsic factors (genetically predetermined cell cessation, chronological aging, hormone depletion, immune suppression) all culminate in what we define as aged skin.

It isn't just oxygen depletion, free-radical damage, collagen destruction, reduced cell turnover, abnormal cell formation, decreased fat content, intercellular deficiency, genetically predetermined cell shutdown, hormone loss, and so on, that affect the way skin ages—it is a combination of all these things and more taking place.

Looking at the issue objectively can help us better understand what is happening to our skin and what can and can't be done for it. Gaining insight into why wrinkle products make the claims they do and why it is most unlikely that they can actually live up to those claims will ultimately benefit our skin and our budget, too. For example, while we know that collagen and elastin, the support structures of the skin, break down and flatten as a result of repeated sun exposure, they also become less pliant and more hardened with age, so the skin becomes less elastic. Some products claim to only build collagen or only improve elastin. That is much like building a house with only cross beams and no support beams. One without the other is useless because the house won't stay erect without both of them.

It would take an entire book to evaluate every element of the skin affected by intrinsic (genetically induced) and extrinsic (environmentally induced) age factors, but it is important to get a basic sense of what is taking place to better understand why most antiaging or antiwrinkle creams can't possibly live up to their claims.

For example, one notable characteristic of older skin versus younger skin is that younger skin has more fat cells in the dermis than older skin. That is one reason older skin looks more transparent and thinner than younger skin and why someone 30 pounds or more overweight tends to have fewer wrinkles. Furthermore, for some unknown reason, the skin keeps growing and expanding as we age, despite the fact that the supporting fat tissues of the lower layers of skin are decreasing. That is why the skin begins to sag: Too much skin is being produced, but there aren't enough bones (remember, bone also deteriorates with age) and fat to shore it up. Simultaneously, the facial muscles lose their shape and firmness, giving the face a drooping appearance.

Certain components of the skin also become depleted with age. The water-retaining and texture-enhancing elements in the intercellular structure such as ceramides, hyaluronic acids, polysaccharides, glycerin, and many others are exhausted and not replenished. The skin's support structures, collagen and elastin, deteriorate or are damaged. Older skin is also more subject to allergic reactions, sensitivities, and irritation than younger skin due to a weakening immune system.

On a deeper molecular level, the DNA and RNA genetic messages to the skin cell for reproduction slows down and the cells stop reproducing as abundantly or in the same way as they did when we were younger. This preprogrammed change makes cells become abnormally shaped, which further changes the texture of the skin and prevents the cells from retaining water. This is why older skin tends to be drier than younger skin. This change in the skin's DNA and RNA seems to happen for a variety of reasons: it is genetically predetermined, a result of sun damage, and a result of an inflammatory response from free-radical damage built up in the skin cells over a period of time (Source: *Annals of the New York Academy of Sciences*, April 2001, pages 327–335).

You have probably connected the dots and noticed that many of these factors of aging are targeted by corresponding cosmetic ingredients that claim to counteract the effect of their naturally occurring depletion. Collagen, elastin, ceramide, hyaluronic acid, polysaccharide, DNA, RNA, and other skin components are popular additions to wrinkle creams. (DNA and RNA are the biggest jokes in this group of ingredients because not only don't you want to mess around with the cell's genetic coding, you can't. If you could, you would have the cure for cancer!)

Putting collagen and elastin in a skin-care product may sound convincing, but they can't bond to the collagen and elastin in your skin, although they can work as moisturizing ingredients. Ingredients like ceramides and hyaluronic acids do work to help support the intercellular structure of the skin, but there is no research demonstrating that they prevent its continuing depletion.

Good old glycerin is also abundant in the layers between the skin cells, and it's just as reliable in helping the skin to feel better, but the cosmetics industry doesn't talk much about glycerin because it is too commonplace to sound distinctive. Unfortunately, the cosmetics industry loves to use phrases such as "replaces what skin has lost" that lead you to believe these kinds of ingredients can affect skin structure in some permanent way. They can't. The point of all of this is that growing old cannot be reversed, much less with a skin-care routine or a handful of specific skin ingredients.

# DRY SKIN DOESN'T CAUSE WRINKLES

I understand how difficult it must be to overcome the bombardment of moisturizers claiming to take care of wrinkles and dry skin, yet it is completely false that dry skin and wrinkles are related. **How do we know dry skin and wrinkles are not associated? Because after slathering on tons of moisturizers and wrinkle creams and lotions over the years, women still get lots of wrinkles regardless of their skin type.** Even women who use expensive products still get wrinkles and make appointments with plastic surgeons. Moreover, kids with dry skin don't have wrinkles, and women with oily, sun-damaged skin do have wrinkles. Scientifically, we know dry skin and wrinkles are not associated because when you look at the skin under a microscope there is no physical evidence that the two are linked. Dry skin may look more wrinkly, but that doesn't mean those wrinkles are permanent.

The dilemma is that, in fact, dry skin does look more wrinkled and—here's the crux of the confusion—wrinkled skin looks better with a good moisturizer on it. That's how we get sucked into this myth about wrinkles and dry skin. A woman with oily skin has her own built-in moisturizer (that's basically what moisturizers are: oils or oil-like ingredients and water), which helps her skin look smoother without the aid of a moisturizer.

The truth is, moisturizing the skin does not have any long-term effect on wrinkles. That doesn't mean moisturizers can't make wrinkles less apparent, because they absolutely do, but the notion that these soothing creams, lotions, gels, and serums do anything to prevent or stop wrinkling in its tracks is wishful thinking fostered by constant reinforcement from the cosmetics industry. We know the cosmetics industry tells us lots of things that aren't true, this myth just seems more believable as we become more worried about wrinkles.

Another important distinction between dry skin and wrinkles is that when the outer layer of skin becomes dry or irritated the surface can literally crack, and something referred to as "fine lines" can appear. These "fine lines" are not the same as permanent lines caused by intrinsic (genetic aging) or extrinsic (sun damage) factors. This type of dry-skin damage can "look" wrinkled, which is why the elusive term "fine lines" is used. That also explains why the cosmetics industry uses the term fine lines, because those are just what moisturizers can easily correct. Fine lines (better described as nonpermament lines) nicely disappear with almost all moisturizers; on the other hand, permanent lines don't go away no matter how much moisturizer you put on them. Extremely dry skin can crack and chafe if it isn't moisturized, causing a parched appearance and a tight, irritated feeling, which is why dry skin is so uncomfortable.

Keep in mind that part of what makes the skin feel parched and dry is that the skin's intercellular matrix is deteriorating. The intercellular matrix is the glue within the skin that keeps skin cells together and helps prevent individual skin cells from losing water. It is actually the intercellular matrix that gives skin a good deal of its surface texture and feel. This matrix is composed of such substances as glycerin, cholesterol, sodium PCAs (NaPCA), and mucopolysaccharides, among many others referred to throughout this book as water-binding agents and natural moisturizing factors (NMFs). Water (as in moisture) doesn't help that part of the skin's health at all. Emollients, lipids, and NMFs do.

## THE BACKSIDE TEST OF AGING

A great many of the wrinkles and signs of aging we see on our face, hands, arms, and chest are a result of sun damage. The amount of evidence supporting this is overwhelming (Source: *Journal of Photochemistry and Photobiology*, October 2001, pages 41–51). However, you can prove this for yourself with something I call the backside test of aging. I've talked before about this indisputable, clear-cut evidence of wrinkling's direct relationship to sun damage, and it is as valid today as it was years ago when Dr. Kligman, the inventor of Retin-A, first described the phenomenon.

Here's how it works. If you are over the age of 40, preferably not more than 20 pounds overweight (fat helps plump up skin and smooth out wrinkles), you need only compare the skin on your face, hands, or the other parts of your body that are consistently exposed to the sun, with the skin on your backside. (If you don't meet the qualifications for this test, you can sneak a peek at women in the locker room at your exercise club and do the test surreptitiously.) Most people who have never, or rarely, exposed their bare backside to the sun will find a radical difference between it and those parts of the body that have been exposed to the sun. What you will notice is crepy skin on the face and hands, some loss of elasticity, lines, furrows, some skin discoloration (usually darkening, redness, or ashiness), and signs of new freckling. However, the skin on your bottom will be smooth, evenly toned (no freckling or discoloration), and elastic (unless there has been a fluctuation in weight, in which case the backside may be out of shape and saggy), without lines, crow's feet, crepiness, or any sign of wrinkles. These differences become more prominent the older you are and the more sun exposure you've experienced.

How does the cosmetics industry account for this difference in skin texture and appearance when it comes to wrinkle products? Or why doesn't your backside or tummy area need wrinkle creams like the face does? The cosmetics industry doesn't have an explanation; they just ignore this fact and so does the consumer. I imagine that if you don't see the contradiction right there in front of you on a daily basis, you might not notice this clear evidence about what causes skin wrinkling.

# CELLULAR RENEWAL AND REPAIR

Cellular renewal and repair are well-established marketing terms used by the cosmetics industry to sell skin-care products. The ability to generate healthy cell growth (in other words, the way that younger skin cells reproduce) is a claim many antiwrinkle and antiaging moisturizers make.

This idea of stimulating healthy cell growth definitely has some basis in scientific research, as I point out throughout this book. But the cosmetics industry distorts the concept of cellular renewal into a great deal of misinformation represented by overpriced products. Here are the facts about what it is possible to do for skin, regardless of the price tag on the product you are buying.

Essentially anything that protects skin can help encourage healthy cell production. This is particularly true for sunscreen and, theoretically, for products that contain antioxidants and anti-irritants. As described in the sections on tretinoin and alpha hydroxy acids in Chapter Six, you can even effect some repair and generation of collagen and elastin.

Skin cell production slows down with age or sun damage. That can leave older, dried-up cells on the skin's surface longer than is normal. Skin cells can become misshapen, sticking together unevenly, causing problems with moisture content, and producing a dry, dull, and extremely flaky layer of surface skin. All of this builds a very good case for exfoliation. Removing dead skin cells helps pave the way for plumper, healthier skin cells to surface, which can make a huge difference in the appearance of the skin. When this takes place, underlying skin density improves, moisture content goes up, and skin functions better (oil flows more easily out of the pores, and blackheads and blemishes decrease now that the dead skin cells that were in the way are gone). All of that can be termed cellular renewal and repair, but it doesn't take an expensive product to gain this kind of benefit. And, as you might expect, many of the other claims circling around cellular renewal make it sound like you can expect 20-year-old skin again, and that is not the case.

For most of our lives cellular renewal and repair is an inherent process all skin goes through. New skin cells are generated in the deepest structures of the skin, then migrate up to the skin's surface, changing their shape and size as they go. At the end of their life cycle, at the surface, the flattened and dried-up cells are shed. Healthy, newly-produced skin cells make this trek to the surface over a period of about 28 to 45 days. As we age, due to both extrinsic and intrinsic aging factors, that process can become impaired, negatively affecting the skin's appearance.

What can go wrong with skin cells as they are born, work, die, and shed? Depending on your age and genetic predisposition, a lot. In most women under the age of 40 with normal skin, new skin cells are generated and move upward through the layers of the epidermis, with a complete turnover taking place every 28 to 45 days. But for some women, particularly older women and women affected by the sun damage, smoking, genetic abnormality, or pollution that causes free-radical damage, the process is not always smooth, and problems occur along the way that can affect the appearance of the skin. When skin cell turnover is sluggish, the turnover process can take much longer, leaving dead skin cells on the surface longer. These dead skin cells that hang around longer than they should have a dull, flat, thickened appearance and a grainy, coarse texture. Doing things to improve this process can also be termed cellular renewal or cellular repair.

Aside from helping skin improve cell production and cell turnover, cellular repair and renewal can also refer to anything that helps reinforce or fortify the skin's intercellular matrix—the substance between the cells that forms the skin's protective barrier. Ingredients in skin-care products such as glycerin, hyaluronic acid, ceramides, glycosaminoglycans, vitamins, amino acids, and phospholipids can help this part of the skin. That's a benefit because keeping the intercellular matrix intact is the skin's first line of defense against many elements that can harm healthy skin.

Inasmuch as many things can help skin with cellular renewal and repair, it is still not the panacea the cosmetics industry makes it out to be. Even if women could use every product recommended for antiaging, there is still a genetically preprogrammed turnoff point where all skin cells stop reproducing the way they did when they were young. Remember, all cells are regenerated again and again. For a good deal of our lives we continue producing new cells, but as genetic aging (over our natural life span) takes place, the process simply slows down, almost to the point of shutting down completely. There are some who would suggest that growth factors can prevent the cells from shutting down, but this research is in its infancy and no one yet knows the consequences of attempting to affect or change genetic aging. After all, having skin cells that don't know when to die is the very definition of cancer.

# FACIAL EXERCISES

I am completely bewildered by the enthusiasm and passion the practice of facial exercises seems to generate. The number of questions I receive asking me if these work to get rid of wrinkles is just astounding. I also get swarms of letters from women telling me that I have my non-exercised head screwed on wrong when I suggest that facial exercises don't work. Banners on infomercials and advertisements that claim facial exercises can achieve something akin to a nonsurgical face-lift with only five minutes of effort a day keep a lot of women making strange faces in the mirror! But is there any information or research that would somehow explain the mania surrounding all this stretching and toning of the face muscles?

For the most part, facial exercises of any kind are more likely a problem for skin than a help. The reason why facial exercises can have little to no benefit is because loss of muscle tone is not a major cause of wrinkles or sagging skin. In fact, muscle tone is barely involved in these at all. The skin's sagging and drooping—and most every facial wrinkle—are caused by four major factors:

1. Deteriorated collagen and elastin (due primarily to sun damage)
2. Depletion of the skin's fat layer (a factor of genetic aging and gravity)
3. Repetitive facial movement (particularly true for the forehead frown lines and for smile lines from the nose to the mouth)
4. Muscle sagging due to the loosening of facial ligaments that hold the muscles in place

It turns out that facial exercise is not helpful for worn-out collagen, elastin, or the skin's fat layer because none of that is about the muscles, it's strictly about layers of skin and fat tissue. It is especially not helpful for the lines caused by facial movement! Rather, facial exercises would only make those areas appear more lined. The reason BoTox injections into the muscles of the forehead, laugh lines, and lines by the temple and eye area work at smoothing out lines in those places is because BoTox *prevents* the muscles from moving! It actually prevents muscle movement of any kind, including movements like squinting and raising the eyebrows that create wrinkles in those areas.

Facial exercises also won't reattach facial ligaments; that is only possible via surgery. One step involved in a surgical face-lift is to actually redrape the muscle of the cheek and the jaw, drawing it back and then literally stitching it back in place where it used to be. So if facial exercise could positively impact the muscle tone of the cheek and jaw it would cause a bulge in the wrong place. This is because exercise doesn't reattach the ligaments, it would just tone the sagged muscle, making it appear fuller lower down, and that would only make skin look more droopy in that area.

The ads for facial exercises often tout the fact that the facial muscles are the only muscles in the body that insert (or attach) into skin rather than into bone. They then use this fact to explain why, if you tone facial muscles, they directly affect the appearance of the skin. What this reasoning leaves out is that skin movement itself is one of the elements that causes the skin to sag and that helps the elastin in skin to become exhausted. If you are doing facial exercises and can see your skin move or frown lines and laugh lines look more apparent, that will only make matters worse.

While every dermatologist and plastic surgeon I've ever interviewed found facial exercises either silly or detrimental, there was one exception. As I was researching this story I found the name of one dermatologist who wasn't part of the crowd and who was repeatedly quoted on Web sites selling facial exercise programs. Dr. Wilma Bergfeld, Head of Clinical Research, Department of Dermatology at The Cleveland Clinic, and the first woman president of the American Academy of Dermatology (1992) was being quoted as someone who thought facial exercise was worthwhile. I had to hear this for myself. I spoke with Dr. Bergfeld and it turns out she isn't quite a supporter of facial exercises. "While there is no research or studies demonstrating facial exercises as being helpful, it is a reasonable assumption that it may be useful," she said. "Though I don't recommend them I do believe they could work in some controlled situations. However, you would never want to do anything that moves the facial skin, especially as it ages, or overmanipulate the skin," Bergfeld added, "because it would create more wrinkling [and] increase the loss of elasticity in the skin."

If facial exercise that moves the skin is problematic, what about electrical stimulation for the facial muscles? Wouldn't that form of involuntary stimulation tone the muscles without causing movement of the skin? The answer to that question is a resounding yes. It would exercise the muscle without moving skin. But there is no research demonstrating that this wouldn't make matters worse by creating surfaced capillaries (after all, electrical shocks to the muscles would zap capillaries, too, and that can be a problem), and it doesn't address the issue of the muscle being toned in the wrong area (given that most women start this treatment only after the muscles have already sagged and stretched). And finally, it won't affect the ligaments that have caused most of the sagging and drooping in the first place.

# Facial Masks for Wrinkles

Lots of facial masks, if not the majority, are little more than clay, mud, or earth minerals. Although there is much ado about the quality of clay from various parts of the world, conjuring images of volcanic ash or minerals derived from exotic waters, the truth is that clay is clay, and its value for the skin is negligible. Clay has some ability to absorb oil, and when the mask is removed it takes a layer of skin with it, which can make your face feel smoother—temporarily. But that doesn't compare in the least with regular use of AHAs, BHA, or tretinoin.

When facial masks don't contain clay, they often contain a plastic-like hairspray ingredient that places a Saran Wrap-like layer over the face. These peel-off masks, when they don't contain other irritants, can be fun. Like the clay masks, they take off a layer of skin when they are removed but, as with the clay masks, the benefit is at best insignificant and very short-term. Some facial masks contain AHAs or BHA. Although these ingredients definitely benefit the skin, they work best when used daily, not once a week or once a month.

You might be thinking, "But facial masks feel so good." As long as facial masks don't contain irritants, they do feel good, and your face can feel nice and temporarily smoother after they are removed because they take off the top layer of skin. You can mimic this effect by placing a layer of glue on the back of your hand, letting it dry, and then peeling it off. The back of your hand will feel incredibly smooth, at least for a short period of time. That's fine, but there is no long- or short-term benefit. There may even be a problem if peeling off these masks also removes some of your skin's intercellular protection.

If you are going to use a facial mask, and you have normal to dry skin, I suggest using only those that are lightweight and soothing—no peeling agents or clay needed.

# Sunscreen, Tretinoin, and AHAs— A Very Good Place to Start

One of the fundamental characteristics of sun-damaged skin is that the outer layer becomes thickened and yellow and the underlying layer, where new skin cells are produced, becomes damaged, generating abnormal cell growth and hypermelanin production. The abnormal cell growth also results in malformed elastin, collagen deterioration, and distorted circulation of the blood and lymph systems. Regular use of sunscreen can slow this damage, allow for some improvement, and prevent further destruction. But topical tretinoin has been shown to partially reverse the clinical and histological (structural) changes induced by the combination of sunlight exposure and chronological aging. A formulation of tretinoin in an emollient cream (as in

Renova, Avita, Tazorac, or generic tretinoin) has been extensively investigated in multicenter double-blind trials and has been shown to produce significant improvement within four to six months of daily use, compared with the vehicle alone, as part of a regimen including sun protection and moisturizer use.

Histological (structural) changes in the epidermis and dermis that were noted after 12 months suggest that tretinoin repairs photodamage by reconstitution of something called the rete pegs (the anchoring structure of skin that binds the outer layer of skin to the lower layer), repair of keratinocyte ultrastructural damage (surface-skin-cell damage), more even distribution of melanocytes and melanin pigment, deposition of new papillary dermal collagen, and improvements in vasculature (arrangement of blood vessels).

Alpha-hydroxy acids (AHAs) have also been widely used for therapy of photodamaged skin, and these compounds have been reported to normalize hyperkeratinization (over-thickened skin) and to increase viable epidermal thickness and dermal glycosaminoglycans content. To sum this all up, recent work has substantially described how the aging process affects the skin and has demonstrated that many of the unwanted changes can be improved by topical therapy. (Sources: *Cutis*, August 2001, pages 135–142; *Journal of the European Academy of Dermatology and Venereology*, July 2000, pages 280–284; *American Journal of Clinical Dermatology*, March-April 2000, pages 81–88; *Skin Pharmacology and Applied Skin Physiology*, May-June 1999, pages 111–119; *Journal of Cell Physiology*, October 1999, pages 14–23; *British Journal of Dermatology*, December 1996, pages 867–875).

There is every reason to consider using the combination of sunscreen (SPF 15 or greater with the UVA-protecting ingredients of avobenzone, titanium dioxide, and/ or zinc oxide), topical tretinoin, and an AHA lotion, gel, or moisturizer as an effective approach for combating wrinkles. A litany of research points to these as being as basic as it gets for your skin when it comes to battling wrinkles.

## HORMONES FOR WRINKLES

A great deal of research has affirmed the notion that hormone loss contributes to wrinkles and changes in the skin associated with aging. An article in the *American Journal of Clinical Dermatology* (2001, volume 2, issue 3, pages 143–150, "Estrogen and Skin. An Overview") stated that "Estrogen appears to aid in the prevention of skin aging in several ways. This reproductive hormone prevents a decrease in skin collagen in postmenopausal women; topical and systemic estrogen therapy can increase the skin collagen content and therefore maintain skin thickness. In addition, estrogen maintains skin moisture by increasing acid mucopolysaccharides and hyaluronic acid in the skin and possibly maintaining stratum corneum barrier function. Sebum levels are higher in postmenopausal women receiving hormone replacement therapy. Skin wrinkling also may benefit from estrogen as a result of the effects of the hormone on the elastic fibers and collagen. Outside of its influence on skin aging, it has been suggested that estrogen increases cutaneous wound healing by regulating the levels of a cytokine [proteins that generate an immune response]. In fact, topical estrogen has been found to accelerate and improve wound healing in elderly men and women." Similar research in *Maturitas,* the official journal of the European Menopause and Andropause Society (July 2001, pages 43–55), concluded that "HRT... regimes significantly improved parameters of skin aging."

There are compelling reasons to consider hormonal treatment as part of a battle plan for wrinkles. It is a multifaceted as well as a controversial issue. The following information will provide an overview to help you create a dialogue with your physician to evaluate all the options available to you.

# SKIN CARE FOR PERIMENOPAUSE AND MENOPAUSE?

It has been said that menopause starts the day you get your first menstrual cycle. I don't know if that's a hopeful comment or a depressing one, but any way you slice it, a woman will have periods for about 40 years after they first begin, and then they'll stop. Though there is still a great deal of research that needs to be done on all the issues surrounding perimenopause (referring to the symptoms in the years before the onset of menopause), menopause (the actual cessation of the menstrual cycle), and postmenopause, there is a lot that is known regarding the health and appearance of skin, hair, the body, and other physical as well as psychological aspects of this challenging and intricate life event.

Perimenopause and menopause are brought about by the body's changes in hormone production. The irksome side effects of menopause are caused primarily by the imbalance between a woman's female hormones (estrogen and progesterone, which become depleted) and her male hormones (like androgens such as testosterone). Because the male hormones decline more slowly, there are proportionately more of them, so they have a stronger impact. This imbalance, for example, can affect hair growth. When estrogen levels decrease, many women experience an increase in androgen production, resulting in varying amounts of dark hair growth on the face—particularly around the chin and moustache area above the lip. Ironically, while the hair on your face may get darker, the hair on your head will have reduced growth and you may experience some balding; even the individual hairs actually become smaller in diameter.

The lessening and eventual loss of estrogen and progesterone also affect skin negatively. Aside from problems caused by sun damage, perimenopausal and menopausal women experience thinner, looser and less elastic skin, reduced production of collagen, cessation of oil gland function, and dry skin. Other parts of the body are also influenced by the diminishing amount of female hormones; the vaginal lining becomes thin and can burn and itch, and the breasts' mammary tissue is replaced with more fat tissue, which can cause sagging.

To make matters even more frustrating, perimenopause and menopause can also bring hot flashes, flushes, night sweats and/or cold flashes, a clammy feeling, intermittent rapid heartbeat, irritability, mood swings, trouble sleeping, heavier periods, flooding, loss of libido, itchy skin, and more brittle nails, just to name a few.

As complex and multifaceted as this all sounds, there are actually some fairly exciting options for addressing the side effects of perimenopause and menopause, and these include both alternative herbal options and conventional Western medical choices. For the purpose of this section I'm going to highlight a few of the current options, but I cannot encourage my readers strongly enough to seek out as much information as they can, or to find a doctor who is an expert in this arena.

**Warning:** Please avoid the Web sites, companies, or physicians who do not offer a balanced approach to this issue. Medical options are not evil or dangerous, as many alternative-based supplement companies assert, and herbal alternatives are not as ineffective (or as unproven) as many medical doctors assert. Both approaches play a role in mitigating some of the more annoying (as well as intolerable) symptoms of perimenopause and menopause.

**Hormone Replacement Therapy (HRT) or Estrogen Replacement Therapy (ERT).** There are many prescription-only hormone replacement options to consider. HRT, taken in pills or skin patches, has been shown to restore some amount of the skin's support tissue and elastic quality. A number of studies have demonstrated that ERT and HRT can increase the thickness and elasticity of skin as well as lessen the appearance of skin's "aging" (Sources: *Skin Research and Technology*, May 2001, page 95; *Maturitas*, May 29, 2000, pages 107–117). The *American Journal of Clinical Dermatology* (2001, volume 2, issue 3, pages 143–150) summed up what all of these reports concluded by stating, "Estrogen appears to aid in the prevention of skin aging in several ways. This reproductive hormone prevents a decrease in skin collagen in postmenopausal women; topical and systemic estrogen therapy can increase the skin collagen content and therefore maintain skin thickness. In addition, estrogen maintains … stratum corneum [skin] barrier function…. Skin wrinkling also may benefit from estrogen as a result of the effects of the hormone on the elastic fibers and collagen…. [I]t has been suggested that estrogen increases cutaneous wound healing…."

There are risks associated with ERT and HRT and there are controversies regarding their effects on heart disease, osteoporosis, and breast cancer. But there seems to be little opposition to the notion that they ease hot flashes, night sweats, mood swings, and vaginal thinning. It is essential to weigh the pros and cons of ERT and HRT to decide if they are the right direction for you.

**Herbal Alternatives (phytoestrogens, also called plant estrogens):** As someone who has been drinking 8 ounces of soy milk per day and eating lots of tofu for the past six years, as well as applying an over-the-counter progesterone cream for the past several months, I can attest to the benefit of both. But that is only anecdotal, and I would never want you to rely on anecdotal information for any health matter. However, there is a great deal of research pointing to phytoestrogens and natural progesterones as valid options for perimenopausal and menopausal symptoms. Research on Dr. Andrew Weil's Web site (http://www.drweil.com) offers a very balanced approach between herbal and medical choices, and includes the medical options of HRT and ERT and herbal alternatives such as soy, black cohosh, dong quai, damiana, evening primrose oil, and borage oil.

Further, a paper on this issue published in the journal *Endocrine-Related Cancer* (June 2001, pages 129–134) stated that "Current descriptive epidemiology data in Asian women and the absence of any obvious harmful effects of soy-rich diets constitute arguments which encourage Western women to adopt a diet low in saturated fats and ... soy supplement." However, this same study discussed the need for more studies to establish the safety of consuming plant estrogens, especially given the American woman's propensity for believing that if a little is good then a lot must be even better. When you add to this the fact that there is no way to measure how much soy to eat or how much progesterone to rub on your body, you find that the alternative supplement world is one of personal experimentation. That isn't bad, but whether or not there are risks is just now being studied.

It is probably wise for women to get a baseline estrogen count around the age of 40 and then again at 45 to determine what normal is for you. That way you can monitor the changes and balancing effect that varying combinations of supplements are having on your body.

There are a lot of believers in "natural progesterone" and it definitely has helped change some of the problematic bleeding I've been experiencing over the past several years. However, it's important to point out that while natural progesterone is absolutely an option, you should be aware that natural progesterone creams are not regulated in any way by the FDA, and so they are, in actuality, merely cosmetics. That means any cosmetics company can put progesterone into whatever product they want to.

**Skin Care Options:** I would love to say that there are skin-care products out there that positively affect the changes that occur in perimenopausal and menopausal skin, but there aren't. There is simply no information suggesting that applying soy extract, black cohosh, or evening primrose oil to the skin can mitigate any of the changes taking place in the epidermis and dermis, and definitely not in comparison to taking those substances orally. None of those substances are a problem if they show up in skin-care products, but their benefits are most likely not any different from those of other anti-inflammatory and antioxidant cosmetic ingredients.

The truth is the real basics for skin care continue to apply to perimenopausal and menopausal women alike: sun protection, treating the skin type you have (not all menopausal women have dry skin), considering using Retin-A or Renova, and using gentle skin-care products. If you have dry skin, use an emollient moisturizer with antioxidants and anti-inflammatory agents (which most products these days contain). The use of hydroquinone or arbutin-based skin-lightening products is another important option. But there is nothing you can apply to skin (other than over-the-counter products containing USP progesterone or prescription-only estrogen creams) that can alter the actual condition of your skin caused by the depletion of hormones.

**Note:** What about the use of effective AHAs and BHA for menopausal women? This depends more on the condition of your skin than anything else. For some women (usually those over 70—well after menopause) the skin can become so thin it can literally tear when gently scratched or rubbed. This thinning is a result of many factors but primarily it is brought about by a combination of estrogen loss, genetic aging, and sun damage. All of these things cause the skin cells to produce "less skin" and less healthy skin. In terms of genetic aging, skin cells seem to have a preprogrammed mechanism that slows down skin-cell turnover, causing a buildup of dead skin cells on the surface of skin. It would be helpful if there were a way to tell skin cells not to slow down production, stay healthy (produce normally), and not build up on the surface of skin. Renova is the only real option we have for producing healthy cells. As for AHAs and BHA, they indeed help the outer layer of skin to shed by removing built-up dead skin cells. For some women in their 70s, 80s, and 90s with extremely fragile skin that may be problematic (they may indeed need the dead skin cells to stick around on the surface for as long as possible). However, for many women who don't have that kind of fragile skin the benefit of removing surface dead skin cells is that it absolutely helps improve the appearance of skin and allows healthier skin cells to come to the surface. It is also thought that AHAs and BHA can stimulate the production of collagen, which also has benefit.

# CHAPTER 9

## BATTLE PLANS FOR DRY SKIN

### UNDERSTANDING DRY SKIN

Before I go about creating a battle plan for dry skin it is essential for you to have a fundamental understanding of what dry skin is all about so you know exactly what kind of problems you are dealing with. Ironically, dry skin does not seem to be about a lack of moisture. The studies that have compared the water content of dry skin to normal or oily skin don't seem to find a statistically significant difference in moisture content between them (Source: *Journal of Cosmetic Chemistry*, September/October 1993, page 249). As mentioned in the earlier discussion of moisturizers, too much water can be a problem because it can disrupt the skin's intercellular matrix, the substances that keep skin cells bonded to each other, ensuring that the outer layer of skin is intact and smooth.

What is thought to be taking place in dry skin is that the intercellular matrix has somehow become impaired or damaged and that creates water loss. It's not that the skin doesn't have enough water, but rather it doesn't have the ability to prevent water loss, or to keep the right amount of water in the skin cell. When the intercellular matrix is disrupted, it impairs the integrity or health of the skin and the skin inevitably becomes dry, literally torn and ruptured.

There are some genetic factors that create this weakened or ineffective outer layer of skin but some of the things we do to our skin cause dryness as well. Perhaps the biggest offense is the use of drying skin-care products such as soaps, harsh cleansers, or products with drying or irritating ingredients. All of these disrupt the outer layer of the skin, destroying the intercellular matrix and causing dry skin. In skin-care products, the ingredients that are the worst culprits are alcohol, witch hazel, fragrance, camphor, menthol, citrus, and peppermint.

Weather and the way we heat and cool our homes, cars, and workplaces are also problematic for creating or worsening dry skin. Constant exposure to arid environments, as well as to air blasting from dry heaters or air conditioners, also destroys or impairs the skin's outer layer and intercellular matrix. Adding a humidifier to your home can make a world of difference to prevent external factors like this from causing dry skin to occur in the first place.

Unprotected sun exposure is another factor that damages the outer layer of skin. Sun damage causes abnormal cell production, resulting in a malformed outer layer of skin. In this situation skin cells adhere poorly to each other and the result is that the surface of new skin being formed is continually unhealthy and unable to provide reliable protection. Removing the damaged outer layer of skin can also make a world of difference in the health and appearance of the skin's surface. AHAs, BHA, and cosmetic skin-resurfacing procedures handle this problem beautifully. Tretinoin is also helpful for its role in improving cell production.

Perimenopause and menopause also factor into the causes of dry skin. Estrogen helps maintain skin's moisture content by increasing mucopolysaccharides and hyaluronic acid in the skin, helping to maintain the function of the skin's outer layer. Loss of estrogen also reduces the lipid content of skin, which eliminates the skin's natural protection against dryness.

## TOO MUCH WATER CAN BE A PROBLEM

While companies love touting how much water their products can put in your skin it turns out that may not be a good thing because too much water can is particularly hard on dry skin. Overhydration can indeed be a problem, and products that brag about increasing water content in skin cells by 180% can be doing more harm than good. Supporting this contention was a recent article in the May 2000 issue of *Cosmetics & Toiletries* magazine. The article on page 18 reviewed a book by Loden and Maibach called *Dry Skin and Moisturizers, Chemistry and Function*. One of the points in this book that impressed the reviewer was the fact that "prolonged water contact is not innocuous. Intense dermatitis can occur simply by prolonged water exposure…. Water alone also disrupts the SC [stratum corneum—the outer, surface layer of skin]…. Their studies show that water can directly disrupt the barrier lipids [protecting skin covering] and are consistent with surfactant-induced intercellular lamellar bilayer disruption." That means water can break down the stuff that binds skin cells together, actually degrading skin in the same way that strong cleansing agents can. (Note: *Cosmetics & Toiletries* magazine is a cosmetics industry journal read by cosmetics executives, formulators, and packaging companies.)

Another article, in *Contact Dermatitis* (December 1999, pages 311–314), stated that "Water is a skin irritant, which deserves attention because of its [pervasiveness].... In occupational dermatology, the importance of water as a skin irritant is especially appreciated. The irritancy of water has been demonstrated by occlusion experiments; occlusion with either closed chambers or water-soaked patches has been shown to produce clinical and histopathological inflammation. Functional damage, as revealed by increased transepidermal water loss, has also been shown.... However, much remains to be done to clarify the risk factors and mechanisms of water-induced irritation."

What this means is that those with dry skin should avoid soaking in a tub or taking long showers. Water is great, but it can be overdone and end up causing more problems than it helps.

# DRINKING WATER

Wouldn't it be great for those with dry skin if just drinking eight or more glasses of water a day could prevent or change dry skin? Drinking water is definitely important for the health of the body but that doesn't translate to getting rid of dry skin. If all it took to eliminate dry skin would be to drink water no one would have dry skin! Attempting to overdrink is always accompanied by an almost immediate need to go to the bathroom, where the excess water is quickly eliminated. So even if the extra water could be delivered to skin cells it would never have the chance to get there.

# BATTLE PLAN FOR DRY SKIN

To prevent or eliminate dry skin, the goal is to maintain the health of the skin's intercellular matrix. Moisture loss is definitely a symptom of dry skin, but simply giving the skin moisture won't repair the intercellular matrix because it has no water content to begin with. Rather the intercellular matrix is made up of substances like glycerin, lecithin, cholesterol, hyaluronic acid, and on and on, but not water.

Without question, moisturizers play a significant role for dry skin, and the number of products aimed at this problem is staggering. Fortunately, almost all moisturizers are wonderfully able to take care of most dry skin conditions. Yet for a number of men and women even a well-formulated moisturizer can't take care of the type of dryness they have and special management must be practiced.

Dry skin does show improvement and feels vastly better when emollients and lipids are used and dry air is kept off the skin. Here are some practical recommendations for winning this battle:

- If you can add a humidifier in your home, bedroom, or workplace, do so. This can make a huge difference in the feel of your skin.

- Use gentle cleansers from head to toe. Harsh or drying soaps or cleansers of any kind will either create dry skin or make matters worse.

- Avoid immersing your skin in water for long periods of time.

- **At night, apply an effective AHA or BHA product.** This is great for dry feet, legs, and arms, as well as the face! You may have to experiment to find out how frequently to apply these types of products, but it is essential to exfoliate the outer layer to get rid of the unhealthy buildup of dry, sun-damaged skin.

- In the morning it is essential to apply an emollient moisturizer with an SPF 15 or greater that has UVA-protecting ingredients avobenzone, titanium dioxide, or zinc oxide.

- At night an emollient moisturizer that's made with lipids (plant oils), natural moisturizing factors (ceramides, hyaluronic acid, vitamins, polysaccharides), and water-binding agents (glycerin) can help a great deal.

- For very dry skin, apply a layer of olive oil or other plant oils such as safflower, almond, or canola, over your nighttime moisturizer as an extra treatment.

- Medical hormone replacement therapy or alternative sources of hormones can also reduce or eliminate dry skin.

# CHAPTER 10

## BATTLE PLANS
## FOR BLEMISHES

## UNDERSTANDING WHAT CAUSES A BLEMISH

There's no way around it: One of the most worrisome and prevalent skin-care problems many women suffer through at some time in their lives is some degree of acne. Whether it's blackheads, whiteheads (milia—hard white bumps that do not contain pus and are not swollen or red), papules (inflamed, red, raised bumps that do not contain pus), or pustules (inflamed, red, raised bumps that contain pus), blemishes are commonplace skin imperfections. The language may not be pretty, but "Acne affects approximately 95% of the population at some point during their lifetime." This common disorder can range from mild to severe forms, can sometimes cause extensive scarring, and can occur somewhere between the ages of 11 and 50 (Source: *Journal of Cutaneous Medical Surgery*, June 2000, Supplemental, pages 2–13).

Regardless of your age, gender, skin color, or ethnicity, what causes acne is the same across the board (Source: *British Journal of Dermatology*, May 2000, pages 885–892). As a result there are certain basics for fighting breakouts that are essential if you are going to have any chance of winning the battle. To create a plan of action—and it does take an organized plan of action—it is essential to let go of the inaccurate but persistent and pervasive information concerning blemishes and instead learn what really can help your skin. You can't choose wisely if you don't know what you're fighting against! If you don't understand all your options and don't focus on what can work and what can't, you will end up making the condition worse than it was to begin with, or find temporary relief, only to have the problems show up time and time again.

First and foremost, you need to get over three myths about treating breakouts—because not only will they fail to prevent or eliminate a blemish, but they can also cause a whole range of additional skin problems.

**The first myth is the notion that you can dry up a blemish.** Water is the only thing you can "dry up" and a blemish has nothing to do with being wet. Skin cells, however, do contain water, and when you dry up the skin you are really drying up the water in the skin cell. Drying up skin impairs the intercellular matrix (skin's protective barrier), which can increase the presence of bacteria in the pore and cause flaking and a tight, dry feeling. None of that stops breakouts but it can lead to irritation and add another predicament to your skin-care woes. What's true is that blemishes can be aggravated by oil production, which needs to be reduced and/or absorbed. Absorbing oil on the skin or in the pore is a radically different process from drying up skin.

**The second myth is that blemishes are caused by dirty skin.** Unfortunately, this mistaken belief causes harsh overcleaning of the face with soaps and strong detergent cleansers. That only increases the risk of irritation and dryness, and doesn't do anything to prevent blemishes. Not only that, the ingredients in bar cleansers and soaps that keep them in a hard bar form can clog pores and actually cause breakouts. The truth is that gentle cleansing and overall gentle skin care are critical to getting breakouts under control (Source: *Cutis*, December 2001, Supplemental, pages 12–19).

**The third myth is that you can spot-treat blemishes.** Sadly, lots of products are based on this concept. However, once you see a blemish, you can't just zap it into oblivion in the hope of changing anything. For most types of blemishes (other than those created by an immediate reaction to a cosmetic or some other topical irritant or sensitizing reaction), by the time it shows up on the surface of the skin, it has been at least two to three weeks in the making. The truth is, it takes time for conditions in the pore to create a blemish. If you don't understand and you don't learn how to deal with that somewhat lengthy process, you can't successfully tackle recurring breakouts. Dealing with only the blemishes you see means that the blemishes that are forming won't be stopped.

Remember, you can't dry up a blemish because it isn't wet, and irritating ingredients not only may make matters worse by creating more redness and swelling, but also hurt the skin's ability to heal. The best course of action is to work on the cause of the blemish, not the aftermath.

## WHAT CAUSES BLEMISHES?

What truly causes breakouts? There are four major factors and one minor one that contribute to the formation of blemishes:

1. Hormonal activity

2. Overproduction of oil by the oil gland

3. Irregular or excessive shedding of dead skin cells, both on the surface of skin and inside the pore

4. Buildup of bacteria in the pore

Less likely to cause problems but still a problem for some is:

5. Irritation or sensitizing reactions to cosmetics, specific foods (rarely), or medicines

Fundamentally, this is how a blemish occurs. Inside an oil gland a type of bacteria called *Propionibacterium acnes* (or *P. acnes*) finds a perfect environment for growth. Dead skin cells and excess oil in the oil gland provide just the kind of conditions that *P. acnes* needs to thrive. As *P. acnes* reproduces, irritation and inflammation occur, which is why most blemishes are red and swollen (Source: *Seminars in Cutaneous Medicine and Surgery*, September 2001, pages 139–143).

Each hair follicle grows from a sebaceous (oil) gland that secretes an oily, firm wax called sebum. The structure that the oil gland and hair follicle share is called the pilosebaceous duct or unit, more popularly referred to as a pore. When things are going well, the sebum smoothly leaves the pore and imperceptibly melts on the skin's surface, helping to keep the skin surface moist and smooth. When things aren't going well, as when the pore becomes plugged with sebum and dead skin cells and bacteria run amok, a blemish is the outcome. Surplus sebum is generated primarily by hormonal activity (Source: *Journal of the American Academy of Dermatology*, December 2001, pages 957–960). When too much oil is produced, it can become mixed with dead skin cells from the skin's surface, with poorly sloughed skin cells from the pore's lining, and with small pieces of hair debris from the follicle. This combination of sebum, dead skin cells, and small pieces of hair can clog the pathway out of the hair follicle/oil gland, creating quite a backup. Now you've got problems.

When your body produces too much oil, and dead skin cells on the surface of skin or inside the pore aren't shed normally, they can join together in blocking the exit from a pore. All this excess oil and dead skin cells solidify as a soft, white substance that plugs the pore. If the surface of the pore is covered by skin, it is called a whitehead (milia). If the pore is open, without any skin covering, the top of the plug is exposed to air and darkens, causing a blackhead.

Whiteheads and blackheads become pimples when *P. acnes* begins growing inside the plug, causing irritation and inflammation. This inflammation and excess oil causes the wall of the oil gland to rupture, spilling the contents (oil, cell debris, bacteria, and all) into the surrounding skin tissue. The body's immune system then responds, sending lymph to the inflamed area to help with repair (and causing swelling), and you now have a pimple.

This still leaves some pretty important questions unanswered. What causes the hormones to increase oil production, and can you slow it down? How do the skin cells build up and clog the pore, and how do you stop that from happening? How do you stop the bacteria that cause the inflammation and redness? And who can break out or get acne, and why?

# WHY ME?

Why my skin? Why another blemish or blackhead? Why can't I have smooth, poreless skin? Why me? Believe me, I know this feeling.

Why do you suddenly, at the age of 28 or 48, have blemishes? Why haven't you outgrown the blemishes and oily skin that have plagued you since you were 14, and that at 35 are worse than ever? Why, at 40, do you have incessant blackheads and breakouts that won't go away no matter what you do, and you've done everything? Why do you still have acne when you're 18 and have tried oral antibiotics, Retin-A, sulfur masks, topical antibiotics, and every cosmetic skin-care routine imaginable? These are great questions and I understand them well.

Regardless of how old you are, breakouts and oily skin are upsetting, and anyone can be a victim! The main culprits in all these scenarios are hormones, because hormones are what affect oil production, and because their levels fluctuate at different times of life.

Breaking out is definitely most prevalent during adolescence. Statistics suggest that three out of four teenagers have problems with breakouts and various forms of acne. That isn't surprising when you consider that adolescence is a time of colossal hormonal changes that stimulate sebaceous (oil) glands and increase sebum production, which in turn increases the chances for breakouts. But acne can happen at any age. More than 40% of all women will experience some form of acne (Source: *Journal of European Dermatology and Venereology*, November 2001, pages 541–545).

Anything that can raise hormone levels—stress, the menstrual cycle, pregnancy, birth-control pills, or certain medications such as corticosteroids, and lithium—can act as a trigger. Specific foods are not responsible for breakouts, but an individual can have allergies to specific foods. There is also speculation that foods with hormone additives (specifically poultry and beef), iodine in food (shellfish), or fluoride in toothpaste may aggravate blemishes.

There's no question that hormone activity is the main thing responsible for oily skin and breakouts. When hormones gush, blemishes can flare, but hormones alone are not enough to create this annoying skin malady. For some unknown reason(s), something goes wrong in the oil gland, blocking the natural flow of oil. Theories about what causes acne generally focus on a genetic predisposition that creates either a defective oil gland, a malfunctioning pore lining that doesn't shed properly, or oil (sebum) that itself is in some way abnormal (too thick or irritating to the skin). In real life, you have to address most, if not all, of these issues if you want to reduce the chances of breakouts.

There are many theories why some people have more severe cases of acne than others. Some suggest that it's increased levels of male hormones, while others say that a genetic abnormality of the oil gland is the culprit. Hypersensitivity to *P. acnes* may also account for the great variation in the severity of acne (Source: *Dermatology*, 1998, volume 196, issue 1, pages 80–81). There is even research showing that the actual fatty acid components of the oil gland may be responsible. Most likely it's a combination of all these that cause the differences between those with mild or severe breakouts.

## YOU CAN'T ZAP ZITS

Most of us have sought relief from the emotional pain and humiliation that often accompany acne, whether it is one blemish or many, by going to drugstores or cosmetics counters where acne products and skin-care regimes line the shelves. Myriad products promise clear skin, and several pledge to zap zits, dry up blemishes, and drink up oil. The commercials and ads sound convincing, but a closer look reveals that many of these products really can't zap zits or dry up oil (you can never really dry up oil). Spot-treating only the blemish you see doesn't prevent other blemishes from forming. It takes consistency (regularly exfoliating, disinfecting, absorbing oil, hormonal balance) to stop breakouts. Further, many of these products that assure you they can zap zits contain drying, irritating, or sensitizing ingredients that actually make matters worse.

If you just pay attention to what you see on the surface without taking into consideration what is occurring underneath, you can't help heal the skin, reduce breakouts, or prevent scarring. Finding solutions that address each problem—hormonal activity, oil production, exfoliating the skin (and the pore), and killing the bacteria that cause the infection—is the only course of action that makes sense. Focusing on that single lesion without keeping the entire picture in mind can result in more breakouts, increased risk of scarring, and additional skin problems such as redness, surfaced capillaries, irritation, and dry skin.

## WHAT YOU CAN DO

Effective blemish treatment works by reducing oil production, eliminating skin-cell buildup on the surface of skin and in the pore, and killing the bacteria, *P. acnes*, that caused the inflammation in the first place. That's why the best course of action for blemishes is twofold: topical (what you put on the skin, whether it's an over-the-counter or a prescription option) and systemic (prescription oral medication that addresses the issue of oil production and bacterial growth).

## TOPICAL OPTIONS

**Clean the skin gently** with a water-soluble cleanser that doesn't contain ingredients that can clog pores or irritate the skin. This helps reduce further irritation and redness, which would make matters worse.

**Remove dead skin cells and encourage healthy skin-cell turnover** from both the skin's surface and inside the pore to help skin shed more normally.

**Absorb or reduce excess oil** to reduce the main cause of clogged and enlarged pores.

**Kill the bacteria** *(P. acnes)* that is causing the eruption, inflammation, redness, and swelling.

## SYSTEMIC OPTIONS

**Oral antibiotics** to eliminate bacterial growth.

**Birth-control pills and hormone blockers** to control oil production.

**Topical retinoids** (Retin-A, Tazorac, Avita, generic tretinoin, Differin) to normalize cell function, allowing the pore to function normally.

**Accutane**, the only prescription medication capable of curing acne.

You need to experiment to discover exactly how to put these various steps together in a combination that works for you. Unfortunately, there isn't one absolutely right way. It is essential to try different options until you find what suits your skin type and your specific condition. If you are consistent and avoid veering from your special battle plan, you stand a pretty good chance of winning a good part of the war against blemishes and blackheads. But the battle plan must deal with all of a blemish's causes.

# WHAT YOU SHOULDN'T DO

**Don't use harsh or irritating skin-care products.** Throughout this book I discuss the need for gentle cleansing for all skin types. This concept is particularly difficult for someone with oily or blemished skin to believe, despite the research backing it up, because the desire to *really* clean the skin is almost irresistible. Yet, a paper published in the *Proceedings of the Fourth International Symposium on Cosmetic Efficacy* (May 10–12, 1999, entitled "The Effects of Cleansing in an Acne

Treatment Regimen") concluded that 52% of the time a hydrating face wash gave better results in reducing comedones, papules, and pustules when used with benzoyl peroxide. **By comparison, this type of gentle cleanser was more effective than either soap or a benzoyl peroxide cleanser alone.**

What is most frustrating is that many of the blemish products on the market actually make breakouts worse or cause more skin problems than you started out with. Products designed to tackle acne often contain ingredients like harsh surfactants and overly abrasive scrub particles, as well as alcohol, menthol, peppermint, camphor, and eucalyptus, lemon, or grapefruit oils. All of these ingredients are extremely irritating, and the resulting irritation can impair the skin's ability to heal or to fight bacteria.

What makes all these standard, harmful "blemish-fighting" ingredients worse is that they don't reduce any of the factors causing breakouts. They can't disinfect, reduce oil production, affect hormonal activity, or help exfoliation. Instead, they kill more skin cells than necessary, which can further clog pores, produce dry skin, cause irritation, and make skin redder. **A blemish by definition is already irritated, red, and swollen, so it doesn't make any sense to use ingredients that will make it even more irritated, red, and swollen.**

Skin-care products with irritating ingredients, such as facial masks, astringents, toners, and facial scrubs (which also contain waxes), are a big no-no. These can all hurt the skin, and that can aggravate acne. If a product irritates the skin, if it tingles or burns, it is not helping. And not only does irritation stimulate oil production, promote redness, increase swelling, and dry out the skin, it can also add small rashlike pimples to the breakouts you're already trying to deal with.

Bar soaps and bar cleansers are often recommended for acne, yet all of them contain ingredients that can clog pores. Soaps contain tallow and bar cleansers contain other heavy, wax-based thickening agents that can clog pores. Shockingly, high-pH soaps and cleansers (those with a pH of 8 or higher) can actually increase the presence of bacteria in the pore! All this makes matters much worse inside the pore, again greatly increasing the risk of breakouts.

Oversqueezing, picking, digging, scraping, or poking at pimples may be hard to resist, and you may think it speeds healing, but in fact it sets you up for more problems. Creating scabs and constantly reinjuring the lesion just increases the chances of scarring. There is nothing wrong with gentle squeezing to remove a blemish's contents, but unless you are extremely careful you will create more problems than you started with.

Many women think they can use hot compresses to bring pimples to a head. Actually, hot compresses severely damage skin by burning it; the heat causes more redness and swelling; and the whole process can also rupture the pore, increasing the possibility of more breakouts. The same is true of steaming the face or using hot water. Hot water burns the skin, impairing the skin's ability to heal and fight bacteria. Tepid water is what you need to help soothe the skin and calm things down. Use tepid water and a gentle, water-soluble cleanser on the face, and do not wipe off makeup. Wiping and rubbing will make the irritation worse, and can also make the skin sag and cause wrinkles.

Be careful that the breakouts you're struggling with aren't a result of hair products getting on the face. Hairspray, mousse, hair gel, and other styling products contain polymers (plastic-like, film-forming ingredients) that can clog pores and cause pimples.

**Don't smoke.** A study in the *British Journal of Dermatology* (July 2001, pages 100–104) concluded, "According to multiple logistic regression analyses acne prevalence was significantly higher in active smokers (40.8%...) as compared with non-smokers (25.2%). A significant linear relationship between acne prevalence and number of cigarettes smoked daily was obtained.... In addition, a significant dose-dependent relationship between acne severity and daily cigarette consumption was shown by linear regression analysis.... Smoking is a clinically important contributory factor to acne prevalence and severity."

## WHEN TO SEE A DERMATOLOGIST

Some women run to see a dermatologist the second they see a blemish. Others put it off well past the time when over-the-counter options have stopped working even when their breakouts are still rampant. Though there are many options for dealing successfully with breakouts outside the realm of prescription medications, if your acne is severe or chronic it may indeed be best to seek medical attention. Dermatologists have a host of options in their arsenal that can be more effective than over-the-counter products in reducing sebum production, creating healthy skin-cell turnover, and fighting bacterial infection.

Most prescription-only options such as tretinoins (Retin-A, Tazorac, Avita, generic tretinoin), Differin (technically adapelene), and azelaic acid (trade name Azelex), plus topical antibiotics, oral antibiotics, and hormone blockers have no nonprescription counterparts. Dermatologists also have one option that can be an absolute cure for acne and breakouts. That option is Accutane, the only medication that has a chance of curing acne as opposed to just keeping it under control. All of these options are discussed in this chapter.

Nonetheless, it is completely acceptable to start with the options available over the counter or from some cosmetics lines. Some of these are similar to what a doctor would prescribe, such as salicylic acid products to exfoliate and benzoyl peroxide products to disinfect. If you select this course of action, it is essential to use only what works and to use it consistently. If after a period of time you find those options don't work or aren't working as well as you would like, you can always make an appointment with a dermatologist.

## WHAT ABOUT DIET?

**There is little, if any, scientific evidence that diet affects acne, although specific food allergies certainly can be a contributing factor—but that depends on what you personally are allergic to. Not everyone has the same food allergies.** Likewise, drinking soda pop, not exercising, popping vitamins, and eating healthy or unhealthy foods will neither help nor hurt acne. Lots of Olympic-caliber athletes have acne-prone skin, and lots of people who don't exercise and are overweight have a flawless complexion. However, if certain foods—such as nuts, shellfish (because of their iodine content), milk products, or wheat—seem to make your acne worse, it is best to avoid them (try omitting them one by one) to see if it makes a long-term difference in your skin.

Incidentally, fluoride in toothpaste may be the source of breakouts around the mouth. The research for this is very old, with a couple of studies published in the '70s and '50s. That is not exactly current information, but if you tend to have acne just around your mouth, it is simple enough to try nonfluoride toothpaste for awhile and see if things improve. If your acne is indeed triggered by fluoride, consult your dentist about alternative cavity-prevention treatments.

## OIL-FREE IS A BAD JOKE

But the joke is on us, because while "oil-free" is a meaningless claim it may mislead consumers into buying products that can actually clog pores. There are plenty of ingredients that don't sound like oils but that can absolutely aggravate breakouts. On the other hand, not all oils clog pores. **Yet, many cosmetics (anything that isn't in a liquid form) contain waxlike thickening agents that may clog pores.** Simple, standard moisturizing ingredients that are great for dry skin can cause problems for someone with oily skin or breakouts. When any product looks like a cream or a lotion (as opposed to a fluid), the ingredients that give it that consistency may clog pores. Despite the problems these ingredients can cause, they show up in lots and lots of so-called "oil-free" products.

Above and beyond the products that claim to be oil-free, label after label promises that the product is "noncomedogenic" or "nonacnegenic." Most of us have bought products with this assurance, only to find that they did cause breakouts. I wish I could say otherwise, but the truth is you can't trust any product that makes the claim that it's not comedogenic because there is no approved or regulated standard for that assertion. Aside from the regulatory aspect of this bogus claim, I'm certain all of us have used products that promised not to cause breakouts and yet we still broke out. What many women already know from experience is that trying to guess how their skin will react based on a product's promises, especially when it comes to blemishes, is truly a lost cause—or at the very least a difficult problem with no easy, slam-dunk answers.

# WILL IT MAKE ME BREAK OUT?

So if you can't trust the terms "oil-free", "non-comedogenic", or "nonacnegenic", how do you know if a product will cause problems? Why does it seem so impossible to find products that won't cause breakouts? It's because *most* ingredients used in cosmetics can cause breakouts, depending on your skin type.

There is evidence that some specific ingredients can trigger breakouts, but there are no absolutes. I wish there were, but there aren't. Several Web sites that showcase lists of comedogenic ingredients have caused quite a stir for many women. The major source of information for these data appears to be *Dr. Fulton's Step by Step Guide to Acne,* published in 1983 by Harper & Row (though credit is not given on any Web site, it is the exact same information presented in the book). At the time (and 1983 is a long time ago), Fulton's research on the causes of breakouts was unprecedented. Fulton applied cosmetics ingredients to rabbits' ears and waited to see what happened. As promising as this research was, it has never been repeated, and is rarely cited in later research (except when it suits a company's marketing agenda). There are many reasons why lists of this kind are unreliable.

First, the methodology involved pure concentrations of the ingredient, not the concentrations that are used in actual cosmetic formulations, which are usually only a fractional percentage. It also didn't address the issue of usage and application. For example, the exposure risks of specific ingredients are very different for a cleanser, which is left on the skin for a few seconds, and a lotion or liquid, which is left on the skin for hours. Beyond this, the research didn't look at the host of plant extracts or sunscreens in cosmetics that were introduced during the early '80s. To call this list out of date and inconclusive would be an understatement!

I have to admit that I'm also to blame for some of the confusion. In my books I have included a list of ingredients that may cause breakouts. I based this list on the emollient or waxlike characteristics of the ingredients and on findings in more contemporary research when it was available. I warned against products that contain ingredient groups such as triglycerides, myristates, palmitates, and stearates, but it was probably not wise to include such a list because in some ways it is misleading information. For example, isopropyl palmitate is a waxy thickening agent used to bind other ingredients together, has an emollient feel on skin, and is used most frequently in moisturizers for dry skin. On the other hand, ascorbyl palmitate is a stable form of vitamin C that is used in small amounts in skin-care products, and is not a problem for skin. So much for following the rule about palmitates. Further, depending on the ingredient, just because it is present in a formulation means nothing if it is toward the end of the ingredient list—while if it's the second, third, or fourth ingredient it may be problematic. But that may not be true if there are many of these kinds of ingredients strewn across a label and, therefore, present in small amounts. Also, keep in mind that even the most notorious ingredients (such as isopropyl myristate) won't cause problems for everyone. Just because an ingredient *may* cause breakouts doesn't mean that it *will*.

Another point these kinds of lists can't account for is that there are thousands and thousands of cosmetic ingredients being used in skin-care and makeup products today! A lot of them are emollients, waxy thickening agents, or irritants that can cause skin problems. Whether they do or not, however, is completely dependent on the amount used and the nature of the individual ingredient (some ingredients cause problems in far smaller amounts than other ingredients, while others cause problems in various combinations). A comprehensive list would not only be impossible, but also would be nothing more than guesswork.

There are no easy answers for this one, but you can understand that trying to research, categorize, classify, and make absolute conclusions about 50,000 ingredients with an infinite number of possible combinations is just not humanly possible. So, what's a woman to do when trying to fend off blemishes and still use skin-care and makeup products? While I still think some ingredients are more problematic than others, the easiest and most reliable quality for a consumer to consider is consistency of the product. The thicker the product (meaning those with a high, thick, or creamy viscosity), the more likely it is to cause problems. That means you can feel safer with a gel or serum (because these have a low or watery viscosity).

What about greasiness? It is safe to assume that a product with plant or mineral oils of any kind listed high up on the ingredient list might make the skin feel greasy. But greasiness doesn't necessarily trigger breakouts.

Finally, it makes more sense to watch out for irritating ingredients than so-called pore-clogging ingredients. It doesn't take much alcohol, menthol, peppermint, balm mint, eucalyptus, camphor, lemon, grapefruit, or lime to cause a negative skin reaction that can impede the skin's healing process by stimulating bacteria production— and that won't help heal blemishes.

# BLEMISH FIGHTING BASICS

Each of the following products and product categories reflects state-of-the-art treatments for blemishes, acne, and blackheads. How to put them all together is addressed in the "Battle Plans for Fighting Blemishes" section at the end of this chapter.

All of the products described below address each of the factors that cause pimples. These are the best options for reducing oil production, for disinfecting the skin, for improving exfoliation, and for controlling hormonal activity, and are a potential cure for blemishes. Finding the combination that works for you is the first goal, and then you must focus on hitting all the steps and carrying them out consistently.

**Gentle cleansing is the first place to start.** I've already elaborated on the need for gentle cleansing, but let me say it one more time for added emphasis. Using a water-soluble cleanser gently cleans your skin without stimulating the oil glands, increasing redness, or creating dryness. This step is standard for any skin-care routine because it makes an instant difference in the appearance and feel of the skin, and it is essential for reducing breakouts. Once you stop using drying, irritating, pore-clogging soaps or bar cleansers, and you realize how nice your skin feels when it is no longer dry and irritated, you will never go back to the old way again. Just be certain the water-soluble cleanser you select doesn't contain irritating ingredients and won't dry out the skin. Using cleansers that contain exfoliating agents, topical disinfectants, or oil-absorbing ingredients is not the best option because the active ingredients would be washed away before they had a chance to have an effect on skin. Save these ingredients for another step.

**Disinfecting.** There aren't many options for disinfecting the skin. Alcohol (when used in the right concentrations) and sulfur can be good disinfectants, but they are too drying and irritating, causing more problems then they help, which can generate more breakouts. Plant-derived disinfectants such as tea tree oil (melaleuca) are an option but there are no products currently being sold that contain a high enough concentration to reliably kill bacteria. Benzoyl peroxide is still the best over-the-counter disinfectant to consider and is available in 2.5%, 5%, and 10% concentrations.

If benzoyl peroxide isn't effective, a topical antibiotic or even an oral antibiotic prescribed by a doctor may be the only option left to kill stubborn, blemish-causing bacteria, but an oral antibiotic should be a last resort because of systemic problems and problems with resistant bacteria. Oral antibiotics can indeed kill blemish-causing bacteria, but they also kill good bacteria in the body, causing yeast infections and stomach problems. In addition, *P. acnes* in your body can develop resistant strains in a short period of time, making the antibiotic you're taking ineffective.

**Exfoliating.** Because blemishes occur inside the pore and involve oil production, an effective 1% to 2% salicylic acid (beta hydroxy acid—BHA) product is a crucial over-the-counter starting point for exfoliating the skin. Salicylic acid is lipid soluble, which means it can exfoliate inside the pore, plus it is extremely gentle. I recommend using BHA in a gel, liquid, or extremely light lotion formula because they are unlikely to contain waxy thickening agents or emollients that can clog pores. Topical scrubs and alpha hydroxy acids (AHAs) can be helpful for surface exfoliation, but they can't affect the pore lining, and it's essential to do that to deal with one of the root causes of a blemish.

**Improving cell production.** Tretinoins, Differin, and azelaic acid are prescription options for generating healthy cell growth that can change the shape of the pore, allowing for normal oil flow. This improvement can eliminate the environment that allows the blemish to develop.

**Absorbing or controlling excess oil.** Clay masks are an option for absorbing oil as long as they contain no irritating ingredients. Using milk of magnesia as a facial mask is a simple and effective way to absorb oil. Birth-control pills and hormone blockers can equalize hormones, reducing or eliminating the source of excess oil production.

**When all else fails.** If your breakouts persist after you've tried these over-the-counter and prescription options then you can still try Accutane, which is the only medication that can essentially cure acne. This is the last option in any lineup concerning blemishes only because of its serious side effects if a woman becomes pregnant while using it and because of other health issues (these are discussed in more detail later in this chapter).

## SALICYLIC ACID

Referred to as beta hydroxy acid (BHA), salicylic acid can be a judicious starting point in the treatment of breakouts for all skin types. This is a multifunctional ingredient that addresses many of the systemic causes of blemishes (Source: *Seminars in Dermatology*, December 1990, pages 305–308). For decades dermatologists have been prescribing salicylic acid as an exceedingly effective keratolytic (exfoliant). Yet, in addition to salicylic acid's incredibly helpful exfoliating properties, it can do even more. Salicylic acid is a derivative of aspirin (both are salicylates—aspirin's technical name is acetyl *salicylic acid*) and so it also functions as an anti-inflammatory (Source: *Archives of Dermatology*, November 2000, pages 1390–1395). Combining exfoliation with reduced irritation has many advantages for skin, especially for someone struggling with breakouts. Diminishing or eliminating the redness and swelling blemishes cause can help skin heal, prevent scarring, and decrease the chance of further breakouts.

Preventing pores from becoming clogged is a requisite key to preventing blemishes. One way to achieve this is to improve the shape of the pore lining. The lining of a pore is made of skin cells (epithelial tissue) that can become thick and misshapen, preventing the natural flow of oil out of the pore. To act on the pore lining it is necessary to exfoliate inside the pore, dislodging excess skin cells. Exfoliants such as alpha hydroxy acids (AHAs) or mechanical scrubs have limitations for blemish-prone skin due to their inability to penetrate inside the pore. AHAs are water-soluble and can't get through the oil. Mechanical scrubs have particle sizes that are too large for them to have any effect below the surface of skin. Salicylic acid is the perfect answer. It is an effective exfoliant, it is lipid soluble (so it effortlessly penetrates into the pore), and it is an anti-inflammatory so it can actually reduce irritation, swelling and redness.

Another notable aspect of salicylic acid for breakouts is that it has antimicrobial properties (Source: *Preservatives for Cosmetics*, by David Steinberg, Allured Publishing, 1996; Health Canada Monograph Category IV, *Antiseptic Cleansers*). That means it can be effective in killing the bacteria that cause acne. Together, all these properties mean salicylic acid is one of the more multifunctional ingredients in combating the causes of acne.

As wonderful as this sounds, salicylic acid is a tricky product to buy. The concentration must be at least 0.5%, but 1% to 2% is more effective. Additionally, the formula's pH is a critical factor. For salicylic acid to work as an exfoliant on skin, it must be in a formulation with a pH of 3 to 4; if it isn't, it loses its ability to exfoliate skin (Source: *Cosmetic Dermatology*, October 2001, pages 65–72). Well-formulated salicylic acid products do exist, and once you've found the right one, it can be a successful part of your battle plan to fight blemishes.

## OVER-THE-COUNTER ANTIBACTERIAL

Some things go hand in hand: bread and butter, love and marriage, Laurel and Hardy. None of these are the same by themselves. That's also true for exfoliants and topical antibacterial agents when it comes to reducing or eliminating blemishes. Cleaning the skin without exfoliating *and* disinfecting is far less likely to have an impact on skin. You can get pretty good results using one or the other, but together they are a formidable defense against blemishes.

Benzoyl peroxide is considered the most effective over-the-counter choice for a topical antibacterial agent in the treatment of blemishes (Source: *Skin Pharmacology and Applied Skin Physiology*, September-October 2000, pages 292–296). The amount of research demonstrating the effectiveness of benzoyl peroxide is exhaustive and conclusive (Source: *Journal of the American Academy of Dermatology*, November 1999, pages 710–716). Among benzoyl peroxide's attributes is its ability to penetrate into the hair follicle to reach the bacteria that are causing the problem, and then killing them—with a low risk of irritation. It also doesn't pose the problem of bacterial resistance that some prescription topical antibacterials (antibiotics) do (Source: *Dermatology*, 1998, volume 196, issue 1, pages 119–125).

Benzoyl peroxide solutions range from 2.5% to 10%. For the sake of your skin, start with the less potent concentrations. A 2.5% benzoyl peroxide product is much less irritating than a 5% or 10% concentration, and it can be just as effective. It completely depends on how stubborn the strain of bacteria in your pores happens to be.

Despite benzoyl peroxide's superior disinfecting and penetrating properties, some bacteria just won't give up easily, and in those situations a different weapon may be necessary. That's when you should consider prescription topical disinfectants (topical antibiotics).

## PRESCRIPTION ANTIBACTERIALS

If your skin doesn't respond to a 2.5% benzoyl peroxide or to the various over-the-counter higher strengths, the next step is a prescription topical antibacterial, meaning antibiotics in a lotion or gel form. Topical antibiotics have limitations. They can have difficulty penetrating the hair follicle and long-term use can lead to antibiotic-resistant strains of bacteria. Erythromycin, tetracycline, and clindamycin are the most popular topical antibiotics.

You can use these antibiotics alone, but a good deal of research points to the greater benefit of combining these with benzoyl peroxide to create a potent and effective treatment. Studies indicate that "Topical clindamycin and benzoyl peroxide have each demonstrated clinical efficacy in the treatment of acne vulgaris. When used in tandem, they promise greater efficacy than either individual agent through their antibacterial and anti-inflammatory effects.... [B]enzoyl peroxide [and] clindamycin demonstrated significantly greater reductions in inflammatory lesions … and significantly greater overall improvement as assessed by physicians … and patients" (Source: *Journal of Cutaneous Medical Surgery*, January 2001, pages 37–42). This same assessment was echoed in the *American Journal of Clinical Dermatology* (2001, volume 2, issue 4, pages 263–266).

Another option, considered to be quite effective, is a prescription product called Benzamycin, which contains 3% erythromycin and 5% benzoyl peroxide. This combination boosts penetration, which benzoyl peroxide does best, and combines that with erythromycin's strong antibiotic action (Source: *British Journal of Dermatology*, February 1997, pages 235–238).

**Basic directions:** *After you have cleaned your face and used a toner, you then apply the BHA over the face (or areas of the neck, back, or chest where you tend to break out). You then apply your topical antibacterial. During the day, sunscreen goes on next; in the evening, if you need a moisturizer, apply it minimally only over dry patches or dry areas around the eye.*

**Warning:** Do not apply benzoyl peroxide and a retinoid (such as Retin-A, Renova, Tazorac, Avita, generic tretinoin, or Differin). Benzoyl peroxide inactivates retinoids (Source: *British Journal of Dermatology*, September 1998, page 8).

## TEA TREE OIL VS. BENZOYL PEROXIDE

Please see the section in Chapter Three, *Miracle, Frauds, & Facts*, on "Melaleuca— Tea Tree Oil."

## TRETINOIN FOR BLEMISHES

Retinoid is the general category name for any and all forms of vitamin A. Tretinoin is a form of vitamin A and, therefore, comes under the general heading of retinoids. The best-known products that contain tretinoins are Retin-A, Renova, Retin-A Micro, Tazorac, Avita, and generic tretinoin. These are all basic treatments for blemishes because they change the way skin cells are formed in the layers of skin as well as in the pore. If skin cells have an abnormal shape, they tend to stick together and shed poorly, often getting backed up in the pore. Tretinoin can transform cell production by improving shedding and by unclogging pores, thereby producing a significant reduction in inflammatory lesions. Topical tretinoins and antibacterial agents have complimentary actions, and they work well together when combined. Tretinoins are not able to kill *P. acnes*, the bacteria that cause the breakouts, but an antibacterial agent can. Meanwhile, tretinoins can improve and restore the shape of the pore, opening a clear pathway for the antibacterial agent so it can be more active (Source: *Journal of the European Academy of Dermatology and Venereology*, December 2001, page 43).

One of the major drawbacks to the use of tretinoin is the irritation it can cause. For some people this can be so severe as to prevent its use. But there are alternatives. There is a great deal of research showing that adapalene (brand name Differin), another retinoid but different from tretinoin, can be just as effective as tretinoin but without the irritation (see the following section on Differin).

Meanwhile, remember that using any tretinoin product can make the skin more vulnerable to sun damage and sunburn. It is essential to wear an SPF 15 sunscreen that contains the UVA-protecting ingredients avobenzone, titanium dioxide, or zinc oxide as the active ingredient. Zinc oxide and titanium dioxide are occlusive and can possibly clog pores and avobenzone can be sensitizing for some skin types. It takes experimentation to find the right sunscreen that works best for your skin type.

**Basic directions:** *After you have cleaned your face and applied a topical antibacterial (though not benzoyl peroxide, which inactivates retinoids), you can spread a tiny amount of Retin-A, Renova, Retin-A Micro, Avita, Tazora, or generic tretinoin over the face. If you are going outdoors in the daytime, it is essential to follow this with a sunscreen to protect the face from sun damage. At night you can apply a moisturizer afterward over dry areas or around the eyes.*

# DIFFERIN

In the world of prescription acne treatments, Retin-A and tretinoins have been in a class by themselves for many years. Now they have some stiff competition in the form of Differin, generically known as adapalene, a prescription-only, topical acne medication from the folks who make Cetaphil.

Remember, if abnormal skin cells in the layers of skin and in the pores are left to do their own thing, they just accumulate there, creating an environment in which blemishes can flourish. Aside from topical and oral antibiotics that primarily address the issue of killing off the bacteria responsible for producing pimples, tretinoin was the only prescription product available that could help exfoliate skin cells (especially inside the pores), literally changing the way the skin cells are produced. It works for more than half of the people who can tolerate the treatment, but therein lies the rub—tolerance—because tretinoin can irritate the skin. Even Dr. James Leyden, an associate of Dr. Albert Kligman, the original patent holder for Retin-A, said, "Retinoid [Retin-A] therapy ... due to the side effects, has always been a double-edged sword, limiting its use in many patients."

I can relate. When I was young, Retin-A left my face so red and inflamed I thought it was going to blister, especially in the days when I also used strong astringents and bar soaps.

Where does Differin fit into this picture? Differin is a retinoid, a form of vitamin A that has been shown in clinical studies to be significantly less irritating than tretinoin. According to a study published in the March 1996 *Journal of the American Academy of Dermatology*, Differin was also significantly more effective in reducing blemishes and was better tolerated than tretinoin gel. Other more recent studies have come to the same conclusion, which is that, by several measures, adapalene cream and gel were less irritating upon multiple dosing than various tretinoin creams and gels (Sources: *International Journal of Dermatology*, October 2000, pages 784–788; *Journal of Cutaneous Medical Surgery*, October 1999, pages 298–301).

It seems that Differin has a radarlike ability to positively affect the skin-cell lining of the pores, substantially improving exfoliation and helping to prevent blockage. Moreover, for those with oily skin, the original Differin comes in a lightweight gel formula that is barely felt on the skin. It contains little more than water and cellulose, a sheer thickening agent. Differin is also available in a cream base for those with dry skin and blemishes.

Should you consider Differin? If you have tried Retin-A or other tretinoins and had difficulty dealing with the irritation, or if you just want to see if Differin can work better for you (which it may), then it is certainly an option.

**Basic directions:** *After you have cleaned your face and applied a topical antibacterial, spread a tiny amount of Differin over the face, or any other part of the body with breakouts. (Do not use benzoyl peroxide with Differin because benzoyl peroxide inactivates retinoids.) If you are going outdoors in the daytime, it is essential to follow this with a UVA-protecting sunscreen to shield the face from sun damage. At night you can apply a moisturizer afterward, over dry areas or around the eyes.*

## AZELAIC ACID

The introduction of new and reformulated prescription exfoliants in more-emollient or nonalcohol bases reflects the demand for medications that meet the needs of older women looking for ways to deal with pre- and postmenopausal acne. Differin, the new tretinoins, and azelaic acid all affect the way skin cells are formed and shed in the skin layers and inside the pore lining. The difference with azelaic acid (trade name Azelex) is that in addition to exfoliating the skin, it also performs an antimicrobial action on the skin.

Technically, azelaic acid is a saturated dicarboxylic acid found naturally in wheat, rye, and barley that behaves like a 5% topical benzoyl peroxide gel, a 0.05% tretinoin cream, or a 2% erythromycin cream (a topical prescription antibiotic), meaning it can exfoliate and disinfect the skin at the same time. There is some research that shows azelaic acid to be well tolerated, and that it may not cause as much overt irritation, redness, or swelling as tretinoin (Source: *Acta Dermato-Venereologica*, November 1999, pages 456–459). However, other research indicates that irritation is a possible side effect.

Unlike the tretinoins, azelaic acid is not likely to cause sun sensitivity. It is most definitely an ally in the battle against breakouts, particularly if skin is naturally sensitive to the sun or if irritation is an issue.

Azelaic acid's efficacy can be enhanced and improved when it is used in combination with other topical medications such as benzoyl peroxide 4% gel, clindamycin 1% gel, tretinoin 0.025% cream, and a gel combining 3% erythromycin with 5%

benzoyl peroxide. Furthermore, another study has shown that azelaic acid plus benzoyl peroxide achieves greater efficacy and higher patient satisfaction ratings of convenience than [single] therapy with erythromycin–benzoyl peroxide gel (Source: *Journal of the American Academy of Dermatology*, August 2000, Supplemental, pages 47–50).

**Basic directions:** *After you have cleaned your face and applied a topical disinfectant, you spread on a tiny amount of azelaic acid. If you are going outdoors in the daytime, it is essential to follow this with a UVA-protecting sunscreen to shield the face from sun damage. At night you can apply a moisturizer afterward, over dry areas or around the eyes.*

# ORAL ANTIBIOTICS

If topical exfoliants, retinoids, and antibacterial agents don't provide satisfactory results, an oral antibiotic prescribed by a doctor may be an option to kill stubborn, blemish-causing bacteria. Several studies have shown that oral antibiotics, used in conjunction with topical tretinoins or topical exfoliants, can control or reduce many acne conditions (Source: *International Journal of Dermatology*, January 2000, pages 45–50). As effective as oral antibiotics can be, they should be a last resort, not a first line of attack. Oral antibiotics can produce some unacceptable long-term health problems. Some dermatologists tend to give the negative side effects of oral antibiotics short shrift and prescribe them as if they were nothing more than candy for their acne patients. Oral antibiotics are anything but candy. They kill the good bacteria in the body along with the bad, and that can result in chronic vaginal yeast infections as well as stomach problems.

A more worrisome side effect is that the acne-causing bacteria can become immune to the oral antibiotic. According to an article in the *American Journal of Clinical Dermatology* (2001, volume 2, issue 3, pages 135–141) "The main cause for concern following the use of systemic antibiotics is the emergence of antibiotic-resistant strains of *P. acnes*." Similarly a paper presented at the General Meeting of the American Society for Microbiology in May 2001 (http://www.asmusa.org/memonly/abstracts/AbstractView.asp?AbstractID=47544) stated that "antibiotic treatment in patients with severe acne causes development of antibiotic resistance.... The prevalence of antibiotic resistance to tetracycline, erythromycin, clindamycin and trimethoprim-sulphamethoxazole..." was found after two to six months. "When patients with acne are treated with antibiotics, the risk of development of antibiotic resistance should be realized. The use of antibiotics to treat acne should be restricted and other regimens should be tested."

This means that if you have been taking an oral antibiotic to treat your acne for longer than six months it can stop being effective. This loss of effectiveness leaves many women puzzled when initially the antibiotic they were taking gave incredible results, but then became ineffective.

An even more serious argument against taking oral antibiotics was discussed in the *American Journal of Clinical Dermatology* (July-August 2000, pages 201–209), which stated: "At a time when there is global concern that antibiotic resistance rates in common bacterial pathogens may threaten our future ability to control bacterial infections, practices which promote the spread of antibiotic-resistant bacteria must be fully justified."

The decision to use oral antibiotics should not be taken lightly. The course of action you take should be discussed at length with and monitored by both you and your dermatologist.

## BIRTH-CONTROL PILLS FOR ACNE?

If you are a woman (sorry, guys) looking for a way to reduce breakouts, you might want to discuss your skin problems with your gynecologist instead of your dermatologist. The FDA has approved low-dosage birth-control pills (Ortho Tri-Cyclen and generic norgestimate/ethinyl estradiol) for use in the treatment of acne. In Canada, Diane-35, a combination of cyproterone acetate and ethinyl estradiol is approved for the treatment of acne (Source: *Skin Therapy Letter*, 1999, volume 4, number 4). Depending on your lifestyle and medical history, you could solve two problems with one prescription.

How does the birth-control pill work on acne? Increased oil production can be caused by the body's androgen (male hormone) production, which can be highest just before menstruation starts. It appears that low-dosage birth-control pills can decrease the presence of excess androgens, thereby decreasing breakouts. They work particularly well when used in conjunction with other therapies such as topical antibacterial agents or tretinoins (Source: *Skin Therapy Letter*, February 2001, pages 1–3). For a lot of women this is no surprise. Many have noticed an improvement in their skin after they started taking birth-control pills.

According to a double-blind, placebo-controlled study published in *Fertility and Sterility* (September 2001, pages 461–468), other "low-dose birth-control pills can be an effective and safe treatment for moderate acne." The double-blind, placebo-controlled, randomized clinical trial found that the birth-control pill containing levonorgestrel (Alesse®) reduced the appearance of acne.

Low-dose oral contraceptives also result in a low occurrence of estrogen-related side effects like nausea, headaches, and breast tenderness, in addition to low, if any, weight gain (Source: Medscape press release, September 7, 2001).

Is taking birth-control pills to control acne right for you? There are risks associated with taking birth-control pills, and these should be taken into account before you make a final decision. These risks include increased chances of heart attack, strokes, blood clots, and breast cancer (and these are compounded if you smoke), not to mention possible side effects such as vaginal bleeding, fluid retention, melasma (dark-brown skin patches), and depression. All that may not be a worthwhile trade-off for clear skin. But if you are already considering or using the pill for birth control, this remedy may be worth looking into.

# ACCUTANE

Looking back, my only regret is that I waited so long. I tried. I really tried. I patiently waited for my skin to clear up. Spent untold dollars on dermatologists and followed their instructions. Diligently wiped antibiotic lotions over my face and took oral antibiotics for years. Exfoliated with baking soda, faithfully used Retin-A, and slathered on sulfur masks. I used milk of magnesia masks twice a week, and sometimes wore it under my makeup to soak up oil during the day. For most of that time my skin did improve, but it never really stopped breaking out and I still had to put up with oily, wet-looking skin. Besides, despite the improvement I saw from using antibiotics and the other treatments, I didn't want to stay on them forever. Adapting to the antibiotics was a risk I wasn't willing to continue taking. Who knew how much longer I would continue breaking out? It had been going on since I was 11, and by then I was 38.

I had known about Accutane for a long time. I knew it had some pretty serious, even dangerous, side effects, and that most dermatologists didn't prescribe it very often, and then only in the most serious cases. My acne and oily skin were serious to me, but not as bad as the pictures I had seen of the cystic acne cases that responded brilliantly to treatment with Accutane. Then, in 1990, a woman I worked with and two of her friends started taking Accutane, and they not only lived through it, their skin looked flawless. More than flawless—radiant (at least in comparison to what it looked like before).

"Considered the biggest breakthrough in acne drug treatment over the last 20 years, Accutane is the only drug that has the potential to clear severe acne permanently after one course of treatment" (Source: *FDA Consumer* magazine, March-April 2001, http://www.fda.gov).

I was convinced that I needed to research the topic for my newsletter, *Cosmetics Counter Update*. What a remarkable decision that turned out to be. A dermatologist I had heard about at my health cooperative, Group Health in Seattle, Washington, told me it was possible, in fact, highly probable, that I could have clear skin for the rest of my life if I took Accutane. I told him I had heard controversial things about Accutane and was hesitant to try yet another prescription drug for my acne.

And this one sounded even more serious than antibiotics. He responded with a fascinating saga.

Accutane (its generic name is isotretinoin) is a drug derived from vitamin A, and is taken orally. It essentially stops the oil production in your sebaceous glands (the oil-producing structures of the skin) and literally shrinks these glands to the size of a baby's. This prevents sebum (oil) from clogging the hair follicle, mixing with dead skin cells, rupturing the follicle wall, and creating pimples or cysts. Normal oil production resumes when treatment is completed and the sebaceous glands slowly begin to grow larger again, but never (or at least rarely) as large as they were before treatment.

**"Because of its relatively rapid onset of action and its high efficacy with reducing more than 90% of the most severe inflammatory lesions, Accutane has a role as an effective treatment in patients with severe acne that is recalcitrant to other therapies"** (Source: *Journal of the American Academy of Dermatology*, November 2001, Supplemental, pages 188–194).

In a large percentage of patients who complete a four- to six-month treatment with Accutane, acne is no longer considered to be clinically significant. In other words, for all intents and purposes, *their acne is cured!* Does this mean if you take it you'll never break out again? You may once in a while, but an occasional pimple here and there is hardly anyone's definition of acne. Especially anyone who, on a daily basis, had numerous breakouts, lots of blackheads, and oily skin.

The remaining percentage of patients who take Accutane do experience recurrences. For this group, when the breakouts return, typically three to six months after treatment, they are often milder and easier to treat, and can on occasion be cured with a second or third treatment with Accutane. Of course, there is a percentage that receive no benefit from taking Accutane, no matter how many treatments they take.

By the way, dosage and duration depend on the severity of the patient's acne, but treatments generally last 16 weeks. If a second treatment is necessary, an 8-week rest period is required between treatments. Interestingly, acne continues to improve even after the course of treatment is completed, although doctors do not know exactly why.

**[Accutane] is the treatment of choice for severe nodulocystic acne. It represents the sole agent that effectively addresses all of the pathophysiological factors in the production of acne"** (Source: *Seminars in Cutaneous Medical Surgery*, September 2001, pages 162–165).

So what's the catch with this "miracle" drug and why don't doctors prescribe it to everyone? Accutane is controversial for many reasons, but principally because of its most insidious side effect: It has been proven to cause severe birth defects in nearly 90% of the babies born to women who were pregnant while taking it. Before physicians knew about this alarming hazard, when it was first prescribed in France back in the 1970s before enough research had been conducted to establish its safety, more than 800 babies out of 1,000 births were born seriously deformed. The only way to avoid this risk is to abstain from sex during treatment or, according to the information provided with every prescription, to use a minimum of two forms of birth control. If you are taking a birth-control pill, you still need to use a condom or diaphragm. You will need to discuss with your physician how long to continue using the extra birth-control precautions after you are done taking Accutane. Generally, Accutane's effects do not last very long once you stop taking it.

If you *aren't* pregnant, are there still risks? Absolutely. Commonly reported, although temporary, side effects of Accutane include dry skin and lips, mild nosebleeds (your nose can get really dry for the first few days), hair loss (I lost a small amount of hair that grew back when I finished the four months of treatment), aches and pains, itching, rash, fragile skin, increased sensitivity to the sun, headaches (mild to severe—mine were fairly mild), and peeling palms and hands.

A study in the *Journal of Cutaneous Medical Surgery* (April 2000, pages 66–70) followed 124 people through their course of treatment with Accutane. "The majority of patients experienced persistent dryness of lips. Dry eyes affected 40% of patients; this continued throughout treatment in 25%. Contact lens wearers were more likely to develop conjunctivitis. Lower back pain was reported early in about 30% of patients and fewer than 10% of patients would develop it later in the course of treatment. Joint pain was noted in 16.5% of patients at the first visit and there was little change with ongoing treatment. Hair loss was experienced in a small percentage but was rarely noted on more than one occasion. Headaches occurred in less than 10% and were occasionally severe, but most often intermittent and recorded at a single visit. Depression occurred in 4% of patients and tended to persist throughout the treatment. All these patients completed the full course of treatment." The study concluded "patients treated with [Accutane] experienced a predictable series of side effects. Some occurred fleetingly, but several persisted for the duration of treatment."

More serious, although much less common, side effects include severe headaches, nausea, vomiting, blurred vision, changes in mood, depression (discussed more in this chapter), severe stomach pain, diarrhea, decreased night vision, bowel problems, persistent dryness of eyes, calcium deposits in tendons (doctors don't know yet whether this is significant), an increase in cholesterol levels, and yellowing of the skin.

Understandably, many people, doctors included, are scared off by these side effects, above and beyond the risk to pregnant women. That's why dermatologists recommend Accutane only to patients with chronic acne (large, recurring cysts or blemishes that can permanently distort the shape and appearance of the skin), or sometimes to people with less-severe acne that has not responded successfully to other forms of treatment. Many doctors won't prescribe Accutane at all.

Although the high risk of birth defects and the other side effects should be taken seriously, it seems a shame that Accutane has been kept away from many acne patients. It is the most effective, short-term drug for acne available today. All other acne treatments require ongoing, tenacious adherence to the program and they don't offer a cure. The public is largely misinformed about Accutane's potential dangers as well as its potential benefit. Many doctors believe that if it weren't for the proven risk of birth defects, Accutane would be prescribed almost as frequently as antibiotics. Not surprisingly, it is prescribed much more frequently to men.

Given what I have learned, I wish somebody had told me about Accutane twenty years ago! It would have saved me a lot of time, money, and heartache. Although oral and topical antibiotics, exfoliants, gentle cleansing, staying away from products that aggravate breakouts, and using milk of magnesia to absorb excess oil can work successfully for lots of people, for many people the question remains, "When will I outgrow acne and how long will I have to struggle with the pain of breakouts?" Sadly, there is no telling if you're *ever* going to outgrow it. People who don't outgrow it, and lots of women don't, are looking at years of applying topical solutions and taking oral antibiotics that sometimes work well and sometimes don't.

## ACCUTANE PREGNANCY WARNINGS IGNORED

Despite warnings and information regarding Accutane's detrimental effect on fetuses, women are still becoming pregnant while taking it. According to an August 17, 2001, FDA press release, the Centers for Disease Control and Prevention (CDC) reported "that despite prevention efforts some women who take Accutane, a prescription medication given for severe acne and known to cause birth defects, still become pregnant while on this medication." The CDC also reported that a symbol intended to remind women that they must not get pregnant while taking these medications is commonly misinterpreted. The two studies, "Continued Occurrence of Accutane-exposed Pregnancies" and "Interpretations of a Teratogen Warning Symbol," were published in *Teratology* (2001, volume 64, issue 3, pages 142–147 and 148–153). (Teratogen refers to a substance or process that causes developmental malformations and birth defects.) Both of these studies indicate that there are serious problems related to women either not understanding or not being fully informed about the risks of becoming pregnant while taking Accutane.

The press release went on to say that "Since 1988, the CDC and the Food and Drug Administration (FDA) have worked closely to help educate health care providers and women of reproductive age who may be prescribed Accutane. The devastating birth defects caused by Accutane include: brain defects, heart defects, and facial defects such as babies born without ears." Women who want to take Accutane are supposed to have two negative pregnancy tests before beginning the medication, use two forms of effective birth control during treatment, and have repeat pregnancy tests every month during the course of medication. It turns out that many women do not follow these recommendations. Moreover, many doctors do not inform their patients that this is required despite the fact that more women are taking Accutane for their acne than ever before.

In response, the FDA has established new restrictions designed to prevent women from becoming pregnant while they are taking Accutane. According to the FDA, the new requirements for being allowed to take Accutane, or for a doctor's ability to prescribe the drug, will include mandatory monthly pregnancy tests. Pharmacists will be allowed to fill only a one-month supply at a time, requiring proof of a negative pregnancy test from the patient. Physicians will have to place an "Accutane Qualification Sticker" on their prescriptions to establish that the patient has had a negative pregnancy test.

You can find more information about the CDC's work on Accutane and birth defects at http://www.cdc.gov/ncbddd/bd/accutane.htm. For more information about the FDA's review of Accutane and birth defects, please see http://www.fda.gov/cder/drug/infopage/accutane/default.htm.

## DEPRESSION FROM ACCUTANE

According to an article in the *Journal of the American Academy of Dermatology* (October 2001, pages 515–519), "The Food and Drug Administration (FDA) has received reports of depression and suicide in patients treated with [Accutane].... [F]rom 1982 to May 2000 the FDA received reports of 37 US patients treated with [Accutane] who committed suicide; 110 who were hospitalized for depression, suicidal ideation, or suicide attempt; and 284 with nonhospitalized depression, for a total of 431 patients. Factors suggesting a possible association between [Accutane] and depression include a [limited time] association between use of the drug and depression.... Compared with all drugs in the FDA's Adverse Event Reporting System database to June 2000, [Accutane] ranked within the top 10 for number of reports of depression and suicide attempt."

In contrast to this report, a paper presented at the 59th Annual Meeting of the American Academy of Dermatology (March 27, 2001, Washington, DC) stated that "Up to the current time, a rate of 12 suicides per 8 million isotretinoin-treated patients has been documented. Half of these patients were on concomitant [other] medications. A small number of patients have reported that depression subsided when isotretinoin was withdrawn and recurred with treatment resumption. In the United States, 64 suicides occurred between 1991 and 1999 in patients who at one time took isotretinoin. Thirty occurred during treatment, 24 after treatment was stopped (6 months—10 years), and 10 occurred in patients whose treatment status was unknown.

"These numbers must be compared with general suicide statistics in the United States. In total, 30,000 suicides occur per year (in the general population, the rate is 11.4 per 100,000). Eighty percent are males. Suicide is the third leading cause of death in the 15- to 24-year age group (6000 per year). So when isotretinoin patients are observed, the 64 total suicides must be compared with an expected suicide rate of more than 10 times that number (670). These data suggest that in these patients the suicides were likely due to factors other than isotretinoin treatment. The isotretinoin suicide rate of 1.8 per 100,000 is well below that of the general population, as noted above. In addition, in the isotretinoin patients, there was no alteration in the typical US pattern of suicide in terms of gender distribution, relationship to depression, underlying psychiatric disorders, or lack of warning signs (typical of youth suicide)."

Despite the controversy, Hoffman-La Roche, the makers of Accutane, is adding a warning about depression to the product information insert. Hoffman-La Roche is also removing copy from their ads that suggests Accutane can relieve the "psychological trauma" and "emotional suffering" associated with acne. The lengthy package insert for Accutane did include warnings about depression but not about possible suicide or psychosis.

As is true with any medication, all the pros and cons must be considered before starting treatment. If you or the teen you are responsible for already have a history of depression, then the potential for exacerbated depression must be taken into account and discussed with your physician.

# HANDLING THE SIDE EFFECTS OF ACCUTANE

How do you deal with some of the side effects when taking Accutane? It helps to be prepared. If you take Accutane, stay out of the sun! This drug makes the skin photosensitive even if you are wearing sunscreen (and you must wear sunscreen). Any prolonged sun exposure can cause severe redness and fever. Treat dry areas of the face with a moisturizer. If your nose becomes dry, apply a thin layer of petroleum jelly on the skin inside the nose, and do it frequently. That will make a big difference. Do not use any skin-care products that can cause irritation or dryness. Avoid bar soaps, washcloths, AHA and BHA products, scrubs, hot water, and facial masks. If you are using tretinoin, Differin, azelaic acid, or topical antibiotics, I suggest you stop using them unless your doctor recommends that you continue. Dry eyes can be treated with artificial teardrops; do not use products like Visine that simply constrict blood flow and can dry out the eyes even more. Headaches and body aches are eased quite nicely with ibuprofen. Be sure to drink plenty of water. If you have any concerns, discuss them at once with your physician.

Pay attention to your mood. If you find yourself feeling excessively depressed, hostile, angry, or have even a fleeting thought of suicide speak to your doctor immediately. It is also essential for your doctor to monitor your blood. Cholesterol can shoot up dangerously high and liver function must be monitored. It is extremely important that you stay in close contact with your physician during the entire time you are taking Accutane.

## HORMONE BLOCKERS FOR ACNE?

Using a testosterone-blocking drug to reduce the hormone levels responsible for activating oil production is controversial; it's also an approach to treating acne and oily skin that is not very well-researched. The most frequently prescribed hormone blocker is known as spironolactone (brand name Aldactone). It is an option only for women, however, because without testosterone men start to develop female characteristics such as enlarged breasts and softer skin. But because testosterone can be one of the primary causes of acne, curtailing its presence in the body may have positive results—namely, acne clears up and oil production slows.

What kind of results can you expect? A study described in the *Journal of the American Academy of Dermatology* (September 2000, pages 498–502) looked at "...85 women with acne treated consecutively with spironolactone.... Results: Clearing of acne occurred in 33% of patients treated with low doses of spironolactone; 33% had marked improvement, 27.4% showed partial improvement, and 7% showed no improvement. The treatment regimen was well tolerated, with 57.5% reporting no adverse effects." Another study, reported in the *Archives of Dermatology* (September 1998, volume 134, number 9) reviewed " ... 38 patients: 4 with severe acne (with cystic lesions), 32 with moderate acne, and 2 with mild acne. Improvement in acne, defined as a lessening in severity of acne classification, was observed in 32 (97%) of 33 patients who continued to follow up while receiving therapy. Of the 32 patients with improvement in their acne, all 4 patients with severe acne improved to moderate acne, 26 of 27 patients with moderate acne improved to mild acne and in 2 the acne disappeared, and both patients with mild acne experienced complete resolution. One patient had no improvement in her acne."

While those statistics aren't exciting, they may be of interest for women who have not responded well to other treatments. But the side effects of Aldactone are as daunting as those for Accutane. The list of adverse effects include abdominal cramping, nausea, diarrhea, headache, reduced sexual drive (libido), dry mouth, excessive thirst, unusual tiredness, unusual muscle weakness, skin rash, deepening of voice, irregular or no menstrual periods, and slowed heart rate, plus enlarged breasts in men, and breast tenderness in women.

Moreover, hormone blockers require long-term use to effectively treat acne. When you stop taking it, the testosterone returns and so can the acne. Because hormone blockers require repetitive, continuous use, at least for treating acne, I strongly recommend trying Accutane before trying hormone blockers. Although Accutane's side effects can be more serious than those of the hormone-blocking drugs, use of Accutane is very short term, involving only a few months, and it can be a permanent cure.

## WHAT ABOUT ORAL SUPPLEMENTS FOR ACNE?

Very little, if any, research points to vitamins, herbs, or minerals of any kind or in any combination as having an effect on breakouts. What little research does exist shows zinc to be a valid option to consider. A handful of studies have compared oral antibiotics to zinc, with zinc showing some benefit. A study reported in *Dermatology* (2001, volume, 203, issue 2, page 40) evaluated "the place of zinc gluconate in relation to antibiotics in the treatment of acne vulgaris. Zinc was compared to minocycline [an antibiotic] in a multicenter randomized double-blind trial. 332 patients received either 30 milligrams elemental zinc or 100 milligrams minocycline over 3 months. The primary endpoint was defined as the percentage of the clinical success rate on day 90...." The study concluded that "Minocycline and zinc gluconate are both effective in the treatment of inflammatory acne, but minocycline has a superior effect evaluated to be 17% in our study."

In conjunction with other treatments, zinc may prove to have even better results. But zinc is not a benign supplement. High doses of zinc can be toxic. Avoid taking more than 100 mg of zinc per day from a supplement (Source: http://www.drweil.com). It is also recommended that you take a daily multivitamin because increased levels of zinc mean that the body requires more copper and manganese.

Of course, zinc is not a cure-all and end-all for your acne, and it probably works best in tandem with other topical agents.

Pantothenic acid (vitamin B5) is touted as being effective for acne. However, there is only one study supporting this notion and it dates from the early '80s (Source: *International Journal of Dermatology,* 1981, volume 20, pages 278–285). There is no current research showing this to be an effective treatment.

Vitamin A is another oral supplement thought to be helpful for acne. In one study, showing it to have a positive impact, the participants were given 300,000 IU per day. Considering that the usual recommended daily amount is 10,000 IU, the 300,000 IU is a large enough amount of vitamin A to be possibly toxic and is not recommended.

At this time there is no reliable research pointing to any oral supplement other than zinc as being helpful in the treatment of acne.

## FACIAL MASKS FOR BLEMISHES

Some facial masks, particularly masks that are part of a skin-care routine for acne, contain sulfur, which can have some benefit as a disinfectant for breakouts. However, it is an unnecessary (compared to other options) and fairly strong substance to use to disinfect the skin, especially when you leave it sitting on your face in a facial mask for a period of time. There are gentler ways to disinfect the skin. Sulfur has pretty much been abandoned as an option for treating breakouts since the '80s, given the other successful and less irritating topical choices available.

Masks are a poor choice for dealing with blemishes anyway, because when breakouts are the problem, the bacteria that cause the eruptions must be killed daily or even twice daily, depending on the severity of the problem. Sulfur masks are usually applied too sporadically to effectively prevent breakouts.

For someone with oily skin, I recommend a mask of plain milk of magnesia (no mint or cherry flavors, please), the kind you buy at the drugstore for an upset stomach. Milk of magnesia is just liquid magnesium. Magnesium, like clay, is an earth mineral, but, unlike clay, magnesium has some disinfecting and anti-inflammatory properties and can absorb more oil for its molecular weight than clay can. Clay masks are an option as long as they contain no additional ingredients that can cause irritation.

## REMOVING BLEMISHES

This isn't a pretty topic, but it is a fact of life and human nature that just leaving a blemish or blackhead alone is almost impossible. Fortunately, gently removing a blackhead or blemish with light-handed squeezing can actually help the skin. Removing the stuff inside a blackhead or especially a pimple relieves the pressure and reduces further damage. Yes, squeezing can be detrimental to the skin, but it's the way you squeeze that determines whether you inflict harm. If you oversqueeze, pinch the skin, scrape the skin with your nails, or press too hard, you are absolutely doing more damage than good. Gentle is the operative word and, when done right, squeezing with minimal pressure is the best (if not the only) way to clean out a blackhead or blemish.

Although I never recommend steaming the face (heat can overstimulate oil production, cause spider veins to surface, and create irritation), a tepid to slightly warm compress over the face can help soften the blackhead or blemish, making it easier to remove. First, wash your face with a water-soluble cleanser, pat the skin dry, then place a slightly warm, wet cloth over your face for approximately 10 to 15 minutes. Once that's done, pat the skin dry again. Using a tissue over each finger to keep you from slipping and tearing the skin, apply even, soft pressure to the sides of the blemish area, gently pressing down and then up around the lesion. Do this once or twice only. If nothing happens, that means the blemish cannot be removed, and continuing will bruise the skin, risk making the infection or lesion worse, and cause scarring. Again, only use gentle pressure, protect your skin by using tissue around your fingers, and do not oversqueeze.

Be sure to use a 2.5% benzoyl peroxide solution after you're done, and if you wish you can follow up with a facial mask of plain milk of magnesia to soothe the skin and reduce inflammation. Do not remove blackheads or blemishes more than once or twice a week or you can cause too much irritation.

## WHAT ABOUT PORE STRIPS?

Pore strips in all their varying incarnations are meant to remove blackheads. You place a piece of cloth with a sticky substance on it over your face, as you might do with a Band-Aid, wait a bit for it to dry, and then rip it off. Along with some amount of skin, blackheads are supposed to stick to it and come right out of your nose. There is nothing miraculous about these products, nor do they work all that well. The main ingredient on these strips is a hairspray-type ingredient. If the instructions are followed closely you can see some benefit in removing the very surface of a blackhead. In fact, you may at first be very impressed with what comes off your nose.

Unfortunately, that leaves the majority of the problem deep in the pore. What has me most concerned about pore strips is they are accompanied by a strong warning not to use them over any area other than the intended area (nose, chin, or forehead) and not to use them over inflamed, swollen, sunburned, or excessively dry skin. It also states that if the strip is too painful to remove, you should wet it and then carefully remove it. What a warning!

Also, despite the warning on the package, I suspect most women will try these strips wherever they see breakouts. If I didn't know better, I know I would. The way these strips adhere, they can absolutely injure or tear skin. They are especially unsafe if you've been using Retin-A, Renova, Differin, AHAs, or BHA; having facial peels; taking Accutane; or if you have naturally thin skin or any skin disorder such as rosacea, psoriasis, or seborrhea.

# YOU STILL NEED SUNSCREEN

There is no way around it: Even if you are battling blemishes, you still need to minimize sun damage by using an effective sunscreen. In fact, it's especially important because, as part of that battle, you should be exfoliating the skin, which can make it more susceptible to the sun's rays.

Unfortunately, the last thing someone with oily skin needs is another product on her skin. Most sunscreens, even those that claim to be oil-free, contain ingredients that can cause blemish flare-ups. The few sunscreens that are indeed lighter-weight tend to be alcohol-based, posing new problems, because alcohol can be an irritant. Plus the sunscreen ingredients themselves can cause breakouts, particularly so-called "nonchemical" sunscreens, which contain titanium dioxide or zinc oxide. Even though titanium dioxide and zinc oxide are superior sunscreen agents, doing their work with little to no risk of irritation, they are occlusive and can clog pores. Other types of synthetic sunscreen ingredients can cause irritation and also result in breakouts. So you're between a rock and a hard place. Yet you still need sunscreen. In my opinion, the best option in this situation is to wear a foundation with a reliable SPF (preferably SPF 15) that uses either avobenzone, titanium dioxide, or zinc oxide as one of the active ingredients.

A foundation that contains sunscreen is less of a problem than moisturizers when it comes to causing breakouts, regardless of the ingredients. Foundations are designed to stay on top of the skin, rather than be absorbed. Additionally, it means using one product instead of two, if you were going to wear a foundation anyway. The fewer products you put on your skin, the better, and this is doubly true for someone afflicted with breakouts or oily skin. And please, if you do choose to wear a foundation that contains sunscreen, don't forget that the other parts of your body that are exposed to sun during the day need sunscreen, too.

The bottom line: It takes experimentation and diligence to find a comfortable sunscreen for any skin type, but even more so for someone with oily skin and a tendency toward breakouts.

# BATTLE PLANS FOR FIGHTING BLEMISHES

The following battle plans are presented in order, starting with the most commonly available products with the least potential for side effects such as irritation, and working up to stronger products, some available only by prescription. The first battle plan may be all you need to help your skin. As you see how your skin responds, you can experiment with the various options for each category. **The most important element for all these skin-care battle plans is consistency. It takes a minimum of three weeks to six months to see a consistent improvement in your skin.** Remember that spot treatment doesn't work. You have to maintain consistent gentle cleansing, exfoliation, disinfecting, and reduced oil production to change the way your skin behaves.

If irritation or skin sensitivity occurs, you may need to cut back on the exfoliant, disinfectant, and/or facial mask you are using. That doesn't mean the skin-care routine isn't working for you (or that it won't eventually work), but perhaps your skin can't handle the frequency of application, at least not in the beginning. In that case you may need to reduce how often you apply the AHA, Retin-A, or Differin from twice a day to once a day or every other day, and the same is true with the disinfectant and facial mask.

**Note:** The following plans include the types of products needed to gently cleanse (without further clogging pores or increasing the presence of bacteria), exfoliate, and then disinfect. (The products are not presented in the order in which you'd apply them.)

**Plan A.** Gentle cleanser; 1% or 2% salicylic acid—exfoliant; 2.5%, 5%, or 10% benzoyl peroxide—disinfectant; and milk of magnesia—facial mask.

**Plan B.** Gentle cleanser; 8% or 10% AHA—for those who can't use salicylic acid for exfoliation; 2.5% or 5% benzoyl peroxide—disinfectant; and milk of magnesia—facial mask.

**Plan C.** Gentle cleanser; 1% or 2% salicylic acid—exfoliant; tretinoin (Retin-A, Tazorac, or Avita) or Differin in the evening; 2.5%, 5%, or 10% benzoyl peroxide—disinfectant, in the morning (do not apply at the same time the Retin-A, Tazorac, Avita, or Differin is applied); and a milk of magnesia facial mask.

**Plan D.** Gentle cleanser; azelaic acid—antibacterial and exfoliant; and a milk of magnesia facial mask.

**Plan E.** Gentle cleanser; tretinoin (Retin-A, Tazorac, Avita), Differin, or azelaic acid; a topical prescription antibacterial; and milk of a magnesia facial mask.

**Plan F.** Gentle cleanser; tretinoin (Retin-A, Tazorac, Avita), Differin, or azelaic acid; a topical prescription antibacterial; oral antibiotic; and milk of magnesia—facial mask. (Please note: Oral antibiotics can eventually result in development of resistant acne bacteria and are therefore best considered as short-term treatment.)

**Plan G.** When all else fails, Accutane.

# BATTLING BLACKHEADS AND LARGE PORES

I understand the frustration of battling blackheads. Insidious and glaring, blackheads make skin look mottled and unclean. The truth about blackheads (usually accompanied by oily skin) and whiteheads (usually accompanied by dry skin) is hard to accept. What is the truth? The truth is they are just hard to get rid of. It is hard to win the battle against clogged pores! However, because there are only a handful of options for dealing with this annoying skin malady, it's relatively simple to explain.

Pores that are functioning normally produce a normal amount of sebum (oil) and easily distribute the oil to the surface of skin. Hormones, almost exclusively, regulate the amount of sebum production. When a normal amount of oil is produced it moves effortlessly through the pore and out onto the surface of skin, where it melts into an imperceptible film that forms a protective barrier over the face.

Hormones can cause too much oil to be produced, or skin cells can block the exit path of the oil, or, when you have pores that are malformed, the oil in the pore can get clogged and then blackheads or whiteheads form. Further exacerbating these conditions is the buildup in the pore of skin-care or makeup products—mixed in with skin cells, they can get trapped in the sticky sebum sitting in the pore. When sebum and skin cells sit in a pore that is not covered over by skin, they are exposed to air, which causes the sebum and skin cells to oxidize and turn black. If the sebum and skin cells are sitting in a pore that is covered by skin, they are not exposed to air and remain clear, forming a slight white bump under the skin.

What's behind all this is primarily a genetic predisposition accompanied by the right conditions (mentioned above) randomly occurring in any one of the thousands of pores we have on our face. Not to mention unknown reactions to the over 50,000 cosmetic ingredients we may come in contact with from products we use.

To clear up the confusion, the following are battle plans against blackheads and whiteheads, because with some effort they can be reduced, and, depending on how your skin reacts, maybe even be reduced a lot.

Other than avoiding products that are too emollient (meaning thick or greasy creams) and not using moisturizers when you don't need them, there are really only four essentials for dealing with whiteheads and blackheads:

1. **Gentle, water-soluble cleansers** (and avoiding bar soap). The ingredients that keep bar soap in its bar form can clog pores, and irritation can cause skin cells to flake off before they're ready and accumulate in the pore. It's actually getting harder and harder to find a cleanser that isn't gentle. Be careful of cleansers that are too emollient and leave a greasy film on the skin, which can cause further problems.

2. **Gentle exfoliants** that can both remove the excess skin cells on the surface of the face (so they don't build up in the pore) and exfoliate inside the pore (to improve the shape of the pore, allowing a more even flow of oil through it). Keep in mind that the inside structure of the pore itself is lined with skin cells that can build up, creating a narrowed shape that doesn't allow natural oil flow. But don't get carried away with this step. Removing too many skin cells (over doing it) can cause problems and hurt skin. Exfoliation is essential for both dry and oily skin when you are trying to eliminate blackheads or whiteheads. The only difference is that someone with dry skin will want an exfoliant that has a more moisturizing base. The best option for exfoliating skin both within the pore and on the surface of the skin is a salicylic acid (beta hydroxy acid—BHA) lotion, gel, or liquid. Salicylic acid can penetrate the pore to help improve the shape of the pore lining, allowing an unobstructed path of oil flow.

3. **Absorbing excess oil.** This step is more for those with oily skin. It's really not an option for those with whiteheads (milia) and dry skin because with milia the problem is more due to trapped oil than it is to excess oil. For those with oily skin, you all know I prefer milk of magnesia (a few companies, including mine, have cosmetic versions of this). Clay masks are an option as long as they don't contain other ingredients that are irritating . The handful of silicone-based oil-absorbing products meant to be worn under makeup, from companies like Lancome and Clinique, get mixed reviews from women but are worth a trial run.

4. **Improving cell production** can help the pore function more normally. Effective considerations for all skin types are tretinoins (Retin-A, Tazorac, Avita, Renova), Differin, and azelaic acid. These can be used by themselves or with a BHA product. Research has definitely established that Retin-A, Renova, and Differin have positive effects on how pores function, and these products should be considered for very stubborn cases or when blackheads are accompanied by breakouts.

For those with oily-skin troubles, certain low-dose birth-control pills may be an option to reduce the hormone levels that create the excess oil that is at the root of the problem. And, when all else fails, Accutane can be considered. Be aware that many doctors are reluctant to prescribe Accutane for "merely" oily skin and blackheads. The fact is, for those with that kind of persistent skin problem it does not feel like a "mere" problem in the least, and Accutane can be a cure.

Blackheads can be made to seem less noticeable with pore strips, but only when the instructions on the box are followed exactly and they are not overused. Pore strips do not affect pore function.

For all skin types, AHA peels, microdermabrasion, and laser resurfacing can significantly affect the appearance of blackheads and whiteheads; however, they don't necessarily improve pore functioning (it depends on the depth of the treatment); rather, they temporarily get rid of the surface problem, making your skin look better.

Topical disinfectants (such as benzoyl peroxide) or topical antibiotics available by prescription are unwarranted and would be wasted in the treatment of blackheads and milia because bacteria are not involved in these conditions.

# WHAT ABOUT EMPTY, ENLARGED PORES?

Once a pore is emptied and the unsightly blackhead is removed it can take a period of time for the pore to heal and close up. Maintaining the regimen of gentle cleansing, exfoliating, and absorbing oil can go a long way toward making this happen. If your skin can tolerate Retin-A, Renova, or Differin, these products can help promote healing by further improving cell production in the pore. However, even after all this, an empty, open, but permanently damaged, pore can be an unattractive, leftover by-product of the original problem. If you have patiently adhered to all the "right" steps, there is very little else that can be done to change the damage. Time will tell if the effects of improving pore function can shrink a pore, but it does take time, and not everyone will have the same results. Microdermabrasion, AHA or BHA peels, and laser resurfacing can improve the appearance of pores, but these are considered temporary fixes and are not noted for actually changing or correcting the problem. Most likely the improvement is caused by the skin's swelling which makes the pores look smaller. Again, it is hard to determine success rates because there are no published results from long-term studies available.

The struggle to cover up large pores is nothing less than maddening. The very nature of a depression in the skin makes it difficult, if not impossible, to keep the indentation from showing. Especially if your skin is still oily, and even if you use an extremely matte foundation, such as Revlon's Skin Mattifying Makeup or regular ColorStay, Lancome's Teint Idole, or Estee Lauder's Double Wear or Double Matte, the oil can still cause some shifting, creating a look of pooled foundation in the pore.

I apologize for sounding dismal about this, but when there are limitations in the skin *and* in the world of makeup, searching for better options or alternatives can waste money and only increase your frustration. Here is a game plan to tackle the problem. It isn't foolproof and it won't work for everyone, but these are the best options available.

1. Avoid moisturizer over the open-pore areas of the face before applying makeup—even if you have dry skin. Any extra "slip" on the skin will cause

makeup to pool in the pore. If the skin is dry and flaky, be more diligent in the evening about treating your skin. Then in the morning use a toner with water-binding agents that can help soothe skin and reduce any dry feeling, yet not add anything that can make skin feel slippery. That means it is essential that your foundation contain your sunscreen, because an additional sunscreen under the foundation will almost certainly cause slippage.

2.  Do use a matte or ultra-matte foundation. Even if you have dry skin, these stay on far better than other foundations, are somewhat impervious to oil production, and, therefore, prevent the foundation from slipping into the pore.

3.  Consider wearing a tiny amount of milk of magnesia under your foundation over the open-pore area. This is a bit like applying spackle that has minimal to no movement. It can absorb oil at the same time and the foundation glides over it, creating an even surface. This works better under matte foundations than under ultra-matte foundations.

4.  For more stubborn problems, touch up your makeup several times during the day with oil-blotting papers. Then dust the face with a pressed powder designed to be worn as a foundation. Pressed powder foundations apply a slightly thicker layer of powder than normal pressed powders do, and can better hide the pore. But do this only with a brush; never use a sponge or pad to apply powder because they can place way too much product on the face, making things look cakey and thick.

# CHAPTER 11

## BATTLE PLANS FOR WOUNDS AND SCARS

### HOW SKIN HEALS

Whether it is a paper cut, scratch, cut, sore, lesion, or a really bad wound that requires stitches, one of the more amazing aspects of skin is its capacity to heal. Damaged skin regenerates and repairs itself. Only in certain circumstances, usually a result of some other illness such as diabetes, is that not true. When skin is injured, a multifaceted, complicated number of reactions take place. Many factors affect how long a wound takes to heal, and the way the wound heals affects how the skin will look, meaning what kind of scar will result. And that's not to say a scar is a bad thing—rather it's a sign that the body's repair system has kicked in so the fissure in your skin, no matter how small or big, closes up and mends.

Basically, skin goes through three fundamental and essential stages of repair. In the first stage, the scab is formed, and it's almost always accompanied by swelling, redness, and some tenderness or even pain. During the next stage, new skin tissue is formed under the scab. The final stage involves the rebuilding and reforming of the outer and inner layers of skin. Each of these stages of skin repair needs different kinds of help to aid in the healing process. What you do during the first days of a wound versus what you do after the scab has formed, or when the scab eventually comes off, is vital to the final appearance of the skin.

**Stage 1, Inflammation.** As soon as a cut or break in the skin has occurred, the body begins its job of preventing further injury. Signals are sent out for the blood to begin clotting and to call skin cells in to start protecting the damaged area. While the skin is working on its initial repair response, the immune system is trying to remove any foreign matter or bacteria that may have invaded the injury.

**Stage 2, Regrowth.** Now the body is busy producing collagen and reforming the substances that constitute the intercellular matrix. Intense collagen growth and the tightening of the surrounding tissue are the reason why we see an edge around wound while a scab is being formed.

**Stage 3, Renewal.** With the inflammatory reaction calmed, and after the new skin tissue, in the form of a scab and then a scar have been achieved during regrowth, it is time for the skin to focus on returning to normal. As time passes the scar becomes less noticeable, redness decreases, and the skin texture normalizes.

How your body goes about this process is genetically determined, but outside influences can also affect the way your skin responds to being injured.

# WHAT TO DO WHEN YOUR SKIN IS INJURED

Does applying aloe, vitamin E, or a variety of marine plants from algae to seaweed help heal wounds, prevent scars, or reduce the scarring you already have? There's no single substance or product that can address the complex issue of wound healing and scars, but there is a battle plan you can follow to minimize scarring as much as possible. Although aloe and algae can't hurt a scar and may indeed be helpful, what is more important is the overall way you treat the wound from its beginning, when the skin is injured, to the end, when the scar has formed.

Skin's unique, but unfortunate, response to injury is scarring. But skin, almost miraculously, also regenerates quickly, essentially renewing itself in two to four weeks. Depending on your genetic makeup and the depth of the injury, scarring can range from a slightly reddish discoloration to a thick, raised red or darkened scar (described as hypertrophic or keloidal), to serious disfigurement. Even so, the way you initially take care of a wound makes all the difference in the world.

Whether it is from acne, getting cut, or an operation, when skin damage first occurs you should allow it to "breathe" as much as possible. Do not gunk up the area with creams, lotions, or vitamin E capsules. Rubbing creams and lotions on a wound can damage fragile skin in the first stages of healing. Keep the damaged skin clean (but don't overclean it); using a gentle cleanser is the best way to do this. If you suspect there is a risk of infection, consider using an over-the-counter antibacterial such as Bacitracin.

At this stage, a little pure aloe vera gel or a very sheer, lightweight moisturizing gel is just fine, but *little* is the operative word here. In the beginning, keep the injured site out of sunlight altogether, as opposed to loading up on sunscreen. Heavy creams will suffocate the skin and prevent it from healing. Once the wound is healed, keep it out of sunlight as much as possible; then, remember it's imperative to protect the area with sunscreen. Sun damages skin and doesn't promote healing. Smoking is a skin destroyer and will also prevent healthy healing of wounds.

Here's what to do when you have a wound:

1. Wounds or lesions that don't require immediate medical attention (that is, if the wound does not require stitches and is not a chronic non-healing ulcer)

should not be completely or heavily occluded when the damage first occurs (Source: *Archives of Dermatological Research*, November 2001, pages 491–499). After cleansing, it is best to cover the wound with a light, thin bandage. In other words, avoid heavy bandages, creams, salves, or oils, that can impair the skin's initial healing process. Depending on where the wound or lesion is, it can be OK to wear a very lightweight bandage during the day or very lightweight moisturizers to protect the skin from getting reinjured, but, if you don't have a lightweight bandage, take the coverings off at night or apply a lotion that lets air get to the wound.

2. Let a scab form and don't pick or touch it—ever! Any manipulation or removal is a serious impediment to the healing that is taking place underneath and can cause scarring that would otherwise not have taken place.

3. Do not soak the lesion in water. Too much moisture saturation prevents wound healing.

4. It is important to keep the wound clean to prevent infection. Using a gentle cleanser is essential. Topical Bacitracin is an option if you suspect a risk of infection, but use it minimally because it is very thick and occlusive and can prevent air from getting to the wound.

5. Do not irritate the skin! The skin's primary, natural reaction to a wound is inflammation, which makes blood surge to the area to aid in healing. However, inflammation must be kept to a minimum and it should not be exacerbated because it can further damage skin. Anything you do to irritate the skin more makes matters worse. That means no soaps (they're too drying), no highly fragrant products (fragrant plant extracts and synthetic fragrances are all irritating), and, as always, no alcohol, peppermint, menthol, citrus, eucalyptus, clove, camphor, or mint.

6. Use sun protection! Leaving a wound unprotected to sun exposure impedes the skin's healing process *and* causes further skin damage.

7. If you do want to apply something soothing to the skin, use a very lightweight moisturizing lotion or pure aloe vera gel. Aloe's benefit for wound healing is mostly anecdotal; however, because aloe allows skin to breathe and can be soothing, it is still a great option to consider in the beginning. A moisturizer with antioxidants is the best way to help the wound continue healing.

# AFTER THE WOUND HAS HEALED

After the wound has healed you can use slightly more emollient products with antioxidants to keep free-radical damage to a minimum. Sunscreens in a light moisturizing base are essential, not only to keep the skin moist, but also to allow the skin to continue healing. There is some evidence, although the relevant studies used small samplings, that AHAs and tretinoins (such as Retin-A, Renova, Tazorac, Avita, and generic tretinoin) can significantly reduce the appearance of scarring by exfoliating the surface skin (using AHAs) and by stimulating normal cell production (using tretinoin). Exfoliation can reduce the thick, discolored appearance of scar tissue. Tretinoins, over time, *may* help generate collagen production to possibly shore up some of what was lost from the injury.

Exfoliation, antioxidants, and sunscreens can all help minimize scarring after the skin has healed. None of them will get rid of a scar, but the possibility of reducing the appearance of a scar is not to be ignored. Basically, there are no miracle skin-care ingredients or products when it comes to healing skin or reducing the appearance of scars. Instead, practice good skin care: don't overmanipulate the site, protect it from the sun, keep the area disinfected, keep heavy emollients off the skin, and, as much as possible, let the skin handle its own healing process.

As to nutritional issues, some of these definitely play a factor in healing wounds and scars. A list and description of oral supplements (i.e., systemic treatments) that have been shown to help heal wounds and scars is presented on the Web site http://www.drweil.com.

The following list describes topical factors for healing wounds and scars. The most important thing, both for healing a wound and trying to improve the scar's appearance is patience. It can take up to two years or longer depending on the depth of the lesion or wound, and it can depend on how diligent you are about caring for your skin with the following steps:

1. Once the skin has healed completely and the scab is gone, you can use nonfragrant plant oils or a lightweight moisturizer to keep the skin moist. The point here is to keep skin pliant and soft to help the skin's healing process (dry skin can fissure and tear, which can cause further skin damage). Topically applied vitamin E has not been shown to be of any special help in healing wounds or scars and may make matters worse.

2. Now that the skin is healed, it is helpful to remove the surface layers of skin where scar tissue may be forming. It is also helpful to improve skin-cell production, which may have been damaged from the wound (which is completely dependent on the depth of the lesion—meaning how many layers of

skin were affected and how well you have left the scab alone). For gently removing the surface layers of skin, consider using an effective salicylic acid product (BHA is preferred over AHA because BHA is composed of salicylic acid, which has anti-inflammatory properties, and reducing or preventing inflammation is essential for the healing process) as well as tretinoin (Retin-A, Renova, Tazorac, Avita) for improving cell production.

3. Once the wound or lesion is completely healed (this can take several months and up to two years), there are several options for dealing with the resulting scar. For surface discolorations and minor irregularities, microdermabrasion is an option. Acid peels (including AHA peels or trichloroacetic acid peels) as well as laser resurfacing are also significant options for reducing or eliminating scars.

4. For a thickened, raised scar, silicone sheets are still a primary option. It is believed that both the silicone and the pressure from the sheets encourage hydration, softening, and compression of the scar. Keep in mind that the silicone sheets may need to be worn for prolonged periods of time to gain the best and most lasting results. For further explanation of this option, refer to the passage below.

## VITAMIN E FOR SCARS?

The simple answer to that question is, "Probably not." A report of research published in *Dermatologic Surgery* (April 1999, pages 311–315), in an article titled "The effects of topical vitamin E on the cosmetic appearance of scars" concluded that the "… study shows that there is no benefit to the cosmetic outcome of scars by applying vitamin E after skin surgery and that the application of topical vitamin E may actually be detrimental to the cosmetic appearance of a scar. In 90% of the cases in this study, topical vitamin E either had no effect on, or actually worsened, the cosmetic appearance of scars. Of the patients studied, 33% developed a contact dermatitis to the vitamin E. Therefore we conclude that use of topical vitamin E on surgical wounds should be discouraged." The study was done double-blind "with patients given two ointments each labeled A or B. A was Aquaphor, a regular emollient, and the B was Aquaphor mixed with vitamin E. The scars were randomly divided into parts A and B. Patients were asked to put the A ointment on part A and the B ointment on part B twice daily for 4 weeks." Antioxidants are definitely an option for skin, but, for preventing scars, vitamin E directly applied on skin does not appear to be one of them.

# SILICONE SHEETS FOR KELOIDAL SCARRING

Even though you've done all you can to help heal the skin, thicker raised keloidal scars can set in. One way to treat this kind of scarring is with a pliable sheet of silicone. Some examples of silicone sheets are ReJuveness *($39.50 to $95, depending on the size)*, Syprex Scar Sheet *($20 to $40 depending on the size)*, and Curad Scar Therapy Cosmetic Pads *($16.99)*. It is not clear how these sheets of silicone oil work. They may increase the amount of water in the scar, and continuous rehydration of scars may soften the tissue, making it more elastic and pliable, thus encouraging the flattening process (Source: *European Journal of Dermatology*, December 1998, pages 591–595). But they do work, and rather successfully (although I use the word "successfully" with caution).

Silicone sheets appear to be most effective for hypertrophic or keloidal scarring. As wonderful as this sounds, there are disadvantages. Users purchase one relatively inexpensive sheet of silicone that is worn over and over again. The sheet must be kept clean, which requires care and maintenance time. The sheet must be worn over the scar for prolonged periods of time, so you might not want to wear one on your face or other exposed parts of your body, at least not during the day. Also, the silicone sheet can stick to the skin and skin reactions such as rashes or irritation can occur.

As mentioned, you must wear the sheet for long periods—for hours at a time, over a span of at least two to nine months—to see a difference. But patience pays off. The longer you wear it, the more likely it is that the scar will dissipate to some extent. Of course, these sheets work best over new scars, but they can make a difference with old ones, too. Even acne scarring—thick, raised scars, not pits—can be reduced if the scars have been present for less than 16 years. As wonderful and hopeful as this all sounds, be aware that the word "reduce" is imprecise. Do not try these if you are hoping for extraordinary results, of the kind the advertising implies. Dr. Loren Engrav, associate director and Chief of Plastic Surgery for the University of Washington burn unit at Harborview Medical Center, explains that the "silicone strips are standard treatment for helping dissipate scars, and though the results may be good, they are absolutely not a miracle."

Some women buy silicone sheets to use over stretch marks, but there is no clinical evidence that this product will have any effect on them whatsoever. These sheets create a flattening process, while a raising process is what would be required for stretch marks.

# Lasers for Scar Repair

"A variety of lasers can be used to treat scars and stretch marks effectively. It is of paramount importance that the type of scar be properly classified on initial examination so that the most appropriate method of treatment can be chosen. Classification also allows the laser surgeon to discuss with the patient the anticipated response to treatment. The 585-nm pulsed dye laser (PDL) is the most appropriate system for treating ... keloids, [red] scars, and stretch marks. The PDL carries a low risk of side effects and complications when operated at appropriate treatment parameters and time intervals. Atrophic scars are best treated with ablative $CO_2$ lasers and Er:YAG lasers; however, [growing or worsening] keloids and [deteriorating] scars should not be vaporized because of the high risk of scar recurrence or progression. The appropriate choice and use of lasers can significantly improve most scars. As research into laser-skin interaction continues, further refinements in laser technology, coupled with the addition of alternate treatment procedures, will allow improved clinical efficacy and predictability" (Source: *Dermatologic Clinics*, January 2002, pages 55–65).

# Options for Keloidal Scarring

Effecting treatment of keloidal scarring is best approached with a multitherapy course of action. Using only one method is not as successful as combining two or more options.

Cryotherapy, or cryosurgery, uses extreme cold, in the form of liquid nitrogen, to get rid of the unwanted tissue. This method doesn't cause bleeding or scarring but it can leave behind a white mark that often doesn't regain normal skin color. It works best on some raised scarring but can be less successful on keloids. Ultrasonic treatment uses high-pulse sound waves to reduce collagen buildup.

Scar massage is not recommended because, while it can break down the material in the skin creating the raised scar, the massage can also stimulate collagen production, which caused the scar in the first place. Corticosteroids can be injected into the raised scar to inhibit production of the cells that are responsible for generating the scar tissue. Interferons are known to reduce the production of major scar-forming growth factors (Source: *Rehab Management*, August-September 2001, http://www.rehabpub.com/features/892001/3.asp).

Topical verapamil hydrochloride is a relatively new option for the prevention and treatment of keloidal scarring. One study showed "keloids were cured in 54% of the cases in the first group ... [and] in the remaining 36% of patients in the first group in whom keloids recurred, there was an improvement in size and above all in consistence" (Source: *Dermatology*, 2002, volume 204, issue 1, pages 60–62).

# STRETCH MARKS

Whether from pregnancy or weight loss, the striated tracks that can show up on skin are frustrating to women. One treatment that seems to show promise for improving the appearance of stretch marks is the use of topical tretinoin, especially if it is applied as soon as the skin alteration is noticed (Sources: *Archives of Dermatology*, May 1996, pages 519–526; *Advances in Therapy*, July-August 2001, pages 181–186). While these studies show promise for improving the appearance of stretch marks, the word "improve" needs to be qualified. These studies were done on a small sampling of women and the improvement was evaluated as good, but the stretch marks did not disappear. What does show the most promise for reducing or even eliminating the appearance of stretch marks is laser resurfacing or chemical peels. These are discussed in Chapter Thirteen, *Cosmetic Surgery*.

**Note:** Some types of laser resurfacing are considered problematic for women with darker skin colors.

# MEDERMA

An article in the *Archives of Dermatology* (December 1998, pages 1512–1514, "Snake oil for the 21st century") from the Department of Dermatology, Harvard Medical School, stated that "With the current promulgation of skin 'products' and their promotion and even sale by dermatologists, and the use of treatments of no proven efficacy, this association between dermatology and quackery is set to continue well into the 21st century. The list of offending treatments includes silicone gel sheets and onion extract cream (Mederma) for keloids ...."

Another study (Source: *Cosmetic Dermatology*, March 1999, pages 19–26) concluded that there were no discernable differences between skin treated with Mederma and skin that was treated with a placebo. Nevertheless, Mederma advertises itself as promising to get rid of scars.

Mederma, which uses onion extract as the scar-changing ingredient, contains water, thickeners, onion extract, fragrance, and preservative. There is no research showing onion extract to be effective as a skin-care ingredient. A customer service representative for Mederma told me that the onion extract "prevents the release of histamines which causes scarring." Even if onions could prevent the release of histamines, however, histamines have everything to do with allergic reactions but nothing whatsoever to do with scarring. The body produces histamines in response to an allergic reaction; the body sends them in to fight the allergen that causes the redness, swelling, and itching. While histamines can cause the skin to react, that reaction isn't related to the breakdown of collagen and elastin that causes scarring. If anything, because onions release a complex mixture of sulfur-containing oils to-gether with sulfur-free aldehydes and ammonia, all of which are more or less in-tensely volatile (that's what makes your eyes burn and tear when you cut into them), onions can be a potent skin irritant.

## WHAT ABOUT SCARS FROM ACNE?

Severe and even mild acne can often lead to some form of scarring. A permanent scar is a defect in the skin caused by an injury to the area, such as an acne lesion. The key word here is "permanent." Most of the acne lesions that people call scars are really not scars at all, but instead post-inflammatory redness—red spots left behind after the blemish heals. What is frustrating about this redness is that it takes time for it go away—anywhere from 6 to 12 months, depending on the depth of the original lesion and how you cared for the lesion. However, there are ways to facilitate heal-ing. Following the guidelines for treating wounds that were presented in previous sections of this chapter will make a huge difference in the way the skin heals.

Permanent scars develop as the skin attempts to heal itself by surrounding the acne lesion with new skin. The epidermis (outer layer of skin) grows in from the sides to the center, and underneath the sebaceous gland. When the acne finally heals, a depressed pit can remain in the skin. Scarring is unpredictable—it's impos-sible to know how much a particular person will scar, if at all. The best way to prevent acne scarring is through early treatment of lesions.

The best way to prevent scars is to not do anything that makes matters worse. Untreated or improperly treated acne is likely to cause the worst scarring because the problem is never mitigated and the skin has no chance to heal. Harshly attacking blemishes and creating deep scabs and sores that take a long time to heal are surefire ways to guarantee a scar will be permanent. Using heavy or irritating facial products will also hinder the healing process. In addition, because many women don't know how to treat acne, they use ineffective topical disinfectants and exfoliants, which can also impede the skin's ability to repair itself. Unprotected sun exposure can exacer-bate scarring, too. Yet, if you are good about not picking and oversqueezing blem-ishes from the outset, scarring can be greatly reduced. Even so, the most meticulous state-of-the-art acne skin-care routine can still result in scars. Most acne scars do fade with time, but that time can seem like an eternity when the face is yours.

Once acne and breakouts have been reduced or eliminated, the brown, pink, or purple discolorations left by acne lesions can fade a great deal in about 6 to 12 months, depending on your skin color. You can speed up that fading by continuing to use a product with AHAs, BHA, or tretinoin (which are all helpful in the treat-ment of acne and breakouts anyway).

Once acne has healed, small areas with shallow scars or pit-type scars can be injected with dermal fillers (various substances used to lift or fill the depression), but these are not permanent fixes and require repeated treatments.

Chemical peels such as salicylic acid (beta hydroxy acid—BHA), alpha hydroxy acids (AHAs), and trichloroacetic acids (TCAs) can improve the appearance of surface scarring. (But these peels are unwarranted for scarring if the acne is still active.) Just don't expect an AHA or BHA peel to improve the appearance of deep scarring. For larger areas of the face, laser resurfacing is absolutely the treatment of choice (Sources: *Facial and Plastic Surgery*, November 2001, pages 253–262; *Aesthetic Plastic Surgery*, January-February 2001, pages 46–51).

Microdermabrasion can improve the texture and color of skin, but it requires deeper microdermabrasion treatments to obtain visible improvement in acne scarring (Source: *Dermatologic Surgery*, June 2001, pages 524–530).

Skin-lightening lotions with hydroquinone or other skin-lightening ingredients do not work well, if at all, on acne scarring. These lotions prevent melanin production; they do not have much effect on what gives acne scars their color.

# CHAPTER 12

# COMMON SKIN DISORDERS

## SPECIAL CONCERNS

As if the issues surrounding skin type (normal, oily, sun-damaged, blemish-prone), skin sensitivities, and allergic reactions weren't enough, a large percentage of the population deals with medical conditions that add to skin-care woes. These problems make selecting the appropriate skin-care routine extremely tricky. It becomes a challenge to find the right combination of products that will benefit the skin and not make matters worse. The most common skin disorders are eczema, psoriasis, seborrhea, and rosacea. Early identification goes a long way toward reducing the symptoms of these skin afflictions because it can help sufferers avoid buying products that are likely to exacerbate the condition. Almost without exception, these skin disorders require a dermatologist's care; they cannot be treated at the cosmetics counter or with over-the-counter products from the drugstore. Finding the right skin-care and makeup routines that work with each of these conditions is important, but it's equally vital that they complement, and not undo, the benefit of the medical treatments for the specific disorder.

## ROSACEA

Rosacea is no fun. It is a stubborn skin disorder that is frustrating and extremely difficult to treat. Thought to afflict at least 30% to 50% of the population, it is frequently misdiagnosed by dermatologists and physicians. Rosacea develops over a long period of time, starting with what first seems like a tendency to blush easily, a ruddy complexion, or an extreme sensitivity to cosmetics. The distinctive redness or flushing, which appears in a characteristic butterfly pattern over the nose and cheeks, is the first likely indication that rosacea may be what your skin is struggling with. Though bothersome, the subtle initial redness is often ignored by women as being just a skin-tone or color problem and not a skin disorder.

Another challenge with identifying rosacea is that pustules (pimples) and papules (red raised bumps) that resemble acne are often present. That makes rosacea look like acne and that means it's often misdiagnosed. Unlike most acne conditions, rosacea is rarely, if ever, accompanied by blackheads. The distinctive flushing and extreme skin sensitivity also differentiate rosacea from acne. The final toll on the face is the presence of flaky patches that may or may not be accompanied by either dry or oily skin, or possibly by both at the same time. Rosacea can be extremely confusing for a woman because the dry, flaky skin responds minimally or not at all to moisturizers and the acnelike bumps and whiteheads respond minimally, or not at all, to typical acne treatments.

Even more confounding, when rosacea first develops, it may appear, disappear, and then reappear a short time later. This fluctuation also makes diagnosis difficult. Yet, despite its evasive beginnings, the condition rarely reverses itself (meaning there is no cure) and almost always becomes worse without treatment.

What usually happens is the skin doesn't return to its normal color and stays persistently red. Other symptoms, such as enlarged blood vessels, flaky patches, oily skin, skin sensitivity, and breakouts, become more and more visible. As rosacea progresses, pimples appear on the face in the form of small, solid red bumps and pus-filled bumps. In more advanced cases of rosacea, a condition called rhino-phyma may develop. Rhinophyma is characterized by a bulbous, enlarged red nose and puffy cheeks. It may also involve thick bumps that develop on the lower half of the nose, spreading to the nearby cheek areas. However, rhinophyma rarely occurs in women.

For years rosacea was referred to as "acne rosacea." That only added to the confu-sion because rosacea is completely unrelated to acne. However, because the papules and pustules that can accompany rosacea look like acne, many doctors misdiagnose it and end up prescribing medications that make matters worse instead of better. Most acne treatments (tretinoin and topical antibacterials) can increase rosacea's red, flaky appearance. That's why the right medication is crucial for relieving the cause of the disorder. You and your doctor need to know exactly what you are dealing with to be sure you are receiving the right treatment. Understanding the difference between acne and acne rosacea can make a huge difference in the health of your skin.

There are only a handful of treatments for rosacea, and they are all available by prescription only, including topical application of MetroGel, MetroCream, MetroLotion, and Noritate. The active ingredient in each of these is metronida-zole, which is considered the primary treatment for rosacea (Source: *Skin Therapy Letter*, January 2002, pages 1–6). Occasionally, azelaic acid and oral antibiotics are also an option. Because you must experiment until you find what works best for your skin, all of these should be considered when creating your own battle plan for treating rosacea.

What causes rosacea? Surprisingly, no one really knows, but it is suspected that some kind of microbe under the skin is responsible for the symptoms. Killing off this microbe seems to be the most helpful way to improve the appearance of skin and, if caught early enough, keep matters from getting worse. The active ingredient metronidazole may work in this capacity due to its antimicrobial activity on the skin. If the microbe is left to flourish, the resulting chronic inflammation (redness, swelling, breakouts, flaking skin) is believed to account for some of the symptoms of rosacea (Source: *Advances in Therapy*, September-October 2001, pages 237–243).

## BATTLE PLAN FOR ROSACEA

Red, flushed cheeks; swollen, almost bulging, oil glands; dry flaky skin, often with an oily layer underneath; overly sensitive skin that reacts to everything; and red, pimple-like lumps—this is what rosacea can look like. It can be a combination of symptoms, or a variety, or just one. Regardless, if left untreated, rosacea almost always gets worse and it just doesn't feel pretty when you have it.

Rosacea is much like any other pervasive skin disorder, from breakouts to eczema, because there are no easy answers. Cosmetics companies looking for your money have a penchant for claiming that their line has the answer to your problems, but these products often have no relation to the needs of someone struggling with rosacea (exfoliants, anti-irritants, antifungal ingredients, and so on). But the hope that the next product can make a difference is just too tempting for most women looking for the magic bullet. In reality, even well-formulated products, meaning primarily those that are free of topical skin irritants, can be a problem for rosacea.

So where do you begin when you're dealing with rosacea? Because rosacea is so often misdiagnosed, the place to start is with a dermatologist who has experience with this disorder. Next come skin-care considerations, to be sure the products you are using aren't making matters worse, and then lifestyle considerations, because what you do can cause flare-ups.

**Treatments:** As stated above, no one really knows what causes rosacea but it is suspected that a microbe under the skin causes the symptoms. Killing off the microbe seems to be the most helpful way to improve the appearance of skin and, if caught early enough, keep matters from getting worse. **Only a handful of treatments exist that can combat the microbe responsible for rosacea. These prescription-only topical medications include MetroLotion, MetroGel, MetroCream, Noritate, and azelaic acid** (Source: *Journal of the American Academy of Dermatology*, June 1999, pages 961–965). The success of these topical medications, when combined with an oral antibiotic, can be significant. (When considering an oral antibiotic you must consider the risk of the microbe adapting to it after prolonged use. If that happens, that specific oral antibiotic won't be effective to help deal with other types of infections you may encounter.)

**Isotretinoin (Accutane).** This medication has been shown in several studies to be effective for those with treatment-resistant rosacea, and it is effective in a low dose of about 0.5 to 1.0 milligram per kilogram of body weight. (Accutane is always prescribed based on the weight of the patient.) No one is quite sure how Accutane works for rosacea but the success rate is good, and after treatment the swelling and distortion of the oil glands are often resolved (Source: *Archives of Dermatology*, July 1998, pages 884–885).

Accutane is also considered an option for treating the occurrence of rhinophyma (nose swelling) that often takes place in cases of advanced rosacea. Rhinophyma is the distorted appearance of the nose resulting from overgrowth of its oil glands. Ironically, rhinophyma has been traditionally associated with alcoholism, yet there is no evidence to support this association. Generally, rhinophyma is best treated surgically, though systemic isotretinoin may also be an effective option (Source: *Facial and Plastic Surgery*, 1998, volume 14, issue 4, pages 241–253). For an assessment of warnings and risks associated with Accutane, see the "Accutane" section in Chapter Ten, *Battle Plans for Blemishes*.

**Gentle skin-care products.** Because redness, irritation, and skin sensitivities are part and parcel of rosacea itself, anything exacerbating those things will cause more problems. Gentle cleansers, a soothing toner with anti-irritants, lightweight moisturizers with antioxidants and anti-irritants, and nonchemical sunscreens (with zinc oxide and titanium dioxide) are the basics. The National Rosacea Society (http://www.rosacea.org) surveyed 1,000 of its members who identified alcohol, witch hazel, fragrance, menthol, peppermint, and eucalyptus as contributing to flare-ups. It isn't always easy to identify those substances on a label when they are listed under the Latin names that are required by the FDA for ingredient labels. Moreover, there are many fragrant components and lots of other potentially irritating skin-care ingredients in many products. Even if you've been diligent in checking your products you can still run into problems because it is often hard to determine what is causing your own specific flare-ups. Yet as difficult as it is to pinpoint exactly what ingredients may trigger rosacea, the ones listed in Chapter Four, *Skin Care Basics for Everyone*, in the section "How to Be Gentle," as problems for irritation give you a good idea about what to avoid. Keep in mind that not everyone responds the same way to any of these ingredients, but avoiding these as much as possible will at the very least reduce the redness and dry flaky skin.

**Salicylic acid treatment.** I feel strongly that anecdotal information is correct when it points to the benefits of using a gentle toner or moisturizer that contains 1% to 2% salicylic acid (BHA) in a base with a pH of 3 to 4. Salicylic acid is an exfoliant that helps to remove the built-up layers of dry, flaky skin on the face and, because salicylic acid is related to aspirin (both are salicylates), it can also have anti-inflammatory properties on the skin, reducing redness and swelling.

**Lifestyle factors to avoid.** Several lifestyle factors can make rosacea worse, although these are not the same for everyone because people have different reactions to the same ingredient or external elements. These catalysts can include hot liquids, spicy foods, exposure to extreme temperatures (including cooking over a hot stove), alcohol consumption, sunlight, stress, saunas, hot tubs, smoking, rubbing or massaging the skin, irritating cosmetics, and anything else that overstimulates the skin and blood vessels.

**Other irritants to avoid.** Rosacea can also be exacerbated by AHAs (though not for everyone), Retin-A, Renova, Differin, exfoliants of any kind (including scrubs and washcloths), and clay-based facial masks. The less you do, meaning the fewer products you use, and the fewer ingredients in each, the happier rosacea-afflicted skin is going to be.

**Ocular rosacea.** This condition refers to rosacea of the eye and, according to an item in the March 2001 issue of *Cosmetic Dermatology*, is significantly underdiagnosed and untreated. They note that "Of an estimated 13 million U.S. adults [with rosacea], 89% of 2,010 rosacea sufferers … indicated they also experienced discomfort or redness of the eyes in varying degrees." Those with ocular rosacea most commonly experience irritation of the lids and eye, as well as sties and chronically red eyes. In rare cases, ocular rosacea can also affect the cornea. This condition can be treated, usually with soothing eye drops (but not Visine) along with oral or topical antibiotics, but it requires a dermatologic evaluation before any action is taken.

The *Rosacea Review*, an online newsletter of the National Rosacea Society, at http://www.rosacea.org./rrindex.html, is an excellent source for detailed and ongoing information concerning treatment and research for rosacea.

# LASER TREATMENT FOR ROSACEA

The following letter I received from a reader sums up the issues around laser treatment for rosacea.

*Dear Paula,*

I have rosacea and have had four PhotoDerm laser treatments by a top dermatologist in the Houston area. After the fourth treatment, I was quite discouraged, as the veins on my nose still showed, and overall I still had a great deal of pinkness. I went to her about it, and she patch-tested the side of my nose with a stronger laser setting. The veins are still there, and I still look sunburned.

I have now moved to a midwestern city. They still seem to be discovering current beauty treatments here and there isn't a PhotoDerm laser to be found. I am also seriously questioning whether this treatment is viable for rosacea. At $1,600 later, I'm not too keen about trying the supposedly magic fifth treatment anyway!

What do you suggest for me? If you say PhotoDerm is still an option, is there a way I can find out (other than the yellow pages) who is professionally certified in it where I live? I don't have a problem with breakouts, so my MetroGel doesn't do a lot for me.

**Frustrated in St. Louis**

Dear Frustrated,

As helpful as PhotoDerm can be for treating rosacea, not everyone gets the great results you've heard about. According to an article in the *Journal of Cutaneous Laser Therapy* (April 1999, pages 961–965), "A total of 200 patients were treated with an intense pulsed light source (PhotoDerm VL) using various treatment parameters. The patients were treated for facial veins (primarily telangiectasia), facial hemangiomas, rosacea and port wine stains. Results: Of the 188 patients who returned for follow-up after 2 months, 174 achieved 75% to 100% clearance in one to four treatment sessions. The post-treatment side effects were minimal and well tolerated by the patients. There were no instances of scarring or other permanent side effects." While that statistic is impressive, there were still 26 people who weren't happy with their results. Statistically it was wise for you to consider this treatment, but after four sessions it is clearly not one that will work for you (assuming of course that the physician you saw knew what she was doing).

There are other options for your skin, but they involve deeper laser resurfacing. You would need to discuss this with a plastic surgeon or dermatologist with a well-established practice in working with lasers. To find one in your area refer to http://www.plasticsurgery.org (The American Society of Plastic Surgeons) or http://www.aad.org/DermProfile/index.html (American Academy of Dermatology).

One other point: You seem to be under the assumption that MetroGel is meant to treat "breakouts," and that is not the case. MetroGel is meant to deal with the symptoms (and theoretically the source of the problem) for rosacea. Whether it is redness, flaking, enlarged pores, or breakouts, MetroGel (active ingredient: metronidazole) should be considered an option.

# PSORIASIS

Psoriasis is a chronic recurring skin disease, identified by the presence of thickened scaly areas and papules (small, solid, often-inflamed bumps that, unlike pimples, do not contain pus or sebum). These bumps are usually slightly elevated above the skin surface, sharply distinguishable from normal skin, and red to reddish brown in color. They are usually covered with small whitish silver scales that stick to the cystlike swelling and, if scraped off, may bleed. The extent of the disease varies from a few tiny lesions to generalized involvement of most of the skin. Often the elbows, knees, scalp, and chest are involved. Psoriasis affects over 7 million people in the United States alone, but for most people it tends to be mild and unsightly rather than a serious health concern, which is probably why fewer than 2 million people seek medical treatment for it (Source: *OTC Journal Newsletter*, October 15, 2001, online at http://www.otcjournal.com/profiles/astr/20011015-1.html).

No one knows for certain exactly what causes psoriasis, although recent studies suggest it may be related to an immune system problem, which triggers inflammation. The resulting intense inflammation causes the skin to shed too rapidly. Psoriasis is the recurring growth of too many skin cells that are not able to shed properly, accompanied by inflammation and redness. A normal skin cell matures in 28 to 45 days, while a psoriatic skin cell takes only 3 to 6 days. Both men and women can get psoriasis at any age, so it isn't unusual to start noticing red, swollen, flaky bumps on your skin late in life.

Psoriasis appears in several forms. The scaly, papule kind called plaque psoriasis is the most common. Other forms include guttate psoriasis, typified by small dotlike lesions all over the body; pustular psoriasis, with weeping lesions and intense scaling; and erythrodermic psoriasis, characterized by severe sloughing and inflammation of the skin. Psoriasis can range from mild to moderate to severe and disabling. On occasion, some people who have psoriasis experience spontaneous remissions, but no one knows why or when that may happen.

Sadly, there is no cure for psoriasis, but there are many different treatments, both topical and systemic, that can clear it for periods of time. Experimenting with a variety of options is essential to find the treatment that works for you, but all require a doctor's attention.

## BATTLE PLANS FOR PSORIASIS

Of the various therapies available to treat psoriasis, it is generally best to start with those that have the least-serious side effects, such as topical steroids (cortisone creams); coal-tar creams, lotions, cleansers, or shampoos; and careful exposure to sunshine. If those methods are not successful, you can proceed to the more serious treatments involving oral medications. More often than not, successful treatment requires a combination of methods.

## TOPICAL TREATMENTS

**Natural sunlight** can significantly improve, or even clear, psoriasis. Ultraviolet (UV) light from the sun suppresses the skin's immune response and, therefore, reduces inflammation, slowing the overproduction of skin cells that causes scaling. Daily, short, nonburning exposure to sunlight clears or improves psoriasis in many people. Therefore, sunlight may be included among initial treatments for the disease (Source: National Institutes of Health, Department of Health and Human Services, *Questions and Answers about Psoriasis*, January 2002, online at http://www.niams.nih.gov/hi/topics/psoriasis/psoriafs.htm).

Regular daily doses of sunlight, taken in short exposures with adequate sun protection, are strongly recommended. Sun protection is vital not only to prevent sunburn, which may make psoriasis worse, but also to reduce skin damage from the sun's UV radiation. This outdoor approach to treating psoriasis is often referred to as **climatotherapy**. Some people travel to Florida, Hawaii, the Caribbean, or the Dead Sea in Israel (where special clinics offer treatment solariums and supervised medical assistance) to use swimming and natural sunlight as their psoriasis treatment (some people believe immersion in salty, mineral-laden water may also have some unknown benefits). In some countries, medical plans actually cover trips to these types of sunny climates and mineral spas for subscribers with psoriasis.

When you can't get to sunshine, medically supervised administration of UVB lamps may be used to minimize widespread or localized areas of stubborn and unmanageable psoriasis lesions. UVB light is also used when topical treatments have failed, or in combination with topical treatments. The short-term risks of using controlled UVB exposure to treat psoriasis are minimal, and long-term studies of large numbers of patients treated with UVB have not demonstrated an increased risk of skin cancer, suggesting that this treatment may be safer than sunlight. (Sunlight has both UVA and UVB radiation; UVA causes skin cancer, while UVB mainly triggers sunburn.) UVB treatments are considered one of the most effective therapies for moderate to severe psoriasis, with the least amount of risk. There are even sources of UVB light therapy, called narrow-band UVB, that give off only the part of the UV spectrum band that is most helpful for psoriasis and reduce the risk of wide-band UVB light.

Treating psoriasis with **coal tar** is a very old and effective remedy. It is a topical medication available both over the counter and by prescription; the difference is in the potency and amount of coal tar the medication contains. Coal tar inhibits certain skin substances that incite cell proliferation, thus reducing the appearance of psoriasis. Coal tar can be combined with other psoriasis medications (like topical steroids) or with sunshine (UV). However, coal tar can make the skin more sensitive to UV light, and extreme caution is advised when you combine coal tar use with UV therapy (or exposure to the sun) to avoid getting a severe burn or causing skin damage. Other downsides to coal tar are the irritation it can cause, the smell, and its tendency to stain clothes.

**Anthralin**, much like coal tar, is a topical prescription medication that has been used to treat psoriasis for decades. Though anthralin's action on skin is not clear, it appears to inhibit cell proliferation. It has few serious side effects but can irritate or burn the normal-appearing skin surrounding psoriatic lesions. Anthralin also stains anything it comes into contact with. It is prescribed in a range of concentrations, but the most effective form is a hard paste that is very difficult to apply, requiring a great deal of patience; also, it can't be used over inflamed lesions, and must not get on the face. There are a variety of regimens for its use, but the negative side effects and cumbersome and time-consuming application process often make it a less-than-desirable option.

A study in the *American Journal of Clinical Dermatology* (2001, volume 2, issue 2, pages 95–120) reviewed the efficacy and studies involving the topical application of **calcipotriene** (trade name Dovonex), a derivative of vitamin D3 used to treat mild to moderate psoriasis. (It is not the same compound as the vitamin D found in commercial vitamin supplements.) Calcipotriene acts not only to inhibit cell proliferation and enhance cell differentiation in the skin of patients with psoriasis, but also appears to have effects on immunologic markers that are thought to play a role in the cause of the disease. In several well-designed, short-term studies in adults, the efficacy of calcipotriene ointment (50 micrograms twice daily) was similar or superior to the efficacy of several other antipsoriatic agents in adult patients with mild to moderate psoriasis. Calcipotriene is generally well tolerated in short- and long-term studies in adult patients, with the major side effect being irritation. In addition, calcipotriene ointment proved beneficial in combination with other topical, phototherapy, or systemic antipsoriatic treatments, reducing the dosage and/or duration of some of these treatments and potentially improving their benefit/risk ratio. Calcipotriene ointment is valuable as a first- or second-line therapy option for the management of mild to moderate psoriasis and also in combination with other antipsoriatic agents for more severe psoriasis. Other forms of vitamin D3 creams include **calcitriol** and **tacalitol**.

**Topical corticosteroids** (cortisones) have been used for years as the first-step approach in the treatment of psoriasis. Cortisones reduce inflammation, itching, and potentially reduce cell buildup. Brands differ in potency, and the more power ful a drug the higher the risk of more severe side effects, which include burning, irritation, dryness, acne, thinning of the skin, dilated blood vessels, and loss of skin color. Less potent drugs should be used for mild to moderate psoriasis, saving the high-potency drugs for more severe conditions. An effective regimen uses high-potency cortisones, such as halobetasol (Ultravate), daily until the psoriasis plaque flattens out, after which they are applied only on the weekends. Another high-potency corticosteroid, mometasone (Elocon), needs to be administered only once a day and is as effective, or more effective than other corticosteroids while having a lower risk of severe side effects. These very potent drugs carry a small risk of causing hormonal problems for a period of time after the drug has been withdrawn. The larger the area treated with corticosteriods, the higher the risk, especially if the area is covered by heavy material or is bandaged. Also, in most cases, resistance to these drugs eventually develops; and the disease can recur after treatment is stopped (Source: http://my.webmd.com/content/article/1680.51881).

**Topical retinoids** such as **Tazorac** (active ingredient tazarotene) have been shown to have a positive effect on psoriasis (Source: *Cutis*, January 1999, pages 41–48), particularly in combination with other treatments (Source: *International Journal of Dermatology*, January 2001, pages 64–66).

**Salicylic acid (beta hydroxy acid)** in strengths of 1.8% to 3% is approved by the FDA as an over-the-counter treatment for psoriasis. Because it is a keratolytic, meaning it softens and removes scaly skin layers of psoriatic lesions. Removing these skin layers is important because it allows other topical medications to better penetrate skin. Also, because of salicylic acid's chemical relationship to aspirin, it has anti-inflammatory properties and can reduce the redness associated with psoriasis. Salicylic acid is available in many forms, and it is often combined with other topical medications to enhance their effectiveness (Source: http://www.psoriasis.org). The primary concern in choosing a well-formulated salicylic acid product is to be sure the concentration is stated clearly on the product, and that the pH of the product is no higher than 3.5.

## SYSTEMIC TREATMENTS

**Methotrexate** is an anti-cancer drug that can reduce the overproduction of cells. It is an established and highly effective systemic treatment for severe psoriasis and has been widely used during the last three decades. For this reason, the long-term adverse effects of methotrexate are well known. The most frequent adverse effects that occur during methotrexate therapy are abnormal liver function test results, nausea, and gastric complaints. The most feared adverse effects are liver damage and the suppression of bone marrow activity. However, liver problems associated with methotrexate are related to a high cumulative dose. This means that rotating types of therapy or using methotrexate intermittently instead of continuously can reduce the risk. Most people tolerate low-dose methotrexate therapy relatively well, provided they work closely with their physician and watch carefully for adverse effects and drug interactions during treatment. The long-term clinical efficacy and relative safety of methotrexate remain impressive (Sources: *American Journal of Clinical Dermatology*, January-February 2000, pages 27–39; *Clinical Rheumatology*, 2001, volume 20, issue 6, pages 406–410).

**Cyclosporin** (trade name Neoral) is a strong immune-suppressant drug and a primary medication used to prevent the rejection of transplanted organs such as liver, kidneys, and heart. In skin diseases, cyclosporin acts by reducing inflammation in the skin and reducing cell proliferation by blocking immune factors that may be generating the problem. Studies have shown cyclosporin to be highly effective and well tolerated in short-term treatment of severe psoriasis (Source: *American Journal of Clinical Dermatology*, 2001, volume 2, issue 1, pages 41–47). However, this is a serious medication. Temporary side effects of cyclosporin can include headaches, gingivitis, joint pain, gout, body-hair growth, tremors, high blood pressure, kidney problems, and fatigue. Of serious concern is the National Toxicology Program's *Eighth Report on Carcinogens,* 1998, which warns that cyclosporin is "known to be a human carcinogen based on studies in humans." All of these factors must be weighed and carefully assessed before deciding on this course of treatment.

**Etretinate** (trade name Tegison), **acitretin** (Soriatane), and **isotretinoin** (Accutane) are retinoids. Etretinate and acitretin are similar to isotretinoin, except that etretinate and acitretin are approved by the FDA for use in the treatment of psoriasis, while isotretinoin is approved by the FDA for use in treating acne. How retinoids work in the treatment of psoriasis is not completely understood, although they are thought to block the overproduction of skin cells. The substantial amount of data on the clinical effectiveness of etretinate was obtained empirically from numerous multicenter trials and individual reports (Sources: *Journal of the American Academy of Dermatology*, December 1992, pages S8–S14; *European Journal of Dermatology*, November-October 2000, pages 517–521).

While none of these retinoids are to be used when a woman is pregnant, the risks associated with etretinate are considered even more problematic. All systemic retinoids have the strong potential to cause major fetal abnormalities, including neurological and skeletal deformities. It is essential that effective contraception be used for at least one month before and throughout treatment. However, because etretinate can remain in the blood for up to *three years* after treatment, birth control must be continued for an indefinite period of time following therapy. It has not yet been determined how long it is necessary to wait before becoming pregnant after you stop taking etretinate to ensure that none of the drug remains in your system (Source: FDA Web site, http://www.fda.gov/cber/bldmem/072893.txt). As a result of the risks associated with etretinate, particularly the length of time it can stay in the system, acitretin and isotretinoin are considered safer, and just as effective choices for severe psoriasis (Source: *Journal of the American Academy of Dermatology*, November 2001, pages S150–S157).

Severe fetal abnormalities do occur if a woman is or becomes pregnant while taking either acitretin or isotretinoin (Accutane), but because these drugs don't remain in the system for long after you are finished with treatment, no long waiting period is required before becoming pregnant. Specifics regarding how long to wait after treatment before considering having a baby should be discussed with your physician.

**Etanercept** (trade name Enbrel) is an antitumor medication that is used in the treatment of rheumatoid arthritis. It has also been found useful in the treatment of psoriasis. Etanercept appears to be a promising agent that can be used in combination therapy for the treatment of psoriasis (Source: *British Journal of Dermatology*, January 2002, pages 118–121).

**5-fluorouracil** (brand name Efudex) is a chemotherapy drug that may be effective in the treatment of psoriasis affecting the nails. Psoriatic-affected nails are quite common for those with psoriasis—up to 50% of those with psoriasis have it in their nails, too. There is no consistently effective treatment for psoriasis of the nail, though there are a handful of studies showing a topically applied 5% 5-fluorouracil cream can be beneficial (Source: *Cutis*, July 1998, pages 27–28). For risks associated with 5-fluorouracil please see the section on "Actinic Keratosis" in Chapter Five, *Sun Sense*.

## COMBINATION THERAPY

The most typical combination therapy for psoriasis is something called **PUVA**. PUVA involves the use of a prescription medication called Psoralen and exposure to ultraviolet light A (UVA)—hence the initials PUVA. It is also called "photochemotherapy." The drug Psoralen, which can be taken orally as a pill or applied topically to the skin, makes the skin more sensitive and receptive to the wavelength of UVA light (320 to 400 nanometers). This combination suppresses the growth of abnormal skin cells. The good news is that PUVA can eliminate or dramatically reduce psoriatic lesions for the majority of people who use it, and there is evidence it can provide extended remissions. The bad news is that Psoralen and UVA light are phototoxic and carcinogenic. Getting rid of psoriasis can mean a lot, but putting your skin at risk for premature aging and cancer may be trading one problem for another. In light of the risks involved, PUVA should be considered only for extreme or disabling psoriasis, after other treatments have failed (Sources: http://www.psoriasis.org; *Cutis*, November 2001, pages 345–347; *Biochemical Pharmacology*, January 2002, pages 31–39).

**All of the above treatments, both topical and oral, are often used in varying combinations for the best results. Frequently, several combination treatments are used in rotation to reduce the potentially harmful side effects of each one.** Discovering whether any of these will work for you, alone or in combination, takes patience and a systematic, ongoing review and evaluation of how your skin and health are doing. Successful treatment, as is true with all chronic skin disorders, requires diligent adherence to the regimen and a realistic understanding of what you can and can't expect. It is also important to be aware of the consequences of the varying treatment levels. For example, continued long-term use of topical cortisone creams can cause skin thinning, stretch marks, and built-up resistance to the cortisone medication itself, so that it actually becomes an ineffective treatment. Exposure to sunlight without adequate protection (particularly from UVA radiation) can cause skin cancer. Oral steroids can have serious withdrawal effects, including increased bouts of psoriasis. Accutane causes birth defects if a woman becomes pregnant while taking it. Several systemic psoriatic treatments can cause liver problems, nausea, and severe irritation. Each option has its own set of pros and cons that need to be researched and discussed at length with your physician.

For more information on the current status of available treatment visit the Web site for the National Psoriasis Foundation (NPF) at http://www.psoriasis.org/.

## SEBORRHEA

Seborrhea is a skin disease of the sebaceous (oil) glands marked by an increased secretion of sebum (oil) or a thickened sebum discharge. It can resemble acne and blackheads. One of the differences between acne and seborrhea is that in seborrhea the increased oil production is often accompanied by a scaly, thickened skin, especially on the scalp, and the oil itself can have a strange, viscous texture. However, in seborrhea—and sometimes in acne—the sebum (a firm waxlike substance in the pore that liquefies into oil on the surface of the skin) in the sebaceous gland accumulates, causing the gland to become swollen and filled to the brim. When this overproduced sebum is covered over by skin, it forms a small, firm mound called a whitehead. When the sebum is exposed to air (not covered by skin) and the duct fills with dead skin cells, the sebum turns dark and the blemish becomes a blackhead. The size of the eruption, the texture of the oil, and the flaky skin are what differentiate seborrhea from acne.

Seborrhea can show up wherever there are lots of oil glands. The scalp, sides of the nose, eyebrows, eyelids, behind the ears, and middle of the chest are the areas most commonly affected. Other areas, such as the navel and the skin folds under the arms, breasts, groin, and buttocks, may also be involved. The swelling, breakouts, and accompanying yellowish, greasy-appearing scales make this skin disorder hard to miss.

Seborrhea is identified by excessive yellowing, thickened scaling, accompanied by excessive oiliness, and is possibly triggered by a yeast organism (yeast is a type of fungus) present in the hair follicle (Source: *British Journal of Dermatology*, March 2001, pages 549–556). Seborrhea can occur at any age, but typically it is seen in infants, when it is called "cradle cap." Because yeast, or some other form of fungus, likely triggers seborrhea, antimicrobial agents capable of targeting this type of organism have been shown to have a high success rate.

Prescription medications for the treatment of seborrhea include ciclopiroxolamine 1% in a cream base. This is an antifungal that has been shown to be effective in a well-controlled study (Source: *British Journal of Dermatology*, May 2001, pages 1033–1037). Topical metronidazole (Noritate, MetroLotion, MetroGel, and MetroCream) also can have significant positive results, and are very effective in the treatment of seborrhea (Source: *Journal of Family Practice*, June 2001, volume 50, issue 6). An oral medication, terbinafine, has been identified as beneficial in the treatment of seborrhea as well (Source: *British Journal of Dermatology*, April 2001, pages 854–857).

Several over-the-counter topical treatments for seborrhea include zinc pyrithione 1% (Dandrex, Zincon, Head and Shoulders, Denorex); coal-tar preparations (DHS, Neutrogena T-Gel, Ionil T, Tegrin, Esorex), ketaconazole (Nizoral), selenium sulfide 1% (Selsun Blue), and selenium sulfide 2.5% (Selsun). As in the treatment of psoriasis, UV light therapy can be of benefit for those who suffer from seborrhea, but it carries the same risks mentioned above for psoriasis. Topical steroids are often of limited use because they can cause thinning of the skin.

Treating seborrhea takes patience and experimenting to find what works for you. All of these medications, either alone or in combination, are options for achieving the best results.

# ECZEMA

On a personal note, I suffered from eczema for many years. At one point in my life almost 80% of my body was affected, and the resulting itching and scratching, sores, irritation, and discomfort were more awful than I can put into words. For years I struggled with medications and a varying assortment of cortisone creams and bar soaps, from Basis to Aveeno, until the day my dermatologist found the right cortisone strength and I started to stay away from topical irritants; then my skin finally settled down—but the problem didn't go away until much later in life.

Eczema, also known as contact dermatitis, atopic dermatitis, irritant dermatitis, allergic dermatitis, and a host of other designations, is without question a difficult, uncomfortable, often painful skin disorder. When you have it, you generally know it by the cracked, abraded, blistered, crusted, weepy, reddened, patchy, dry skin surface, accompanied by persistent, almost unbearable itching and the tendency for everything you touch to make matters worse. A simple act like washing your hands, applying eye makeup, or wearing scratchy material can instigate a flare-up that feels interminable.

Almost anything can trigger eczema, and sometimes nothing at all can precede a bout of oppressive itching, scratching, and rashes. Wool (from clothing to carpets), shampoos, hair dyes, nail polish, jewelry, plants, undergarments (elastic waistbands and spandex bras are special villains), deodorant, tight socks, nylons, pet allergies, excessive heat or air conditioning (which increases dry and itchy skin), bathing too often (which leaches moisture out of the skin), using harsh or mild soaps, hot water, vigorous rubbing or massaging, chlorinated water, salt water, and even sweat (this triggered my eczema almost instantaneously) are all possible offenders. In the world of cosmetics, preservatives, irritants (such as peppermint, menthol, alcohol, camphor, eucalyptus, fragrance, and essential oils), bath salts, bubble bath, scrubs, AHAs, BHA, and loofahs are all potent eczema triggers.

Despite this daunting list, everyone is different, and what irritates your skin might not irritate someone else's. There is no exact science to discovering what causes your skin to react; rather, it is a process of paying attention to what you come into contact with, seeing what makes things worse for your skin, and then eliminating or avoiding those things at all costs.

Generally, dry skin (an impaired surface skin barrier) is more prone to the sensation of itching and chapping, so finding a reliable way to deal with dry skin is almost always the starting point for the treatment of eczema. To this end it is important to keep bathing time short, avoid bath salts or bubble baths, use lukewarm to warm water (avoid hot water most of all), and avoid bar soaps of any kind (they all contain potential irritants). Using fragrance-free, gentle liquid cleansers that also contain moisturizing agents, and applying and reapplying moisturizers quickly afterward, can help a lot.

Unquestionably, moisturizers minimize dryness and are a mainstay in treating mild to chronic dermatitis. It is believed that regular and frequent use of emollient moisturizers can reduce the amount of topical steroids needed in the maintenance treatment of eczema. The more emollient the cream the better, and when fatty acids are included in the formula it's particularly helpful. Fatty acids are ingredients such as triglycerides, oleic acid, linoleic acid, evening primrose oil, borage oil, fish oil, flaxseed oil, coconut oil, and palm oil (Source: *Skin Pharmacology and Applied Skin Physiology*, March 2002, pages 100–104). While using a moisturizer twice daily is considered adequate, it is essential to keep a moisturizer with you at all times so that you can reapply it every time you wash your hands. During the day it is essential that you apply an emollient moisturizer with an SPF 15 or greater that contains UVA-protecting ingredients on exposed areas of your body. In the case of eczema, because of the risk of irritation and skin sensitivity, the UVA-protecting ingredients should be only titanium dioxide and zinc oxide with no avobenzone or other synthetic sunscreen agents of any kind. Synthetic sunscreen agents have a potential to cause skin irritation.

For years topical corticosteroids (cortisone) have been the drug of choice for treating eczema. These products are available in a vast range of strengths and molecular structures that allow for varying skin penetration and potency. The risks associated with prolonged use of a potent corticosteroid are that it may result in skin deterioration and adaptation (that means it stops having an effect on the skin). Because of these risks, newer nonsteroidal treatments for eczema have been formulated and have been approved by the FDA. However, if these newer treatments are not effective for you, concerns about skin breakdown (which happens with any long-term cortisone use) and adaptation should not limit your use of a good potent steroid. It is still a valid way to get control of the dermatitis. As much as possible, try to minimize the frequency of cortisone application, using it only as necessary to keep the irritation abated. But don't cut back too far because there is a point of no return where if you don't use enough your skin becomes an itchy, rashy mess.

## BATTLE PLANS FOR ECZEMA

An announcement in the December 2000 *FDA Talk Papers* reported the approval of a new drug for the treatment of a form of eczema called atopic dermatitis. For anyone struggling with this itchy, red, oozing, sensitive-skin condition, this is definitely worth looking into. The drug is called Protopic and contains the active ingredient tacrolimus in a 0.1% and 0.03% concentration ointment for adults and a 0.03% concentration ointment for children two years of age and older. It is a nonsteroidal (meaning not cortisone) ointment indicated for patients with moderate to severe eczema and for whom standard eczema therapies such as cortisone creams have not worked or are not considered healthy. (With repeated use, cortisone can cause thinning of the skin and prematurely aged skin.) According to the *FDA Talk Paper*, "The FDA based its approval on the results of three 12-week studies which indicated that 28–37% of patients using Protopic experienced greater than or equal to 90% improvement of their skin condition, as measured by physicians, and two one year studies that indicated that the drug is safe for intermittent long term use." In addition, the drug has been tested in 28 worldwide trials on more than 4,000 adults and children. What makes tacrolimus unique is that it has been used primarily orally to prevent transplant rejections due to its action as an immunomodulator. In other words, by suppressing the immune system it prevents the body from rejecting a transplanted organ. It is thought to work in some cases of moderate to severe dermatitis because of its effect in preventing the skin's own immune reaction from causing red, itchy, inflamed rashes. (In other words, in this form of eczema, it's as if the person's own immune system is attacking the skin, causing the itching, blistering, and irritation.) By stopping this immune reaction, it eliminates the problem.

The study goes on to note that "Common side effects associated with this drug include temporary stinging or burning sensations where the drug is applied, which may lessen if the diseased skin heals. There was evidence from an animal study that Protopic may accentuate the adverse effects of ultraviolet light on the skin. Therefore sun protection at all times is vital" (but you already know that sun protection is vital all the time regardless of what else you put on your skin).

Another interesting study on eczema, presented in the *Archives of Dermatology* (January 2001, pages 42–43), reported research in Japan that demonstrated that two-thirds of the patients with eczema improved after a month of drinking a liter of oolong tea daily. According to the study "118 patients ... were asked to maintain their dermatological treatment. However, they were also instructed to drink oolong tea made from a 10-gram teabag placed in 1000 milliliters of boiling water and steeped for 5 minutes. After 1 month of treatment 74 (63%) of the 118 patients showed marked to moderate improvement of their condition. A good response to treatment was still observed in 64 patients (54%) at 6 months." The study concluded that "The therapeutic efficacy of oolong tea may well be the result of the antiallergic properties of tea polyphenols." While the study didn't look at the effect of tea drinking if the topical treatments were stopped, the patients did receive some benefit. So by combining topical treatments (moisturizers and possibly Protopic) with some oolong tea, perhaps the positive effects of both will add up, and those with eczema can breathe a sigh of relief.

# CHAPTER 13
## HAIR REMOVAL

### HAIR-BRAINED IDEAS?

From the onset of adolescence, the desire to get rid of unwanted body hair becomes an almost daily obsession. Whether it is shaving legs or underarms, struggling with dark hair above the lip or on the chin, or dense hair growth on the arms, finding a way to effectively and efficiently deal with this problem is a recurring issue. Most of us realize that if a beauty need exists, lots of cosmetics companies are more than willing to manufacture products with claims to solve it. However, most of these end up sounding far more effective than they actually perform. Infomercials and ads in fashion magazines seem to have the answer for the hair you're longing to get rid of, but alas, these products either can't live up to their claims or they are just standard depilatories or waxing options that offer little to no improvement over what has been around for years. Believe me when I say I would love to find an easy way to achieve a smooth bikini line or a hairless upper lip without trouble or bother, but hair removal just isn't that simple. Here are all the available options, each with its own pros and cons. Depending on your budget, available time, and the area you want to make hair-free, you can check these over and choose what works best for you.

### DEPILATORIES

Depilatories literally melt and dissolve hair with strong ingredients like calcium hydroxide and sodium or calcium thioglycolate. There are many reasons why this group of products is not great for everyone: the most compelling is they risk causing serious irritation or (in the extreme case) possible burns to the skin and eyes. It is essential to test the depilatory on your arm first as a precaution against allergic reactions or skin sensitivities. Hair and skin are similar in composition, so chemicals that destroy the hair can also destroy the skin.

Depilatories, much like shaving, remove only the hair on the surface, which means the hair comes back in just a few days. To get the best results from your depilatory, first apply warm to hot (but not too hot) compresses, which help soften the hair and open the pores (where the hair is growing), allowing the depilatory to be absorbed better. Then apply an extremely thick, generous layer of the depilatory completely over the entire length and base of the hair shaft and let it stay on for the full recommended time, but no longer than between 4 and 15 minutes, depending on how fine or coarse the hair is. Because depilatories dissolve the hair, applying pressure can help remove more of the shaft. Instead of simply washing the depilatory away, use a washcloth and wipe the cream off, using a firm back-and-forth motion.

Depilatories should never be used for the eyebrows or other areas around the eyes, or on inflamed or broken skin.

The FDA issued a recall on September 13, 1997, for The Art of Beauty Epil-Stop Hair Removal Cream *($49.95 for 4 ounces)*, manufactured by International Chemical Corporation, Amherst, New York. Previously, on September 4, 1997, the California Poison Control Office had issued a press release warning that Epil-Stop "is adulterated in that it has high pH levels which may cause skin irritation and burning." Check out the FDA home page at http://www.FDA.gov for more information.

Epil-Stop (not to be confused with EpilLight, a pulse-light laser device) was advertised on television, magazines, and over the Internet, with claims about removing hair and stopping hair growth naturally and painlessly. It turns out that Epil-Stop worked like any other drugstore depilatory—by dissolving hair with a high-pH ingredient base. Unlike other drugstore products, however, Epil-Stop took their pH to a still higher level, so that it ate away not only the hair but also the skin.

# HAIR-GROWTH-INHIBITING PRODUCTS

**Ultimate Hairaway** *($39.95 for 2 ounces)* is a prime example of how the cosmetics industry doesn't need to relay honest information. This is supposed to be a hair-growth-inhibiting product and it claims to be all-natural, yet the ingredient list is as far from natural as you can get. It contains water, extractable fruit derivatives (whatever that's supposed to mean), polypropylene glycol, glycerol, disaccharides, urea, dithiothreitol, EDTA, methylparaben, and propylparaben. What could be inhibiting hair growth in this product? It isn't the natural-sounding fruit derivatives. It's probably the dithiothreitol. Dithiothreitol is related to thioglycolic compounds, standard and highly alkaline ingredients that can dissolve hair and potentially irritate skin, similar to any depilatory.

Depending on your sense of humor, you may find it terribly funny that Ultimate Hairaway suggests that you "first remove hair from the roots, as with waxing, sugaring, tweezing, or electrolysis" before you apply their product. They claim Ultimate Hairaway isn't a depilatory, which is why the hair has to come off first. Rather, it is supposed to inhibit hair growth, eventually letting you phase out the need for hair-removal procedures. Given the variable cycle of hair growth and the fact that you are supposed to use another method to remove the hair, it would be a long time before you had any idea this product wasn't working. Tweezing and waxing already make hair growth seem slower because when hair has been removed from the root, it has to grow longer to get back to the surface. Moreover, electrolysis has long been a hair-removal method known to stop hair growth because of the impact of the treatment on the hair follicle, but Ultimate Hairaway fails to mention that.

Another claim Ultimate Hairaway makes is that it works like "male pattern baldness, inhibit[ing] hair growth." While that comment simplifies the issue, the description in the brochure is much more complicated and hard to follow. According to the booklet, "the top of a healthy papilla ['papilla' is a term that refers to the bump or bulge where a hair grows] is naturally cornified ... ['cornified' refers to the conversion of skin cells into a keratinized material, such as hair or nails]. When the hair is removed, the sides of the papilla are exposed and susceptible to the treatment. [That may be true, though I doubt it; but regardless, the papilla isn't where the hair grows from.] . . . Male pattern baldness is caused by renegade type apocrine glands, which develop and connect to the duct of the sebaceous gland and introduce naturally occurring secretions into the hair follicle. The opening of hair follicles at the skin's surface is often blocked by shampoo, conditioner, gels, hair spray, sweat, oils, sebum, etc. This blockage disallows these natural secretions to escape. These acidic secretions, having no place to go, seep their way to the base of the hair follicle and slowly cornify the sides of the papilla, preventing penetration of hair cells. Ultimate Hairaway can duplicate the cause of baldness on the desired area." Wow!

Let me try to interpret this mumbo jumbo. First, male pattern baldness is caused by the hormone dihydroxytestosterone (DHT), which binds to the base of hair follicles and causes them to shrink and deteriorate. "Apocrine glands" refers to any glandular secretion, anywhere in the body. I have no idea what that has to do with the hair shaft because it isn't how the hair follicle functions (unless they are referring to DHT, but they don't say that). Then they start talking about how some hair-care products can clog a hair follicle and, I suppose, cut off its blood supply and reduce growth. Now, that is true, but hardly something you would want to encourage, because you would also be clogging the pores at the same time. The rest of the stuff I can't decipher. I've never heard of this acidic secretion issue that cornifies the hair follicle itself. It sounds like their product is supposed to block the pilosebaceous unit (the hair follicle and oil gland combined are the pilosebaceous unit) to stop unwanted hair growth. Are they suggesting that you can artificially create acidic secretions in the hair follicle (secretions I haven't seen any evidence of) to stop hair growth? Does that mean AHAs (which are highly acidic) can stop hair growth?

None of this is substantiated by one ounce of published research, and none of the dermatologists I spoke to confirmed or even understood what the company's statement means.

Perhaps the final joke is the last statement in the Ultimate Hairaway brochure: "If you prefer to shave to control unwanted body hair, simply apply [Ultimate Hairaway] twice a day for one week and then once a day thereafter until the desired results are acquired. Shave as necessary." See, they were talking about mechanically removing hair by shaving (or any other method) all along; it just took them a very long time to say that.

There are many more products boasting hair-inhibiting ability, such as Derma Nude Advanced Moisturizing Spray *($39.95 for 4 ounces)* and Hair No More Advanced Hair Growth Inhibitor Soothing Gel *($29.95 for 2 ounces)*. These two are representative of many I've seen. While they don't seem to contain anything irritating or painful, the claims that they are all pure and natural is purely nonsense. Both include water, propylene glycol, glycerin, aloe vera, green tea extract, enzymatic plant extracts, EDTA, and DMDM hydantoin. DMDM hydantoin is a form of formaldehyde (Source: *Contact Dermatitis*, April 1988, pages 197–201) and propylene glycol is also a synthetic ingredient. Further, enzymatic plant extracts are not a legal or approved ingredient description name. The FDA requires all cosmetic ingredient lists to comply with Cosmetic & Toiletry Fragrance Association (CTFA) rules or the International Nomenclature Cosmetic Ingredient (INCI) names. With vague wording like this, there is no way consumers can actually know what they are putting on their skin. Enzymes sound natural, so the consumer assumes it must be gentle, but that is a leap of faith you might want to think twice about before you jump into this quagmire of misleading and invalid information.

# WAXING

Waxing is an excellent and inexpensive way to deal with most hair removal on the body or face. Waxing leaves the area smoother than shaving does because it pulls the hair out below the top layer of skin, which makes it grow back slower and less uniformly. You can do waxing at home by yourself, and beauty supply stores sell all the equipment you need, from the wax to spatulas, strips of cotton, and anti-inflammatory lotions. There are even hair-remover kits with strips of wax or waxlike ingredients that you just peel off, place on the skin, and then rip off. No heating or mixing. This is by far the most convenient and easiest way to peel off hair from large areas such as the legs, bikini line, and arms. For smaller areas such as the upper lip, a wax that is melted in the microwave (instead of on the stove) and applied with a small spatula offers the most control.

In hot waxing, a thin layer of heated wax is applied to the skin in the direction of the hair growth. The hair becomes embedded in the wax as it cools and hardens. The wax is then pulled off quickly in the opposite direction of the hair growth, taking the uprooted hair with it. Cold waxes work similarly. Strips pre-coated with wax or a cool, sugar-based substance are pressed onto the skin in the direction of the hair growth and pulled off in the opposite direction.

Before you consider doing this yourself, visit an aesthetician with experience in this method of hair removal. It's tricky to get the technique right, and getting it wrong can mean a sticky mess on your body, in your kitchen, and around your bathroom. It also smarts a bit when the hair is ripped off. You can't wax again until the hair grows out to a noticeable length.

## SUGAR FORMS OF WAXING

The best known "sugaring" method of hair removal is Nad's Gel Hair Removal (*$29.95 for one kit*). Thanks to its many reruns in late-night and early-morning infomercials, this is a product many women are now familiar with. What makes this kind of hair removal different is that it literally uses sugar instead of wax. With its thick, caramel-like consistency, it works identically to regular waxing, only instead of spreading a wax substance over the skin, you're spreading caramel.

I have to say this is one of the first products I've ever run into where the claim of being 100% natural and organic is 100% true. Nad's ingredients are honey, molasses, fructose, vinegar, lemon juice, water, alcohol, and food dye. Now that's what I call natural. But does that make it better than waxing, as the company claims? First, waxing isn't unnatural—after all, wax is a natural substance. And as far as hair removal is concerned the effect is identical. You spread the Nad's caramel gel over the hair you want removed (there needs to be some hair length or there won't be anything for it to grab). Then you rip it off and out comes the hair, same as waxing.

However, there are two main positives to sugaring over waxing. First, sugaring's mess washes away while wax has to be peeled or scratched off (and that isn't easy). Plus sugaring doesn't require heating while waxing often does, and adding heat is far more damaging to skin! Easy cleanup and a relatively easier application (no risk of burn) are the incredible benefits of sugaring.

But before you jump on the Nad's or other sugaring hair-removal system bandwagon, you should know a few more details about the claims that accompany the sugaring method, as some aren't true. Nad's states, "when you use Nad's, the hair is extracted, including the roots so re-growth is softer, finer and slower." That isn't true. Hormones and genetics determine hair growth and hair thickness, not the hair-removal method. What does happen when you "tweeze" out hair is that because it has been removed closer to the root the new hair takes longer to grow back to the top of the skin, unlike with shaving, where the hair is removed only from the surface, so the hair pops back out faster. Also, because each hair follicle has a different rate of growth, there will be less of it as it grows back than what was present when you first waxed or sugared, making the hair seem softer.

There are also claims that sugaring prevents ingrown hairs. Ingrown hairs are unrelated to the way hair is removed. Ingrown hairs occur when a hair that has been removed below the skin's surface has trouble finding its way back to the surface. That applies to hair removal in general, regardless of whether you shave, tweeze, sugar, or wax.

Another claim: "Because of the natural substances in Nad's, there is little chance of irritations. Redness for a short time is normal, depending on how sensitive your skin is." Natural or not, ripping out hair hurts, and for some skin types that can be a problem. What is better about sugaring, however, is that the stuff doesn't have to be heated and so, as a result, it's less irritating—but that isn't because it's natural.

## TWEEZING

Tweezing is not only a painful option, but also an extremely time-consuming one. It is OK for occasional stray hairs or very small areas, but it is not the best for large areas or areas with dense hair growth. Tweezing works virtually the same way as waxing—pulling the hair out from the root—which means the effects last far longer than shaving. Some women worry that tweezing will increase the growth or make the texture of the hair heavier, but it won't. If plucking (or waxing and shaving) altered hair growth, we would all have bushy eyebrows! Actually, pulling out hair can eventually shut down the hair follicle by causing repeated shock and injury, though this takes a very, very long time. For the most part, any texture change is a result of the initial grow-back phase, when the hair reemerges from the pore.

## BLEACHING

Bleaching is a great, inexpensive option if the issue is not the density of the hair but its darkness. This method is particularly effective for the upper lip or other parts of the face, neck, and arms. There are many options for facial bleach products at the drugstore or on the Internet. One of the best Internet sources for a range of inexpensive options is http://www.folica.com. Please be aware that this site also sells an array of products that exaggerate their claims or simply mislead as to what they can really do for skin.

# ELECTROLYSIS

Electrolysis is the only permanent form of hair removal, at least so far, but it requires repeated treatments that can take up to a year and it can be pricy, especially when you take into consideration the time commitment. The biggest hurdle is finding an extremely skilled technician to achieve satisfactory results. Before you see someone, check out the clients who have had permanent success with this tricky, but effective, method of hair removal.

There are two types of devices that use electric current to remove hair: the needle epilator and the tweezer epilator. (Tweezer epilators are discussed in the next section). Needle epilators introduce a very fine wire under the skin, and into the hair follicle. An electric current travels down the wire and destroys the hair root at the bottom of the follicle. The loosened hair is then removed with regular tweezers. Every hair is treated individually. Needle epilators are used in electrolysis because this technique destroys the hair follicle. Thus, this is considered a permanent hair-removal method. The hair root may persist, however, if the needle misses the mark or if insufficient electricity is delivered to destroy it. However, the stimulus for hair growth can never be permanently removed. For instance, you can't control hormonal changes that may cause new growth (Source: FDA *Consumer* magazine, September 1996).

The major risks of using electrolysis include electrical shock, which can occur if the needle is not properly insulated; infection from a non-sterile needle; and scarring resulting from improper technique. In addition, there are no uniform licensing standards regulating the practice of electrolysis. Only 31 states require electrologists to be licensed, and among those the license requirements vary from as few as 120 hours to 1,100 hours, which means that to set up shop many electrologists only need a machine and very little else.

The American Electrology Association and the Society of Clinical and Medical Electrologists have certification programs based on a written exam. A list of licensed and certified electrologists is available from the International Guild of Professional Electrologists, 202 Boulevard Street, Suite B, High Point, NC 27262; (800) 830-3247 or on the Web at http://www.igpe.org/.

# HOME ELECTROLYSIS

Technically, these devices work the same way as those that the professional use (they also carry the same health risks). However, the risks for the home-use machines are not very great because the voltage and current output are not very high, and that means they aren't as effective. I know we've all seen those little machines you can buy via mail order (for about $100) that claim to remove hair painlessly and permanently. They've been advertised for years and years. I remember them from when I was a kid. The chances of operating these successfully yourself are at best slim. You probably would end up just tweezing instead of zapping the hair because getting the device to work right is extremely tricky and incredibly time-consuming. Given the time it takes for a hair to grow back, it could take months before you knew if it was really working (Source: FDA *Consumer* magazine, September 1996).

Perhaps the most advertised at-home product is IGIA's Hair Removal System *($119)*. It is supposed to be a "painless home electrolysis system that helps keep hair from growing back! Unlike common [tweezing] and depilatory devices that can cause skin irritation, this system uses mild radio frequency pulses that is absolutely safe and is delivered through the tweezers to remove hair without touching the skin." Well, that much is true. This overpriced machine delivers low-voltage radio waves through the hair shaft. Does that kill off a hair follicle? There is no research indicating that these machines do anything but tweeze the hair. The low voltage makes these machines extremely low risk, but they are also ineffective. What a waste. Still, in comparison to the other IGIA products, this one is the safest of the bunch. Keep in mind that even though these kinds of self-electrolysis machines have been advertised for years and years, there are other truly effective options to try.

## SHAVING

Shaving is fine, but we all know the problems associated with it. Shaving is the method most of us go back to for our legs and bikini line, but the hair grows back way too fast and the stubble or redness it can cause on the thigh and crotch is obnoxious. There are ways around the redness, such as shaving with a good topical lotion like a hair conditioner or body wash and applying a nonfragranced moisturizer afterward. Also, one of the best options for preventing red bumps is applying aspirin topically to the skin. Aspirin has potent anti-inflammatory properties even when applied to the surface of skin. Simply dissolve one or two aspirins in about 1/4 cup water and then apply the solution with a cotton ball to the area you just shaved! This works on any part of the body you shave. You will be impressed by the results.

On the legs, using a mild scrub of baking soda mixed with Cetaphil Gentle Skin Cleanser can help keep flaky skin at a minimum, which means you can get a closer shave. Skin should never be shaved while dry; wet hair is soft, pliable, and easier to cut. Contrary to what many believe, shaving does not change the texture, color, or rate of hair growth. Hair density is genetically and hormonally determined; it has nothing to do with what you do topically to the skin (unless you traumatically damage the hair follicle via injury or burns).

# LASER HAIR REMOVAL

Since the advent of the first FDA-approved laser hair-removal system in 1995, its popularity has made laser hair removal a financial cornerstone for many dermatologists and plastic surgeons. The original laser hair-removal machine was **The Soft Light Hair Removal System** developed by Thermolase Corporation. Since then the growing popularity of and demand for this treatment from eager consumers reading ads and articles in fashion magazines has prompted many laser manufacturers to seek FDA clearance for their laser hair-removal machines. The market is growing so quickly that the FDA cannot maintain an up-to-date list of all laser manufacturers whose devices have been cleared for hair removal, as this list continues to change. However, to learn if a specific manufacturer has received FDA clearance, you can check the FDA Web site at http://www.fda.gov/cdrh/databases.html. You will need to know the manufacturer or device name of the laser. You can also call FDA's Center for Devices and Radiological Health, Consumer Staff, at 1-888-INFO-FDA or (301) 827-3990, or fax your request to (301) 443-9535 (Source: FDA Center for Devices and Radiological Health, *Laser Facts*, May 2001, online at http://www.fda.gov/cdrh/consumer/laserfacts.html).

One of the significant FDA regulations regarding all companies that promote approved laser hair-removal systems is that "… manufacturers may not claim that laser hair removal is either painless or permanent…. The specific claim granted is 'intended to effect stable, long-term, or permanent reduction'…. Permanent hair reduction is defined as the long-term, stable reduction in the number of hairs regrowing after a treatment regime, which may include several sessions. The number of hairs regrowing must be stable over time—greater than the duration of the complete growth cycle of hair follicles, which varies from four to twelve months according to body location. Permanent hair reduction does not necessarily imply the elimination of all hairs in the treatment area." That is a very convoluted way of saying that laser hair removal is not permanent and that there are no studies showing it to be so even after several treatments. However, the consumer is usually not told what the FDA's regulation is.

When laser hair removal arrived on the scene, many exaggerated, largely unsubstantiated claims about its efficacy, risks, side effects, and long-term effects were asserted (Source: *Journal of Cutaneous Laser Therapy*, March 2000, pages 49–50). Far more research has taken place since then and there's much more data (both clearer and more precise) regarding statistical analysis of performance and adverse outcomes. For example, a study reported in *Dermatologic Surgery* (November 2001, pages 920–924) used a "… 755 [nanometer] alexandrite laser equipped with a cryogen cooling…. Eighty-nine untanned patients … in the study underwent a minimum of three treatment sessions spaced 4-6 weeks apart [each patient had an average of 5 treatments].... Treatment sites included the [armpit], bikini, extremities, face, and trunk. RESULTS: The patients had a mean 74% hair reduction.... The best results are achieved in untanned patients..." Several studies have looked at various other laser systems, including some showing more promise for darker skin tones (Source: *Annals of Plastic Surgery*, October 2001, pages 404–411).

The risks in laser hair removal can include skin discoloration (either darkening or lightening of skin), swelling, inflammation, and infected hair follicles. Laser hair removal is particularly problematic for those with tans or darker skin colors (Source: *Cosmetic Dermatology*, November 2001, pages 45–50). Because of the potential for complications and the plethora of hair-removal machines available, it is essential to have this procedure performed by a physician who is familiar with the research and who can make the correct choice about which procedure is best for you.

# VANIQA

Manufactured by Bristol-Meyers Squibb, Vaniqa *($37.50 for 1.05 ounces)* is FDA-approved as a prescription-only topical cream for reducing and inhibiting the growth of unwanted facial hair (it has not been studied for its effect on hair on other parts of the body). On the surface, Vaniqa might sound like a depilatory (those nonprescription, drugstore products that topically "eat" away hair), but Vaniqa's effect on hair and skin is unrelated to the way a depilatory works.

The active drug in Vaniqa is eflornithine hydrochloride, which has been used as an oral medication for certain cancers and to treat African Sleeping Sickness. Many disconcerting side effects are associated with this drug, ranging from anemia to diarrhea, vomiting, and hair loss. The notion that topical application of eflornithine hydrochloride could also effect hair loss probably stems from its hair-loss side effect when taken orally. However, the product information insert for the medication states that, when applied topically, eflornithine hydrochloride, "is not known to be metabolized and is primarily excreted unchanged in the urine with no adverse systemic side effects."

The information insert for Vaniqa explains, that eflornithine hydrochloride affects the skin because it "interferes with an enzyme found in the hair follicle of the skin needed for hair growth. This results in slower hair growth.... [However] Vaniqa does not permanently remove hair or 'cure' unwanted facial hair.... Your treatment program should include continuation of any hair removal technique you are currently using.... [Further] Improvement in the condition occurs gradually. Don't be discouraged if you see no immediate improvement. Improvement may be seen as early as 4 to 8 weeks of treatment ... [and] may take longer in some individuals. If no improvement is seen after 6 months of use, discontinue use. Clinical studies show that in about 8 weeks after stopping treatment with Vaniqa, the hair will return to the same condition as before beginning treatment."

There are warnings that accompany this cream and there is still research to be done. Note that the insert warns, "You should not use Vaniqa if you are less than 12 years of age…." Plus, there are animal studies that showed definite fetal problems. That means pregnant women should not use this drug, and lactating women probably should not either, though there is no research about that risk. Also, "Vaniqa may cause temporary redness, stinging, burning, tingling or rash on areas of the skin where it is applied. Folliculitis (hair bumps) may also occur", as well as acne.

So, should you consider Vaniqa? Well, that depends on how you look at the statistics, because clearly for some women it may work well to reduce the amount of facial hair. In addition, you must consider how often you have to use other methods such as tweezing, shaving, or waxing. And it sure beats the expense of laser hair-removal treatments.

What about those statistics? Vaniqa does not work for everyone. "In two randomized double-blind studies involving 594 female patients, approximately 32% of patients showed marked improvement or greater after 24 weeks of treatment compared to 8% [with a placebo]." It is important to note that 42% to 66% of those women in the study showed no improvement or actually believed their condition got worse. If you think it's worth it to find out if you fall into the group of those who might have success with Vaniqa, it may be worth the risk. Just keep in mind that this isn't a slam dunk. More than half of those who use it won't be happy with the results.

## HAIR GROWTH SCAMS

An article in the October 25, 1999, issue of *The Rose Sheet* reported that the National Advertising Division (NAD) of the Better Business Bureau was taking action on unsubstantiated claims for hair-regrowth products being sold by Dr. Adam Lewenberg. Full-page ads in the *New York Times* stated astounding results and a "90% success rate" from using Lewenberg's products, which each sell for around $70 for 2 ounces. "NAD found the study used by Lewenberg not to be adequate for the claims. It was not a controlled clinical study, but rather the advertiser's anecdotal reports of personal observations…." What is particularly dismaying is that Lewenberg's formula is merely minoxidil with tretinoin! Both of these are readily available, either over the counter (in the case of minoxidil) or from a dermatologist (in the case of tretinoin, which is the active ingredient in Retin-A and Renova). Tretinoin and minoxidil are indeed options for hair growth, but the statistics are incredibly overblown. Regardless, if you want to give these a trial run, it doesn't require Lewenberg's products, and you'll spend far less money to boot.

## HAIR-REMOVAL WARNING!

All treatments for hair removal are contraindicated after any facial peel or laser procedure. It can take six to eight weeks for the skin to completely heal after a peel. Any trauma to the skin during the recovery period can cause discoloration or even scarring.

Hair removal is also extremely problematic if you are using AHAs, BHA, topical retinoids, azelaic acid, or taking Accutane. These treatments can make skin more susceptible to tears, wounds, and irritation. This can all prove damaging and uncomfortable.

# CHAPTER 14

## COSMETIC SURGERY

## CUTTING AND PASTING

Sometimes money is the root of expensive mistakes. Just because celebrities are doing something doesn't mean you should jump in and do it, too. Yes, lots of celebrities have had their looks altered by cosmetic surgery, but often you can tell at a glance who got a bad face-lift because their faces have been cut and pulled so tight they look constantly surprised or incessantly half-smiling. Michael Jackson is a classic example of facial cosmetic surgery gone amok, but we've all seen others who seem shockingly unattractive, or strangely altered as a result of having had skin pulled too tight, or overfilled with dermal implants, or BoToxed into an expressionless-looking zombie. A number of famous women have had their chests augmented and enlarged to the point that their breasts seem to enter the room a full minute before they do, or stand out like rocks from the chest, but that doesn't mean you should too.

In short, what you don't know about plastic surgery (namely, the pros and cons and all your options) can hurt you—not just your appearance, but also your health and your pocketbook. To help you think about this, I'd like to give an overview of what is available, along with what you need to know about the risks and/or benefits of different procedures.

Before I get to the details involving the various corrective medical procedures available, I want to address the most important consumer challenge of all: Who should do your surgery, regardless of what you decide to have done. Given the growing number of doctors with cosmetic or plastic surgery practices (and if you live in Southern California or Florida, their advertisements are about as prevalent and insufferable as those for car dealerships), it is very difficult to know where to go and how to get started.

Most women use one of four methods to select a cosmetic surgeon: articles in fashion magazines, finding out where celebrities went (everybody loves knowing where the "stars" are going for anything and everything, regardless of how they look), getting a referral from a friend or a friend of a friend, and, last but not least, checking out the doctors who advertise their services.

Though I wouldn't call these the worst plans of action, they should just be the beginning of the process. You need to know more before you can make an informed final decision. Take the time to gather detailed consumer information. Draw up a comprehensive list of questions to ask so you'll know what all your options are, which procedures will meet your needs, what are the risks or disadvantages, and which doctors are performing the safest and most reliable current procedures. The latest method doesn't necessarily mean the best when it comes to surgery—you don't want to be someone's test case.

Shockingly, many physicians downplay any risks. A quick review of several cosmetic surgery Internet sites reveals a scarcity of information regarding what can go wrong during or after a procedure. Yet each and every medical or cosmetic corrective procedure has risks. Yes, the risks are few and far between, but an average of about 1% to 4% (depending on whose statistic you use) of all patients have some sort of problem or negative outcome. When you consider that over 7.4 million procedures were performed in 2000, that would mean there were at least 74,000 problems. It is wise for you to decide if you want to chance being one of those who may fall in that statistic.

Being proactive about any surgery is incredibly important, but let me reiterate that it is even more vital with cosmetic surgery. After all, this surgery is usually elective and completely up to you; there is (or ought to be) nothing life-or-death about these procedures. Furthermore, cosmetic surgery is a very lucrative business— most surgeons get paid up front before you go under the knife or laser. So, before you hand over your hard-earned money, your very appearance, and your well-being, you have to be knowledgeable about every detail.

## COSMETIC SURGERY VERSUS PLASTIC SURGERY

What is the difference between a cosmetic or plastic surgeon and a board-certified plastic surgeon? A lot! Training and credentials in surgery are the issues in contention. Although a doctor may offer cosmetic, plastic, or aesthetic surgery, he or she may not be board-certified to perform that surgery. The person could literally be a gynecologist, pediatrician, or dermatologist with no training in cosmetic surgery whatsoever. Board-certified means the doctor has gone through very specific and extensive training in a specialized field and passed a difficult examination by a board of experts in that field. A non-board-certified cosmetic or plastic surgeon may be self-taught and may lack formal training in that field. Board-certified plastic surgeons consider this an issue of public safety, and I think that's an understatement. They suggest that going to anyone but a board-certified plastic surgeon is a huge mistake, asking, "Would you want your plastic surgery performed by someone who has never had any formal plastic surgery training?" Good question.

According to the American Society of Plastic and Reconstructive Surgeons (a professional association), many physicians who today practice plastic or cosmetic surgery received their formal training in another specialty—often a nonsurgical specialty—or had surgical training for another area of the body. One clear distinction with board-certified plastic surgeons is that they will have privileges to perform plastic surgery at an accredited hospital. Though most cosmetic surgery procedures are done in a doctor's office, you want to be assured that your surgeon has the level of skill accepted by an accredited hospital. It is completely fair to ask any doctor you see for cosmetic surgery whether he or she is board-certified and which hospitals he or she is affiliated with. Then check to be sure the hospital is accredited and the doctor's certification is current and recognized by the American Board of Plastic Surgery (ABPS), the only board recognized by the American Board of Medical Specialties (ABMS) to certify physicians for the full range of plastic and reconstructive procedures. To verify a surgeon's certification status, contact the American Board of Plastic Surgery at (215) 587-9322 or visit the board's Web site at http://www.abplsurg.org or the American Board of Medical Specialties at http://www.abms.org or by phoning (800) 776-2378 (Source: American Society of Plastic Surgeons, online at http://www.plasticsurgery.org).

Of course, there are great dermatologists and lousy board-certified plastic surgeons practicing plastic surgery. But the odds of getting someone who is inexperienced are greatly reduced when you take the time to find out if that person is board-certified. To be certified by the ABPS, a physician must have at least five to six years of approved surgical training, including a two- to three-year residency in plastic surgery. He or she must also have been in practice for at least two years and pass comprehensive written and oral exams in plastic surgery.

For more information about a physician in your area who provides these kinds of services, call the Society for Dermatologic Surgery at (800) 441-2737 or the American Society of Plastic Surgeons (888) 475-2784.

## WHAT TO ASK

Once you've dealt with the issue of board certification, ask lots of questions, and look for answers that make you feel comfortable and make the most sense to you in light of the research you have done. Not all cosmetic surgeons will come up with the same game plan for your face. Each surgeon has techniques he or she prefers, sometimes regardless of whether they represent the best or most current technology. That's not necessarily bad. Some surgeons use the latest technology not because it is better or has proven more effective but due to pressure from their "elite" clients, who expect what's new regardless of the risks.

One of the most important questions you can ask the surgeons you interview is how often per month they perform the specific procedure or procedures you are considering. It is best (but not essential) to get a doctor who specializes, as opposed to a doctor who tries to do it all.

Likewise, it is also imperative to ask how many surgeries the doctor performs in a day. If the doctor schedules more than three procedures a day, most likely another doctor or nurse will do the prep work and/or the finishing work. That may not mean poor results, but it does mean the doctor is not giving you his or her full attention. Make sure the doctor you are consulting will be the only doctor working on your face or body, and that he or she will never leave the operating room during your procedure.

It is also valid to ask if the doctor charges for redos and touchups. Though it isn't something doctors like to admit, going back in for fine-tuning or to correct mistakes is common, and you don't want to be charged to have the doctor repair what you don't like.

Be insistent about understanding every nuance of the postoperative procedure. Many complications can occur when the patient doesn't realize her part in the healing process. For example, scar tissue can cause problems for a breast implant. One of the ways to minimize that risk is to keep your breasts tightly bound and your arms firmly at your side, with little to no movement and no lifting for four to seven days.

## WHAT CAN GO WRONG

Negative outcomes are another complex issue. Both patients and physicians have a tendency to ignore the downside of cosmetic surgery. Paying attention to the risks of cosmetic surgery takes the glamour out of the process, so dangers are downplayed almost to the point of being entirely ignored. Even when a doctor does broach the perils of cosmetic surgery, they are often mentioned in an offhand style or glossed over completely in a vague and patronizing manner. Do not turn your face over to a surgeon who doesn't discuss, at length, all the risks involved with the cosmetic procedure you are interested in!

For example, if you are interested in a $CO_2$ ablative laser peel, you should be told about the risk of scarring or skin discoloration. About 2% of the patients who have a laser peel may develop some amount of scarring (Source: *FDA Consumer* magazine, May-June 2000, http://www.fda.gov). You may also not be told that, in one study, 22% of the patients who underwent laser resurfacing considered their results to be disappointing and 77% of the patients (even those who had good results) stated that they would be unwilling to undergo another resurfacing procedure (Source: *Facial Plastic Surgery*, August 2001, pages 187–192).

Another fascinating article in *Facial Plastic Surgery* (2000, volume 16, issue 3, pages 215–229, "Prevention and Correction of the 'Face-Lifted' Appearance") discussed some of the known problems of various facial cosmetic surgery procedures. "The unopposed tension of lateral vector face-lifts [traditional face-lifts] allows the cheek tissues to descend eventually over the tightened jawline, creating a "lateral sweep" or pulled appearance of the face…. Following conventional blepharoplasty [plastic surgery of the upper and lower eyelids], the lower eyelid contour becomes deeper, and often a hollow appearance develops…. Unwanted and unattractive results are not the fault of the surgeon or the patient but are caused by the surgical technique. As a primary rejuvenative procedure, a composite [face-lift] will deliver an impressive result that will disallow the ultimate lateral sweep and hollow eyes. In patients that have the unhappy signs of surgery this procedure can effectively correct the face-lifted appearance."

Cosmetic corrective or plastic surgery procedures can produce amazing results and literally erase years off your face or create the appearance you've always wanted, but do not assume there aren't risks, because there are. What you don't know means you can end up unhappy and, in plastic surgery, you won't get your money back.

## WHEN TO DO IT

The options for changing your body and face are almost limitless, and the results can be stunning. Traditional surgical procedures that cut off leathery, thick, lined, and sagging skin long abused by the sun can subtract years from a person's appearance. Laser resurfacing can create smooth skin and remove skin discolorations. Dermal fillers can plump up wrinkles and acne scarring. Endoscopic face-lifts can rejuvenate the face using tiny incisions without any cutting and pasting of the skin.

In the past, most people waited until they were well into their late 50s and 60s, with noticeably aged skin, before they jumped into the fray of cosmetic surgery. All that has changed with the advent of relatively noninvasive, low-cost procedures such as laser resurfacing, BoTox, and dermal fillers. Indeed, having some procedures done at a younger age, before you "need it" means having healthier-looking skin for years as opposed to an abrupt change when you finally decide you can't take it any more and search out a plastic surgeon.

Women in their early 40s and 50s may want to undergo cosmetic surgery to deal with sagging corners of the mouth, slight pouching or sagging of the chin and jawline, and folds along the forehead. Though hardly aging by some standards, these irksome signs of middle age are easy to modify. Cosmetic surgery at this relatively young age slows the way skin will continue to age.

There are also endless options for cosmetic procedures that are just about maintenance or reshaping the face. Whether it is acne scarring, excess fat or skin, surfaced face veins, skin discolorations, hair removal, or changing the appearance of your nose or lips, facial enhancement has a plethora of options to offer.

Some cosmetic surgeons suggest that when you are younger, laser resurfacing, endoscopic face-lifts, and mini-tucks (doing a section of the face as opposed to an overall face-lift) are the best ways to put off the need for a full face-lift or eye tuck until you're much further down the road. They claim that if you do things as they crop up there's less trauma, better healing, and, because younger people generally have more elasticity and fat in their skin, the results should last longer. Whether or not less-invasive procedures or minor procedures decrease the need for eventual major surgery is not yet known, but there is something to be said for having the face you want now as opposed to later.

We are in a new era of accessibility to cosmetic surgery. Some people are pleased to know their face doesn't have to look as old as they really are, and that they can have a choice about what to do about it. As long as the results are impressive (and they are), people will want to stay young-looking via any procedure that is relatively nonrisky and permanent (although all cosmetic surgery has duration limitations). That's not bad or good, it is just a legitimate option for creating the look you want. Plus, it beats wasting money on creams and lotions that do nothing for the wrinkles. As one plastic surgeon I spoke with noted, "Women have been buying wrinkle creams by the truckload, and yet they still get wrinkles and I'm still in business because none of those cosmetic products work to stop or change wrinkling."

## PRETREATMENT

Some women have been told that before they have a chemical peel, laser resurfacing, or any cosmetic surgical procedure they need to purchase special products weeks ahead of their treatment. The claim is that these will prepare the skin, improving the outcome and healing process. Most typically you will have been sold an AHA solution of some type, a skin-lightening product (hydroquinone-based), and a vitamin C concoction, along with the recommendation to pick up a prescription for Retin-A or Renova. However, an article published in *Cosmetic Dermatology* (March 2000, "Pre-Treatment of Skin for Laser Resurfacing: Is It Necessary?") states: "Retinoic acid derivatives [tretinoin such as Retin-A or Renova] have been studied most thoroughly and have been shown to accelerate wound healing. On the other hand, the preoperative use of AHAs, hydroquinone, and ascorbic acid [vitamin C] has proven to be of no apparent clinical benefit. Since these compounds appear to affect only superficial epidermal melanocytes [skin cells] (which are vaporized upon … laser irradiation)… they have no effect on the lower layers of skin." That means you can save your money on expensive pretreatment products being sold by the physician.

However, you will want to consider using a topical tretinoin cream. A study published in the *Archives of Dermatological Research* (November 2001, pages 515–521) concluded that wound healing is greatly improved with the pretreatment of topical tretinoin, but that is different from the cosmetic products many doctors are selling these days.

Although cosmetic skin-care products are not helpful for use as a pretreatment, at least in terms of helping your skin handle the procedures better, the ongoing use of well-formulated AHAs, BHA, skin-lightening products, and sunscreen can go a long way toward helping you keep the results you achieved and also ensuring that your skin is as healthy as it can be all the time.

# POSSIBILITIES FROM A TO Z

The first section that follows includes procedures from the neck up, the second section includes procedures from the neck down. Both lists are alphabetical. The risks and gains are best contemplated cautiously and from a consumer's point of view (weighing the pros and cons), not by how your friend looks after she had it done. These procedures are not a guarantee of happiness, just a way to buy the kind of body and face you want. (If that designer suit didn't make you happy, don't expect new breasts or a face-lift to provide peace of mind!) Every plastic surgeon I spoke with suggested that the patients most pleased with the results of their surgery were the ones who had the most realistic expectations. What are unrealistic expectations? Expecting to end up looking like a supermodel or believing you will now find the perfect relationship. Plastic surgery should be about your self-esteem associated with societal standards of beauty—nothing more and nothing less.

Important details: Keep in mind that everyone scars differently, and it often has little to do with the skill of the surgeon. You could be left with lines wherever an incision was made. In general, the paler your skin, the more prone you may be to red, welt-like scarring, and the darker your skin, the more prone you may be to thick, dark, keloidal scarring.

There are serious risks with all surgical procedures, and recovering from the more serious operations such as face-lifts, tummy tucks, and breast implants can be a daunting, frightening experience. Studies indicate that 97% of people who experience some kind of cosmetic surgery are quite pleased with the results. However, the

3% who are unhappy can be devastated. For example, eye tucks can damage the tear ducts or permanently destroy eyelashes, face-lifts can leave painful scars and pockets of dimpled flesh, laser or chemical peels can render skin tone uneven, and breast implants can leak or become encapsulated and painful.

Many doctors love to use computer imaging to "close the sale" on the cosmetic procedure they are recommending. A picture of your face or body is taken and scanned into a computer program, allowing the surgeon to then demonstrate how you would look pulled a little here, tucked a little there, and lifted a little all over. As impressive as this is, it is only a computer image and not real life. It is a great tool for getting an idea of what you can expect, but it isn't an exact blueprint. Don't let it be the deciding factor in your final decision.

All cosmetic surgery procedures have limitations as to how long the change will last, depending on skin type, age, the surgeon's technique, and postoperative care (including using sunscreen). Do not expect any cosmetic surgery to be permanent, especially laser peels, dermal filler injections, chemical peels, and BoTox (discussed later in this chapter).

**Note:** As indicated below, prices for these procedures vary widely. The region of the country you live in, the popularity of the surgeon, the specific techniques used (the more invasive or complex, the more expensive), the combination of techniques, and discounts given for doing more than one procedure can all greatly affect price.

# FROM THE NECK UP

### BoTox (Botulinum Toxin A) ($300 to $1,000)

The following section on BoTox is the only place where I share my personal experience with a cosmetic corrective procedure. I believe my experience was extremely representative, and after all the research I've seen, I thought it would be helpful and maybe a bit fun. What happened, to mention just one thing, was that for a period of time I couldn't look too surprised. At least not for three to four months after I had it done. BoTox is the brand name of the nontoxic form of botulinum toxin type A. In 2001 botulinum toxin type B (see next section) was launched, with the trade name Myobloc. When injected into specific muscles, both these treatments prevent movement by partially and almost completely paralyzing them. The resulting inability to use particular face muscles causes certain wrinkles to disappear completely. This helps eliminate almost all of the wrinkles of the forehead, in the crow's feet area (by the eyes), and the lines that run from the nose to the mouth (the naso-labial folds). As outlandish and frightening as this sounds, in reality it is no more bizarre than any other cosmetic corrective procedure. It is also important to mention that the results from BoTox are truly astounding, and I mean really astounding, which explains the growing popularity of this medical procedure for the treatment of wrinkles. Over 800,000 BoTox treatments were administered in 2001.

BoTox is not anything new. Since 1973 it has been used by ophthalmologists to treat patients with disabling eye ticks, as well as to treat crossed eyes. It is also used by other medical specialists to treat spasmodic neck muscles, spasmodic laryngeal muscles, multiple sclerosis, cerebral palsy, some post-stroke states, spinal cord injuries, nerve palsies, Parkinson's disease, facial spasms, and, most recently, migraine headaches. This extensive use (and the corresponding research) has shown that BoTox has a great success rate, with minimal risk of detrimental side effects. In rare cases, depending on what parts of your face were injected, you may experience temporary facial or eye drooping, bruising, or jaw and neck weakness, but it lasts only for the duration of the BoTox, so it goes away in three to six months.

From my own experience, the BoTox injections, about ten of them in various points of my forehead, did hurt. One injection site bruised and two others were sore for three days. The bruising was completely gone after five days and so was the soreness. I did have a consistent, though mild, tension headache for several days. I think this was from repeatedly testing the results by trying to raise my eyebrows or frown. I couldn't look in mirrors often enough, straining to raise my eyebrows to see how it was going, plus my friends and those in my office wanted to see the results. Though everyone could tell my forehead wrinkles and the wrinkles between my eyes were gone they couldn't tell the difference when it came to the way I use my forehead and eyebrows. It was amazing to me that no one could tell I wasn't able to squint or look surprised. Once I stopped my facial demonstrations the headaches seemed to disappear.

After the first day I couldn't raise my eyebrows. It took several days before I could no longer furrow my brows. After the first injections, I had a consistent feeling of heaviness in my eyes and I thought they looked somewhat puffy under the eyebrow area (that did not happen on subsequent injections). This feeling lasted about a week. One interesting and unexpected side effect is that putting on eye makeup is now a little tricky because I can't raise my eyebrows to adjust my eyelid and crease area to get a flat area to apply eyeshadow.

The bottom line, or should I say the bottom un-line, is that my forehead is unusually smooth and the wrinkles are practically gone! It is the most amazing thing I've ever experienced. Studies have shown that repeated injections can create a buildup effect, making the results last longer. This one is too tempting to ignore—which explains its rise in popularity.

**Note:** The physician who performed the procedure on me warned that there are physicians advertising or offering inexpensive BoTox treatments for under $400. He feels strongly that, given the raw material cost of BoTox (over $300 to treat the forehead area alone), if a physician isn't charging enough they could very possibly be using a watered-down BoTox solution, resulting in poor or extremely short-term results. It takes just a little mathematics to realize that a doctor would be operating at a loss if he didn't charge appropriately for the BoTox treatment. If the solution costs $300, you have to add in the doctor's expenses like rent, assistants, liability insurance, equipment, and on and on. There are no doctors providing cosmetic BoTox treatments as a charity. As is true in any cosmetic or medical procedure, this is not an arena where you should expect to get both good results and a bargain.

## MYOBLOC (BOTULINUM TOXIN B) ($300 TO $1,000)

Myobloc (botulinum toxin type B) was approved by the FDA in December 2000 "for the symptomatic treatment of patients with cervical dystonia (CD) to reduce the severity of abnormal head position and neck pain associated with CD." Cervical dystonia is a neurological movement disorder in which a person's neck and shoulder muscles are subject to contractions that force the head and neck into abnormal and sometimes painful positions, making it difficult for some people to function normally in their daily activities.

For those receiving Myobloc treatments for CD, the side effects may include dry mouth, dysphagia, dyspepsia, and injection site pain. These adverse effects are generally mild to moderate, transient, self-resolving, and more common only with higher doses. The side effects are also related to the location of the injection site and the muscles involved and not the drug itself. Myobloc was formerly known as BotB and is marketed outside the United States as Neurobloc.

For facial wrinkles, people who are resistant to BoTox might find Myobloc more suitable and effective. However, the question of whether to choose BoTox over Myobloc is not a simple one. According to Mike A. Royal, MD, in an online research paper entitled "The Use of Botulinum Toxins (BT) in the Management of Myofascial Pain and Other Conditions Associated with Painful Muscle Spasm," (http://www.pain.com), "The recent addition of the Elan Pharmaceuticals product, Myobloc™ (BTB—Botulinum Toxin Type B) also raises the important issue of choice. Although the net effect of each BT is to block acetylcholine release, one cannot take data derived from clinical studies of BTA (Botulinum Type A) and apply it to BTB by making some adjustment for potency differences. Each BT has a different structure, different mechanism of action (although the net effect may be the same), different formulation, different storage and handling guidelines, different FDA-approved uses, different dosing concerns, and possibly different antibody development concerns. BTA has been around much longer and all of the published pain and headache clinical research used BTA."

The same holds true for wrinkles. Clearly, Myobloc can be effective for wrinkles but the information for this is limited. As this book goes to press, we know far more about the success of BoTox (BTA) for wrinkles than we do about Myobloc. I would wait to jump on the Myobloc bandwagon. You don't need to be the guinea pig for this one.

## CHEEKBONE (MALAR) AUGMENTATION ($2,000 TO $3,500)

Improving the shape of the face is an option separate from the issue of facial rejuvenation. For many women a more sculpted face is an aesthetic goal, and, therefore, cheekbone augmentation is a more common procedure in facial plastic surgery practices. Cheekbones are reshaped and built up by placing a plastic implant over them. This procedure is considered a safe, relatively simple technique with generally good results (Source: *Facial and Plastic Surgery*, February 2000, pages 35–44). The implant is usually inserted via an incision within the mouth, but it may be done through a lower eyelid or brow incision. Perhaps the biggest mistake made during this procedure is overcompensation which causes a fake-looking visage because of cheekbones so enlarged that they look like they belong on someone else (think Disney's Cruella de Vil.

Alternatively, the buccal fat pads, which are located above the jawline near the corners of the mouth, just below the cheekbone, can be removed in individuals with an excessively round face. This procedure imparts a more contoured look, sometimes referred to as the "waif look," à la Kate Moss. However, plastic surgeons warn that, in many individuals, removal of the buccal fat pads can lead to a more drawn, hollow-cheeked look as aging progresses something that naturally occurs to the face as it grows older.

## CHEMICAL PEEL ($500 TO 2,700 DEPENDING ON THE TYPE OF PEEL)

Peel solutions may contain alpha hydroxy acids, beta hydroxy acid, tricholoracetic acid (TCA), or phenol as the peeling agent. Each of these are categorized by the concentration and the resulting depth of the peel on the skin. Fine lines and wrinkles, skin discolorations, reduction in the appearance of skin discolorations and scars, along with overall improvement in skin texture and subtle rebuilding of the skin's collagen are all possible outcomes of chemical peels. There are definite drawbacks to consider, but this is largely dependent on the depth of peel. The risk of complication is directly related to the amount of benefit desired. Superficial peels have little to no associated risks, although prolonged redness, swelling, and increased skin sensitivity do occur. When more significant results are desired, the complications increase proportionately. Skin discoloration in medium and deeper peels (called hypopigmentation) is typical for most Caucasian patients. Many more complications and scars are recorded from TCA peeling than from phenol, perhaps because of the care with which phenol peels must be performed and the implied safety of TCA (Source: *eMedicine Journal*, February 14, 2002, volume 3, number 2).

Chemical peels are performed by the application of the specific solution that peels away the skin's top layers, either on the entire face or on specific areas. Often, several shallow to medium-depth peels can achieve results similar to one deep-peel treatment, with less post-procedure risk and a shorter recovery time.

**Alpha hydroxy acids (AHA) use glycolic acid** as the chemical ingredient. Various concentrations can be applied, but most commonly 30% to 70% concentrations are used. The lower the concentration, the less impressive the results. AHA peels are effective in improving skin texture, causing some collagen and elastin rebuilding, somewhat reducing the appearance of acne scarring, and reducing the appearance of skin discolorations (Source: *American Journal of Clinical Dermatology*, March-April 2000, pages 81–88).

AHA peels are not medical procedures and as a result are not regulated by the FDA. A physician usually performs higher-concentration peels, but this is not always the case. In lower-concentration peels, often performed by aestheticians, repeated treatments are necessary to achieve and maintain the results seen immediately after the peel is performed.

**Beta hydroxy acid (BHA) or salicylic acid peels** are not as popular as AHA peels, yet they are equally as effective and have specific advantages for some skin types. A solution of salicylic acid can work in a way that is similar to a glycolic acid peel, but irritation is much reduced. Salicylic acid is a compound closely related to aspirin (acetylsalicylic acid), and it retains its aspirin-like anti-inflammatory properties. A deep BHA peel can be superior for many skin types because the irritation and inflammation are kept to a minimum due to the analgesic action of the BHA compound. Salicylic acid is also lipid soluble; therefore, it is a good peeling agent for blemish-prone skin with blackheads. The most common concentrations used today are 20% to 30% (Source: *Dermatologic Surgery*, March 1998, pages 325–328).

**Trichloroacetic acid (TCA) peels** in concentrations of 10% to 35% have been used for many years and are considered effective and safe (Source: *Dermatologic Clinics*, July 2001, pages 413–425). It can be used for peeling the face, neck, hands, and other exposed areas of the body. It has less bleaching effect than phenol (see the next paragraph) and is excellent for "spot" peeling of specific areas. It can be used for medium or light peeling, depending on the concentration and method of application. TCA peels are best for fine lines but are minimally effective on deeper wrinkling (Source: *eMedicine Journal*, December 5, 2001, volume 2, number 12). However, at higher concentrations, such as 50% and above, TCA has a tendency to scar and is less manageable than other agents used for superficial peels.

**Phenol** is sometimes, though rarely, used for full-face peeling when sun damage or wrinkling is severe. It can also be used to treat limited areas of the face, such as deep wrinkles around the mouth, but it may permanently bleach the skin, leaving a line of demarcation between the treated and untreated areas that must be covered with makeup. "Although phenol produces the most remarkable resolution of actinic damage and wrinkling among the various [chemical peels] … it also possesses some of the more significant [serious side effects]. Many have abandoned phenol in favor of other agents or laser resurfacing…. Hypopigmentation may occur in all skin types, noticeably lightening patients with darker skin and making lighter-skinned patients appear waxy or pale. A clear line of demarcation may be present between treated and untreated skin" (Source: *eMedicine Journal*, July 20, 2001, volume 2, number 7). Given the positive results that can be achieved with other resurfacing procedures and the extreme risks associated with phenol, this method is actively discouraged and rarely used.

**Buffered phenol** offers yet another option for severely sun-damaged skin. One such formula uses olive oil, among other ingredients, to diminish the strength of the phenol solution. Another, slightly milder formula uses glycerin. A buffered phenol peel may be more comfortable for patients, and the skin heals faster than with a standard phenol peel, but it is still a risky procedure that can depigment the skin.

## CHIN AUGMENTATION (MENTOPLASTY), CHIN REDUCTION
### *($1,700 to $5,000)*

Chin augmentation can strengthen the appearance of a receding chin by increasing its projection. (Look at pictures of Michael Jackson when he was young, then look at a recent picture; it's hard to ignore his mega-chin implant.) The procedure does not affect the patient's bite or jaw, and can be done using one of two techniques. One approach is to make an incision inside the mouth, move the chin bone, and then wire it into position; the other requires the insertion of an implant through an incision inside the mouth, between the lower lip and the gum, or through an external incision underneath the chin. Hydroxyapatite granules, a bone substitute made from coral, can also be used to enhance facial contours, such as forming a more prominent chin or cheekbones. The substance also has reconstructive uses in craniofacial surgery.

From another perspective, even if the shape of the chin may not be an issue, but excess skin can start pouching along the jawline, creating the appearance of a double chin or a turkey neck. A chin tuck can help shore up this sagging by cutting away surplus skin and using liposuction to remove the excess fat. The scar is hidden just under the jaw.

## COLLAGEN INJECTIONS ($325 TO $1,400)

See Dermal Fillers in this chapter.

## COSMETIC TATTOOING ($750 TO $1,500)

Cosmetic tattooing, or micropigmentation, can be used to create permanent eyeliner, eyebrow color, or lip color. It can also be used for permanent blush or eyeshadow, though this is uncommon. Other uses include re-creating the coloration of the areola around the nipple following breast reconstruction; restoring the color of dark or light skin where natural pigmentation has been lost through such factors as vitiligo (a whitening of the skin from an autoimmune response), cancer, burns, or other scarring; and eliminating some types of birthmarks or previous tattoos.

As a general rule, I do *not* recommend tattooing as a cosmetic way to create permanent eyeliner, eyebrows, colored lips, and especially not for blush. As seductive as permanent makeup sounds—who wouldn't love to avoid drawing on eyebrows and eyeliner, or constantly reapplying lipstick—remember that fashions change and the face ages. Permanent eyebrows that look nice and even when you're in your 40s can sag as your skin ages, and the same is true for the eyeliner and blush. Additionally, your personal style preferences can change. A pink or red lip color imprinted on your mouth may look good today, but in five or ten years it can look strange and out of date. Many cosmetic surgeons I've interviewed have commented that removing tattooed-on lip liner, eyebrows, and blush has become a lucrative business due to the large number of botched applications.

## DERMABRASION ($1,000 TO $2,500)

Dermabrasion is a procedure in which a high-speed wheel, similar to a rotary sander using fine-grained sandpaper, is used to abrade the skin. As a method of resurfacing, dermabrasion can provide effective treatment for treating deep acne scars and deep facial wrinkling. Its benefit is the absence of heat damage that lasers and chemical peels can cause. However, some expected side effects, both transient and long-term, are considered normal and do occur. Transient effects can include spot bleeding for several days after surgery, swelling, breakouts, and hyperpigmentation. Hypopigmentation, the more permanent loss of skin color, occurs in 20% to 30% of patients. Possible scarring can also occur but that is true for any of the deeper chemical peels and ablative laser resurfacing (Source: *eMedicine Journal*, October 17, 2001, volume 2, number 10).

Despite these daunting considerations dermabrasion may still be recommended for deep acne scarring, providing there is a real understanding about the risk of depigmentation.

## DERMAL FILLERS

Whether it's called tissue augmentation, injectable fillers, soft-tissue fillers, implants, or filler injections, one of the more popular ways to improve the appearance of wrinkles or acne scars is to fill them in with a variety of substances. These fillers work by literally being injected or implanted into a wrinkle or a scar where the material (either synthetic or natural) then fills in the depression (temporarily or semi-permanently), creating a smoother impression. Almost all fillers can also work to plump up lips or alter the shape of the face, but their primary use is to fill in wrinkles and acne scars.

Filling in wrinkles or scars using any form of tissue augmentation is often done in combination with other cosmetic procedures. These can range from BoTox injections to laser or chemical peel resurfacing (as well as face-lifts) to achieve optimal results in obtaining the smoothest looking skin you can get. If you're considering injectable fillers of any kind the following information will help give you a realistic guideline for comparisons, risks, and expectations. It is vital to understand that with any cosmetic corrective procedure that there isn't one *best* option. Quite the contrary—there are many excellent alternatives available, with the final decision determined by your doctor's skill, your budget, how much risk you're willing to take, and what kind of realistic results you're looking for.

When it comes to filling in wrinkles with injectables or any filler substance, each type has its own limitations and benefits. Once again, there isn't a single best or foolproof method. Injectable fillers and tissue augmentation are not reliable options for extreme wrinkling, particularly the criss-crossed or interwoven wrinkles that appear on the cheeks or the lines around the mouth. The effects are also rarely permanent, requiring subsequent procedures at different intervals (typically three months to a year). Some of the fillers can feel hard or look noticeable under the skin, while others can distribute unevenly and look lumpy. In addition, many of the fillers being used today are new and there isn't a great deal of information about long-term results.

I know it's a lot of work trying to understand such a confluence of complicated information regarding all your options. But weighing the pros and cons of each alternative and then discussing them with your doctor *is* truly the best way to get the results you want and not be disappointed.

**Note:** One of the risks that all injectable or tissue fillers present is a possible reaction to the needle or device used to place the material in the skin. Side effects can include pain, bruising, inflammation, discoloration, and swelling. These often resolve within a few days to a few weeks. On rare occasions discoloration can last for up to year if a blood vessel was affected.

## ANIMAL-DERIVED COLLAGEN INJECTIONS

**Brand names:** Zyderm, Zyplast, Fibrel
**Major risks:** Allergic reactions can occur. It can have a hard feel under skin, and may look lumpy or uneven under the skin.
**Stability:** Benefits can last three to six months.
**Results:** Appearance improves immediately.
**Cost:** $300 to $800 (subsequent injections may cost less).

Collagen is found in all living tissue, and its basic function is to provide support and structure for the skin. The FDA approved injectable collagen in 1981. For most of the 1980s and 1990s, collagen injections were one of the primary methods used to fill in wrinkles. Zyderm and Zyplast are derived from cow collagen; Fibrel is derived from pig collagen. Injectable animal collagens are used less frequently in Europe than in the United States due to the risk of their association with bovine spongiform encephalopathy (Mad Cow Disease). Collagen injections derived from animal sources are now used less frequently than other dermal fillers in the United States, but that is largely due to a substantial risk of allergic reaction (according to the FDA, "about 3 percent of the population is allergic to collagen") and the short duration of the results.

Because of the potential for allergic reaction (particularly for cow collagen), it is essential to have a pretest at least four to six weeks prior to treatment. A small amount of the collagen is injected into the arm or thigh and the area is monitored closely for any signs of inflammation, swelling, irritation, rashes, or itching. Once it has been determined that you are not allergic to the material it can be injected into the wrinkle underneath the skin. Repeated injections may be necessary until optimal results are achieved.

## HUMAN-DERIVED COLLAGEN INJECTIONS

**Brand names:** Dermalogen, Autologen, Isolagen
**Major risks:** Minimal to no risk of allergic reaction, but the area injected can have a hard feel under skin and may look lumpy or uneven.
**Stability:** Benefits can last three to nine months and possibly longer, though there is no research establishing exact length of time.

**Results:** Appearance improves immediately.

**Cost:** $500 to $1,000 (subsequent injections may cost less).

Dermalogen is derived from human cadaver collagen, Autologen is derived from your own skin's collagen, and Isolagen is made of cells that are actually cloned from your own skin. The primary benefit of human-derived collagen injections is that there is almost no chance of having or developing an allergic reaction.

Autologen can be harvested during cosmetic surgery procedures such as tummy tucks, face-lifts, and breast augmentation or reduction. The skin removed from those procedures is sent to a laboratory where it is processed to become injectable collagen filler. Depending on the results you are trying to achieve you may receive a series of injections over a period of a year. Some doctors claim that Autologen achieves permanent results, but that has not been proven, and for many women is definitely not the case.

Isolagen, as futuristic as it sounds, is made of cells cloned from your own skin. It's done by simply removing a small piece of skin (about the size of a dime) from your neck or behind your ear. The skin is sent to a lab that, in about four to six weeks, can grow your own injectable collagen from it. Generally, three to four injections are delivered over a two-month period. Each subsequent injection produces increased improvement. After the last injection, continued improvement may still be seen because, unlike all other injectable procedures, Isolagen uses live cells and that stimulates further smoothing out of wrinkles for a period of time.

**Note:** Isolagen was available in the United States from 1996 to 1999. During that time the FDA categorized Isolagen as a graft, and it was, therefore, not subject to any regulatory scrutiny. In 1999, the FDA reclassified Isolagen as a drug, which meant it could no longer be used in regulated surgical medical procedures. The company that makes Isolagen has filed a New Drug Application with the FDA, and clinical trials are pending. That process can take up to four years before it meets the FDA standards for drug acceptance. However, there are patients currently involved in clinical trials who are receiving Isolagen injections (Source: *Skin & Allergy News*, May 1999).

The process of creating Dermalogen is similar to that for creating both Isolagen and Autologen. Dermalogen, however, is derived from skin tissue removed at the time of death, much as other organs are removed from human donors. All three—Autologen, Isolagen, and Dermalogen—are thought to last longer than animal-derived collagen, but that is yet to be proven. A primary benefit of Dermalogen over Isolagen and Autolagen is that it doesn't require any skin removal (at least not from you); and there's no waiting time for preparation.

## FAT TRANSFER INJECTIONS

**Technical names:** Autologous Fat Transplantation, fat injections, Microlipo-injection, Fat Grafting

**Major risks:** There are risks associated with liposuction procedures. From the injection itself there can be some local swelling, redness, and bruising. Scar-tissue buildup is possible, and it is possible to temporarily lose sensation in the treatment area due to nerve damage or swelling. Long-term or permanent loss of sensitivity is possible. There is also the risk of an asymmetrical appearance.

**Stability:** Your body will absorb about 65% of the fat within the first six months. The remaining 35% can remain in place for longer, but exactly how much longer varies greatly from person to person. For some reason some people's bodies just can't hold on to the injected fat, even when it's their own.

**Results:** Appearance improves immediately, though doctors often overfill the area to improve the chances of long-term results.

**Cost:** $450 to $3,000.

Getting rid of your own fat and then injecting it into your wrinkles to eliminate them does sound like the best of all worlds, but fat injections are a more complicated process than other injectables. So even though the concept of redistributing fat from an area where you don't want it (like the thighs and buttocks) to areas where it may be of better use (like wrinkles) is very appealing, the benefit of fat transplantation is limited by the dramatic re-absorption of fat grafts.

The first step is to remove fat from your own body, and it's usually taken from the abdomen or buttocks. It is important that the fat being used has a soft texture so it can more easily adapt and be contoured to the shape of the face. Once the fat is extracted it is processed to make it usable, so it can be injected precisely underneath the wrinkle to fill in and reshape the area. This injection process is repeated until the desired enhancement is attained.

Another added benefit of fat injections is that when physicians extract fat from a liposuction procedure, breast augmentation, a tummy tuck, or some other reduction surgery, they can store the fat in a freezer to be used in future fat-injection procedures.

Because of the amount of absorption that takes place within the first few months of treatment; many physicians overfill the treated area to help improve the long-term results. This overfilling can create a strange appearance by making the face look swollen and puffy. The puffiness does diminish over a period of weeks, but be aware that this is a potential problem for the short term.

### HYALURONIC ACID DERIVED FILLERS

**Brand names:** Restylane, Hylaform, Perlane, Rofilan Hylan Gel

**Major risk:** Hypersensitivity can occur in 1 out of every 2,000 treated patients. There have also been cases of persistent inflammation and noninfected abscesses, which may persist for up to a year, or until the injected material is fully reabsorbed.

**Stability:** Benefits can last three to six months and occasionally for one year.

**Results:** Appearance improves immediately.

**Cost:** Still in trial stages so pricing is not available.

Restylane, Hylaform, Perlane, and Rofilan are not yet approved by the FDA for use in the United States. However, a handful of doctors have been selected to test them on patients willing to sign a waiver while the products go through the FDA's process of being accepted as approved medical treatments for wrinkles. All of these fillers are derived from nonanimal sources of hyaluronic acid. Although hyaluronic acid is a part of human skin, these injectable substances are synthetically modified. Even though a pre-test is thought not to be necessary, it is generally best to go through the process anyway to be certain you do not have a special or unique reaction to this substance. None of these new fillers are permanent and they are eventually reabsorbed into the body.

Hylaform, Perlane, Rofilan, and Restylane have many similarities. The primary difference is in their consistency: Hylaform, Perlane, and Rofilan are viscoelastic gels, which means that they are more viscous and pliable than Restylane. This makes them better for treatment of deeper lines than for superficial wrinkles, where they can feel thick and be visible under the skin. Restylane, on the other hand, is better for treatment of superficial wrinkles.

## HUMAN DONOR TISSUE IMPLANTS

**Technical name:** Acellular Cadaveric Dermis

**Brand names:** AlloDerm, Micronized AlloDerm, Cymetra

**Major risk:** There can be some local swelling, redness, and bruising (mainly from the injection itself), but this is usually short lived. The implant area can feel hard for a period of months and even longer for some patients.

**Stability:** Benefits can last one to two years, though maybe less for areas of the face that have the most movement.

**Results:** Appearance improves immediately, but continued improvement takes place as production of your own body's collagen is stimulated.

**Cost:** $1,000 to $1,500.

Acellular Cadaveric Dermis is essentially the use of donor tissue obtained from dead bodies. Much as donor organs are removed from cadavers at the time of death, skin tissue can also be surgically removed and then processed to be used as filler material for wrinkles or to improve facial contours. The donated human tissue goes through a treatment process until it is finally freeze-dried in a way that preserves the integrity of the dermal matrix. When it is ready to be used it is rehydrated and surgically inserted under the skin where recontouring is desired. Once implanted, AlloDerm merges with your own skin and stimulates your body to produce its own collagen until it essentially becomes a part of your skin. Although Alloderm is not widely used as a filler for wrinkles, it has been successfully used in thousands of skin-graft operations and is considered exceptionally safe, stable, and reliable for creating natural-looking results.

## FASCIA INJECTIONS

**Technical name:** Irradiated Human Cadaveric Preserved Fascia Lata
**Brand name:** Fascian
**Major risks:** Depending on the amount of material and the size of the needle used, the injected site can become swollen or bruised. The area may also feel thick or lumpy, though typically this softens in time. Allergic reactions are rare.
**Stability:** Benefits can last three to six months.
**Results:** Appearance improves immediately.
**Cost:** $800 to $1,000.

Fascian, much like Alloderm (reviewed above), is obtained from donor tissue from dead bodies. In this case the donated material is fascia, the substance covering your muscles (and some organs) in large, thick, white sheets, keeping them compact and supported yet limber. Fascia's unique property is that it is a firm yet pliable type of human tissue, with qualities that make it adaptable for use in improving the appearance of skin. The main drawback of this procedure is its expense when compared with the length of time results remain, which is not much longer than other injectables.

## SYNTHETIC IMPLANTS

**Brand names:** Gore S.A.M., Softform
**Major risks:** Unpleasant firmness and risk of the implant breaking through the skin. Thinner strands of Gore S.A.M. (Subcutaneous Augmentation Material) and Softform may reduce the risk of over-firmness. Synthetic implants are not recommended for lip enhancement due to the potential for an uneven or hard, unnatural appearance of lips. Your body can reject the implant. Scarring can occur.
**Stability:** Benefits can be permanent.
**Results:** Appearance improves immediately, but as your own skin tissue meshes with the implant further improvement is often seen.
**Cost:** $1,000 to $4,000.

For those of us who live in the Northwest, Gore-Tex is a well-known, durable, synthetic fabric that works well in all weather conditions. It is essentially a form of Teflon. Gore-Tex has remarkable flexibility, and in the form of Gore S.A.M. created by the same company that developed Gore-Tex—W. L. Gore and Associates), it can be used for cosmetic corrective procedures. The actual implant material is called expanded polytetrafluoroethylene (ePTFE). Implanting threadlike strips of Gore

S.A.M. under the skin around the lips or along the naso-labial folds (the lines that run from the nose to the mouth) can improve the appearance of the face.

Gore S.A.M. is porous, and therefore allows the body's own tissue to attach itself to the implant, creating a very durable, stable implant. However, Gore S.A.M has limited uses. For example, those with thin skin would find that the implant can easily be felt or even seen under the surface. It also should not be used on the lips because of the risk of stiffness, making the mouth look unnatural.

The Softform implant is made from the same material as Gore S.A.M. The major difference between Softform and Gore S.A.M. is that Softform threads are hollow, as opposed to Gore S.A.M., which is porous. Softform's hollow form allows your own tissue to grow through the cylinder to help make it more stable and durable.

### ARTECOLL

**Brand name:** Artecoll

**Major risk:** Artecoll has the same potential for allergic reactions as collagen injections.

**Stability:** Benefits can be permanent, but this is still under investigation.

**Results:** Appearance improves immediately, but continued improvement takes place as your own body's production of collagen and connective tissue is stimulated.

**Cost:** Still in trial stages so pricing is not available.

Artecoll is a combination injectable made up of a synthetic substance called polymethylmethacrylate (PMMA) and collagen (similar to Zyderm and Zyplast, reviewed above). Artecoll is not approved as an implant material in the United States. The FDA has only recently accepted it for research as an Investigational Medical Device (IDE) for wrinkles, which means that only a handful of doctors are approved to use it. While Artecoll is relatively new in the treatment of wrinkles, it has been around for the past 50 years as a bone substitute and it is approved in Canada and Europe as an injectable filler for wrinkles. It is thought to have fewer reactions than other injectables, but this is yet to be established definitively.

Artecoll is injected in the same manner as collagen, and has the same initial results. With Artecoll, however, after the collagen is absorbed or broken down by the body, the synthetic material PMMA remains, stimulating the formation of new collagen and connective tissue in the area surrounding the PMMA. One or two applications are enough to obtain good results. The results are thought to be permanent, but this is yet to be proven.

### SILICONE INJECTIONS

**Brand name:** Dermagen

It is amazing to me that silicone injections are still being used to fill in wrinkles.

According to the FDA, silicone injections are approved only for limited ophthalmic use and are prohibited for any other purpose. We tend to think of silicone in relation to breast implants or breast augmentation. Dow Corning has settled some very sizable lawsuits due to complications resulting from their medical-grade silicone breast implants. However, there are some doctors who still use injectable silicone as a wrinkle filler for the face. While the exact potential for damage to the body is an extremely controversial question, there is no doubt that silicone in the body can become encapsulated as the body tries to reject it, creating a serious and persistent inflammation that has strong potential for becoming infected and destroying surrounding skin tissue. I would not encourage anyone concerned with filling in wrinkles to pursue this procedure.

## EAR SURGERY (OTOPLASTY) *($2,000 TO $3,000)*

If you've worn heavy earrings for most of your life, your earlobes may be swinging down closer to your shoulders than you ever thought possible. A simple, 30-minute earlobe reduction can be performed in a plastic surgeon's office or at the same time as a face-lift. Aesthetically speaking, or at least to be sure your earlobes don't wobble, the earlobe should not be more than 25% of the total length of the ear. If it exceeds this, an L-shaped wedge can be cut away, and the earlobe edges can be brought together and sutured.

The earlobes can also protrude from the head. This protrusion can be part of the entire ear sticking out or be caused by an oversized ear shape that looks out of proportion to the shape of the head. Earlobe surgery can achieve an appearance that makes the ear more in balance with the face. One way to accomplish this is to position the ears closer to the head by reshaping the cartilage (supporting tissue). Otoplasty can be performed on children as early as age five or six.

## EYELID SURGERY (BLEPHAROPLASTY) *($2,500 TO $5,000)*

Eyelid surgery is one of the more popular cosmetic surgeries because it is relatively simple, it requires minimal postoperative recovery, and the results can be stunning. This operation involves cutting away the fat that causes bags beneath the eyes and removing wrinkled, drooping layers of skin on the eyelids. Blepharoplasty is often performed along with a face-lift or with other facial rejuvenation procedures, especially forehead lifts. Incisions follow the natural contour lines in both upper and lower lids, and the thin surgical scars are usually barely visible and blend into the eyelids' natural lines and folds, although it depends on how your skin scars. A talented surgeon can avoid some of the typical mistakes, such as creating a scar that sits above the fold of the upper eyelid, overpulling the skin, or removing too much of the fat pad areas, which would create a sunken, drawn appearance (Source: *Facial Plastic Surgery*, 1999, volume 15, issue 3, pages 173–229).

Transconjunctival blepharoplasty, a variation of eyelid surgery, is performed by making an incision inside the lower eyelid. It avoids any scarring on the lower lid and may reduce the possibility of the eyelid pulling down, a postoperative complication in some patients. It is a useful technique when fat only, and not skin or muscle, needs to be removed from the eyelid area.

It is important to note that eyelid surgery may not be indicated if a forehead lift (of the endoscopic type) can produce a more positive effect without risking the eye area or obvious scarring. This option should absolutely be discussed with your surgeon.

## ENDOSCOPIC FACE-LIFT *($2,500 TO $5,000)*

An endoscope is a small surgical instrument that can be inserted under the skin through small incisions, allowing a surgeon to perform a cosmetic corrective procedure via microsurgery. The endoscope itself is a miniature camera with a light fitted on one end of a long tube. When inserted under the skin the camera transmits magnified images to a television monitor. During the procedure the surgeon watches the screen as the endoscope functions as the doctor's under-skin eye. Simultaneously, the surgeon inserts and uses other surgical instruments, including scalpels, scissors, or forceps to actually perform the operation. Endoscopic face-lifts are an optimal way to minimally impact the skin and yet achieve impressive results similar to the results of traditional face-lifts. But without cutting and pasting sections of skin how does an endoscopic face-lift work?

It turns out that a good deal of the skin's tendency to sag over time is a result of the face's muscles and fat pads shifting down and in toward the center of the face. This is what happens with the deepest furrowed lines on the face, particularly the forehead and the naso-labial folds from the nose to the mouth.

Let's say your jawline is beginning to sag. Using the somewhat simple surgical procedure called endoplasty, the surgeon makes a mere quarter-inch cut underneath the chin and at each edge of the jaw, and then, via microsurgery (the surgeon watches what is being done via a television screen), sutures the platysma muscle, which extends from jawline to jawline under the chin, back where it belongs.

Similar to the reason skin sags, the deep frown lines and vertical creases in the mid-forehead result from a literal slippage of the forehead muscles downward and inward, as well as just simple frowning and movement of the forehead. The same endoscopic technique used to anchor the platysma muscle can be used on the forehead muscles, and an additional separating of the muscles between the eyebrows can reduce the fold lines there. This operation can be done via three tiny incisions inside the hairline, allowing the surgeon to anchor the slipped muscles back in place and to cut away a small section of the muscles between the eyebrows.

There is a great deal of research showing that endoscopic face-lifts not only achieve impressive results—as good as, if not better than traditional cut-and-paste face-lifts—but also have minimal to none of the risks associated with traditional surgical procedures (Sources: *Facial Plastic Surgery*, 2000, volume 16, issue 3, pages 283–298; *Plastic and Reconstructive Surgery*, January 2002, pages 329–340; *Facial Plastic Surgery Clinics North America*, August 2001, pages 439–451; *Aesthetic Plastic Surgery*, January 2001, pages 35–39).

**Note:** While reanchoring the muscles of the jaw and forehead can eliminate or decrease sagging, forehead lines, and the naso-labial folds (the fold of skin from the nose to the mouth), laser surgery is the treatment of choice for smoothing out fine lines all over the face, principally around the eyes and the mouth. Laser surgery can also slightly decrease sagging, but its main function is to smooth out lines. Although laser surgery can take three weeks to heal, endoscopic surgery takes only about 48 hours, although it is often accompanied by a postoperative headache that can last for a few days.

## FACE-LIFT (RHYTIDECTOMY) *($5,000 TO $10,000)*

Here's what one respected source has to say about this procedure: "Although there are a multitude of techniques currently used for performing face lifts, there is no general agreement as to which, if any, of these techniques is most effective. There may never be a definitive answer to this issue because of the highly subjective nature of aesthetics, variability among surgeons, differences in patient anatomy, and specific patient desires" (Source: *Plastic and Reconstructive Surgery*, 1998, volume 102, pages 878–881).

An article in the *Journal of Plastic and Reconstructive Surgery* (October 2000, "National Plastic Surgery Survey: Face Lift Techniques and Complications") stated that "... 15 percent of [cosmetic] surgeons perform ... [superficial] skin-only procedure[s], and 74 percent said they address the SMAS [superficial musculoaponeurotic system]. Nine percent of surgeons prefer a composite or deep-plane lift. Only 2 percent generally perform a subperiosteal-lift; about half of those use the endoscope." (See the section above on endoscopic face-lifts.)

The art of the face-lift is extremely complicated and the choices read like a menu with too many entrees. A traditional face-lift can dramatically reduce sagging skin on the face, neck, and jaw. As impressive as this cosmetic procedure can be in creating a youthful, taut visage, it can also create an overly pulled, masklike appearance, with the face drawn up in a stretched, permanent smile (à la The Joker of *Batman* fame). This is one cosmetic procedure where you want to see the doctor's work on someone else up-close and personal.

During this complicated, elaborate procedure, incisions are made in the hairline both in front of and behind the ears (the exact design of the incisions may differ from patient to patient, and surgeons' personal techniques can vary widely). For younger patients, more-limited incisions may be appropriate. When necessary, fatty deposits beneath the skin are removed or repositioned, and sagging muscles are tightened. The slack in the skin itself is then taken up and the excess cut away. Scars can usually be concealed, but when things go wrong thick, obvious scars may be seen or the hairline behind the ear or along the forehead may be altered in such a way that it creates an unnatural, strained appearance.

Most face-lifts also involve repositioning the muscles and fat pads of the cheek that have slipped forward, causing deep lines near the mouth (laugh lines), as well as sagging the muscle along the chin. Face-lifts that tighten only the skin without repositioning the muscles and fat pads can cause the face to look gaunt and unnatural. Face-lifts also have limitations as to the areas of the face they can affect. Other areas require a forehead lift, chin tuck, or endoscopic repositioning of those muscles and fat pads. Likewise, wrinkles by the eyes and mouth are not affected by a face-lift alone and require additional procedures (such as laser resurfacing) that are often done at the same time the face-lift is performed. Here is a menu of options for face-lifts a doctor can select from:

**Classic or Traditional Face-Lift:** This is what most of us think of when we think of a face-lift. Sagging, wrinkled skin is cut away and repositioned to create a smoother and tighter visage. Cutting skin is only one part of this procedure; to create the most natural finished appearance, the muscles and fat pads under the skin need to be repositioned so the realigned skin is formed over a youthful base.

**SMAS-Lift (Superficial Musculoaponeurotic System):** The SMAS face-lift is a term that has become familiar to those looking into plastic surgery. SMAS refers to the superficial musculoaponeurotic system. The skin on the face is composed of the superficial layers of skin, both the top and lower layer as well as the underlying layer of fat. Beneath the skin, fat, and muscle is a gliding membrane composed partly of connective tissue and partly of muscle. This gliding tissue is the SMAS, which is responsible for our ability to have facial expressions. Realigning this structure is considered a valid option for re-creating a youthful appearance for the face. However, when you cut under the muscle layer you can negatively affect nerve endings, and that is the major risk of this procedure. However, if you pulled only the top layer of skin and fat layer, the muscle layer (which also sags and causes an aged appearance to the face) would not be corrected. Many surgeons feel that addressing the SMAS layer of skin is necessary to avoid giving a flat or unnatural appearance to the face (Source: *Plastic and Reconstructive Surgery*, 2000, volume 105, pages 290–301).

## SUBPERIOSTEAL LIFT

Periosteal refers to the thick membrane that covers the surface of bones. The subperiosteal lift is a technique used for the mid- and upper-face area, an area that is not helped by the typical face-lift (cutting and pasting skin around the ear area) or by endoscopic face-lifts (that reposition fat tissue and muscles without cutting and pasting). This is an aggressive technique that removes all the tissue and muscles attached to the bone and reshapes it into a more youthful position over the face. The benefit of the subperiosteal approach to the midface is the ability to lift the center of the face, improving the appearance of the naso-labial folds, smoothing the cheek area, and tightening the eye area (Source: *Plastic and Reconstructive Surgery*, September 1999, pages 842–851). However, any time work is done deeper under the skin the risk of impairment to nerve endings increases.

## NECK LIFT

A woman's neck area is often the place that can look the most aged. Traditional face-lifts do not address this area. Sagging of the neck results when the platysma muscle loosens and becomes elongated. Typically, when an SMAS-Lift is performed the platysma muscle is reshaped and repositioned at the same time. Excess skin and fat can also be cut away at this time (Source: *Plastic and Reconstructive Surgery*, 1999, volume 104, pages 1093–1100).

## S-LIFT OR MINI-LIFT

This technique may be helpful for minor jowling or sagging skin. One source describes its objective this way: "To develop a safe and effective method to lift the jowl either as a single procedure or combined with other rejuvenation methods, S-shaped incisions are marked and then cut from the area just in front of the tragus [the front part of the ear]" (Source: *Dermatologic Surgery*, January 2001, pages 18–22). Once the small S-shaped flap of skin is cut and lifted away from the face it is tightened and repositioned along with the underlying muscles and fat tissues. If necessary, excess fat can be removed from this area at the same time.

## TEMPORAL LIFT

The temporal face-lift refers to the area along the sides and top of the forehead. This technique is also referred to as a brow-lift. It is meant to smooth out the lines of the forehead and some of the eye area by repositioning the forehead skin along the hairline. At the time of the cutting and pasting for this area, the muscles of the forehead would also be repositioned (Source: *Facial Plastic Surgery*, February 2001, pages 57–66).

### DEEP-PLANE LIFT

A deep-plane face-lift simply refers to how deep under the skin the surgeon works to perform any given face-lift procedure. Although it is similar to the SMAS-lift, the deep-plane face-lift goes even deeper. It involves lifting and repositioning the various layers of the face—skin, fat tissue, muscles, and other structures—as a single unit rather than separating and lifting them individually. Because of its complexity, this procedure is not widely performed. However, while it is technically demanding, the results are considered more satisfactory than those of a traditional or more superficial face-lift (Source: *Ophthalmology*, March 2000, pages 490–495).

## FAT IMPLANTS

See Dermal Fillers, above.

## FOREHEAD LIFT (BROW LIFT—TRANSBLEPHAROPLASTY BROW LIFT) *($3,000 TO $5,000)*

The forehead lift is designed to correct or improve wrinkling, as well as sagging of the eyebrow area that often occur as part of the aging process. The procedure may also help to smooth horizontal expression lines in the forehead, smooth vertical frown lines between the eyebrows, and reduce the sagging appearance of the eyelids. Behind the hairline, incisions are placed above the ear and over the top of the head, although in some cases incisions may be made in front of the hairline. Forehead lifts are often (and usually should be) accompanied by repositioning the muscles of the forehead, which are partly responsible for the furrowed lines of the brow. The major downside of this procedure is that the hairline may be pulled farther back than desired.

## LASER RESURFACING PROCEDURES *($1,200 TO $7,500)*

Issues involving cosmetic corrective surgical procedures are complicated as it is, but when the topic turns to laser resurfacing what you find is a large tangled mess—one that's almost impossible for the consumer to wade through. An article in the *Archives of Facial Plastic Surgery* (January-March 2002, pages 6–7, "Laser Madness in Facial Plastic Surgery") summed up the problem beautifully: "In facial plastic surgery, many articles written by physicians promoting … facial resurfacing lasers appear in both peer-reviewed and non–peer-reviewed journals. These articles may read more like advertisements than science, overestimating the advantages of laser surgery, while underestimating the disadvantages and complications. Furthermore, the public's fascination with high-tech procedures related to cosmetic surgery has further exacerbated the unchecked outbreak of laser madness…. Promoters [of facial resurfacing with the $CO_2$ laser] have greatly exaggerated the advantages of laser facial resurfacing over other methods of resurfacing. A better result is not guaranteed simply by using a laser, despite suggestions to the contrary by advertisers. Laser facial resurfacing may be appropriate in patients with severely photodamaged skin and deep wrinkles who are willing to have a prolonged painful healing period and accept the risks of permanent pigmentation changes…. Currently, it is unclear who is benefiting from laser madness in medicine. Is it the patient, the physician, or the laser company?"

Why the controversy? It will become clear in just a moment!

Lasers and light-emitting machines are all about electrical wavelength, energy output, and pulse-width variations. The length of each of the waves used relates to the structures it will affect, such as blood (veins), melanin (skin pigment), and water (found in skin cells). The energy output tells you how powerfully that wavelength will impact the targeted structure. Pulse width indicates how long the wavelength will be in contact with the structure. Each machine has variations on each of these parameters, and can, therefore, target different aspects of skin.

There are basically two types of laser resurfacing options, ablative and nonablative. Nonablative laser treatments use lasers that are noninjurious and do not cause damage to skin tissue. Nonablative lasers include the N-lite laser, Nd:YAG laser, Flashlamp laser, the Pulsed-Light laser, and the CoolTouch laser. Ablative laser resurfacing uses extreme heat generated by laser pulses that can injure and damage skin even as they may benefit it. In fact, part of the effect that ablative lasers have is a direct result of the damage they cause. Ablative lasers include the $CO_2$ Pulse laser, the Er:YAG laser, and the Q-Switched Ruby laser.

Ablative laser resurfacing can absolutely make a remarkable difference in the appearance of skin, particularly in terms of long-lasting improvement in the appearance of deep wrinkles, surface wrinkles, and skin discolorations. But as wonderful as that sounds there are risks and complications that can occur with ablative laser resurfacing. These include swelling, scabbing, oozing, bleeding, flaking, redness, and irritation that can last for an extended period of time, and there is also a definite risk in terms of even longer-term skin discoloration and scarring.

Nonablative laser resurfacing is performed by plastic surgeons and dermatologists alike, and has none of the side effects associated with ablative laser resurfacing. That means no downtime and none of the risks associated with ablative laser resurfacing. However, nonablative resurfacing doesn't produce the same dramatic results as ablative resurfacing can. According to an article in the July 2000 issue of *The Journal,* online at http://www.lasernews.net, "Non-ablative [laser resurfacing] leads to improvement in photodamaged skin and rhytids (wrinkles) without any obvious wound.... However, at the present time, the clinical improvement seen with such techniques is less than that following the inelegant ablative laser resurfacing techniques." Not only are the results of nonablative laser resurfacing subtle, but it requires multiple treatments to achieve any kind of noticeable outcome.

For ablative resurfacing involving a laser peel, the quality of the postoperative techniques is almost as important to the success of the procedure as the skill of the physician performing the peel. In fact, one complication of laser surgery is improper or inadequate home care. The side effects of a laser peel can be daunting. The skin oozes, crusts, and needs to be cleaned and dressed for about two weeks before you look even vaguely normal. Because the top layer of skin has been stripped away, the raw, exposed skin must be cleaned and treated very carefully. The patient can easily do this wrong, causing infection, delayed healing, and irritation.

Although it may sound weird, some physicians require patients who have undergone a laser peel to wear a clear silicone bandage (much like Saran Wrap) over the entire treated area for five to seven days. The silicone bandage prevents any interference from the patient except for gentle cleaning around the mouth, eyes, and nose, which are understandably left unbandaged. But there are problems with this type of wrapping. It can be uncomfortable for the patient, oozing can occur at the edges of the bandage, and it just plain looks strange. (On the other hand, peeled skin looks strange no matter what you do to it.) Antibiotics, special cleansing procedures, and general skin-care instructions are of vital importance in reducing the risk of complications.

To help you make more informed decisions when interviewing a dermatologist or plastic surgeon about laser resurfacing (also called photorejuvenation), you need to have a better understanding of the various laser and light-emitting machines available and their preferred functions on the skin. If a doctor has only limited access to a variety of machines or has only one or two at his disposal, he might not be inclined to let you know each machine's limitations.

The following is a list of the more popular lasers and light-emitting machines in use and their known or ideal benefit for skin, along with their associated risks.

### ABLATIVE LASER RESURFACING

**$CO_2$ Pulse Laser (trade names Feather Touch and Ultra Pulse):** This is one of the oldest ablative laser-resurfacing machines around. While it can deeply resurface skin, creating more lasting and noticeable results than any other laser, it is also associated with the most severe damage and risk to skin. After treatment, skin can take one to two weeks to heal and can be red for one to two months. Risks of scarring, skin discoloration, and uneven texture can occur, though many doctors would insist that this happens less than 2% of the time and rarely when a doctor is experienced in the use of this kind of procedure.

**Erbium:YAG Laser (or Er:YAG Laser):** This ablative laser has a far less invasive effect than the $CO_2$ Pulse laser. The skin may take only four to five days to heal and the redness usually dissipates after one to two weeks. There is minimal risk of scarring and minimal risk of skin discoloration. While all lasers can be used around the eye area, the Erbium:YAG laser can be used to spot treat the eye area for dark circles because it doesn't affect skin colors (it won't cause hypopigmentation or hyperpigmentation).

**Q-Switched Ruby Laser:** This laser is minimally ablative, especially in comparison to the $CO_2$ Pulse and Erbium:YAG lasers. Its primary use is to selectively remove skin pigment, such as freckling, sun-damage spots, and actinic keratosis (precancerous brown skin lesions) without damaging the surrounding skin tissue. It is also especially useful for removing tattoos and some birthmarks. The Q-Switched Ruby laser was the original machine used for temporary hair removal. It can take several treatments to see the desired results.

It is interesting to point out that one of the popular uses for the Q-Switched Ruby laser is to remove cosmetic tattoos. Many physicians believe that the incidence of poor work from inexperienced or poorly trained aestheticians who tattoo lip liner, eyeliner, and eyebrows is so rampant that eliminating their mistakes constitutes a large portion of the laser work many doctors do.

## NONABLATIVE OR COBLATIVE LASER RESURFACING

**Pulsed Dye Laser, Short- and Long-Pulsed:** This nonablative laser gives impressive results in eliminating surfaced capillaries on the face, port wine marks, hypertrophic scarring (thick or raised scars), and hemangiomas (red dots on the surface of skin). Because the Pulsed Dye laser is nonablative it doesn't cause skin damage, but it almost always causes temporary bruising. It can take several treatments to see the desired results.

**Long-Pulsed YAG Laser (trade name Lyra):** This nonablative laser's unique feature is that it has a built-in cooling device that protects the top layer of skin. It is especially suited to those with darker skin tones because it will not affect pigment. It can take several treatments to achieve the desired results. The laser is currently the laser of choice for hair removal.

**CoolTouch Long-Pulsed YAG Laser:** This nonablative laser is noted for its ability to build collagen. It is typically used for wrinkles and acne scars, and it can take several treatments to achieve the desired results. The results for this are very subtle and result in only a slight improvement.

**Long-Pulsed Alexandrite Laser (trade names GentleLASE and Cool Pulse):** This nonablative laser is another option for hair removal, but it is best suited for those with light skin and dark hair. This machine also more easily and quickly covers large areas of skin. It can take several treatments to achieve a subtle improvement.

**Intense Pulsed-Light Device or Flash Lamp (trade names PhotoDerm and Quantum):** This is not a laser, but belongs in this category because of its place in "photorejuvenation" procedures. The Flash Lamp creates a pulse of intense light that is used most frequently as a method to reduce or eliminate surfaced capillaries or veins, port wine marks, hemangiomas (red dots on the surface of skin), and brown spots, as well as to tighten the skin. The number and degree of side effects are considerably less than with laser treatment. It can take several treatments to see desired results.

**1064 Nanometer Long-Pulsed Nd:YAG Lasers (trade names Vasculite, CoolTouch, Varia, and CoolGlide):** These lasers are noted for their treatment of surfaced leg veins. Although bruising can occur, there is no associated skin damage or risk with these devices. However, it is extremely painful and the outcome can vary from person to person. It takes multiple treatments to achieve the desired results. Although new surfaced veins can emerge, the ones that were zapped are gone forever.

The following is a summary covering a range of laser machines and the skin conditions they address:

| Skin Condition | Laser or Light-Emitting System |
|---|---|
| Wrinkles and lines | $CO_2$ (carbon dioxide) |
| | Erbium:YAG |
| | CoolTouch Long-Pulsed YAG |
| Brown spots | $CO_2$ (carbon dioxide) |
| | Nd:YAG |
| | Q-Switched Ruby |
| Deep pigmented lesions | Q-Switched Ruby |
| | Nd:YAG |
| | Pulsed Dye |

| | |
|---|---|
| Scars and stretch marks | $CO_2$ (carbon dioxide)<br>Pulsed Dye<br>CoolTouch Long-Pulsed YAG |
| Tattoos | $CO_2$ (carbon dioxide)<br>Nd:YAG<br>Q-Switched Ruby |
| Hair removal | Nd:YAG<br>Long-Pulsed Alexandrite<br>Intense Pulsed Light (PhotoDerm)<br>Long-Pulsed YAG |

## LIP AUGMENTATION OR REDUCTION *($2,500 TO $4,000)*

While thin lips may not seem like a cosmetic issue, for some women looking for perfection, fuller lips are considered more attractive. Aside from dermal fillers (reviewed above), one of the more interesting methods for augmenting the lips is to surgically advance the lip forward via incisions placed inside the mouth. Fat implants or collagen injections (see the Dermal Fillers section above) may then be positioned under the lining of the lip to add additional plumpness. Neither collagen nor fat is permanent, however, and the procedure must be repeated periodically to maintain results.

A lip lift is a technique that surgically lifts the corners of an aging mouth to eliminate the pronounced droop and unhappy facial expressions that often develop with advanced age. Cutting away small diamonds of skin just above the corners of the mouth raises the border of the lips into a slight smile.

If thin lips have a fashionable downside, it isn't hard to imagine that overly full lips can also be viewed as unattractive. In lip reduction, a small section along the top lining of the lip is surgically removed to narrow the lips to the desired proportion. The small scars on the outside of the lips are often barely noticeable, though it all depends on how you scar.

## MICRODERMABRASION *($300 TO $1,000)*

Microdermabrasion machines require the lowest level of approval from the FDA for a medical device because they are considered Class 1 medical devices, which means they are subject to the least amount of regulatory control. Type 1 devices can be sold and used without any supportive clinical efficacy data (Source: FDA Classification of Medical Devices, http://www.fda.gov/cdrh/dsma/dsmaclas.html#class_1). Often, consumers are given a range of erroneous information regarding microdermabrasion's credentials that just isn't true.

For all intents and purposes microdermabrasion, both "superficial" and "deep" treatments, is similar to an intense topical scrub. The machine delivers a flow of aluminum oxide crystals onto the skin that are then suctioned off the skin through the same tube that was used for delivery. The process produces varying levels of mechanical exfoliation. Superficial microdermabrasion is completely noninvasive (no downtime), readily available, and reasonably quick and safe, which probably explains its increasing use. Deep microdermabrasion disturbs the surface of the skin and can cause oozing, redness, swelling, and discomfort. Because of the risks, only a physician should perform deep microdermabrasion treatments, though that is not always the case.

What makes superficial microdermabrasion a "lunchtime" process is that in most cases the redness and irritation caused by the treatment fade in a matter of minutes to just a few hours. Though the irritation can be minimal, there is some tightness, skin peeling, and, rarely, the skin can appear swollen and red, which can last from a few hours to a few days for more sensitive skins. All this can make skin look somewhat less wrinkled or scarred, at least for a short period of time. Superficial microdermabrasion requires repeated treatment to see results and the results are not long-lasting. It can take from four weeks to three months before the improvement diminishes.

How effective is any of this? There is no easy answer for this one because the studies don't agree. For example, a study published in *Dermatologic Surgery* (November 2001, pages 943–949), "quantified the effects of microdermabrasion on photodamaged skin in 10 individuals. Their subjects underwent once-weekly microdermabrasion for a series of 5-6 treatments (using the *Parisian Peel* device…). During the 5- to 6-week treatment period, patients were assessed at each visit…." The study concluded, "In general, quantifiable results were modest and transient…. Seven of 10 patients showed at least mild (1%-25%) improvement of their photodamaged skin after completing 5-6 treatments… Seven of 10 patients reported subjective improvement; intriguingly, all 3 patients who reported no improvement had the most severe baseline wrinkling…."

However another article, in *Skin & Allergy News* (November 1999), stated that "Microdermabrasion's versatility and potentially destructive power was demonstrated in a histologic study presented at the annual fall meeting of the American Academy of Facial, Plastic, and Reconstructive Surgery…. Used conservatively, the system works well in treating basically, anything that's minor…. Under the microscope, a low number of passes equated with negligible histologic evidence of meaningful skin changes. But increasing passes resulted in extreme damage down to the dermis [deep microdermabrasion]. Of note, deep ablation with the microdermabrasion machine produced serum exudate [oozing] and bleeding, and left histologic evidence of aluminum oxide crystals embedded in the dermis...."

That's not to say there can't be some noticeable results from microdermabrasion. But to suggest it doesn't have risks or that you will end up with wrinkle-free smooth skin is either deception or ignorance on the part of the person performing the service. And it goes without saying that the results are under no circumstance permanent.

It is useful to distinguish a bit more clearly what the differences between superficial and deep microdermabrasion procedures are. Superficial microdermabrasion is the procedure that we commonly call microdermabrasion. It is the procedure performed at spas, as well as physician's offices, by aesthetic, paramedical, and medical personnel alike. It involves superficial abrasion of the skin's surface (the nonliving skin cells that occupy the top 3 to 5 layers of skin only). This cell layer has no capillaries and is nonpigmented, hence its disruption causes no bleeding, crusting, or skin discoloration. It is known that normal skin can take on a dull or thick appearance and fine lines seem more apparent because the surface skin cells slough unevenly. Regular superficial microdermabrasion treatments with an appropriate system can even out and slough skin. This can modestly improve skin texture and some superficial scarring and discoloration.

Deep microdermabrasion should be performed only by physicians and involves disruption of part of or the entire epidermis. Because the skin cells of the epidermis have capillaries and varying degrees of melanin, their disruption can cause bleeding, crusting, and skin discolorations, particularly in darker-skinned individuals. It was believed, when microdermabrasion technology was newer, that this deeper disruption of the skin, akin to traditional dermabrasion, causes dermal remodeling of collagen and should, therefore, reduce the appearance of acne scars, pits, and deeper wrinkles. But as I mentioned, confirmation of this has yet to be established and clinical correlation remains controversial.

## NOSE RESHAPING (RHINOPLASTY) ($4,000 TO $6,000)

Rhinoplasty is usually performed to alter the size and shape of the bridge and tip of the nose. Reshaping is generally done through incisions inside the nose, but sometimes an incision across the central portion of the nose between the nostrils is also made. Narrowing the base of the nose or reducing the size of the nostrils involves removing small wedges of skin at the base of the nostrils. The nose is reduced, or sometimes built up, by adjusting its supporting structures, a process that involves either removing or adding bone and cartilage. The skin and soft tissues are then redraped over this newly created structure.

An open rhinoplasty technique can sometimes benefit patients who need more complex correction or who are undergoing a secondary rhinoplasty procedure. A small incision is made outside the nose across the columella (the tissue that divides the two nostrils). This enables the plastic surgeon to turn the outer tissue of the nose back, providing a view of the structures inside. Additional incisions, like those used in the traditional closed approach, are made inside the nose as well. The scar from the incision on the outside of the nose eventually becomes barely visible.

# FROM THE NECK DOWN

## ABDOMINOPLASTY (TUMMY TUCK) *($4,000 TO $8,000)*

Sometimes, after multiple pregnancies or major weight loss, a person's abdominal muscles weaken and the skin in that area becomes flaccid and hangs below the pubic bone. Abdominoplasty can tighten the abdominal muscles and, in some instances, banish stretch marks (because they are cut away, never to be seen again). In both men and women, the procedure removes excess skin and fat. Generally, an incision is made across the pubic area just above the bikini line and around the navel. The skin is lifted up and away from the sides of the body and up to just under the breasts, then pulled down and reshaped firmly along the body. Liposuction may be used to remove excess fat along the back area just in front of where the skin is lifted away from the body. Often the stomach muscles, which may have separated and pulled apart, are stitched back together, re-creating the natural girdle you had when you were younger. The excess skin is then cut away, and what remains is stitched back together at the original incision above the pubic bone.

The complication rate for this type of surgery is significant. Primary problems include wound infection, the wound splitting open, blood-filled swelling, blood clots, and intestinal obstruction. It is a serious operation with potentially excellent results, but it is not a procedure to venture into lightly without taking all the risks into consideration (Source: *Plastic and Reconstructive Surgery*, 2001, volume 107, pages 1869–1873.)

## ARM LIFT (BRACHIOPLASTY) *($3,000 TO $6,000)*

All the weight-lifting in the world won't build up enough muscle to pick up the excess skin that can hang and flap under the arm, particularly if you have lost a great deal of weight or have a tendency to gain weight in that area. Excess fat in the upper arms can sometimes be reduced through liposuction alone, but loose, drooping skin may need to be excised. To that end, an arm lift is an impressive way to shore up that area, making the skin smooth and taut again. Incisions are hard to hide for this operation, because they can run lengthwise from the armpit to just above the elbow. The risks for this operation are the same as for the tummy tuck procedure.

## Breast Implants, Breast Augmentation
### (Augmentation Mammoplasty)
#### ($4,500 to $8,500)

In 2000, over 187,000 women had breast augmentation, 78,000 had breast reconstruction, 83,000 had breast reduction, and 54,000 had their implants removed. Those are interesting numbers. Since the advent of breast implants in 1962 it is estimated that over 2 million women have had breast augmentation (Source: American Society of Plastic Surgeons, http://www.plasticsurgery.org). I'm going to attempt to sort through the stacks of information in this topic because it is essential that you understand all the options (and the risks) associated with this popular form of cosmetic surgery.

Breast augmentation is typically performed to enlarge small breasts, underdeveloped breasts, or breasts that have decreased in size after a woman has had children or lost weight. It is accomplished by surgically inserting an implant behind each breast. The implant is soft and pliable, and is something like a plastic bag filled with water. An incision is made either under the breast, around the areola (the pink skin surrounding the nipple), or in the armpit. A pocket is created for the implant either behind the breast tissue or behind the muscle between the breast and the chest wall.

Textured-surface breast implants are made with the same silicone material used for the shell of other types of breast implants, but a special manufacturing process creates a textured surface. Some studies have suggested that this surface texture may help reduce the incidence of capsular contracture—tightening of the scar tissue that forms naturally around the implant—which can make the breast feel heavy and hard.

The controversy surrounding implants over the past several years has to do with serious health risks associated with the contents of silicone gel–filled implants leaking into the body and causing autoimmune disorders. Large-scale epidemiological studies conducted independently by leading research institutions have provided some reassuring data. One large-scale study of this kind conducted by the Mayo Clinic and published in the June 16, 1994, issue of the *New England Journal of Medicine* found no connection between silicone breast implants and connective tissue diseases such as rheumatoid arthritis and lupus. Similar conclusions were reached in an extensive study reviewed in the November 2001 issue of *Arthritis and Rheumatism* (pages 2477–2484).

A press release from the National Cancer Institute (http://newscenter.cancer.gov/pressreleases/siliconebreast.html) on Monday, October 2, 2000, stated that "In one of the largest studies on the long-term health effects of silicone breast implants, researchers from the National Cancer Institute (NCI) in Bethesda, Md., found no association between breast implants and the subsequent risk of breast cancer.... Of the implant patients in the study, 49.7 percent received silicone gel implants, 34.1 percent double lumen implants, 12.2 percent saline-filled implants, 0.1 percent other types of implants, and 3.8 percent unspecified types of implants.... The participants had cosmetic surgery during a time (between 1962 and 1988) when a great number of changes were taking place in the manufacturing of breast implants such as the shell thickness, the type of shell coating, and the gel composition. However, the researchers found there was no altered breast cancer risk associated with any of the types of implants."

Due to the controversy regarding implants a new version was launched for clinical trials in 1994. Called the Trilucent™ implant, it was filled with a soybean oil derivative that developers hoped would allow for better results and less risk. Despite the natural sound of the soybean material, this implant has since been withdrawn from the market and it has been recommended that all women who received the Trilucent implant have it removed. It turns out that the breakdown of the soybean oil filler resulted in substances that had a toxic effect on the body (Sources: FDA Center for Devices and Radiological Health, http://www.fda.gov/cdrh/breastimplants/biquest.html; *British Journal of Plastic Surgery*, December 2001, pages 684–686).

There are a wide variety of options when it comes to implants. These now include round or anatomical pre-filled saltwater implants, adjustable implants (that are filled with salt water at the time they are placed in the body), and double-lumen or "stacked" implants (this implant has two layers, an inner sac filled with silicone gel and an outer sac filled with saltwater). Each has its own set of positives and negatives, so the choice depends on what you and your surgeon prefer.

A review published in the *Aesthetic Surgery Journal* (July 2000, pages 281–290) concluded that "... the round and anatomical saline implants have similar teardrop shapes and essentially the same proportions relative to height and volume when the patient is in an upright position, but that round implants behave more like a natural breast when the patient is lying down. When both the upright and the recumbent implant shape is considered, the round implant is the more [natural in appearance]."

Another review in the same issue of the *Aesthetic Surgery Journal* (pages 332–334) stated that "Adjustable breast implants allow women to adjust their breast size up or down within a certain time period following breast augmentation surgery. They also give surgeons the ability to improve breast shape and symmetry, and may be useful in treating capsular contracture (breast firmness), the most common problem associated with breast implants. The technique involves overfilling the implant to stretch the breast tissues, then removing some of the saline solution to obtain the final result." Stacked implants were also discussed in this issue (pages 296–300): "The stacked implant has two compartments, each able to be filled to a different volume, so that greater fullness can be achieved at the base of the breast with a gradual slope in the breast's upper portion." This can also be helpful when breast reconstruction is done, allowing the operated breast to be filled to match the other side more precisely.

Although having large, full breasts can be tempting, be sure your physician is sensitive to your body type and will veto your preconceived notion of what a desirable body looks like if it is not appropriate for your size and shape. It is best to have breasts that look like they are a part of you, not two huge lumps pointing straight out and up from your chest.

Be sure the physician you see is familiar with the differences between saline, silicone gel, and textured-surface implants. Also, your physician should be aware of the need for strict postoperative treatment and should explain it to you at length. For example, it is essential that there be no movement of the hands or arms above the waist for several days after surgery. Also, the breasts must be bound for from several days to three weeks after surgery. All this ensures healing and minimizes the chances of the implant being encapsulated.

There are significant risks with breast augmentation surgery, which can include any and all of the following:

**Capsular contracture**, the most common problem associated with breast implants, occurs when the body rejects the implant or when scar tissue builds up and pushes against the implant, causing a hardening of the area. The result of this encapsulation around the implant can produce hard breast tissue. It is not a health concern, but depending on the extent of the encapsulation it can be extremely painful as well as make mammography screening more difficult. The likelihood of capsular contracture is fairly high, occurring in more than 54% of breast implants.

**Deflation, rupture, and leakage are highly probable. It is very important to understand that breast implants are not lifetime devices and cannot be expected to last forever.** Some implants deflate or rupture in the first few months after being implanted and some deflate after several years; others are intact ten or more years after the surgery, though the incidence of rupture is less likely with saltwater-filled implants than with silicone gel–filled implants.

**Other physical complications** can include pain, infection, swelling, and changes in the physical sensation of the breast and nipple.

**Cosmetically undesirable side effects** can include wrinkling or puckering of the skin around the implant, asymmetry, implant shifting, thickened or noticeable scarring, and an obvious movement of the sac content. Also, the breast tissue can shrink around the implant.

Perhaps the most serious associated problem is that breast implants can **interfere with mammography.**

## BREAST LIFT (MASTOPEXY) *($3,000 TO $5,000)*

Frequently, a woman elects this surgery after losing a considerable amount of weight or when she has lost volume and tone in her breasts after having children. The plastic surgeon relocates the nipple and areola (the pink skin surrounding the nipple) to a higher position, repositions the breast tissue to a higher level, removes excess skin from the lower portion of the breast, and then reshapes the remaining breast skin. Scars occur around the areola, extending vertically down the breast and horizontally along the crease underneath the breast. Variations on this technique, in some cases, may result in less noticeable scarring.

## BREAST REDUCTION (REDUCTION MAMMOPLASTY) *($4,000 TO $8,000)*

Perhaps no other form of elective cosmetic surgery is more life-changing than a breast reduction procedure. A woman with massive breasts struggles with the extra bulk, which is extremely uncomfortable and awkward and curtails physical activity. Additionally, because of the substantial extra mass, detection of breast cancer is compromised and the skin tissue under the breast area can be incessantly lacerated and infected by rubbing, irritation, and perspiration. With the development of successful reduction mammoplasty procedures, there is no reason for any woman to struggle with this kind of physical distortion.

Unlike most other types of cosmetic surgery, breast reduction is normally classified as a reconstructive procedure because oversized breasts greatly interfere with normal daily activity and physical activity, not to mention health issues such as infection and breast cancer screening. Depending on your insurance company's policy regarding breast reduction, the entire procedure may be paid for in full by your health insurance provider. Generally, the determination is made according to how much tissue (by weight) is removed. A certain minimum gram weight must be met to prove to the insurance company that the procedure is corrective and not just aesthetic. However, regardless of the insurance company's position, there is an important aesthetic component to the operation because the plastic surgeon can improve the shape of the breasts and the nipple area, and enhance a woman's physical profile.

Breast reduction involves removing excess breast tissue and skin, repositioning the nipple and areola, and reshaping the remaining breast tissue. Some of the risks are fairly serious, including noticeable scarring, loss of sensation, and the inability to breastfeed. But for women with heavy, pendulous breasts, a breast reduction can be a godsend. Women who wear double or triple D or E bras often experience chronic back and shoulder problems, and because the skin under the breast is never exposed to air, it can become raw and prone to skin infections.

## BREAST RECONSTRUCTION (TRAM FLAP OR PROCEDURE) (*$8,000 TO $10,000*)

Usually as a result of breast cancer, a woman may have one or both breasts removed. Other traumas to the body can also take place that result in a loss of breast tissue. In these instances, rebuilding one or both breasts can return the body to its original condition or even a perceived enhanced appearance. This involves a fairly complicated procedure that uses the muscles of the abdomen. The abdomen has two large parallel muscles, called rectus abdominus. When only one breast is reconstructed, relinquishing one of these poses no risk of impairment to a woman's health or physical activity. However, when both breasts need to be constructed, using both muscles can cause abdominal weakness, so that some movements (such as sitting up from lying down) are harder to do.

During breast reconstruction, the abdominal muscle is used to move the skin and fat from the abdomen to the chest for the construction of a new breast. This flap is referred to as the TRAM flap: Transverse Rectus Abdominus Muscle flap. The skin, fat tissue, and the muscle are cut away intact from the abdomen while remaining attached to the body. Because the TRAM remains attached to the body, blood vessels remain unbroken, allowing the tissue to remain vital and functioning. The TRAM is then repositioned underneath the skin and adjusted and shaped via an opening where the original breast used to be. It is an amazing operation, and many of the same risks associated with abdominoplasty (a tummy tuck, reviewed in this chapter) can occur. However, once complications are resolved, a woman has the benefit of a more natural looking body shape and a tummy tuck at the same time.

## BUTTOCK LIFT (*$4,500 TO $7,000*)

Excess fat and loose skin in the buttock area can be reduced by performing a buttock lift in combination with liposuction (see the Liposuction section below). Incisions required for skin removal can often be hidden in the fold beneath the buttocks. Though the results are impressive, the scarring can be quite noticeable, meaning you'll look great in pants but in the buff your backside might look like a road map.

## CALF AUGMENTATION *($3,000 TO $5,000)*

Increased fullness of the calf can be achieved by using hard silicone implants, which are inserted from behind the knee and moved into position underneath the calf muscle.

## CELLULITE TREATMENTS

See Endermologie and Liposuction.

## ENDERMOLOGIE
### *($750 TO $1,000—FOR A SERIES OF 6 TREATMENTS)*

Struggling with cellulite is a frustrating battle many women fight for most of their lives. Products ranging from diets to magical pills cover an array of options, and are sold to eager women who dream of solving the problem. Spas, salons, and some doctors' offices offer endermologie as a way to conquer the dimpling and puckers that line the thighs and backside. However, almost all of the claims surrounding endermologie are misleading and erroneous. These machines simply massage the skin, and quite roughly at that, but they can't reshape the body, change the structure of skin, or break up fat. Nevertheless, while the machine is doing its thing your cellulite will look reduced because the skin on your leg will become swollen, and that will make things look temporarily improved. But nothing—absolutely nothing—will have changed.

Endermologie machines are medical devices that have the lowest level of approval from the FDA. They are considered Class 1 medical devices, meaning they are subject to the least amount of regulatory control, and they can be sold and used without any supportive clinical efficacy data (Source: FDA Classification of Medical Devices, http://www.fda.gov/cdrh/dsma/dsmaclas.html#class_1).

The comments about how endermologie works sound impressive, but the studies do not back up the claims asserted for the procedure. A study published in *Plastic and Reconstructive Surgery* (September 1999, pages 1110–1114) found "Little scientific evidence exists to support any of the many advertised treatments for it [cellulite]. A total of 52 of 69 women, who were divided into three groups, completed a 12-week, randomized, controlled trial in which the effectiveness of two different treatments for cellulite was assessed. The patients acted as their own controls. The treatments investigated were twice-daily application of aminophylline cream and twice-weekly treatment with Endermologie ES1. Group 1 (double blind) received aminophylline to one thigh/buttock and a placebo cream to the other. Group 2 (singly blind) received Endermologie to one thigh/buttock. Group 3 received Endermologie to both sides and used the same cream regimen as Group 1. Results were assessed subjectively by the patient and by clinical examination and photographic assessment by the surgeon (before and after the trial). Morphologic assessment included body mass index, thigh girth at two points, and thigh fat depth measurement by ultrasound. No statistical difference existed in measurements between legs for any of the treatment groups…. The best subjective assessment, by the patients themselves, revealed that only 3 of 35 aminophylline-treated legs and 10 of 35 Endermologie-treated legs had their cellulite appearance improved. The authors do not believe that either of these two treatments is effective in improving the appearance of cellulite." In addition, any positive result experienced was transient.

Before you invest your hard-earned money on these treatments, understand that you are going more on blind faith that this will have an effect than you are on fact.

## LIPOSUCTION *($1,000 TO $2,000)*

Liposuction allows the plastic surgeon to remove localized collections of fatty tissue from the legs, buttocks, abdomen, back, arms, face, and neck by using a vacuum device that literally cuts up and then sucks up fat tissue. Depending on the area treated, the procedure leaves only minute scars, often as short as one-half inch in length or less. The use of refined equipment allows removal from delicate areas such as calves and ankles. Liposuction does remove fat, but it cannot eliminate dimpling (cellulite) or correct skin laxity, which are the result of the skin's structure and are not caused by the presence of the fat itself. For some patients whose skin has lost much of its elasticity, the plastic surgeon may also recommend a skin-tightening procedure such as a thigh lift, buttock lift, or arm lift, all of which leave more extensive scars. Ultrasonic liposuction uses high-pulse sound waves to liquefy excess fat, which is then removed. The procedure has its advocates and detractors, with complaints that the equipment is cumbersome and considered time-consuming to use. Currently it is believed that ultrasonic liposuction doesn't differ from traditional liposuction except for the initial healing process. For the first months of healing traditional liposuction had better results, but after six months no differences existed (Source: *Annals of Plastic Surgery,* March 2001, pages 287–292).

Liposuction is considered a low-risk procedure that offers impressive results. It is believed that if there is any downside to this procedure it originates on the part of surgeons who do not screen their patients. Liposuction does not take the place of a diet. If someone is obese, gains and loses weight frequently, or has an eating disorder, he or she is not a candidate for liposuction. An article in *Plastic and Reconstructive Surgery* (November 2001, pages 1753–1763) reviewed 631 liposuction cases over 12 years and found "Results showed the majority of patients to be women, aged 17 to 74 years old. Of the preoperative weights, 98.7 percent were within 50 pounds of ideal chart weight.... Cosmetic results were good, with a 2- to 6-inch drop from preoperative measurements, depending on the area treated. Ten percent of patients experienced minor skin contour irregularities, with most of these patients not requiring any additional surgical procedures. One year after surgery, 80 percent of patients maintained stable postoperative weights. No serious complications were experienced in this series. The majority of the complications consisted of minor skin injuries and burns, allergic reactions to garments, and postoperative [swelling]. The more serious complications included four patients who developed mild pulmonary edema and one patient who developed pneumonia postoperatively. These patients were treated appropriately and went on to have [successful] recoveries. The results show that large-volume liposuction can be a safe and effective procedure when patients are carefully selected and when anesthetic and surgical techniques are properly performed. Meticulous fluid balance calculations are necessary to avoid volume abnormalities, and experience is mandatory when performing the largest aspirations. Cosmetic benefits are excellent, and overall complication rates are low."

It is important to keep in mind that scraping fat out of your body is an intense medical procedure. Liposuction can be painful, and the pain can last for several weeks. Adhering to postoperative guidelines is essential for success. "Touchup" work may be necessary because even the best techniques can remove fat unevenly, resulting in unwanted bulges and contours. Moreover, if you gain weight, depending on how your body distributes fat, it can all be added exactly where the liposuction was performed. Now that is some fat to chew on!

## SCLEROTHERAPY *($250 TO $1,000)*

The most typical treatment for surfaced red and blue veins on the legs is sclerotherapy, a procedure that involves injecting a solution into veins of the leg or thigh. The solution causes the walls of the veins to collapse, destroying the source of the problem. One solution used for sclerotherapy is polidocanol (aethoxysclerol), which was originally developed as a local anesthetic. Polidocanol turned out to be undesirable as an anesthetic because it shut down veins wherever it was injected, but it was perfect for sclerotherapy. It is virtually painless. It is also one of the few drugs you can inject into the skin that doesn't leak into the other veins, so it affects only the vein it is injected into. That means there is little to no risk associated with this treatment. Your doctor will want to choose the best option for your condition, but make sure he or she is familiar and skilled with all available options. For more serious, larger varicose veins, a more potent choice is sotradecol. It is similar to polidocanol, but sotradecol can cause sores (ulcers) if it leaks.

Deciding whether to choose laser removal of surfaced veins or sclerotherapy may not be a simple matter. The method the physician prefers is usually what makes the difference, and not the methodology as such. Both laser and sclerotherapy have a place in treating small leg veins. A study in *Lasers in Surgery and Medicine* (2002, volume 30, issue 2, pages 154–159) compared "a long pulsed Nd:YAG laser with contact cooling to sclerotherapy for treating small diameter leg veins by evaluating objective and subjective clinical effects…. Patient surveys show 35% preferred laser and 45% chose sclerotherapy."

Aside from types of treatment, it is best to determine the underlying cause of a problem to prevent recurrences. A surfaced vein is distended and visible because it is connected to a high-pressure system that has gone wrong. You can visualize what happens with these surfaced veins as being similar to the experience of driving along and all of a sudden finding heavy traffic backed up several miles from the actual problem. When veins work normally, they collect blood from tissues and pump it around the body in an even flow, without hitches, stops, or sudden starts. When things go wrong, the blood can actually go in the wrong direction. This occurs because the valves in the vein no longer function properly or because blood volume in the vein increases (often because of trauma); usually both conditions occur together and are interrelated. This misdirected blood flow can build up pressure, creating painful swelling and protrusions. A vein that becomes permanently dilated is called a varicose vein. Theoretically, any vein can develop varicosity, but certain veins, such as those in the legs, are more likely to. This can be due to an injury; pregnancy hormones (which make the valves in the veins soft and floppy, causing damage); being overweight; or just bad veins. And the problem can spread from even one bad vein, affecting a multitude of veins.

Varicose veins that become raised, swollen, and painful should not be ignored. This is more than just a cosmetic problem. Venous thromboses (blood clots), which are tender and painful, may develop and break off and become obstructions elsewhere, particularly in the pulmonary arterioles, causing heart failure.

## THIGH LIFT *($5,000 TO $7,500)*

Losing a lot of weight or suffering a lot of sun damage can cause the thigh area to sag, making cellulite look worse and excess weight more noticeable. Liposuction alone won't lift up the skin that hangs down and causes pouching and folds. Thigh lifts can be performed, along with liposuction, to tighten sagging muscles and remove excess skin in the thigh area. However, because a thigh lift leaves noticeable scars in the inner or outer thigh area, it is not a frequently performed procedure.

# CHAPTER 15

## MEN'S SKIN CARE

## FOR THE MEN

Most men are about as comfortable dealing with skin care, hair care, or any subject related to beauty as they are holding a woman's purse while she shops. The aversion to these topics determines in advance that most men aren't going to be reading this book. That means I have to rely on you, my female readers, to share this section with the men in your lives. Men have faces, too, and they definitely have skin-care needs, but you could never convince the vast majority of men to put even a fraction of the attention and energy into the issue that women do. One positive result of this lack of interest is that most men don't waste their money on wrinkle creams or unnecessary products for their skin. While this monetary savings is significant, it probably means most men don't use sunscreen on a consistent basis, leaving their skin at risk for certain cancers, not to mention wrinkles and other signs of sun damage. It also means most men don't know to stay away from irritating skin-care ingredients in their shave products and end up with red, rash-like bumps and razor burn (which is really, more often than not, product burn).

Men wrinkle as much as women (any notion that they don't is a myth, and a bias about how much better men look with wrinkles than women do) and they, too, can have dry skin, breakouts, skin disorders (rosacea, psoriasis, seborrhea, eczema), skin discoloration, and oily skin. Men also have the additional concerns involving facial hair. Shaving can cause red, irritated spots, and ingrown hair. So why don't men seem to care as much as women do about taking care of their skin? Probably because it is one of the last vestiges of legitimate machismo left to a man. In fact, the very marketing angles used to sell skin-care products to women are the ones that are left almost completely off of men's products.

The morning shave is a characteristic feature that starts the typical man's day. Most men's shaving creams and pre-shave products contain a high concentration of irritating ingredients such as alcohol, menthol, mint, potassium or sodium hydroxide, as well as camphor. These skin irritants make the hair follicle and skin swell, forcing the hair up and away from the skin. While this does make the hair stand up to some extent, supposedly allowing for a closer shave, the irritation and resulting swelling cause some of the hair to be hidden by the swollen follicle and skin. So while it might get the hair to rise to the occasion, it really doesn't make for a better shave because the swollen skin prevents the razor from getting close to the base of the hair. Additionally, after you shave, because some of the facial hair is hidden beneath swollen skin (which temporarily gives the impression of a close shave) the stubble will have a harder time navigating its way back out to the surface. Once the hair begins to regrow (which it does almost immediately) before the swelling is reduced; the likelihood of ingrown hairs is increased.

Moreover, a razor gliding over the face abrades the skin—granted not all that much, but enough to cause havoc when an innocent-looking aftershave with irritating ingredients is splashed over the broken skin. Think of splashing an aftershave on a cut or scrape on any other part of your body where you have an abrasion. Now, why would you want to do that to your face? Basic skin-care rule number one for both men and women: If the skin-care product you're using repeatedly burns, irritates, tingles, causes the skin to become inflamed, or hurts, don't use it. What should men use to take care of their skin or when they shave? Well, aside from shaving, just about everything on the list of skin-care dos and don'ts mentioned throughout this book applies to men, too.

## BEFORE AND AFTER YOU SHAVE

Speaking to men now, the rules and steps for cleansing and every other aspect of your skin-care regime are exactly the same as they are for a woman; the only difference is the shaving foam, cream, or gel used. As is true for every skin-care step, gentle is the supreme rule. A gentle shave product is one that contains no skin irritants of any kind; preferably it is fragrance-free and does not contain any menthol, peppermint, alcohol, lime, lemon, orange, grapefruit, eucalyptus, camphor, or mint. Your skin will feel and look better once you keep away from ingredients that can hurt and damage your skin.

Along with the need to use a gentle shaving foam, cream, or gel, it is equally essential to use a gentle aftershave. At the point when you're finished shaving, it's even more important to avoid the same ingredients listed above (and in Chapter Four, *Skin Care Basics for Everyone*, "How to Be Gentle"). Now that the skin has been abraded with a razor it is critical to not cause further irritation. The entire concept of razor burn is actually a misnomer, the burn does not come from the razor, but rather from the skin-care routine most men use on a daily basis.

What is a gentle aftershave? The bad news is that there are virtually no men's aftershave products that are free of irritants. They are all filled to the brim with fragrance, alcohol, and almost every other irritating ingredient you can think of. To that end, the best aftershave product a man can use (and this may surprise you) is a traditional irritant-free toner. Any of the toners recommended in my book *Don't Go to the Cosmetics Counter Without Me* are excellent options that you can apply after you are finished shaving.

After you are done shaving it is best to follow the general guidelines for the skin-care routine for your skin type. However, as a basic routine, regardless of skin type, everyone needs a gentle, water-soluble cleanser, a gentle shave product (foam, cream, or gel), followed by a gentle, nonirritating aftershave or shaving lotion (which for all intents and purposes is a gentle toner). Then, during the day, use a well-formulated sunscreen with an SPF 15 or greater that contains the UVA-protecting ingredients of avobenzone, titanium dioxide, or zinc oxide, and at night use a lightweight moisturizer wherever you have dry skin.

# DO MEN NEED AHAS OR BHA?

On and off over the years I've heard people say that men don't age the way women do. It isn't true. Yes, there is some validity to the notion that in our society wrinkles and other visible signs of aging—like a less-than-perfect physique or thinning hair—are more socially acceptable for men than for women. Social custom suggests age can make a man look distinguished, while a woman the same age may just look over the hill. Men's clothing styles never reveal as much skin as do women's, nor are they as form-fitting. All that makes physical flaws far more obvious and thus, less socially acceptable, for women than for men.

But when it comes to sun exposure and genetic aging, men and women age in the exact same way. Visible signs of aging have no respect for gender! It is determined primarily by how much time a person has spent in the sun without adequate sun protection and because we naturally do grow older. For most of us, men *and* women, given how little we have known about sun protection over the years, that adds up to a lot of sun damage.

Speaking just of the face, the only advantage men have over women relates to shaving and the resulting cell turnover (exfoliation) it produces. Men who shave have an advantage in that arena because shaving removes the top layer of dead skin cells, thus improving cell turnover. That's good, but it only accounts for a certain amount of surface smoothness and then only over the shaved areas. It doesn't help the areas of the face where men don't shave.

Men who shave daily are probably best off not using AHAs on the bearded area of the face. Shaving exfoliates the skin more than adequately, and it isn't necessary to do more by using an AHA product. However, cell turnover is not stimulated in nonshaved areas. Using an AHA product over the nonshaved areas of the face would be a good addition to a man's skin-care routine.

For blackheads and blemishes, a well-formulated salicylic acid (beta hydroxy acid—BHA) product is an excellent option, and it can be used over shaved areas as well. A BHA product can exfoliate not only the skin inside the pore, thus eliminating the blackhead and the blockage that creates the blemish but also the surface skin. In addition, because BHA is related to aspirin (both are salicylates) it has anti-inflammatory properties that reduce redness, swelling and irritation wherever it is applied.

All the other aspects of skin care that I've discussed earlier in this book, from acne treatments (topical antibacterial or topical antibiotics) to antiwrinkle products (topical tretinoin such as Renova and moisturizers with antioxidants and anti-irritants), sunscreens, treatments for skin disorders, and just about everything else, all apply equally across the board to men just as they do to women.

# CHAPTER 16

## BABY SKIN CARE

It probably won't come as a shock when I tell you that a baby's skin is extremely sensitive and vulnerable. Your first response might be that cleansing and moisturizing your children's skin probably seems not just logical but obvious. Based on the anatomical and functional characteristics of a baby's skin, it is accepted and relatively self-evident that their skin is more delicate than an adult's and, therefore, more prone to irritant and allergic skin problems. The ideal cleansers, moisturizers, powders, and sunscreens should be very mild to avoid irritation, allergic, or sensitizing skin reactions (Source: *Journal of the European Academy of Dermatology and Venereology*, September 2001, Supplemental, pages 12–15).

Despite this fairly intuitive, commonsense information, it turns out that most skin-care products aimed at children are formulated to be anything but gentle and soothing. They are often an irritation waiting to happen.

For all the women who are trying to clean, soften, and soothe their child's skin (or the skin of any child in their life), let me warn you again about baby products. There are an alarming number of expensive and inexpensive baby products that are marketed as better for young, delicate skin—yet, for the most part, they aren't.

I know the baby section in the drugstore—and at a growing number of cosmetics counters and health food stores—have sweet, adorably packaged shampoos, moisturizers, cleansers, and sun products. You assume the manufacturers have taken special care to use only ingredients that will be the most gentle to your baby's skin, but that assumption is not accurate. Think about the wafting, appealing fragrances emanating from most baby products you've shopped for. Right there you've recognized a major problem—fragrance—one serious enough that it makes me leery of using baby products for anyone's skin, let alone a baby's!

Products for babies and young children are usually highly fragranced. That delicious, recognizable aroma you could smell a mile away is nothing more than added fragrance, which we know can cause irritation. Moreover, baby products almost always have a pretty yellow or pink tint, which is contrived by coloring agents, another group of problematic skin-care ingredients for sensitive skin. If baby products were really gentler than those that adults put on their skin, they would be fragrance free and contain no coloring agents. Sadly, few of those exist.

Cosmetics and hair-care companies know that mothers have an impulsive emotional pull toward scents that trigger the image of their babies. That subconscious pull is difficult for a marketer to ignore, given the way women gravitate to the fragrance generated by other perfume-laden products. In other words, hair and skin-care companies don't have much motivation to take these problematic ingredients out. That means you, the mother and consumer, as an advocate for your child, need to pay attention to this issue and choose fragrance-free and color-free products whenever you can!

Aside from the issue of fragrance and coloring agents, it is even more shocking when baby products contain such skin irritants as peppermint, menthol, and citrus. The very idea of their presence is disturbing because these are all problematic for an adult's skin and, thus, so much more for a child's. It is essential to avoid products for your child's skin (and yours for that matter) that contain any unnecessary irritants. Just paying attention to the ingredient label will give you far better information than the product description or claims on the package. Ignore the picture on the label of the sweet innocent child, especially when it can disguise a formula that is anything but sweet and innocent.

## WHAT TO USE?

In general, a child's delicate skin is better served with products that are fragrance- and color-free, and completely gentle, with no added sources of irritation or sensitizing ingredients. The basics for any child's skin are:

- Gentle cleanser
- Gentle shampoo
- Fragrance-free baby wipes

**Lightweight, soothing, nonirritating moisturizer.** Most of the fragrance-free versions are those at the drugstore packaged for adults, such as Cetaphil Moisturizer, Eucerin Daily Replenishing Lotion Fragrance-Free, and Lubriderm Seriously Sensitive Moisturizing Lotion, but these are also excellent for children.

**Zinc oxide- and petrolatum-based diaper rash ointment.** Definitely fragrance-free—it hurts to put fragrance on red, rashy skin.

**Talc-free dusting powder.** Never use talc on a baby's skin. Plain cornstarch is an excellent alternative. It is the primary ingredient in most talc-free baby powders anyway, and plain cornstarch from your kitchen cupboard doesn't contain fragrance.

**Sunscreen with SPF 15 or greater and UVA-protecting ingredients.** During the day, if the child's skin is going to be exposed to the sun, a sunscreen is essential.

The UVA-protecting active ingredients should preferably be titanium dioxide and zinc oxide. (Avobenzone does protect from UVA rays, but it can be a skin irritant and the goal here is to eliminate all sources of irritation as much as possible.) Formulations with only titanium dioxide or zinc oxide as the active ingredient are best because of their reduced risk of irritation compared to other sunscreen ingredients. Besides, babies don't mind the white cast these kinds of sunscreens give to the skin. (For more information about sun care for children and babies refer to Chapter Five, *Sun Sense*.)

Remember: It's important to be alert in the defense of a baby's sensitive skin. There is no reason for a baby to put up with fragrance just because a mother thinks it smells better.

## BABY SHAMPOO

When it comes to cleansing products, the group of ingredients considered the most gentle are called amphoteric surfactants. According to the *Cosmetic Science and Technology Series* (volume 17, *Hair and Hair Care,* by Dale H. Johnson) (Allured Publishing), "amphoteric" describes a category of cleansing agents that do not cleanse or foam as well as others. Nevertheless, they have one unique property, which is a very low potential for irritation. Amphoterics are so gentle that they can even reduce the irritation potential of other surfactants known for their sensitizing possibilities, such as sodium lauryl sulfate. *Hair and Hair Care* states, "The skin irritancy of sodium lauryl sulfate in the presence of cocamidopropyl betaine [an amphoteric surfactant] is reduced substantially."

This explains why Johnson & Johnson's Baby Shampoo was such a phenomenal success when it launched in the '60s. Johnson & Johnson's 1967 patent established the mild, nonirritating capacity for the amphoteric group of cleansing agents. As it turns out, the primary ingredient in Johnson & Johnson's baby shampoos is an amphoteric called cocamidopropyl betaine, which now shows up in most shampoos (adults deserve gentle cleansing, too). Just using amphoterics alone, that is, when they are not combined with other cleansing agents, explains why, when a mother tries to use baby shampoo on her own hair, it doesn't work very well. The amphoteric surfactants simply can't clean like other surfactants can, and given the styling products and conditioners most adults use, it is essential to have a shampoo with good cleansing properties. Nowadays, most baby shampoos use a combination of cleansing agents to lower irritancy and improve cleansing, but they are still almost always more gentle than adult versions.

The following are considered the most gentle cleansing agents for any skin type: cocamidopropyl betaine, cocamphocarboxyglycinate-propionate, sodium lauraminodipropionate, disodium monoleamide MEA sulfosuccinate, disodium monococamido sulfosuccinate, disodium cocamphodipropionate, disodium capryloamhodiacetate, cocoyl sarcosine, and sodium lauryl sarcosinate. Now you'll be able to recognize these on an ingredient list. They are all considered extremely gentle, but do not have good cleansing ability.

Along with the gentleness of the shampoo formula, making sure it's fragrance-free, irritant-free, and coloring agent–free is still a primary concern for the health of your child's skin.

## CRADLE CAP

The crusty, yellowish, thick layer of built-up skin on your baby's scalp is commonly called cradle cap, yet it has nothing to do with the cradle, how your baby sleeps, or what kind of sheets you use. Cradle cap is really seborrheic dermatitis, and it is a typical skin problem for infants that usually disappears by the first birthday. It is always important to discuss any of your child's skin problems with your pediatrician before using anything on your baby's skin. A home remedy for cradle cap you can discuss with your doctor is to gently massage a small amount of olive oil or plain, fragrance-free mineral oil all over the scalp (baby oil is just mineral oil with fragrance and your baby's skin doesn't need the fragrance). Leave the oil on overnight and then wash it off the next day with a gentle, fragrance-free baby shampoo. If several applications of this don't help, you should talk to your doctor about using an over-the-counter shampoo containing ketoconazole (Nizoral) for infantile seborrheic dermatitis. There is research showing this to be an effective option for resolving cradle cap in children (Source: *Pediatric Dermatology*, September-October 1998, pages 406–407).

## MOISTURIZER FOR CHILDREN

Over and above the issue of fragrance-free skin-care products for children, it's important to use a moisturizer to help soothe skin and deal with any potential dry skin. Dry skin can be a precursor to, or early warning sign, of skin rashes and general skin irritation. For the most part, it has always been believed that an extremely emollient, creamy moisturizer is best for a child's skin regardless of the condition. However, there is research showing that a lightweight lotion or gel formula might be preferred (Source: *American Journal of Contact Dermatitis*, December 2000, pages 222–225). It may be helpful to start with a lightweight lotion and see how your child's skin responds. If you find that it is still looking or feeling dry, you can try a more emollient version, which may be better for your child's specific skin-care needs.

# SUNSCREEN

Sunscreens are essential for babies and children, and extensive general information that applies to people of all ages is discussed at length in Chapter Five, *Sun Sense*.

# DIAPER RASH

If you can be sure of anything with a new baby, it's that there is a strong chance he or she will develop diaper rash at some point. In some ways this is a confounding problem, because the very nature of diapering your baby and hoping he or she sleeps through the night sets up the perfect environment for developing diaper irritation. Urine and feces trapped next to a baby's bottom for long periods of time is a problem, but are there really other practical options? "The primary goals of preventing and treating diaper dermatitis include keeping the skin dry, protected, and infection free. Frequent diaper changes with the superabsorbent disposable diapers may be the best tactic for infants' skin, if not the environment. Also, the more time that infants spend without diapers, the less dermatitis they experience, but a practical balance must be struck. Gentle cleansing and barrier creams are beneficial, and [fungus or yeast] infections must be treated" (Source: *Pediatric Clinics of North America*, August 2000, pages 909–919).

Frequent diaper changes, fragrance-free baby wipes (to not add to the irritation), gentle cleansing, and allowing your baby to go diaper free whenever it is practical are essential for getting diaper rash under control. When a child is wearing a diaper it is also extremely helpful to use an occlusive diaper ointment that prevents skin contact with urine or feces. One of the best options is a traditional zinc oxide–based ointment, or a zinc oxide and petrolatum-based formulation, or just plain Vaseline (Source: *Journal of the European Academy of Dermatology and Venereology*, September 2001, Supplemental, pages 5–11).

Even if you are diligent in following all the options for treating diaper rash, you may find your child still suffers from the irritation, redness, and swelling the condition produces. Pediatricians can offer prescription options that may settle matters. These can include any of the following: Nystatin, a topical antifungal (trade name Mycostatin); clotrimazole, another topical antifungal ointment (trade name Lotrimin); a combination product of nystatin and triamcinolone that blends an antifungal with a topical hydrocortisone to reduce inflammation); or just plain hydrocortisone to reduce or eliminate the irritation (Source: *Archives of Pediatric and Adolescent Medicine*, September 2000, pages 943–946).

# Chapter 17

## Body and Nail Care

### From the Neck Down

It may be simplistic to say this, but it is absolutely true that every aspect of skin care for the face discussed in this book applies to the body, too. Even the section on shaving in Chapter Fifteen, *Men's Skin Care*, applies to a woman's body when it comes to shaving legs and underarms. Yet amazingly, when it comes to body care women often neglect their skin from the neck down. Many women tell me they would never tan their face because they want to prevent sun damage and the inevitable wrinkling and discoloration it can cause, yet they happily brown and bake the rest of their body. Somehow there is a disconnect between head and body—or perhaps there is a misconception that the legs, arms, and chest are tougher or aren't subject to the same ruination caused by sun damage. Nothing could be further from the truth. Unprotected skin anywhere on the body develops the same thickened, brown-spotted, lined, and rough texture as skin on the face does, and is subject to the same skin cancers. There are women who fly into a tizzy at the appearance of one facial blemish, but who ignore breakouts on their chest and legs, never thinking of applying the blemish-fighting basics to any other part of the body. This is also misguided. Skin is skin, head to toe—so why accept artificial boundaries between parts of the body?

The number of products dedicated to bathing and body care is growing, but they tend to be all about pampering and indulging ourselves rather than addressing concerns about blemishes, wrinkles, sun damage, exfoliation, and reducing irritation from shaving. A veritable deluge of moisturizers, cleansers, bath salts, exfoliants, bubble baths, hand creams, massage oils, and aromatherapy products in every aromatic combination imaginable promises to soften, scent, stimulate, smooth, and soothe your body. Occasionally, a company puts out a laughable cellulite cream that promises to undimple dimpled thighs, or, and even more laughable, a bust cream that claims it can raise sagging breast tissue, but these products are far outnumbered by the horde of preparations offering more sensual pleasures.

You can't find a square inch of the body that has been neglected by the cosmetics industry. Large cosmetics companies, small cosmetics companies, prestigious lines, simple lines, and even businesses to whom body care is just a sideline, such as Victoria's Secret and The Gap—all want us to soak, scrub, and moisturize everything from dry skin to stress and emotional woes out of our lives with bath oils, bath salts, loofahs, body masks, fragrant moisturizers, and perfumes. And we love buying the stuff. Bath and body-care products and fragrances account for more than 33% of all cosmetics sold! Yet more often than not, these products are poorly formulated, don't contain sunscreen, are overly fragranced, or contain other skin irritants, and generally just don't measure up to the quality of products we put on our face.

## SPA TREATMENTS

One interesting wrinkle (no pun intended) is the number of body-care lines that include the word "spa" as part of their name. **Marketing finesse gives spa lines an authoritative aura and healthful image when it comes to skin care, particularly from the neck down. This misperception can waste money and also cause skin problems.** Spa products are not the result of any particular enlightenment, nor are they specially formulated in any way. In fact, spa products sold at cosmetics counters and specialty spas are notoriously similar to the ones sold in drugstores. I think most women would be shocked to discover that the "spa" formulations for various body washes, bath salts, body moisturizers, and bath oils are really almost identical to the drugstore formulations. Moreover, spa lines, like most body-care products, are highly fragranced, and fragrance is no better for the body than it is for the face.

Far be it from me to deny anyone the pleasure that can be derived from pampering, soothing body care. Taking care of the body should include relaxing in deliciously warm water or being gently massaged. But skin-care problems can occur all over the body, and they require more than sweetly scented bath salts and oils, the very same things that are often responsible for red, flaky, irritated skin. Despite the allure of spa treatments, the products used rarely, if ever, seriously address the issues of sun damage, blemishes, skin sensitivity, antioxidants, anti-irritants, or skin disorders such as rosacea or psoriasis.

Doing all they can to appear more natural and superior to other product lines, spa lines tend to add an eccentric flare. In marketing their services and products, one line boasted their products contained truffles that were handpicked and mixed into their treatments. While handpicked truffles (is there another kind?) might be great for a salad or steak, the skin can't tell the difference. What does matter is whether or not truffles can have a positive effect on skin. It turns out that there is a small amount of research showing black and white truffles to be effective for inhibiting melanin production and for some antibacterial properties (Sources: *Federation of European Microbiological Societies (FEMS) Microbiology Letters*, April 2000, pages 213–319; *Pigment Cell Research*, February-April 1997, pages 46–53). However, there are many different products that contain other effective skin-lightening or antibacterial ingredients.

Caviar is often touted as an especially extravagant ingredient in some products. Exclusivity aside, what is caviar's benefit for skin? It turns out that caviar does contain essential fatty acids similar to the ones found in skin. But lots of living substances, from fish to animals and plants, are replete with identical or better fatty acids (phospholipids and triglycerides). Caviar is not a superior or even desirable source for this skin-care ingredient. Plus, only a tiny amount of caviar is included in these kinds of products, meaning it's almost impossible for it to have any effect on skin.

The herald for almost all spa treatments is the ever-popular mud mask. *Foreign* mud is the concept that gets the consumer's attention, because how could mud from the United States or Canada be worth $50 to $100 a jar or per treatment? How appealing would mud from Idaho be in comparison to mud from Ishia or Austria? "Parafango" mud gets a lot of attention in spa treatments, but "parafango" is merely Italian for "protecting mud"—it isn't a kind of special earth from some distant, far-off land. But could there be parts of the world where the dirt is better for your skin than it is from somewhere else? Well, I have looked for the evidence, and to tell you that there is no research showing mud that is beneficial for skin is an understatement. Further, having a mask applied once a month at a spa is similar to dieting once a month; it ends up being of little help in keeping your body healthy day in and day out. It may feel good to be wrapped or to soak in mud, but the benefit is purely emotional and unrelated to any real effect on your skin.

# THE JOY OF BATHING

I think it is appropriate to start with the luxurious, sensual side of body care, and there is no denying the relaxation you can derive from a quiet interlude in a serene, carefully prepared bath. By adding just a few cosmetic preparations to the tub (and locking the bathroom door), you can create a tranquil refuge right in your own home. And none of these products have to be expensive or contain irritants. In fact, the less expensive ones (like pure almond, olive, or sunflower oil, Epsom salts, or nonfragranced body moisturizers) all work beautifully. Where the body is concerned, fragrance can be a serious skin irritant. If you use fragranced oils and salts in the bath, the perfume component can be especially sensitizing for the vaginal area as well as other parts of the body.

But back to indulgence. Simply feeling beautiful and tranquil is the main goal of a leisurely bath. Imagine steamy water, drizzled with oils or foaming rich bubbles accompanied by scented candles flickering in the mirror (that way you don't need to put fragrance in the bathwater, and your olfactory senses can still participate), and at least a half hour to an hour of spare time. Even the thought is gratifying. Later, when you're done soaking, after gently exfoliating your skin, shaving unwanted hair from your legs and underarms, and applying a moisturizer, your body will feel silky in a way it doesn't after your usual morning ritual of shower and moisturizer.

Without trying to burst anyone's bubble, because my job is to tell you what I know to be true from current research, I must mention that, as blissful as all this can be, the only benefits are psychological. Regularly soaking for long periods, especially in hot water—and that includes Jacuzzis—is actually not best for the long-term health of the skin. **Oversaturating the skin with water can break down its immune/healing response and can actually make it drier** (Source: *Contact Dermatitis*, December 1999, pages 311–314). The best approach is to keep the temperature of your bathwater warm but not hot, and, if you bathe regularly, soak for no more than five to ten minutes. Occasionally it is fine to soak for longer periods, but make that the exception instead of the rule. Whether it's for five or ten minutes, or the infrequent twenty- to thirty-minute soak, the repose and quiet serenity of a bath can give you the time to feel the texture changes in your skin and to calm stressed-out, responsibility-weary nerves.

What is the best way to go about this indulgent ritual? It is definitely easier and far less expensive if you use something other than the products lined up at the cosmetics counters and specialty salons, that's for sure.

Following is one scenario for how to enjoy a relaxing bath.

- Start running the bath using **water that's only slightly hotter than normal**, but only slightly; water that is too hot can be hard on the skin and may cause problems over the long haul.

- If you have normal to dry skin, **drizzle in some almond, olive, or sunflower oil** (but use only a teaspoon or two or you'll feel like you're soaking in an oil spill). If you have oily, blemish-prone skin from the neck down, oils of any kind are not the best idea. Bubble bath is best, and the dish detergent in your kitchen will produce lots of it and you only need a drop.

- Add a teaspoon of bubble bath or bath salts. As I mentioned above, these should preferably be fragrance-free to avoid irritation and breakouts. **Epsom salts are a great, incredibly inexpensive addition to any bath.**

- Rather than pouring fragrance into the bath, which can be irritating for the skin, you can **light a scented candle or two** and place them in strategic locations so the light can flicker on the water and in the mirror. You can also buy tiny oil lamps that help radiate fragrance throughout the room.

- If you plan to give yourself a manicure or pedicure after your bath, take the time now to **file your nails into the shape you want.** Filing nails when they are wet can damage them and cause splitting. If you plan to cut your nails, wait until after you are done soaking, when they are softer and less likely to be damaged.

- Turn down the lights or turn them off altogether and **bathe by candlelight.**

- **Enter the bath slowly**, even gracefully, trying hard not to disturb the water or bubbles.

- **Prop a towel or bath pillow behind your head**, and stretch out.

- While you're soaking, take the time to **gently, and I mean gently, buff a washcloth over your body.** (Be careful with loofahs—they can be hard on most skin types and if they are not cleaned regularly can be a source of staphylococcus infection.)

- **Use a body cleanser or body wash** alone or with a gentle washcloth. Soap can be too drying on skin.

- For obvious reasons, **save shaving your legs till the end**, when the water is going down the drain. Use shave cream or your hair conditioner for the smoothest results. (Shaving the legs is much easier and causes far less irritation and fewer bumps if the legs have been soaked for at least two or three minutes, and preferably more. Also, sitting in water filled with used shaving cream is hardly luxurious.)

- You may want to **shower off as your final step.** If you don't like the feeling of bath oils left on your feet, underarms, or genitals, this is the time to wash those areas again to remove the oil or bath salts from your skin.

- When you're done, **exit as slowly as you entered.** This is still part of the ritual, so keep the candles lit.

- Dry your skin with a fresh **towel, dabbing your skin lightly.**

- If you haven't used a body exfoliant in the bath, you can **use your towel to give your legs and arms a good but gentle rubdown.** But take it easy; hard rubbing can irritate the skin.

- **Next apply a moisturizer.** (Do not apply moisturizer to areas of the body that tend to break out.)

- **If you haven't shaved, you can apply an AHA or BHA moisturizer over your legs and arms, especially on your knees, elbows, and heels.** The exfoliation prevents dead skin cells from building up, which can cause rough texture and dry flaky skin.

- **If you bathe in the morning it is essential to apply an effective sunscreen over those parts of the body that will be exposed to daylight.**

- Finally, **slip on something very soft**, like cotton leggings and a cotton top, or a silky robe, and enter the world slowly, refreshed and renewed. **Don't forget to blow out the candles.**

- If you have extra time, this is the perfect opportunity to give yourself a **pedicure and manicure.**

## BODY WASHES

Body cleansers, body washes, and body shampoos are just what they sound like—they use the detergent cleansing agents typically found in hair shampoos to clean the body—and they are excellent for all skin types. They tend to be less drying than bar soaps and cleansers, they leave no "bar" residue on the skin, and the chance of irritation or dryness is greatly reduced. (A moisturizing body wash can leave a slight film due to oils left behind on the skin, but that's how these cleansers moisturize.) **Bar soaps and bar cleansers can be problematic for the body, just as they are for the face.** Body washes are just as effective as soaps are, without any of the problems soaps can stir up.

Many body washes designed for dry skin claim all kinds of moisturizing properties. What they contain is simply some kind of oil. Vitamins, proteins, amino acids, and other fancy water-binding agents may be in there, too, and while these ingredients can be good moisturizing agents in a cream or lotion you leave on the skin, in a body wash they are just rinsed down the drain. Oils tends to stick around a bit longer and are not easily washed away, so they do provide some emollient benefit for dry skin. Personally, I don't feel quite as clean after using a moisturizing body wash. I prefer the gentle cleaning effect of a regular body wash, followed by a moisturizer applied after I get out of the shower, but the choice is yours.

Here's a list of great body washes to consider: Aveeno Skin Relief Body Wash, Fragrance-Free *($6.99 for 12 ounces)*; Calgon Shower & Bath Gel In the Rain *($4.99 for 8 ounces)*—this also comes in several other fragrant options; Caress Moisturizing Body Wash *($3.99 for 12 ounces)*—also in several different fragrances; Dial Moisturizing Body Wash *($3.49 for 12 ounces)*; Jason Natural Satin Shower Body Wash or Bubbling Bath, Apricot *($9.99 for 34 ounces)*; Jergens Skin Firming Body Wash with Seaweed Extract *($4.99 for 20 ounces)*; Neutrogena Rainbath, Shower & Bath Gel, Unscented *($5.99 for 8.5 ounces)*; Neutrogena Rainbath Shower and Bath Gel *($5.99 for 8.5 ounces)*—this version is scented, and Neutrogena Fresh Body Herbal Body Wash *($6.99 for 6.7 ounces)*; Nivea Bath Care Moisturizing Body Wash, 2 in 1 Cleanser & Moisturizer, Enriched Care *($6.59 for 10.5 ounces)*; Olay Sensitive Skin Body Wash Unscented *($4.59 for 12 ounces)*; and White Rain Moisturizing Body Wash, Sensitive Skin *($2.19 for 10 ounces)*.

# BODY SCRUBS

Exfoliating skin from the neck down provides the same benefits it does from the neck up: It helps the skin absorb moisturizer better, unclogs pores, and allows healthier skin cells to surface. There are lots of ways to help get dead skin cells off the body. You can use anything from a gentle washcloth to a well-formulated AHA or BHA product. Topical scrubs are also an option, but are no better than a washcloth. Even though the skin on the body can handle mechanical scrubbing a bit better than the skin on the face can, you still need to be gentle with this kind of physical scouring. If you're careful, scrubbing can be a good way to immediately exfoliate elbows, heels, and knees.

Loofahs have one major drawback you need to be aware of. Because they hang around in the shower and are often not cleaned or rotated with a new one, they are an ideal breeding ground for bacteria such as staphylococcus. **Overscrubbing or scrubbing over blemishes and cuts with an old loofah that has not been properly cleaned is unwise.** Washcloths are easy to throw in the laundry and tend to be less rough and less irritating on the skin and that is always a benefit.

**Unequivocally and without exception, no amount of scrubbing or beating at the skin will change or eliminate one dimple on your thighs.** The only benefits from exfoliation are those discussed earlier in this book and above, and that's really it. You might feel your thighs look better after you have scrubbed them and applied various lotions and gels, but all these products do is temporarily swell the skin on the thighs, making them look momentarily smoother.

# ANTIBACTERIAL CLEANSERS

It's hard to imagine that the popularity of antibacterial cleansers is a cause for concern, but for many reasons it is. While antibacterial cleansers are usually effective against some bacteria on the skin, they end up causing problems for just that very reason. The widespread use of antibacterial agents suggests that it has already led to the appearance of resistant organisms that will compromise the usefulness of triclosan, the most typical antibacterial agent in these products (Source: *American Journal of Infection Control*, October 2001, pages 281–283). The national Centers for Disease Control and Prevention (Source: CDC, http://www.cdc.gov) states that hand-washing in warm water with plain soap for at least ten seconds is sufficient in most cases (even for healthcare workers) to eliminate germs.

There are now more than 700 antibacterial products available to the consumer. According to the CDC, "The public is being bombarded with ads for cleansers, soaps, toothbrushes, dishwashing detergents, and hand lotions, all containing antibacterial agents. Likewise, we hear about 'superbugs' and deadly viruses. Germs have become the buzzword for a danger people want to eliminate from their surroundings. In response to these messages, people are buying antibacterial products because they think these products offer health protection for them and their families.... Besides resistance, the antibacterial craze has another potential consequence. Reports are mounting about a possible association between infections in early childhood and decreased incidence of allergies. In expanding this 'hygiene hypothesis,' some researchers have found a correlation between *too much* hygiene and *increased* allergy. This hypothesis stems from studies that revealed an increased frequency of allergies, cases of asthma, and eczema in persons who have been raised in an environment overly protective against microorganisms. In one rural community, children who grew up on farms had fewer allergies than did their counterparts who did not live on farms. Graham Rook, University College, London, has likened the immune system to the brain. You have to exercise it, that is, expose it to the right antigenic information so that it matures correctly. Excessive hygiene, therefore, may interfere with the normal maturation of the immune system by eliminating the stimulation by commensal microflora [normal and safe bacteria that live on the skin]."

Even if the hypothesis that antibacterial products help create strains of resistant bacteria doesn't prove out and the theories about "exercising our immune system" fail to be true, antibacterial products may not be the help many think they are. Antibacterial products are marketed under the notion that they will lower the risk of disease. However, flus and most colds are viral infections, not bacterial ones, so antibacterial cleansers are useless to protect against them.

# BATH OILS

Bath oils are primarily just that: oils derived from all sorts of sources, including sunflower, almond, coconut, and jojoba—a virtual plethora of plants and flowers. Some bath oils contain volatile (fragrant) oils that can potentially cause allergic reactions. Other bath oils are formulated with slip agents (ingredients that help the oils move over the skin) as well as with mineral oil (mineral oil can be more soothing for the skin than plant oils because it poses minimal to no risk of irritation). Some even contain water-binding agents, which are hardly necessary, because the skin will be water-laden regardless of their presence and their effect is washed down the drain.

If there is any distinction between oils, it has more to do with how greasy they feel and how much irritation they can cause than with any healing benefits they may have. **Plain mineral oil can be an excellent bath oil because it is fragrance-free, gentle and emollient, and unlikely to cause irritation or breakouts. However, it is also not absorbed by the skin.** Plant oils tend to be a bit more problematic in terms of clogging pores, but they are absorbed far better than mineral oil. Safflower, sesame, almond, avocado, and even olive oil can add the slip and emollience needed by dry skin.

# BATH SALTS

Bath salts can be beneficial for many skin types. **Salts and minerals, regardless of their source, can soften water and, depending on the specific salts used, reduce inflammation and swelling. Epsom salts are probably the best-known type; they work quite well and are wonderfully inexpensive.** Most of the salts added to bath products are just fine, although ingredients such as borax, sodium sesquicarbonate, sodium carbonate, and phosphate can cause irritation and probably should be avoided. Table salt and sea salt can also be a problem, because if they don't get rinsed off well they can pull water from the skin and cause dryness and irritation.

Many cosmetics lines, particularly spa lines, brag about how their products contain minerals from all kinds of sources: mineral springs in France, volcanic waters in Italy, Dead Sea salts from Israel, and on and on. The question is whether minerals and salts from exotic sources have any special effect on skin. In the long run, unless you have a skin disorder such as psoriasis or seborrhea, those salts and minerals have no positive effect. Epsom salts are preferred both for their skin-softening and anti-inflammatory properties, and because they pose a minimal risk to sensitive skin.

# AROMATHERAPY?

Fragrance is one of the most important aspects of body care, at least to many consumers. Ironically, it is one of the least important for the health of the skin. For some people, fragrance can be as much a problem from the neck down as for the neck up. Although the body is generally less susceptible to sensitizing reactions than the face, that can vary from person to person, and there can be a problem even if you don't feel a reaction. Yet, with the advent of aromatherapy, scent has taken on new prominence in the world of body care, and it can be difficult to avoid. Despite the risk to the skin, most body and bath products are highly fragranced, and things are getting worse, not better. While women are becoming more and more aware that fragranced skin-care products can cause problems for the face, they are nevertheless likely to purchase bath and body-care products because of their scent.

Can a particular scent or blend of scents provide special benefits for your skin or your emotions? When it comes to skin, fragrant oils are not helpful for any part of the face or body because they can cause irritation, skin sensitivities, rashes, inflammation, and allergic reactions. Fragrance is especially problematic for the genital area (Source: *American Journal of Contact Dermatitis*, December 2001, pages 225–228).

However, as far as your emotions are concerned, only you can know for sure. Lots of women indeed feel less stressed out after indulging their senses with interesting fragrant blends, but they are also taking time out from their busy day while doing it. Does the fragrance cause the effect or the time out? That's hard to say. What is easy to say is that scent has more to offer for the nose than it does for the skin.

Most people are greatly affected by pleasing aromas, and almost everyone feels invigorated or supremely relaxed after a good long soak. Because fragrance can play such a significant role in this experience, there is no reason not to partake. **However, I would encourage you to find other ways to please your olfactory sense than putting fragrant products in the bath water or all over your skin.** Scented candles, plain candles drizzled with fragrant oils, and oil lamps or diffusers (you can purchase the latter at most health food stores or specialty body-care shops) are a great way to fill the air with sublime scents and leave your skin unaffected.

## PERFUME

Women the world over use perfume and have been doing so for eons. When it comes to buying perfume or cosmetics, one of the first things a consumer does is smell the product. Why? Because a pleasing scent can make a woman feel confident, sensual, and happy. With all that, who cares if it helps the skin?

Buying perfume is an entirely sensory experience. Minute drops applied to the "warm" spots on the body—behind the ears, along the cleavage, inside the thigh, and on the pulse points on the wrist, neck, inside elbow, and behind the knee—can provide all the radiating scent you need to attract someone's attention. Perfume is almost exclusively about love and sex, and not necessarily in that order.

Unless you've been visiting another planet for the last 30 years, you won't be surprised when I say that sex is used as a sales tool for almost every product from shoes to deodorant (if advertisers could figure a way to make the Pillsbury Doughboy into a sex symbol, they would do it to sell more biscuits). Perfume ads almost always feature young, sultry, long-legged, breathless women; half-clothed, hard-bodied men; or both, in couples who can barely keep their hands, lips, or low-lidded eyes off each other.

Most of us throw logic out the window when confronted with the hope of increased desirability, and that's what sells perfume, because there is nothing utilitarian, professional, or rational about it. In short, perfume is a difficult subject for a consumer reporter because it defies logic, and that's as it should be. But let me throw in just a little information to help you in making your selection. Other than allergic reactions, there are no risks when it comes to wearing perfume. How much you like a scent and how it affects the people around you, specifically the people who get close to you, are all that count.

Speaking of the people around you, it is a complete mystery to me why some women or men feel a need to saturate themselves with a conspicuous amount of fragrance. The air around women who have generously anointed themselves with their favorite perfume or eau de toilette is so thick and pungent that their presence is announced by an overpowering hit of fragrance. This is definitely one of those beauty steps that can be overdone and lose its original purpose, which in this case is to exude a subtle scent for those you want to be close to. Perfume should not be so pungent an emission that it overwhelms strangers in an elevator or business associates around a conference table. In addition, an overpowering scent can trigger allergic reactions in others. I suspect many women put on extra fragrance in the morning to make it last longer. Yet it is simple enough to touch up fragrance as the day goes by, just as you would makeup. Most women who overdo their perfume would never apply 20 layers of makeup to make sure it stayed on all day!

While we're on the subject, the endurance of a fragrance has nothing to do with natural ingredients versus synthetic ones or with how many products you apply. If anything, synthetic ingredients take the unreliability of plant extracts and oils out of the equation to create more stable products. Yet there is no way to know which ingredients are used in any perfume or eau de toilette because this is the sole area where the cosmetics industry doesn't have to reveal formulas. Consequently, fragrance recipes truly are secrets (Source: http://www.fda.gov). Several master perfumers have told me that most fragrances are created from a vast combination of fragrance components that are both natural and synthetic. The art of creating a nuanced, resplendent bouquet involves bringing together varying aromas in a cohesive, unified scent that pleases the olfactory sense. **The secrecy and complexity is**

**why fragrance knock-offs and inexpensive imitations just don't work.** Some perfumers have blended hundreds of flower oils, plant extracts, and synthetic scents to create one perfume. How can a formula that complex be duplicated? It can't. And that's why a cheap version of the perfume you like won't make your nose as happy.

Without ingredient lists to turn to, there are only two ways to determine how long a fragrance will last on your body: product type and testing. In terms of product type, you can count on cologne (which is about 1% to 3% fragrance) and eau de cologne (about 3% to 5% fragrance) lasting two to three hours; eau de toilette (about 5% to 7% fragrance) lasting two to four hours; eau de parfum (about 12% to 18% fragrance) lasting four to six hours; and perfume (about 15% to 30% fragrance) six to eight hours or more. Consider purchasing perfume (which is oil-based) instead of cologne or eau de toilette (which are water- and alcohol-based) if longevity is an issue for you. Perfume is more expensive, but it does have a better potential for lasting the whole day because the oil and the fragrance concentration cling better to skin, so it tends not to wear off as easily as alcohol- and water-based fragrances.

Testing is the next step. Body chemistry can greatly affect any fragrance a person applies. How long any fragrance, regardless of type, will last or how well it will retain its scent during the day is anyone's guess. A fragrance can smell different at the beginning of the day than it does by the end. Trying on a fragrance (only one at a time) is the best way to determine how well it endures and which one you prefer. Do not choose a fragrance based on the way it smells in the bottle or on a card because that is not usually representative of what it will be like on your skin.

Should you buy body products that all have the same fragrance as your perfume? In a word, no. As you already know by now, I would rather you *not* apply scented skin-care products of any kind all over the body. It is best if your fragrance comes from a perfume or cologne applied to the inside part of your elbow, knee, neck, and cleavage. That's plenty. You do *not* need an additional bath product, powder, body cream, perfume, or cologne to make a fragrance stick around longer; that's fragrance overkill.

One more point of interest: The most expensive part of any fragrance is the bottle (about 40% of the cost). Then comes the advertising (another 30% of the cost) and the celebrity endorsement or designer insignia (another 10% to 15% of the cost). That leaves about 15% to 20% actual fragrance cost. Now that stinks!

## SMOOTHEST LEGS IN THE WORLD

Shaving is one of the primary ways women remove hair from their legs. Before I get into the discussion about how best to tackle this often-daily event, you might want to read Chapter Thirteen, *Hair Removal* which presents the various options for this repetitive task.

Most women barely get out the door on time with their teeth brushed, their kids off to school, and their makeup on evenly before they commute to the office, so shaving is a luxury that gets put on the bottom of the to-do list. But when the long, cold days of winter are a memory and the shorts and no-nylons time of year begins, there is no more hiding. Women, bring out your razors!

Several lines of cosmetic products are dedicated to the art of shaving. A brochure for one of these lines says a perfect shave requires an understanding of the fundamental principles of wet shaving and the use of five easy products (their products, of course). But what's easy about applying five of anything to the skin? Shaving should take no more than four steps (getting the legs wet, applying shaving cream, shaving, and rinsing) and two shaving products (the razor and a shaving cream or gel), followed by one moisturizer (a sunscreen for daytime if your legs are going to see daylight, and well-formulated moisturizer for night if your skin is dry).

There is no real trick to shaving. We all know how to do it, but not everyone knows how to get the best results and the softest legs. The following tips are the basics of a great, smooth shave:

- It is essential for your legs to be wet for at least two or three minutes before starting. Nothing is as irritating or chafing as shaving dry or slightly damp legs.
- Finding a razor that works well for your skin, given the pressure you use while shaving, the texture of your skin, and the density of hair growth, takes some experimentation. No single type of shaver works well for everyone. After that, the main thing is to change the blade frequently—dull razors make for poor shaving results.
- When it comes to shaving creams, for both men and women, those that contain emollients (usually those identified as being good for sensitive dry skin) work perfectly on the legs! There is absolutely no reason to buy shaving gels or creams in pretty pink containers when in truth they are virtually identical to those in more masculine or unadorned packages.
- Avoid shaving products that contain irritants. Used over newly shaved skin, irritating ingredients can cause red bumps and ingrown hairs. When I find myself without shaving cream in the shower, I use hair conditioner or body wash instead, which is far easier on the legs than bar soap or bar cleanser.
- For best results, shave against the growth of hair and be careful.
- After you are done, do not use a loofah or washcloth. They can cause irritation and create problems.
- Once you are out of the shower or bath, gently dab your legs dry.

- At night apply a moisturizer, and during the day, if your legs are going to be exposed to sun, apply a moisturizer with sunscreen (SPF 15 or greater) that contains the UVA-protecting ingredients avobenzone, titanium dioxide, or zinc oxide.
- Do not use an AHA or BHA lotion over newly shaved skin; they can be unnecessarily irritating then.

## PREVENTING RED BUMPS

As many women know, in addition to the occasional nicks and cuts incurred during shaving, it isn't unusual to also have an aftermath of uncomfortable and unattractive razor bumps (red, inflamed blemishes), particularly along the bikini line. Hair follicles are attached to oil glands, and both are attached to nerve endings. Shaving can easily irritate the skin, the hair follicle, and the oil gland, causing a rash-like breakout of annoying bumps. Ingrown hairs can also be a dilemma. Ingrown hairs are curly, wiry hairs that turn, curl, and dig into the adjacent skin as they grow out, or hairs that grow back in the wrong direction, causing a bump that can become infected.

As widespread a beauty problem as this can be, for women and men alike, the lack of products addressing the issue is surprising. The only product I know of that is aimed specifically at reducing or preventing these red bumps is called **Tend Skin** *($35 for 8 ounces)*. It contains isopropyl alcohol (70%), propylene glycol, acetylsalicylate, and glycerin. This is a very interesting formulation that is ridiculously overpriced, and the alcohol part of it is self-defeating! Alcohol causes irritation and redness, the very problems this product is supposed to address. How absurd! As it turns out, Tend Skin is nothing more than aspirin (that's what acetylsalicylate is) suspended in alcohol with a slip agent (glycerin). Aspirin is an anti-inflammatory, and a very effective one at that. The notion that you can put it on your skin to reduce irritation is valid and completely worth trying. However, the $35 is best kept in your pocket because there is no reason why you can't put this concoction together yourself with a small bottle, one or two aspirins, a quarter cup of tap or distilled water, and perhaps a touch of glycerin (which can be purchased at a drugstore; just ask your pharmacist). The drawback to creating this yourself is guessing at the proportions, but with a little experimenting you should be able to produce an interesting toner for ingrown hairs and for areas that get inflamed after shaving, including the face (for men), bikini line, legs, and underarms. You can apply your moisturizer after the aspirin solution is absorbed into the skin.

If you find the bumps do not respond well to the aspirin, try occasionally using an over-the-counter cortisone cream to reduce the redness and irritation. However, if the bumps get infected you will need to disinfect them with an over-the-counter antibiotic like Neosporin, Polysporin, or Bacitracin. All three are excellent for quick relief from a small topical infection.

## WHAT ARE ALL THOSE BUMPS ON MY ARMS AND LEGS?

Some people have a troublesome inherited skin problem called keratosis pilaris. This is the technical name for a condition in which hundreds of hard, clogged pores cover a person's shoulders, upper arms, buttocks, and upper thighs. It can seem to be a persistent case of acne, but these lesions rarely become inflamed and rarely become a pimple—though they will become inflamed if you pick at them. On darker skin the plugs can look like a sea of blackheads. What to do?

Gentle cleansing, exfoliating, and disinfecting can cause a huge reduction in the number of bumps. First, wash the skin gently with body wash (avoid soap, which can not only be too harsh but also may leave behind a film that can clog pores). If you like, you can use a clean washcloth gently over the bumpy areas. Do not overscrub. You can't rip these bumps off, and inflaming the area will only make matters worse.

After bathing, dry the area gently. When the skin is dried, apply a BHA lotion, gel, or toner over the problem area. BHA (salicylic acid) is the perfect option because it is lipid soluble. Lipid soluble means it can exfoliate inside the pore where the plug exists, improving the shape of the pore to allow a normal flow of oil. That makes it the best choice for reducing and potentially even eliminating the problem. If the bumps you have tend to become pimples or are infected after the BHA, apply a topical disinfectant of either 2.5% or 5% benzoyl peroxide. Do not apply moisturizer to these areas unless they are dry. During the day it is best to keep the area covered by clothing to avoid the use of sunscreen, which can make the problem worse. However, if the skin is going to be exposed to sun then it is essential to apply a well-formulated sunscreen. It will take some experimenting until you find the sunscreen that works for you.

## AHAS, BHA, RETIN-A, AND RENOVA FOR THE BODY

Treatments for dry or sun-damaged skin on the face can also be used on the body. AHA, BHA, Differin, Retin-A, Renova, and azelaic acid are all excellent choices for taking care of sun-damaged skin, dry skin, and areas that break out. AHA, Retin-A, and Renova are superior options for parts of the body such as the neck, chest, and arms that have been exposed to the sun and are showing signs of sun damage. BHA can also be excellent for reducing or eliminating roughness on elbows, knees, and heels, and for minimizing dry skin. (It is completely unnecessary and useless to use AHAs, Retin-A, or Renova on areas of the body that have no sun damage or are not dry.) Tretinoin, which is found in Retin-A, Renova, and Tazorac, can also improve the appearance of stretch marks.

In regard to application, follow the same course of action for the body as for the face. During the day, after cleansing, apply an AHA or BHA lotion, cream, or gel over skin and then Retin-A or Renova over the sun-damaged areas. You should then apply a sunscreen over areas of the body that will be exposed to daylight. At night, if necessary, you can apply an additional moisturizer over particularly dry areas.

If you are struggling with breakouts on any part of your body, follow the information outlined in Chapter 10, *Battle Plans for Blemishes*.

Just one more reminder: If you are going outside, it is absolutely essential to wear a sunscreen with a SPF 15 or greater that contains the UVA-protecting ingredients avobenzone, titanium dioxide, or zinc oxide. Apply it to any and all areas of the body that will be exposed to the sun for any length of time, no matter how brief. Sunscreen can and should be worn over AHA gels, lotions, or creams as well as over Retin-A or Renova. Sunscreen should be applied liberally, and it is the last thing you apply to your skin.

## SERIOUSLY DRY HANDS

Struggling with dry hands can be painful. Even if you are diligent about keeping them protected when doing housework or gardening, and unfailingly apply moisturizer whenever the opportunity arises, you can still suffer from bone-dry, cracked, parched hands. Clearly, it is essential to protect your hands from dish detergent, laundry detergent, excessive washing (medical professionals have a rough time with this one), and irritating ingredients, and also when doing potentially irritating manual work. Wearing gloves to prevent contact with these types of products and ingredients is of the utmost importance. However, a significant number of women may find they are allergic to latex gloves. About 10% of the population have negative reactions, ranging from mild to severe, if they come in contact with latex. If this turns out to be a problem, ask your physician or pharmacist where you can find nonlatex gloves.

The faster you get an emollient moisturizer on your hands after washing, and the longer you can keep it on, the better. It helps to keep small tubes or bottles of emollient moisturizer all over the house, including near the kitchen sink, in the bathroom, at the bedside, and in the garage. Keep more in your car, purse, briefcase, and desk drawer. That way it is never out of reach for a quick application. The best moisturizers for daytime are moisturizing sunscreens whose active ingredient is either avobenzone, titanium dioxide, or zinc oxide. However, titanium dioxide and zinc oxide provide an occlusive barrier that can act as a protective layer to retain moisture in the skin while keeping the sun's rays off the skin. (Bear in mind that brown "sun spots" on the back of hands and arms are a direct result of relentless, daily, unprotected sun exposure.)

Moisturizers such as Palmer's Cocoa Butter Formula, Eucerin Dry Skin Therapy Plus Intensive Repair Cream or Lotion, Curel Extreme Care Body Lotion, Jergens Advanced Therapy Lotion, and countless others are all excellent for use at night. The best approach is to apply moisturizer every chance you get. It is also incredibly helpful to purchase an over-the-counter cortisone cream such as Lanacort or Cortaid to help treat cracks and fissures that may occur, but cortisone creams are only to be used intermittently, not on a regular basis.

## BODY ITCHES

If you find that every time you shower your entire body begins to itch and the problem lasts for either a brief span of time or longer, you may have an allergy to the bath or hair-care products you are using. It will take experimentation to find out exactly what the culprit is, but the best strategy is to switch to products that have no fragrance whatsoever. However, you may also want to check out the possibility that the laundry detergent or fabric softener you use for your clothes or linens may be the real offenders. Fabric softener sheets pose an interesting chemical problem. These sheets are heat-activated in the dryer. When you shower and towel dry, a little of the fabric softener residue comes off on your skin. Then, the next time you take a hot shower, the residue is heat activated on your skin, causing the itching. The itching stops after about twenty or thirty minutes, as your body cools down again. Laundry detergent can also be a problem. Using laundry detergents that have less potential for causing skin irritation, such as Cheer Free, All Free & Clear, Arm & Hammer Free, or Tide Free, can make a huge difference. Sleeping on pillowcases and sheets that have detergent or fabric softener residue can be a serious problem when you have dry, sensitive, or acne-prone skin.

Hot water and showering can also cause problems for sensitive skin and can stimulate itching. I have advocated the use of tepid water for some time, particularly for the face, and it can make a difference for the body from the neck down if itching and rashes are an issue.

Another source of body itches can be the extremely irritating and drying salts that get deposited on the skin when you sweat. Instead of washing with bar cleansers or soaps, consider using a fragrance-free body wash. You will also want to avoid scrubs, loofahs, washcloths, bubble baths, and bath salts, all of which can trigger itchy skin.

Tight clothing such as jeans, nylons, tights, and leggings can also stimulate itching. The only way to prevent that is to loosen things up or do without. Nylons may be hard to give up, but for those with itchy thighs, wearing pants and cotton socks may be the only way to solve the problem.

# HARD AS NAILS

While some women have naturally great nails, others search endlessly for anything that will help make their nails strong, thick (but not too thick), and long (sometimes too long). Sadly, you can't fool Mother Nature. What is genetically predetermined cannot be permanently transformed. If you are lucky enough to have strong, fast-growing, perfectly shaped nails with smooth, even cuticles, only trauma and damage to the nail bed will change the health and appearance of your nails. If you have naturally brittle, soft nails and thick cuticles, there is also no way to alter what you've inherited. There is a lot you can do to make your nails look and feel better (there's plenty you can do to make matters worse, too), but changing the way your nails naturally grow is as impossible as changing the way your hair grows.

I know there are dozens of nail products made by everyone from Revlon and Sally Hansen to Barielle, Orly, and Cutex, plus new ones being introduced monthly, all claiming they can repair the irreparable. Don't any of them work? If they did, we'd all have long, beautiful nails. Yet millions of women have struggled with weak, brittle, soft nails, trying an endless assortment of strengthening, lengthening, and fortifying nail products, only to give up in frustration. It is almost impossible for a woman who wants to improve the appearance of her short, fragile nails not to wonder about all of the products that claim to feed the nails, engorge them with vitamins, or build them up from the outside in. **I would love to say those claims are legitimate and tell you which ones perform the best, but all the claims are bogus; changing the way a nail grows can't be done by putting something on it topically. Also, there's no research showing that vitamin supplements such as biotin can change the way the nails grow either.**
Physiologically speaking, the nail is simply a protective covering composed of dead cells filled with a thick protein called keratin, quite similar in essence to the hair. Although the part of the nail you can see is dead, the matrix (the part of the nail under the skin) is very much alive. The white crescent area of the nail is called the lunula and is part of the matrix. The nail grows out from the matrix and as the growth of new cells builds up and dies it is pushed forward and out toward the

surface. The cuticle is the protective layer of skin between the outside environment and the matrix. Keeping the cuticle intact is perhaps the single most important element in preserving the health of the nail.

Despite the nail's basic attributes, several long-standing myths about getting the talons of your dreams make the coffee-klatch rounds every now and then. Perhaps you've heard some of these nail delusions before, such as that tapping your nails on a hard surface will help nails grow and make them stronger. That isn't true in the least. You can't strengthen the nail by exercising it, assuming the nail needs the same training as a muscle. If anything, tapping will do just the opposite of what you want. Repetitive pressure or strain on the nail will lead to breakage and splitting. Another inane nail fiction is the notion that eating gelatin makes nails healthier. Gelatin probably got its reputation as a nail builder because of its relationship to protein. Like your nails and your hair, gelatin contains protein, but no form of food goes directly to the nail or hair to help it grow. There are no studies or data demonstrating that eating gelatin will improve the condition of anything. Eating a balanced, low-fat, nutritious diet (meaning lots of fresh fruits, vegetables, and whole grains) is certainly an important factor in overall good health, but feeding the nail directly isn't feasible.

## FLUORIDE

Several nail-care products want you to believe that "What's good for your teeth is great for your nails," so you can "Harness the power of fluoride with strengtheners, base and top coats, and cuticle care." If only that were possible! It would be a dream come true to have a product that could make nails as strong as teeth, or even relatively as strong. Alas, unless you were born with naturally strong nails, fluoride isn't going to help your nails the way it helps teeth.

First, teeth are unrelated to nails. Teeth are made of a bony substance composed of various mineral compounds, mostly calcium phosphate. Nails have no mineral content but rather are composed of hardened keratin, basically the same substance that comprises skin and hair. Further, fluoride doesn't "strengthen" teeth, but rather, according to the American Dental Association, has varying influences that work with saliva and the growth of developing teeth to prevent decay. One function of fluoride is to reduce the constant reaction taking place between the tooth's surface, saliva, and bacteria in the mouth. When we eat sugar or starchy foods the number of bacteria in the mouth increases, which raises the acidity of our saliva, which in turn slowly, over time, demineralizes the surface of the tooth. As the acidity subsides, the tooth's surface becomes remineralized. Fluoride reduces the presence of bacteria in the mouth, which reduces the acidity of the saliva and in turn reduces or eliminates tooth decay. None of that, to put it mildly, has anything to do with nail growth or nail problems.

One more point: Given that almost all of us drink and wash with fluoridated water, our nails are constantly exposed to fluoride. If fluoride were important for healthy nails—which it isn't—the amount we get in our drinking water would be more than enough.

The nail-care industry has tried to build up many ingredients in the effort to convince us that we can grow stronger nails. For years protein was a big one that showed up in nail-care products, though protein can't feed the skin or nail from the outside in. Diligently applying most nail-care products does help, but it is the protective coating they provide that does the trick, not these impressive sounding, do-nothing special ingredients.

## CALCIUM

Perhaps the last piece of nail improbability is the belief that applying calcium to your nails will make them strong. Calcium, along with lots of other minerals and vitamins, shows up in many nail-care products owing to the assumption that you can feed the nail from the outside in. You can't feed the nail directly, though even if you could, calcium and other minerals are unlikely ingredients for this purpose. Calcium and minerals may help build strong bones (bones are primarily calcium), but that is unrelated to the content of nails. The notion of having nails as strong as bone does make calcium sound appealing. However, even by itself calcium can't build bone; the body needs other minerals to use the calcium. Moreover, there is virtually no calcium in nails; they're made of keratin and that's about it.

# CUTICLE CARE

Although trying to affect the matrix and change the inherent growth of the nail with nail-care products is a waste of time and money, there are many things you can do to improve your nails. Without question, the most important element to pay attention to is the skin around the nail, namely the cuticle. **The best way to keep your nails healthy, whole, and as free from problems as possible is to push your cuticles back as little as you can. The less you manipulate and cut your cuticle the better off your nails will be.** Aside from inherited problems and physical trauma (getting smashed by a hammer or door can permanently alter the physical attributes of the nail), damage from overpushing or overtrimming the cuticle is the number one cause of nail problems. I know this may seem shocking and contrary to much of what you've heard, but excessively pushing back the cuticle and cutting it off is a huge no-no. Removing too much cuticle can damage the nail.

Overtrimming the cuticle can destroy the integrity of the matrix, which is the source of healthy nail growth. There is no way around this one. The cuticle is the body's form of protection for the area between the exposed dead part of the nail and the living matrix where the nail grows from. Anything that damages this seal puts the nail at risk.

If you cut too much cuticle away it can result in weak, brittle, ridged, dented, peeling, or unevenly growing nails (where one part of the same nail grows at a different rate), and once these problems occur, they won't go away until the nail grows out and that can take anywhere from three months to a year. Orange sticks and metal cuticle tools, even when padded with cotton on the tip as most manicurists do, can cause damage to the nail if they are not used carefully.

Almost every dermatologist I interviewed agreed that cuticle damage negatively affects nail growth. You can test this for yourself. Stop manipulating, pushing, or overtrimming your cuticles. For the next six months, simply take care of your nail shape (I'll explain more about that later in this section) and only minimally trim hangnails or excess skin around the nail. Do not overmanipulate the cuticle in any manner whatsoever. Within a relatively short period of time you are likely to see a radical change in the growth of the nail. I know this is a hard one to get used to but it will pay off in the long run.

Another thing you can do for the cuticle is to moisturize it as often as possible, and during the day be sure you use a moisturizing sunscreen with avobenzone, titanium dioxide, and/or zinc oxide. It doesn't have to be a special nail or hand moisturizer with sunscreen—as long as the SPF is 15 or greater and the active ingredients are the ones I've been mentioning it will do just fine. If the cuticle becomes dry and flaky (or sun damaged), the protective barrier for the matrix will break down, which can absolutely and quickly hurt nail growth. In some ways it is almost impossible to keep the cuticle moist and healthy. Think about how often you wash your hands and use them every day for everything from office work to housework to sports. Also, the hands are incessantly exposed to the sun and it is difficult to keep them constantly protected with sunscreen. Yet doing so is essential. **In short, don't overdo trimming cuticles, keep nails protected from the sun, and use a moisturizer to prevent dryness.**

# MANICURES AND PEDICURES

While leaving the cuticle alone is the best thing you can do for the growth of the nail, leaving the length of the nail alone is also a wise part of nail care. The part of the nail that extends past the quick is long dead and vulnerable to damage. Overfiling can tear at the nail's structure, and that can never be replaced. Once filing tears or starts lifting the fibrous nail material, it can begin a cycle that is hard to stop. Nails are softened by water, and soft nails are more susceptible to damage and tears. Shape the nails only when they are completely dry. It is also essential to avoid metal or extremely coarse nail files. Use the gentlest file with extremely gentle pressure to achieve the shape you want. You'll use up more nail files faster than you did before, but stronger nails will be the result of the extra expense and trouble. You've probably heard the one about filing in one direction only. That is completely unnecessary. Regardless of the direction you file, if you don't do it gently you will damage the nail.

When you do take the time to indulge in a full manicure or pedicure, it is essential to **keep it simple.**

The following is a great system for creating the perfect manicure or pedicure:

- First, remove any previously applied nail polish. **It doesn't matter whether you use a nail-polish remover that contains acetone or not. It also doesn't matter whether the nail-polish remover contains moisturizing ingredients. If a nail-polish remover can remove nail polish it is going to be harsh stuff, but that is the price of nicely painted nails.** Use as little nail-polish remover as necessary to remove the polish. Never soak the nail in nail-polish remover! Nail-polish remover is extremely drying and damaging to the entire nail, especially the cuticle. Keeping contact with nail-polish remover to a minimum is crucial for the well-being of the nail and cuticle.

- Gently file the nails into the shape you want, using the least-abrasive emery board you can find. **Avoid shaping your nails into long talons or severe shapes (too square or pointy).**

- Softening the cuticle around the nail is necessary only if you plan to remove just a tiny bit of excess cuticle. Soak the nails in plain warm water for no more than three minutes. **Oversoaking hurts the nail and the cuticle. Avoid soapy or detergent-filled water, which only dries the skin and damages the cuticle.** If the hands or feet are dirty, wash them first and that's it. Minimal contact with cleansers is best for any part of your body, including the nails!

- **Trim the cuticle and avoid pushing it back as much as possible, being exceedingly careful not to pull, lift, tear, rip, force, or cut into the cuticle in any way.**

- **Trim the nails carefully, using sharp manicure scissors or nail clippers.** Nails are definitely easier to trim after bathing or soaking. Fingernails should be given a slightly rounded edge to protect the nail growth; toenails should be trimmed straight across, slightly above the quick. Avoid cutting nails too short because doing so increases the chance of developing ingrown toenails.

- **Moisturize the cuticle with an emollient moisturizer.** Almost any moisturizer for dry skin will do. It is not necessary to purchase special cuticle creams: They contain absolutely nothing special for the nail or cuticle.

- Before you polish your nails it is essential to remove the moisturizer from them. **Moisturizing ingredients prevent nail polish from adhering to the nail.** Use nail-polish remover just over the nail's surface to take off any moisturizer. Avoid getting nail-polish remover on the cuticle; that's the area you want to keep the moisturizer on.

- Polish your nails in layers, allowing them to dry between coats. A minimum of three coats is standard. **If you have weak or brittle nails, place one or two coats of ridge-filling nail polish on the nail as the base coat.** This is the best way to shore up the nail. Two coats of a colored nail polish are next, followed by a top coat to add shine and luster.

- **Allow plenty of time for the polish to dry.** Quick-dry polishes and some quick-dry top coats of polish often contain alcohol, which can cause the polish to peel and chip more easily, so you want to avoid those. Using a quick-dry oil or spray after you're done polishing is a great way to ward off smudges, but these won't prevent nicks or dents in the polish, so be careful.

- **Do not dry your nails with a blow dryer or any other heat source.** Heat causes the polish to expand and lift away from the nail.

- **Touching up polish every other day with a layer of top coat can help make a manicure last longer.** Carry a bottle of top coat in your purse, and when you have a moment or break in your day, quickly do a once-over. A single layer dries quickly and makes all the difference in keeping up appearances.

## NAIL POLISH THAT LASTS

After spending way too much money on nail-care products and nail polishes, many women complain that for this kind of money their nails should be ten times stronger and the polish should last ten times longer. A nice thought, but that isn't the case. Price has no relation to how long a nail polish will last. Nail polishes are produced by only a handful of manufacturers, so there are no secrets, and the formulations vary only slightly because only a handful of ingredients will stay on the nail.

Lots of women complain that if they want their nails to look good it takes practically a full-time effort, and they can't live life like a normal person. I myself have gone around walking like a surgeon to be sure my nails don't come in contact with any surface anywhere. Though it doesn't take money to improve the appearance of your nails, it does take diligence and care. Those two things can't be avoided. Unfortunately, some polishes do tend to chip more than others (but this is determined by formulation, not cost). I wish I could offer some insight into which formulations work best, but no matter how many surveys I do or how many cosmetics chemists I interview, I have found no consensus as to which products last better. More often than not, polish longevity has to do with the process of applying the layers in the right order, including base coat (preferably a ridge-filler-type product), color, and top coat; applying layers that are thick enough but not too thick; allowing plenty of time for drying; and then treating your nails carefully (wearing gloves, avoiding water, having minimal contact with soaps or cleansers, and not using the nails as tools).

Polishes are often given names like SuperWeave Base Coat, Color Lock No-Chip Sealer, Strong Wear Nail Strengthener Polish, Extra Life Top Coat, Nail Building Base Coat, Color Shield, Fortifier Hydrating Base, or Nail Protector. They are all great names that promise wonderful things they can't even begin to deliver. Take Markron's Five Minute Nail Miracle, for example. This product isn't even a minor miracle. It contains standard nail-polish ingredients and tiny amounts of protein and amino acids, as well as formaldehyde. Nails are dead, and all the protein and amino acids in the world won't help them live. Formaldehyde can toughen nails, but it can also seriously dry them out and damage the cuticle. What kind of miracle is that?

I wish I could find a line of nail polishes that last, but it doesn't exist. So many factors affect how well your nail polish holds up. For example, Do you wear gloves when you clean? What kind of daily work do you do with your hands? Are your nails oil- and cream-free before you start polishing? I also get frustrated trying to separate one nail product from another because they have so much in common. The resins, lacquers, and basic products are all essentially the same. Most women experience about the same amount of wear from product to product, and it's about one to three days. All nail polishes begin to chip on the third to fourth day after application, regardless of the claim on the label (but you already knew that, didn't you?). Reapplying your top coat daily and avoiding fast-drying nail polishes will increase the chances of having your polish last. Finding the discipline to do that isn't easy, but it is the cheapest and most reliable way to make a manicure stick around until the end of the week.

By the way, it is completely unnecessary and actually a bad idea to store nail polish in the refrigerator. Condensation and cold negatively affect nail polish, making it too thick to use reliably.

# DIBUTYL PHTHALATE

Dibutyl phthalate (DBP) is a very common ingredient in almost every nail polish being sold. It is used as a plasticizer and is a key component in giving nail polish its unique properties. But a lot of women are giving their nail polishes a second look since the Centers for Disease Control and Prevention (CDC, http://www.cdc.gov) published the *National Report on Human Exposure to Environmental Chemicals—Results for Mono-butyl phthalate* [which is] *(metabolized from Dibutyl phthalate)*. Basically the CDC found measurable levels of phthalate in the urine of the participants in a study looking at the issue of phthalates. However, the CDC stated that "Finding a measurable amount of one or more phthalate metabolites in urine does not mean that the level of one or more phthalates causes an adverse health effect. Whether phthalates at the levels of metabolites reported here are a cause for health concern is not yet known; more research is needed" (Sources: CDC, http://www.cdc.gov/nceh/dls/report/results/Mono-butylPhthalate.htm; *Environmental Health Perspectives*, December 2000, volume 108, issue 12).

In animal tests, dibutyl phthalate has been shown to produce detrimental effects. The Environmental Working Group (EWG, http://www.ewg.org), a nonprofit environmental research organization, found that "DBP is a developmental and reproductive toxin that in lab animals causes a broad range of birth defects and lifelong reproductive impairment in males [when] exposed in utero and shortly after birth. DBP damages the testes, prostate gland, epididymus, penis, and seminal vesicles. These effects persist throughout the animal's life."

There are no similar studies or research showing any of that to be true in humans. In 1985, the Cosmetic Ingredient Review (CIR) board (http://www.cir-safety.org/) deemed dibutyl phthalate safe for use in cosmetic products. More recently, a press release issued on November 30, 2001, titled "Statement by the Phthalate Esters Panel of the American Chemistry Council on the Cosmetic Ingredient Review Expert Panel Assessment of Phthalate Esters," noted that "The Cosmetic Ingredient Review (CIR) Expert Panel is reviewing the use of three phthalate esters (also known as phthalates) in cosmetics. It is anticipated that the Expert Panel will complete its review in the first half of next year."

As this book goes to press, phthalates in general are still under investigation, and the jury is still out on whether or not phthalates are really harmful when used in cosmetics. In checking every line of polish I have ever seen, from Dior and Hard Candy to Lancome and Chanel, I have yet to find one that didn't contain it, so unless you give up polish there is no way to avoid this ingredient. I wish I could be more definitive about what to recommend, but for now I will continue to monitor the study results as they become available and report on what is published in my print and online bimonthly newsletter *Cosmetics Counter Update*, and my online biweekly Beauty Bulletin.

# FAKE NAILS—REAL PROBLEMS

The long and short of artificial nails is that there are risks associated with having them applied. I won't get into the aesthetic issue here, though it is a mystery to me why women can consider this a valid expenditure of their hard-earned money or believe that anyone thinks these are real—that's another story altogether. What is of more concern is the number of women every year who see a physician because of nail-related disorders that are directly related to the application of artificial nails. The most typical problems are horizontal nail grooves that develop close to the cuticle. This abnormality, according to an article by Dr. Zoe Draelos in the January 1998 issue of *Cosmetic Dermatology*, is seen in chemotherapy patients and women who wear artificial nails. When it's unrelated to chemotherapy, this nail damage is probably a result of the drill used by the manicurist to buff out the acrylic nail, or to rough up the real nail to allow better adhesion of the fake nail. It is far less damaging to use an emery board to file the nail, but salons are using the drill procedure to speed up an otherwise time-consuming process.

The thinning of the nail plate is another problem that occurs, especially when the acrylic nails are finally removed. To address this, it is quite typical for the manicurist to recommend oils, vitamins, or other treatments ranging from calcium to oxygen infusions, none of which will improve the appearance of the nail. The weakened, fragile part of the nail is long dead, and there is nothing that can be done to change the damage that took place when the artificial nail was applied and then repeatedly damaged with each reapplication. The only option is time, enough of it to grow out the damage, assuming that you are not doing anything else to your nails to cause more damage to the nail or cuticle.

Inflammation of the nail area is almost always a direct result of the chemicals used to apply artificial nails, but it can also be an allergic reaction to the acrylic material. However, if the inflammation persists or swells, it is essential to use a topical disinfectant such as Bacitracin. If the swelling continues or becomes more painful, it is imperative to see a physician who can treat the possible infection.

Another typical and more painful problem is something called onycholysis, which is the separation or loosening of a fingernail or toenail from its nail bed. What makes acrylic nails often more amazing than your own nails is, according to Dr. Draelos, "that the adhesion between the artificial nail and the natural plate is stronger than the adhesion between the natural nail plate and the nail bed." If you twist your nail, it is far easier to have your own nail become detached from your skin than it is for the artificial nail to pop off your natural nail. This means you need to avoid misuse (and not think the artificial nail can withstand any amount of pressure). It is imperative to pay attention to any loosening of your own nail and to be careful how you use the artificial nail. Because the artificial nail may be stronger than your own, it can put your real nail at risk.

One other possible problem for fake-nail wearers is infection. If you see a yellow or green discoloration, you can attempt to treat it yourself with Bacitracin. But if this doesn't produce any improvement then it is essential you contact your physician.

## NAIL STRENGTHENERS

If only nail-strengthening products really existed! What I wouldn't give for that, and I've tried them all. As it turns out, many of the products that claim to strengthen nails contain extremely drying ingredients such as formaldehyde or toluene, which do toughen the nail temporarily, but also make it more brittle. Formaldehyde goes by other names on ingredient lists, so watch out for names like toluene, toluene sulfonamide, and toluene sulfonic acid. Toluene and toluene-like ingredients are illegal in the state of California because of the serious health risks they pose, including cancer and respiratory problems.

Some formaldehyde-free nail strengtheners just coat the nail, like the ridge-filling products. So-called strengthening creams contain thick, waxy ingredients, like lanolin, that smooth over the nail and are hard to wash off. If you are good about reapplying these several times a day (sans polish, of course, because they can't penetrate polish), you might just see a change in your nails because they help protect the cuticle and prevent the nail from drying out, but it takes discipline. Keep in mind that you can't wear polish over any kind of moisturizing product because polish won't adhere to a moist, lubricated surface. You can apply these products over polish; but then they won't help the nail, although they can moisturize the cuticle.

## NAIL DO'S AND DON'TS

Surprisingly, there are more don'ts than do's when it comes to taking care of your nails. Most dermatologists will tell you that what you don't do to your nails is by far more important than what you do to them when healthy, strong nails are what you want. This list summarizes some of the things I've mentioned above, but the information bears repeating, given the amount of deceptive nail information and the number of nail products being sold and advertised all over the cosmetics world:

**Do coat the outside of the nails with nail polish or ridge fillers**, which can help protect the nail and prevent breaking and splitting, at least while the manicure lasts.

**Do moisturize the cuticle area** to prevent cracking and peeling, which can hurt the matrix.

**Do wear gloves** to protect nails and cuticles from housework, gardening, and doing dishes.

**Do be cautious when doing office work.** Nails and cuticles can take a beating from filing, opening letters (use a letter opener), typing (use the flat of your finger pads on the keyboard instead of the tips of your nails), and handling papers.

**Do apply a hand cream frequently** especially after you're done washing your hands, and pay attention to the cuticle area.

**Do wear a sunscreen** during the day on the hands and cuticles to prevent sun damage, which can hurt the nail, and reapply every time you wash your hands.

**Do meticulously clean all nail implements** and change nail files often. Bacteria and other microbes can get transferred by the nail tools you use, causing infection or harm to the matrix.

**Do disinfect any tears or cuts to the cuticle, and treat ingrown nails as soon as possible.** Nail infections are not only unsightly, but also can cause long-lasting damage to the nail. Any drugstore antibacterial ointment, such as Polysporin, Neosporin, or Bacitracin, will do.

**Don't use nail products that contain formaldehyde or toluene.** They pose health risks for the nail and for your entire body as well.

**Don't use fingernails as tools** to pry things open.

**Don't use your fingers as letter openers**. That destroys the cuticles, which destroys the nail matrix and affects nail growth and strength.

**Don't soak nails for long periods, and never use any kind of soap or detergent when soaking.** Nails and cuticles that become engorged with water weaken, and the longer soap or detergent is in contact with skin and nails (despite the advertisements for Palmolive dish detergent) the greater the potential for damaging the nail and cuticle structure.

**Don't overuse any kind of nail-polish remover.** Use a minimal amount on the nail and avoid getting too much on the cuticle and skin.

**Don't push the cuticle back too far.** Leave the cuticle alone as much as possible. Trim only the part of the cuticle that has started to lift away from the nail.

**Don't allow any manicurist to touch your hands with utensils that have not been properly sterilized.** The importance of this step cannot be stressed enough. Risking your health and well-being for a manicure is just not worth it, and that is a definite possibility with bacteria-laden nail instruments!

**Don't pull or tear at hangnails.** Always gently cut them away, leaving the cuticle intact and as untampered with as possible.

**Don't ignore nail or cuticle inflammation.** Disinfect the skin as soon as you can with an antibacterial or antifungal agent. Any change to the nail's appearance (see the next section) needs to be checked out by a dermatologist.

# WHEN THE NAIL GETS SICK

There are times when nail care requires a dermatologist. Fingernails and toenails are extremely vulnerable to infection and damage. If you have been diligent about leaving your cuticles alone and avoiding all the don'ts and performing most of the do's in the list above and you are still having nail problems, make an appointment with your dermatologist. Nails that are brittle, discolored, dull, abnormally thick, distorted, crumbling, loose, or subject to unusual debris under the nail are a medical problem not a cosmetic one.

It is quite normal for the skin to host a variety of microorganisms, including bacteria and fungi. Some are useful to the body. Others can multiply rapidly and lead to infections. Specifically, fungal infections are caused by microscopic plants (fungi) that thrive on the dead tissue of the nails and outer skin layers, particularly the cuticle.

Fungal nail infections are most often seen in adults, can be difficult to treat, and often recur. Toenails are affected more often than fingernails. People who frequent public swimming pools, gyms, or shower rooms; people who perspire a great deal; and people who wear tight, occlusive shoes are most likely to develop toenail infections because the fungi flourish in warm, moist areas. Prolonged exposure to moistness on the skin, minor nail injuries, and damage to the cuticle area can also increase susceptibility to fungal infection. Please be aware that fungal and bacterial infections are extremely contagious and can be spread through direct contact with another person who has the problem, and even through contact with contaminated towels, shower and pool surfaces, and nail implements such as cuticle clippers, nail clippers, orange sticks, and cuticle pushers.

Nail infections can be cleared with the persistent use of a prescription antifungal or antibacterial cream or lotion. Because nails grow slowly, treatment must be continued for 3 to 6 months for fingernails and 6 to 12 months for toenails (the time it takes to grow a new nail). There are oral medications for these problems, but they are best discussed with your doctor.

In terms of preventing problems for the feet, it is essential to keep them clean and dry. Change shoes and socks frequently. Dry the feet and hands thoroughly after bathing. Powders such as baby powder or talcum may help keep the feet dry. Of course, avoiding any damage to toenails and fingernails is of utmost importance.

To minimize the risk of damage to the nails, keep them smooth and properly trimmed. Trim the fingernails weekly. The toenails grow more slowly and may be trimmed as needed, about once a month. Nail-polish remover of any kind can weaken and dry the nails. Nail polish may coat and protect the nails slightly, but if you choose to use it remember that all polishes are basically identical, despite advertising claims to the contrary. Nail strengtheners can discolor or break the nails and damage the nail, too. Artificial nails may produce allergic reactions under the nail and can create a perfect environment for bacterial or fungal growth.

## INGROWN NAILS

Ingrown nails are another inelegant but typical nail problem. Often they are the result of cutting the nail too deeply or filing the nail too much, setting the scene for abnormal growth. Pain, swelling, infection, and discharge can result when the nail edge then grows into the surrounding skin. Many women love to wear shoes that crunch their toes into unnatural positions, and this, too, can interfere with nail growth and impair a normal healing process.

How can you prevent ingrown nails? Give your toenails plenty of room. That means wearing shoe styles that do not force the foot into an unnatural shape. Also, when you trim your fingernails and toenails, it is essential to avoid radically changing the natural shape of the nail by overfiling or by cutting the nail below the tip of the finger or toe. Also, do not cut or push the cuticles; damage there can significantly affect the nail's growth.

If an ingrown nail does become infected, thoroughly clean the area and try to minimally trim away the portion of the nail that is digging into the skin. Overcutting can simply re-create the problem, so be cautious. Disinfect the area with an over-the-counter antibacterial ointment like Polysporin, Neosporin, or Bacitracin. If the problem does not improve, it may require medical care.

## CORNS, CALLUSES, AND BUNIONS

Taking a closer look at our feet can be depressing. Statistically, eight out of every ten adults have calluses, bunions, and corns to deal with. Blisters are a common occurrence as the latest shoe fashions are broken in. Athletically-inclined adults (or adults with athletically-inclined family members) run a high risk of struggling with athlete's foot. Depending on how careful you are with pedicures, you can also be subject to painful ingrown nails that can become infected and swollen! There are ways to prevent these problems from occurring and there are solutions to most of these foot infirmities, but some are going to be hard to adopt and adapt to your lifestyle. Try to stick with it though, because soft, smooth feet, without squished toes and lumps and bumps, are definitely the way to go!

There is nothing glamorous about corns and calluses but they are abundant and occur more often than just about any other foot malady. Corns are thickened lumps formed on the outer layer of skin and occur over bony areas such as toe joints, especially on the tops or sides of toes. Corns are most recognizable by a small, tender, and painful raised bump that has a noticeably hard-textured center. Corns can be tender and painful, depending on how large they are and how much pressure shoes put on them.

Calluses are larger and almost always a painless thickening of skin caused by repeated pressure or irritation on the heels or balls of the feet. Calluses can become painful when they become so dry and cracked that the area becomes sore and tender to the touch.

In essence, corns and calluses are the body's way of protecting the feet from injury. For women, the most typical source of injury is from the shoes they wear. The pressure exerted on the foot, especially the toes, when it is forced into high heels or narrow shoe widths is nothing less than torture for the toes, heels, and arches of the feet. Your feet respond to this burden by growing skin cells at a faster rate to form a protective covering as a way to cushion the bones of the foot. It's this overgrowth that forms calluses and corns.

Our feet would almost be picture perfect if we, as women, wore better shoes. High heels, narrow toes, tight fits, and strange shapes (that don't match the proportions of the foot) are all disasters waiting to happen. If stopping the growth of calluses and corns isn't enough of an incentive, it also turns out that wearing high heels can cause back, hip, knee, and ankle pain brought about by a change in one's gait due to severe discomfort and it can also cause degenerative changes in the joint (Source: *Lancet*, May 1998, pages 1399–1401).

A study reported in *Health News* (June 1998, page 5) established that regular walking in high heels may also cause arthritic knees and hips (conditions that affect twice as many women as men). High heels prevent the ankles from functioning as they should, causing added strain to the hips and knees. For those of you who are saying "I don't have severe discomfort wearing heels; heels are just part of my life and I'm used to them," you are only fooling yourselves. Consider Chinese women at the turn of the century who had their feet bound. For some of them, the inevitable, daily pain was just part of their life, too.

As you may have guessed, it is really useless to try and treat corns and calluses until you remove the source of the problem. Once you do that, you can use good old-fashioned corn and callus pads to reduce pressure on irritated areas in your new, comfortable, well-fitting shoes. Many women try to peel or rub the thickened area with a pumice stone, but irritation and pressure will only make things look slightly better temporarily, and probably only exacerbates the problem in the long run. It is also a big no-no to try and slice away the offending areas with a razor or use scissors or clippers to cut them off. That's a sure way to cause injury or infection. A better fix is to exfoliate with a high-concentration beta hydroxy acid product designed for warts. First soak your feet in warm water and then apply a 5% or 10% salicylic acid cream (which may need to be specially compounded by your pharmacist). In general, if you see any signs of infection developing around a corn or callus, such as redness, swelling, pain, heat, or tenderness, see your doctor immediately.

Bunions are another story altogether, except that wearing ill-fitting shoes can also be (and often is) the cause. The technical name for a bunion is "hallux valgus." If you have a lump or bump on the inside edge of your foot around the big toe, especially one that's red, swollen, or hurting, you probably have a bunion. Another telltale sign is the direction your big toe points. If your big toe is angling inward and the joint is jutting outward, you're probably looking at a bunion.

There's no way around this one—you've got to change your shoes or you will never get rid of the bunion. The toes of any shoes you wear should be round or square, not pointy. And think flat! Heels are just asking for trouble. If you're experiencing pain, it is best to see your doctor, but you can try icing down the area or taking aspirin or ibuprofen to reduce the inflammation. Really severe bunions, however, may require surgery.

## ATHLETE'S FOOT

The fungus among us, or at least among our feet, are nasty critters that cause the problem called athlete's foot. The damp, dark area between toes is just heaven for these fungi, which are what cause those spots to tear, ooze, itch, burn, and just feel downright uncomfortable. The most common way to catch athlete's foot is by walking barefoot in public showers and locker rooms. Even if you're good about wearing sandals or thongs in gyms and spas, if someone in your family isn't, it is almost a slam-dunk they will pass athlete's foot on to other family members when they come home and walk around barefoot in the bathroom. Nevertheless, there is a cure, it just takes persistence and reapplication (and reapplication and reapplication) of an antifungal medication even several weeks after the cracks and tears between the toes disappear. Over-the-counter products containing tolnaftate, such as Aftate or Tinactin, or products containing miconazole nitrate, such as Micatin, are sure-fire successes when used in excess and frequently. The other issue is moisture. Athlete's foot fungi can't survive without that, so you must find creative ways to keep your feet as dry as the desert. You can try Zeasorb-AF (found at most drugstores), an absorbent foot powder that can keep your feet bone dry. It also helps to wear cotton socks (nylons are out) to be sure moisture doesn't get trapped and enhance the environment the fungi crave.

For more information about feet or to find a podiatrist in your area, contact the American Podiatric Medical Association at (800) FOOTCARE (366-8227) or visit their Web site at http://www.apma.org.

# CHAPTER 18

## MAKEUP APPLICATION STEP BY STEP

### MAKEUP: A PHILOSOPHICAL APPROACH

A documentary produced by the British Broadcasting Corporation went into entertaining detail and analysis of this salient point. *The Human Face* was written and directed by comedy legend John Cleese and features some rather candid comments from dermatologist Dr. Vail Reese on how we perceive skin flaws while watching films, and the way we make character assumptions based on things like facial asymmetry or scarring. According to Reese, "you'll have the clear complected individual as the hero, while any skin defect can be used by film makers to identify to audiences: Watch out for this one. So skin becomes a reflection not just of health, but of moral content. It is true that people with bad skin are not evil. We know that rationally. But studies have shown that subjects who interacted with those with clear skin and then those with facial scarring showed that there was more hesitation, more avoidance, more fear associated with the people who did not have good skin." In terms of cosmetic adornment, Vail commented that "Makeup is used to minimize any discoloration of the skin, any irregular contours, and then better allow attention to be drawn to certain features such as the eyes or the mouth, which we as humans want to accentuate" (Source: http://www.skinema.com *Skinterview,* March 2001).

History Professor Arthur Marwick, Open University, Milton Keynes, England, maintains that "There are many types of beauty (and with modern travel and the mass media we have become increasingly flexible): there is Chinese beauty, African beauty, Latin beauty, Nordic beauty, etc.; [yet] only a tiny minority within each type is beautiful. Beauty is what the overwhelming majority, on sight, recognise as beautiful: 'beauty is in the eye of all beholders.'" *The Human Face* goes on to reveal how studies from all over the world found that certain similar qualities about women are considered most attractive. It seems that people everywhere rate smooth skin, big eyes, and plump lips as signifying beauty. Interestingly, women and men of all sexual persuasions also rate the same faces as beautiful. The documentary also goes into detail about the way makeup has been used throughout history, showing how today's makeup is no longer the utilitarian tool it once was (think of "war paint" or camouflage), but rather is now sought more for artifice and empowerment. Women's desire for self-appointed personal enhancement is as strong as ever, and although the reasons we use makeup have evolved, looking beautiful continues to involve using makeup, and it has for eons (Source: http://www.bbc.co.uk/science/humanbody/humanface/index.shtml).

I have always believed that beauty is more than skin deep and that physical beauty has little meaning compared with the importance of an individual's positive contribution to the world we live in. A capacity for compassion, kindness, creativity, and an enduring respect toward each other, the environment, and all living creatures is infinitely more meaningful than how we look. Yet, it would be foolish to ignore that personal appearance has an enormous consequence in life. Whether you can or should judge a book by its cover, for the most part, most everyone does. I don't know if Brad Pitt, Jennifer Aniston, Tom Cruise, or Julia Roberts are good people, but they are simply stunning to look at. Looking beautiful has power in our society and often determines the way people relate to each other. Ignoring the significance of that impact may be virtuous, but it is utterly unrealistic.

**Applying makeup can be about looking well-groomed and feeling more beautiful and it can be exciting and fun. When done right, it can also express a great deal of personal power and élan.** In the following pages I explain how to apply makeup with panache and sophistication so you can, if you choose, add to or improve this concept of beauty in your life. I personally feel less is best when it comes to makeup, but I know women's choices and tastes range from no makeup at all to the whole nine yards. Whatever your choice, if you do want to wear makeup, applying it deftly can make the difference between looking attractive and looking out of date, out of place, or just plain unattractive.

Throughout this chapter, I try to guide you through the maze of options and help you create a beautiful makeup look for yourself that feels comfortable and fits like a glove. **Although fashion statements can be taken to extremes—from following the whims of everything the fashion magazines portray or your favorite celebrity decides to get into, to holding on to looks that are long gone—ignoring fashion is a mistake. Finding your own balance between fashion, comfort, and personal style is the most logical and beautiful choice.**

## DRESSING YOUR FACE—WHAT'S IN FASHION?

In many ways, makeup application is infinitely less complicated than skin care. Caring for your skin involves sorting through complex technical, medical, and physiological issues, while makeup is a more subjective and introspective art form. Makeup has little to do with hard facts and everything to do with skill and fashion. Discovering your personal preferences and honing your application technique are the essence of makeup application. **For the most part, makeup application is about experimentation and self-determination, because there are essentially no dos or don'ts, no have-tos or must-nots, no absolute rights or wrongs.** By way of illustration, you may decide that blue eyeshadow, dark brown lipstick, white foundation, and false eyelashes create the fashion statement you want to make, while I unequivocally recommend you avoid doing any of that. Yet wearing that makeup combination won't hurt you in the least. It may prevent you from being taken seriously or from getting the job you want, but that depends on what you want in life or what your career choices are.

When fashion is the topic, there are enough opinions and viewpoints to fill thousands and thousands of pages in hundreds of women's magazines every single month, 12 months a year. With such a storm of possible options screaming at us from the pages of *Vogue, Glamour, In Style,* and all the rest, choosing a direction may seem impossible. One model may wear a minimal sweep of tan blush on her cheeks, a hint of lipstick, taupe eyeshadow used both on the lid and crease, and a thin coating of mascara. Another model may have on an elaborate blend of contour shading; blush on top of that; an array of eyeshadow colors; dramatic, thick liner across the upper lashes and another thick sweep of liner along the lower lashes; and lots of mascara. The variations are endless. To make things even more confusing, each month there are new announcements about what is fashionable and what isn't. One month red lipstick is hot, the next month it's mauve, and the next pink, and then you read that blue eyeshadow is coming back and you have to avoid wearing anything more than a hint of blush. Following these dictates can be maddening, not to mention expensive and perhaps inappropriate for you.

So where do you fit in? There are no hard and fast rules, though I know that's what we all want to hear—a clear path of exactly what to use to make us look picture perfect. In the long run, the final decision is yours amongst an array of choices. **I will show you how to build a basic and classic makeup application, one that most, if not all, makeup artists use repeatedly in one form or another.** Once you get these basics down—how to choose and apply concealer, foundation, powder, contour (if you want), blush, eyeshadow (one is plenty, but you can choose more), eyeliner (optional), eyebrow color (if needed or desired), mascara, lip liner (optional), and lipstick—wearing as little or as much color or using as many of these steps as you feel comfortable with is completely up to you. That's not to say I won't be throwing in my opinions of what I think works and looks best. If you use lip liner that smears, eyeshadows that streak and flake, mascara that clumps, blush that goes on choppy, eyeliner that smudges, or concealer that creases into the lines around your eyes and mouth, you and your makeup will not look beautiful in the least—and the goal is to look and feel more beautiful.

As you look at fashion magazines and study the various makeup applications, styles, and images portrayed, decide which ones will help you with your career or any other aspect of your life that is important to you. The world is complicated enough—who needs to waste time wondering what to wear every season? It is far more powerful and beautiful to stick with classic looks that facilitate and enhance your ability to handle job interviews, get ahead in your career, raise a family, and concentrate on financial matters than it is to chase every new trend that comes along. The fashion headlines and headshots may look beautiful, but if they don't fit with your lifestyle and goals, let them be beautiful for someone else who has time and money to burn.

The pictures in this chapter demonstrate a full makeup application, and depict a progression of colors—neutral tones across the cheeks and eyes going from light to dark—that can fit almost any face. Makeup professionals the world over use this pattern time after time, and you can see it on the covers of most fashion magazines and on news anchors, TV personalities, and celebrities. It can be adjusted to include a wide variety of colors and intensities to achieve the look you want. This type of makeup application has been around for more than 25 years (it was established by makeup artist extraordinaire Way Bandy back in the early '70s, who was my guru when I started) and it's used today by most professional makeup artists, including Kevyn Aucoin, who not only cites Bandy as his main influence but often uses Bandy's style as a blueprint for his own makeup applications.

## DOES MAKEUP CHANGE WITH AGE?

Whether or not you choose a new approach to your makeup based on your age is entirely dependent on what you're doing at the moment and how that makes you feel. Just because more and more candles are finding a way onto your birthday cake, you don't have to hightail it to the nearest cosmetics counter for a makeover. If you have reached a point where you truly feel comfortable and confident in your own skin, what you adorn it with should reflect this. For most women, this may mean a sheer foundation that matches their skin exactly, a neutral-toned, creaseless concealer that does not play up wrinkles, a light dusting of sheer, non-shiny powder, soft matte eyeshadows in a variety of neutral hues, lightly defined and shaped brows, a great mascara that makes the most of your eyelashes, a softly blended blush color that adds vibrancy and color to your cheeks, and a lipstick color that seems "just right" no matter what other makeup you use. Sticking with well-chosen, adeptly applied and blended makeup in flattering shades gives a timeless look that can make ordinary features stunning.

However, if you breezed through your teens and twenties choosing makeup on a whim or enjoyed using bold, shiny eyeshadows, obvious blush, overly greasy or glossy lipsticks, heavy or mismatched foundation and too-thick concealer, and a kaleidoscopic array of eyeshadows and liners that were "out" as soon as you discovered they were "in," then you really should consider making adjustments to your routine. The same holds true if you feel as if you've been a slave to the latest makeup fads or styles, be they a retro Marilyn Monroe look with liquid-lined bedroom eyes and pouty red lips or the Crayola crayon–colored eyeshadows and spiky mascara seen in countless ads for sephora.com. You may discover that changing to a classic, well-blended finish where no one aspect of your makeup is more important than another is a refreshing, freeing style you can make your own. I'm all for self-expression—and when you're younger the limits of this are justifiably something to test—but as an adult, if your goal is to be taken seriously and be respected, why not think twice before heading to the office or grocery store wearing taxicab-yellow eyeshadow, clumpy mascara, and blue lipstick?

**Being a certain age—be it 30, 40, 50, or beyond—doesn't mean you have to overdo or undo your makeup. Regardless of how the years add up, you need to find a style that makes you look and feel beautiful, and that means finding colors that enhance your appearance and practicing blending techniques that make it all look natural and smooth instead of contrived and painted on.**

## WHERE TO BEGIN

**Three of the most difficult aspects of makeup are choosing the right colors, discerning the differences between products, and learning the correct application techniques.** Though these major issues need to be addressed, they are still only part of the picture. Wondering where to put your blush or how to blend your foundation before you know what type of foundation or what color of blush you should wear is putting the cart before the horse. Before you even choose specific makeup colors, discriminate between products, or deal with application, it is important to have a clear idea of the makeup look and style you want to create. Just as you would choose clothes to wear that are appropriate for where you are going—you wouldn't put on a jogging suit to go to a formal dinner or wear a long gown for a grocery run—the same guidelines are true for makeup.

Color, style, and fashion are all essential elements in clothing, and they are also essential to putting together a great makeup look. Too often women shop for or apply makeup with only one of those things in mind. Shopping for a lipstick or eyeshadow color without taking into account the other items in your makeup wardrobe is a mistake. Instead, decide what kind of makeup wardrobe you want to create and then go about choosing compatible colors, products, and application techniques to fit that concept. Think of the makeup staples you will need, such as black mascara, a healthy blush color, taupe or tan eyeshadow, and a suitable red lipstick. These items are akin to wardrobe staples such as a crisp white shirt, blue jeans, or the standard black dress—always fashionable and classic.

The way you see yourself, the way you want to be seen, what you do for a living, what you do in your leisure time, what colors are in your wardrobe, what style of clothing you are comfortable in, and how much time you are willing to spend creating a particular look all affect the way you choose and wear makeup. Those elements should set the course for choosing the right colors and products. So let's think a bit about the image you want to create.

## CHOOSING MAKEUP ACCORDING TO YOUR IMAGE

The first part of this makeup self-analysis is to take a close look at you. How do you want to be seen? What do you do for a living? What occupies most of your time during the day? The external image you want to project in your business life and personal life is what wearing makeup is all about. Too often we dress our face without thinking about how it affects our image. My favorite example of this is in the movie *Working Girl,* which stars Melanie Griffith, Sigourney Weaver, and Harrison Ford (it's a great rental if you haven't seen it). Griffith's appearance changes dramatically as her character decides to become more "professional" in order to fulfill her career aspirations. In addition to changing her wardrobe, she changes the way she wears her makeup and hair. To look more polished and put-together, she *softens* her makeup look. Griffith goes from wearing strong pastel-colored, heavily applied eyeshadows to softly applied, neutral taupes and browns. She stops wearing heavy black eyeliner on the lid and lower lashes in favor of a more subtle shade of dark brown. Her lipstick changes from cranberry red to a neutral coral-tan, and her boldly applied blush is replaced by a soft neutral tone. The striking difference in her looks is a beautiful example of how makeup can affect the image you project—and how others perceive you.

Rather than just randomly selecting a lipstick, stop and consider not only whether it's the right color for your skin tone, but also whether it is too soft, too sheer, too noticeable, too sexy, not sexy enough, or has enough flair or subtlety to support the image you want to project. **Problems with how you apply makeup can be solved with technique, but understanding how you want others to see you comes from a sense of purpose and an understanding of what you want out of life.**

# BEFORE YOU START

Because makeup goes on poorly over skin that isn't perfectly clean and smooth, the first step in applying beautiful makeup is to start with a clean face. Following the skin-care recommendations described in the first part of this book will help you get your skin closer to where it needs to be. Women with dry skin should also wear moisturizer under their foundation (preferably a moisturizer with a good SPF if the foundation doesn't contain one). Women with normal to oily skin should avoid wearing moisturizer under their foundation. Moisturizer of any kind only adds to an active oil flow, and will make skin look greasy that much sooner. (It is, however, completely acceptable to wear a minimal amount of moisturizer over dry areas such as the under-eye area or cheeks.)

**The only reason to use a moisturizer is to smooth and lubricate dry skin or dry areas. In spite of what you hear from cosmetics salespeople, moisturizer does not and cannot protect the face from a foundation, nor is that necessary.** It's a good sales gimmick, but it's not the truth. There is nothing "bad" inside a foundation that your face needs to be protected from. Moisturizers are absorbed into the skin, and once they are, for all intents and purposes, they're gone, and they can't prevent anything else you put on your face from going where it wants. Besides, whatever protection you think you're applying when you put on a moisturizer is likely wiped away as you apply your foundation (including sunscreen, which should be the last thing applied to the face).

I know this idea of wearing a moisturizer only when you have dry skin borders on heresy, but in the long run it makes the most sense for your skin, especially if you wear a water-based or emollient foundation. What you might not know is that most water-based foundations (and definitely emollient foundations) contain many of the exact same ingredients as your moisturizer, so it isn't necessary to double up products. If you're wearing a moisturizer (with or without SPF 15) and a water-based foundation at the same time, your face can become too slippery and the rest of your makeup will tend to slide right off by lunchtime.

If you believe a moisturizer does help your foundation go on more smoothly, the problem might actually be a different one—such as the way you apply your foundation, the type of foundation you're using, or your skin-care routine, which may be drying out your skin and leaving a rough feeling rather than a smooth one. Before you reach for the moisturizer, make sure another product you're using isn't negatively contributing to the way your foundation applies. And remember, it may not be a single product but a combination of products that's contributing to a less-than-smooth skin surface.

A good way to judge whether your skin needs moisturizer during the day is to notice how long your skin feels dry after you wash your face. A slight amount of dryness immediately after you wash your face is typical. However, if this feeling lasts longer than 15 or 20 minutes, you should wear a lightweight moisturizer under your foundation. If your skin tends to feel extremely dry after you wash your face with a gentle, water-soluble cleanser, wear a more emollient moisturizer under your foundation. If your skin tends to become drier as the day goes by, that, too is a good reason to wear a moisturizer.

**Note:** Either your daytime moisturizer or your foundation must be rated SPF 15 and contain UVA-protecting ingredients of avobenzone, titanium dioxide, or zinc oxide. There is no reason to wear two products, a sunscreen and a moisturizer, when so many products combine both beautifully. An exception to this point is that if you opt to use a foundation with effective sunscreen and intend to spot-apply or use it minimally, it is essential to pair this with a sunscreen for proper UV protection.

Now you can start applying your makeup.

## LESS IS BEST!

**Never use more than you have to—either in the intensity of the colors you choose or the number of products you wear. Many steps in applying makeup can be consolidated or eliminated without affecting your overall makeup look in any way.**

Frequently a salesperson at the cosmetics counter insists that you need an absurd number of products to be properly and attractively made up. Yet more complicated doesn't mean you will look any better. If anything, a more complicated makeup routine can mean more chances for mistakes, which can cause you to look overdone as well as waste your valuable time and money.

Speaking of doing too much, so-called foundation primers, eyeshadow bases, blemish cover-ups, and color correctors—to name just a few—are, with few exceptions, completely unnecessary. They complicate the process of applying makeup by requiring additional blending and allowing too many colors and products to interact on the skin at the same time, leaving a thick, gunky mess and sometimes contrasting colors on the face. Your SPF 15 foundation (or foundation with an SPF 15 sunscreen/moisturizer underneath) and/or concealer can quite nicely accomplish all the functions those extra products are supposedly designed to perform, without any of the extra fuss and expense.

**Foundation Primers** are seen in many of the newer makeup artistry lines, such as Laura Mercier, Vincent Longo, and NARS. Basically, these "primers" are nothing more than lightweight, silicone-based moisturizers. The silicone allows the product to spread easily over the skin, and to some extent can help smooth the skin's texture and remedy mild dry patches that could spell trouble when you apply most types of foundation. These primers also tend to have a soft matte finish on the skin once they dry down, and that can make your foundation a bit easier to control and blend because the skin will be much less slippery than if you had applied an emollient moisturizer. Still, primers are truly optional and their benefits do not outweigh the extra step and expense. The only reason to consider one is if you have normal to oily skin and need the extra smoothness these can provide in order to make your foundation look its best. It is best to test these out via sampling before investing in a full-size tube so you can be sure you're making the purchase because you like what it does for your skin—not because you get suckered into the marketing pitch that makes it sound so important for skin.

**Eyeshadow Bases** are sold to the consumer to help eyeshadows stay in place longer. The eye area is indeed a tricky place to get color to last, but there are ways to make it stay without specialty products. Besides, most eyeshadow bases are very similar to cream-to-powder concealers or foundations. Placing a matte or semi-matte face foundation on your eyelid and applying loose powder over it works just as well. Also, if your eyeshadows tend to smear or slip into the eyelid crease, you can greatly reduce the problem by not placing a moisturizer or greasy foundation on your eyelid.

**Blemish Cover-ups** are sold to consumers solely on the basis of something I call "acne anxiety." The promise conveyed by the word "cover-up" is that this product really can hide a blemish, but nothing could be further from reality. Most cover-ups are heavier than your foundation, and they look thick and obvious over a blemish. And if the blemish cover-up doesn't match your foundation exactly (and most don't), it will look like a different layer of color (usually a shade of peach or ash) placed over the blemish, bringing still more attention to the very problem you are trying to hide. Even if the cover-up is the same color as your foundation, you will probably place too much extra makeup over the lesion. Your foundation by itself is more than sufficient to cover the redness without bringing more attention to the area. I totally understand the desire to want these facial sore spots to disappear. Unfortunately, there is only so much you can do to cover up a blemish before you start making matters more obvious by layering on too much makeup.

It is especially problematic to apply concealer only over blemishes and nowhere else, without any foundation. The natural color and texture of your skin just doesn't resemble most foundations or concealers. Spot application looks, well, spotty! That doesn't hide anything, and it can look particularly strange in daylight.

Some concealers and cover-ups are dubbed "medicated" and are meant to cover and heal blemishes, but they are not effective for this purpose. I have yet to find one that contains ingredients that can disinfect, exfoliate, or absorb oil, all critical components for controlling breakouts. Plus, these types of products don't cover any better than normal concealers.

**Color Correctors** are those bottles of pink, mauve, peach, green, or yellow liquid meant to be worn under your foundation to alter skin color. Thankfully, these impractical, useless products are becoming harder to find, though some cosmetics lines are steadfast in making you believe you need them. The notion is that if your skin is pink or ruddy, you need to tone it down or counteract it with a yellow-tinted color corrector. If your skin is olive or sallow, you would change it with a pink or mauve color corrector. It's an interesting concept, but a waste of time.

The ingredient lists for most color correctors are very similar to those for moisturizers, which means they are easily absorbed into the skin. Once they are absorbed, you are left with a slight tint of pink, green, mauve, or yellow on the face. Supposedly this means you have now changed your skin tone for the better. In fact, once the liquid has been absorbed, the result is often so minor as to have little to no real effect on skin tone at all. For the sake of argument, though, let's say there is a noticeable change. The tint of the color corrector on your skin would mix with your foundation and you could end up with a very strange shade of foundation. A good foundation in a neutral, soft yellow-tone base should be able to correct and even out all skin tones without adding another layer of makeup on your face.

## THE CLASSIC FACE

Classic makeup encompasses all of the following elements: concealer, foundation, powder, contour (optional), blush, eyeshadow, eyeliner, eyebrow color (if needed), lip liner (optional), and lipstick. For each of these steps, you want to find a corresponding product that is best for your skin type and the coverage or look you want. Each step also requires an application and blending tool so you can achieve a smooth, flawless appearance. **Along the way, you can eliminate steps that seem excessive or too complicated, and decide how much makeup you want to wear and what colors are suitable to your needs.**

The first two steps in applying a complete makeup are to reduce the darkness under the eyes and to apply a foundation to even out the skin (it's sort of like putting on panties and a bra). Once that's done, the eyeshadows and blushes can blend on smoothly over an even palette instead of over varying skin textures and colors. Whether you start your application with the concealer or the foundation depends more on personal preference than anything else, although the color of the concealer is another factor. For the sake of organization, I'll start with the concealer.

# CONCEALER

Generally, a concealer is thought of as a product that covers blemishes or facial imperfections, as well as dark circles under the eyes. Concealer can also be used to highlight certain areas of the face, especially if it is a lighter texture and color. Concealers with thicker consistencies are best for covering problem areas such as dark circles under the eyes or extreme redness on cheeks or noses. Concealers with a lighter or thinner consistency are better for minimal coverage and for highlighting areas of the face you want accented. Throughout the rest of this book I refer to all products that provide extra coverage (over and above what foundations can do) or make certain areas of the face lighter as concealers.

The primary purpose of concealers is to offset the natural shadows that occur under the eyes, and, in more elaborate makeup applications, to highlight certain areas of the face such as the center of the nose, forehead, top of the cheekbones, or center of the chin. Principally, the under-eye area needs concealer most because the eye is set back in its socket, which lies in a shadow created by the surrounding bone structure. In addition, the skin around the eye tends to be thinner than the skin on the rest of the face, so pigment discolorations and surface veins show through easily, making the under-eye area look dark and dull. The first thing you need, then, is a lightweight, flesh-tone concealer that is a shade or two lighter than your foundation (see the photograph on page 461).

**However, if you don't have dark circles under the eye area, you don't need a concealer.** If your foundation is opaque enough to even out the skin tone under the eyes, you don't need an extra product for that area.

The logic behind using a lighter flesh-tone color is the same basic rule you learned in Art 101: When you need to make paint a lighter color, you add a lighter color than you started with. Any other color, or the same color, or a darker color would defeat the purpose. Blue, yellow, or shades that are the same as your foundation color will not make the under-eye area lighter. Standard shades can cover discolorations, which is fine, but applying a lighter shade is the only way to correct the darkness caused by shadows. Also, a slightly lighter under-eye area can make the face look brighter and more awake. **Foundation may be all you need to even out minimal discolorations under the eye, cheeks, nose, or for minor facial discolorations.**

When you shop for an effective concealer, it is critical that the concealer be the same basic, natural skin tone as your foundation, only one or two shades lighter. That way you can be assured that the foundation and concealer will blend together under the eye. If you choose a concealer that is a very different color than your foundation, you will simply end up with a third color where they overlap and intersect.

The only time you wouldn't use a lighter concealer is when the area under the eye is naturally lighter or the same color as the rest of the face. In that case, it's fine to apply your foundation with no concealer. In fact, it may sometimes be necessary to apply a concealer that is slightly darker than your foundation to reduce having a whitish goggle effect around the eye.

I prefer to apply concealer first and then the foundation. If you are using an ultra-matte foundation, the concealer blending on first prevents streaking and staining. (It's hard to blend anything over ultra-matte foundations.) You can apply your concealer in a small arc around the inside corner of the eye or, for a more involved makeup application, you can apply it in a sweep under the entire eye and out on the upper cheekbone. Blend this out evenly, taking care not to spread it onto areas where you don't want it. Be sure you are using a pat-and-blend method of application, as this will ensure that the concealer covers where it is supposed to and is not inadvertently wiped away. The foundation is then applied lightly over this area and blended out over the face. You may also want to try applying your foundation first and then sparingly applying concealer to the under-eye area if it is still dark. The trick is to make sure the foundation and concealer edges merge imperceptibly on the skin.

The most typical problem with a concealer is applying it smoothly over the under-eye area without making it look too white. It is important to always blend the edge of the concealer away from the eye until it disappears. Also, try to concentrate the concealer along the inside corner of the eye and down, as opposed to out. The less concealer you put at the back corner of the eye (unless that area is dark), the lower your chances of looking like a raccoon with a white mask over the eyes.

At times when you wish to wear as little makeup as possible, try using only a minimal amount of concealer that is closer to your true skin tone than the concealer you normally use. Or try a lighter shade of foundation than you normally wear and apply it only in the under-eye area. This can make a world of difference in making you look rested and polished, but not made up. Again, the trick is to blend extremely well so that there is no discernible edge between the concealer area and the part of the face where there is no makeup.

In the past it was almost impossible to find concealers in a good selection of colors that also didn't crease into the lines around the eyes. Now the tide has turned, and many cosmetics lines have excellent shades and textures to choose from. When shopping for a concealer, the primary things to look for are (1) a neutral skin tone that is one or two shades lighter than your foundation, but not so light that it looks obvious when blended on in the under-eye area, (2) a smooth texture to ensure easy blending, (3) coverage that suits your needs, and (4) staying power, so it doesn't crease into the lines around the eyes.

## TYPES OF CONCEALERS

Concealers come in six different forms: stick concealers, creamy liquid concealers, cream concealers, matte-finish liquid, matte-finish cream-to-powder, and finally the ultra-matte liquid concealers, which blend on smoothly and creamily and dry quickly into an unmovable layer.

**Stick concealers:** Stick concealers come in swivel-up tubes like lipsticks.

**Examples:** Cover Girl CG Smoothers Concealer *($5.69)*, NARS Concealer *($16)*.

**Application:** Stick concealers are applied to the under-eye area much the way a lipstick is applied to the mouth. They can be applied over or under your foundation, depending on how much coverage you want—under the foundation provides less coverage and over the foundation provides more. Dab the stick over the area in dots and then blend with clean fingers or a concealer brush. Avoid wiping it on from the stick in an opaque streak of color. That tends to build up too much makeup and it also pulls the eye area, causing sagging. If the skin under the eye area is dry or wrinkled, it does help to first apply a lightweight moisturizer and then apply the concealer. Be careful the moisturizer isn't too greasy and that you don't put it on too heavily to ensure that the concealer doesn't slip into facial lines. If you have applied too much moisturizer, use a tissue to dab off any excess before you apply the concealer.

**Pros:** Depending on their consistency, stick concealers can provide more complete coverage and control for very dark circles under the eye. They tend to go on thickly and don't spread easily, which means you can better control the application.

**Cons:** The texture of many stick concealers is rather dry and thick, which makes them difficult to blend without overpulling the skin under the eye. They also go on too heavily, which can create an obviously made-up look. Other stick concealers are quite greasy; they can look less obvious because they blend so easily, but the texture often causes slippage into the lines around the eyes. For these reasons, this is the least common type of concealer you will encounter.

**Creamy liquid concealers:** Creamy liquid concealers generally come in small squeeze-tube containers or long, thin tubes with wand applicators.

**Examples:** Prescriptives Camouflage Cream *($16.50)*, Lancome Effacernes *($21)*.

**Application:** Use your finger or the wand applicator to transfer the liquid concealer in small dots or to place a light coat of color under the eye area. Blend gently along the under-eye with either your finger or the sponge applicator, concentrating the largest amount of concealer over the darkest areas. If the skin under the eye area is dry or wrinkled, it helps to first apply a lightweight moisturizer and then apply the concealer. Be careful the moisturizer isn't too greasy and that you don't put it on too heavily or it will ensure that the concealer slips into facial lines.

**Pros:** Depending on their consistency, creamy liquid concealers provide very light, even coverage and have the least tendency to crease into the eye area. They can also be easily layered if more coverage is needed, and they tend to not cake up on the skin.

**Cons:** Depending on their consistency, creamy liquid concealers can have too much movement and be hard to control. It is important when applying an under-eye concealer to keep the color and coverage just where you want it. If the concealer is too greasy or loose, it can spread too easily, highlighting parts of the face you don't want highlighted. Some liquid concealers go on too thinly, offering very little coverage, but if you don't want a lot or don't mind building coverage, these are the way to go.

**Cream concealers:** Cream concealers usually come in small pots and typically have a smooth and creamy texture. Occasionally these may have a dry, thick texture.

**Examples:** M.A.C. Studio Finish Concealer SPF 15 *($12.50)*, Stila Eye Concealer *($16)*.

**Application:** Depending on their consistency, cream concealers can go on easily with your fingertips, a concealer brush, or a sponge, placing the color in dots under the eye area. Blend the concealer out under the eye area, concentrating the application over the darkest areas. If the cream concealer has a dry, thick texture, it can be very difficult to blend and can look heavy and obvious on the skin. If the skin under the eye area is dry or wrinkled, it does help to first apply a lightweight moisturizer and then the concealer. If the cream concealer is very emollient, use minimal moisturizer under the eye area and dab off the excess. Most moisturizers can make cream-type concealers slip even more easily into facial lines. The emollient cream concealers should be set with loose powder immediately after blending to help promote crease-free wear.

**Pros:** Cream concealers can have a very pleasing creamy and moist consistency, but they can also be rather thick and heavy. Depending on the consistency, they can go on well and provide even, often opaque, coverage. They are especially good for someone with very dry skin who wants more coverage. Cream concealers can also be used as foundations in a pinch.

**Cons:** If the cream concealer is too thick or greasy, it will crease into the lines on your face. If it is dry and thick, it can be difficult to blend and can also easily crease into facial lines. This is never the type of concealer to use over breakouts.

**Matte-finish liquid concealers:** Matte-finish liquid concealers typically come in a squeeze tube or a tube with a wand applicator.

**Examples:** Paula's Select No Slip Concealer *($7.95)*, Elizabeth Arden Flawless Finish Concealer *($14)*.

**Application:** Use your finger or the wand applicator to transfer the liquid concealer in small dots to the under-eye area, then quickly blend using a soft patting motion. If the skin under the eye area is dry or wrinkled, it helps to first apply a minimal amount of lightweight moisturizer and then apply the concealer. Although these are not as tricky to apply as ultra-matte concealers, they still demand adept blending for the best results.

**Pros:** Depending on their consistency, matte concealers can provide light to full coverage. They typically do not crease or migrate, and they tend to outlast cream and cream-to-powder concealers. They also work well as a base for eyeshadow if you have trouble with your eyeshadows fading or creasing. Matte-finish concealers work well over blemishes.

**Cons:** If you have prominent lines around and under the eyes, matte-finish concealers can make them look more pronounced. Some matte concealers go on quite thick and dry, and are difficult to blend easily or dry too quickly.

**Matte-finish cream-to-powder:** Matte-finish cream-to-powder concealers usually come in compact form and often look like small versions of cream-to-powder foundation.

**Examples:** Clinique City Base Compact Concealer SPF 15 *($13.50)*, Lancome Photogenic Concealer SPF 15 *($20)*.

**Application:** Use your finger, a concealer brush, or a sponge to dab the concealer on to the undereye area or over other discolorations.

**Pros:** This type of concealer is very easy to apply. It provides the glide and blendability of a cream concealer with the long wear of a matte concealer. Concealers like this work well anywhere on the face, especially if more extensive coverage is needed. Some versions contain effective sunscreens.

**Cons:** Despite the initial matte finish, the ingredients that create the creamy texture tend to cause it to eventually crease—and to keep on creasing. The powder finish can make wrinkles look more pronounced, and this type of concealer is not the best to use over blemishes or dry, flaky skin.

**Ultra-matte liquid concealers:** Ultra-matte liquid concealers generally come in thin tubes with wand applicators. Although these were once easy to find, many of them have fallen out of favor and have been discontinued because they are so difficult to work with and can make lines under the eye more pronounced; however, they rarely, if ever, crease.

**Examples:** Revlon ColorStay Concealer *($9.49)*, Maybelline Great Wear Concealer *($4.69)*.

**Application:** Use your finger or the wand applicator to transfer the liquid concealer in small dots to apply a light coat of color in the under-eye area. You must blend these on very quickly and accurately because they dry in seconds. Once these ultra-matte concealers dry in place, they don't budge, and there is no way to adjust the blending, so you could end up with streaks or patches of color. Once ultra-matte concealers dry, they do what they say they'll do! If the skin under the eye area is dry or wrinkled, it helps to first apply a lightweight moisturizer and then apply the concealer. Concealers like this should always be applied before foundation. Applying them over foundation is just asking for trouble! However, in most cases you don't have to use an ultra-matte concealer if you're using an ultra-matte foundation because the foundation usually provides enough opaque coverage to cover just about anything.

**Pros:** Depending on their consistency, ultra-matte concealers provide light-to-medium, even coverage and, if blended on correctly, they absolutely will not crease into the lines around the eyes. They are great if you tend to lose makeup during the day or have problems with makeup slipping. They also make excellent, long-lasting eyeshadow bases for those who have a problem with their eyeshadows fading or creasing throughout the day.

**Cons:** Because ultra-matte concealers stay so well and are so matte, they can make lines under the eyes look more noticeable. It doesn't always help to apply moisturizer underneath because that can sometimes make the concealer streak and look stained. It is important when applying under-eye concealers to keep the color just where you want it and to blend quickly.

## TECHNIQUES FOR BLENDING CONCEALER

Regardless of the type of concealer you use, the application remains basically the same. Dab the color on with your fingertips, the wand applicator, or the tube concealer itself in a half-inch crescent from the inside corner of the eye out to approximately one-third of the way under the eye. Apply the concealer only where the eye area is dark. If it's dark all the way out under the eye, then that's where the concealer should go. You can apply concealer to the eyelid too if that area is also dark and could use some lightening. Unless you are using a matte or ultra-matte finish concealer, set the concealer with a light dusting of loose or pressed powder. This will ensure a smooth finish and longer wear (but be careful not to overdo powdering under the eye area because this, too, can make lines look more pronounced).

If you want a more elaborate makeup application, you can apply the concealer along the flat bridge of the nose, along the laugh lines, out along the entire under-eye area, on the top of the cheekbone, and in the center of the forehead and chin for accent and enhancement. These options tend to be complicated and time-consuming, even for women adept at applying their makeup, and you can get almost the same results by applying the rest of your makeup correctly. I used none of those techniques with my makeup as it appears on the cover of this book, and all those areas appear nicely highlighted because of the way I applied the rest of my makeup. If you do choose to highlight these areas, place your highlighter in dots over or under your foundation in these areas and blend well, controlling the color so it does not spread all over your face. Keeping the color contained is the goal if you wish to try this extra step (see photograph on page 461).

**Whether you apply the concealer first and then the foundation or the foundation first and then the concealer, carefully blend the concealer out and under the eye in a dabbing motion, with either your finger, a concealer brush, or sponge (I prefer to always use a sponge), making sure you cannot see the edge where the concealer stops and the foundation starts.** The trick is to keep the concealer blended only over the area where it is needed. If you have to ask whether or not a concealer brush is really necessary, then chances are you do not need one!

## Concealer Mistakes to Avoid

1. **If you have noticeable lines around the eyes, do not wear a concealer that goes on too thickly or is too dry; it can cake under the eye and exaggerate wrinkles.**

2. **Consider my recommendations in *Don't Go to the Cosmetics Counter Without Me* for specific concealers that don't crease into the lines around eyes. If you can't find these, be sure to test the concealer first by wearing it under your eyes for awhile to be sure it doesn't crease and to find how it works with your foundation and skin tone.**

3. **If the concealer is obvious, you've chosen the wrong shade, applied it too heavily, or didn't overlap blending with your foundation.**

4. **Do not wear a peach, orange, green, rose, or ash shade of concealer.**

5. **If the skin is dry, apply a lightweight moisturizer under the eye to prevent the concealer from caking or making the wrinkles look more noticeable. A moisturizer that is too heavy or emollient can make almost any concealer slip into the lines around the eyes. Be careful using moisturizer with an ultra-matte concealer, because streaking or splotches of color can result if the moisturizer is too heavy or is applied too thickly.**

6. **Do not forget to blend the foundation and concealer together so there are no edges where one stops and the other starts. This is best done with a makeup sponge.**

# FOUNDATION

Personally, I've never been fond of the whole process of smearing foundation all over my face or even part of my face. I totally understand when women complain about feeling "made up" when they wear a foundation. So why do I recommend using foundation at all? Because of the flawless, even base a foundation can provide. If the skin has a uniform color, texture, and appearance, the blush and eyeshadow colors you apply will look smooth instead of choppy. However, and here's the tricky part, **to the extent possible, the face should never look like it has a layer of foundation on it.**

If you are already blessed with a totally even, perfect complexion, you will nevertheless want to consider wearing a foundation because of how it helps eyeshadows and blushes go on more evenly. If you try to blend blushes and eyeshadows without foundation, they will most likely go on choppily or wear unevenly during the day. Foundation keeps those powdered colors in place. Skin itself has no real adhesive properties (think about what would adhere to it if it did!). Foundation, therefore, gives the rest of the makeup something to hold on to evenly. By themselves, blushes and eyeshadows have some ability to cling, but not all that much. Besides, today's foundations offer some incredible options for creating the illusion of even, flawless skin without looking like makeup, and many of the best ones contain effective sunscreen.

## FINDING THE PERFECT FOUNDATION COLOR

I cannot stress this point enough: Your skin and foundation should match exactly. If you are pale, that's OK—accept the fact that you are pale and buy a light foundation that matches exactly. **Whether you have red hair and fair skin or black hair and dark ebony skin, the foundation must match your underlying skin color exactly. Do not buy a foundation that will make your face look even a shade or two darker or lighter or change its underlying color in any manner.** Even with a difference that slight, you run the risk of a more obvious makeup application than you really want, particularly for daytime wear. Find a foundation that matches your skin perfectly and goes on softly and smoothly.

When I tell you to match the foundation with your underlying skin color, you may be asking yourself, "Exactly what is meant by skin color?"

Traditionally, skin color has been defined by the basic underlying tone, described as olive, when the skin appears ashen or green in color; sallow, when the skin has a yellow or golden shade; and ruddy, when the skin has overtones of pink or red. These categories hold true for all women, including women of color; your underlying skin color will always relate to one of those skin tones. You may have been told that you are a particular "season" and your wardrobe and foundation color should be a specific undertone, either cool (blue tones) or warm (yellow tones). Unfortunately, all that information surrounding skin tone can be misleading when it comes to choosing a foundation color.

If you are told your face has cool undertones, meaning blue undertones, should you wear a blue-toned foundation? Of course not. If your skin color is ashen, choosing an ashen foundation will just make you look greener. If your face is strongly pink or red, applying a pink foundation all over will make you look like you're wearing a pink mask. If you have a sallow skin tone, applying a strong yellow-looking foundation will make you look more sallow. None of those would look natural and flawless the way foundation should look, and none of them would come close to matching your skin's underlying, basic color.

So what to do? When you're purchasing a foundation, it is important to identify your overall, exact skin color and find a foundation that matches it, regardless of the underlying tone. **For the most part, regardless of your race, nationality, or age, your foundation should be some shade of neutral ivory, neutral beige, tan, dark brown, bronze brown, or ebony, with a slight, and I mean very slight, undertone of yellow but without any orange, pink, green, or blue. There are no orange, pink, green, or blue people, and buying foundations in those colors is absurd.**

Why a slightly yellow undertone? Because skin color, more often than not, always has a yellow undertone: that's just what the natural color of melanin (the pigment in the skin) tends to be. There are a few exceptions to this rule. Native North American or South American women, a tiny percentage of African-American women, and some Polynesian women do indeed have a red cast to their skin, and in those instances this information about neutral foundations should be ignored. Because their skin has a slightly reddish cast, they need to look for foundations that have a slightly reddish cast to them—but that's only a hint of brownish red, and not copper, orange, or peach.

A few makeup lines are aimed at Asian women. These boast a "unique collection of yellow-toned foundations" appropriate for all skin types, but most specifically, Asian women. I concur that most skin types, including those of Asian women, are better served by yellow/neutral-based foundations and powders. However, plenty of lines have awesome yellow/neutral-based foundation colors. The same principle holds true for African-American women. There are many lines claiming to meet the needs of darker skin colors, but often these lines actually have poor color selections or poor foundation types (the exception to this is Iman foundation colors, http://www.i-iman.com). It is best to find a foundation color and type that works for your skin type rather than limiting yourself to a special line claiming to serve a specific skin color.

Question: If all the fashion magazines and makeup experts talk about foundations being sheer and matching the skin exactly, why do so many women of all ages wear heavy-looking, obvious foundations? It may be confusion about skin tone and foundation color; it may be failure to check the foundation in daylight; or, in some cases, it may have something to do with the fact that many women hate their skin and think a layer of foundation looks better than what exists naturally. Rather than going into the emotional ramifications of disliking your skin, let me just say that covering your face with an obvious layer of foundation only makes matters worse. **What's essential to an attractive makeup application of any kind is to begin with a good, light-textured foundation that blends impeccably; otherwise you will look as if the makeup is wearing you.** Even if you feel that you are in need of a foundation that provides good coverage, *obvious* coverage is a monumental mistake and can negatively affect the entire makeup application. Of course, all foundation is about coverage, but it is also your personal key to enhancing—not masking—your complexion.

## EXCEPTION TO THE RULE OF MATCHING SKIN COLOR

Although you are attempting to exactly match the skin color of your face when you choose a foundation, in some cases it is more important to match the foundation to the color of your neck. If your face is darker than your neck and your foundation matches the face, it will look like a mask because of the difference in color. The opposite is also true. If your face is lighter than your neck and you put on a foundation that matches the face, it will still look like a mask because of the difference in color. In situations like this, match the foundation more to the neck color or to a color in between the color of the neck and the face.

For some women who have serious facial discolorations or scars it can be hard to ignore the need for a heavy foundation application that provides opaque, full, concealing coverage. Unfortunately, a heavy or thick foundation is the only way to achieve this effect. Foundations that make claims about superior coverage that also looks natural are not telling the truth. You can't cover your face with foundation and camouflage the imperfections without seeing what is providing the coverage. But that doesn't mean you shouldn't consider a heavier foundation—just be aware that you are essentially exchanging one problem for another. The advantage is you do get to choose between two options, and even if that's a dilemma, you are still the best judge of what works and feels best for you.

## THE FINAL DECISION

Once you have selected a foundation color, there is only one way to be absolutely sure it is right for you: Apply the color all over your face and check it outside in the daylight. Check it from all angles and decide if it matches your skin exactly. If you applied it carefully but there are lines of demarcation at the jaw area; or if it looks too thick or too greasy, or gives the face an orange, pink, rose, or ashen tint; or if it looks heavy and opaque instead of sheer and light, go back to the testers. In fact, you may need to test several types before you find the right foundation.

One practical guideline to narrow down your choices is to test many different colors at once. Begin with several that look like good possibilities and place stripes of each one in a row over the cheek area. The best choice is the one that blends almost perfectly with your skin color. The wrong choices will stand out, with obvious edges that don't disappear into your skin. This technique is a reliable way to eliminate some choices, but I've also seen it go wrong more times than I can count because it doesn't go far enough. Use it only as an elimination process; it does not replace the need to check out the color on your face in the daylight, nor the need to blend the foundation shade over a larger area of your face.

Keep trying on foundations until you find the best one. **Once you've made a selection you feel good about, apply it all over your face, wait at least two hours, and check it again in the daylight. How a foundation wears during the day—does it change color or become too greasy or dry as the day passes?—can be evaluated only after you've worn it for awhile.** Once you've assessed all these details, in the daylight, you can safely make a final determination as to whether this is the right color or type of foundation for you. Please take the time to follow this procedure. This advice will guide you in the right direction, and, ultimately, it is the only way to guarantee that you'll find the right foundation. If you rely only on the salesperson and the lighting at the cosmetics counters, it will be pure luck if you end up with the right color. And if you get the foundation wrong, regardless of how perfectly you choose and apply everything else in your makeup wardrobe, those will all look wrong, too.

## WHERE TO SHOP

Although there are many wonderful foundation options available at the drugstore, the almost universal lack of testers is incredibly frustrating. For budget-conscious consumers looking for a reasonably priced foundation, this can be quite a challenge, as you're often left standing in the aisle (under horrendous lighting and with no mirrors in sight) to guess which shade is best for you. For this reason, I encourage you to begin your foundation search at a department store or cosmetics boutique (like Sephora) where testers are the rule, not the exception. You will end up spending more for foundation, but the convenience of testers, mirrors, takeaway samples, and (at times) professional guidance is worth it. Once you become more skilled at knowing which shades work for you and which do not, you can venture back to the drugstore to try again. It can be helpful to bring along the foundation you are currently using—assuming the color is a great match—to compare with the drugstore options. Last, since you will still not be able to see the color on your skin until you purchase it and test it at home, be sure you buy only from drugstores or mass merchandise stores that allow you to return opened cosmetics. Safe bets in this regard are Rite Aid and Walgreens.

## TYPES OF FOUNDATION

Now that you know how to go about finding the right foundation color, the next hurdle is figuring out the type of foundation best suited to your skin type. Cosmetics counters carry a mind-boggling assortment of foundations these days, including oil-free and matte foundations, water-based foundations, oil-based foundations (these are few and far between), pressed powder-based foundations, cream-to-powder foundations, liquid-to-powder foundations, stick foundations, so-called self-adjusting foundations, and foundations that have shine. Given this range of options, narrowing down your choices can be tricky.

**Note:** Many of the following foundation types have effective sunscreen protection with an SPF 15 or greater and UVA-protecting ingredients of avobenzone, titanium dioxide, or zinc oxide. That means you can rely on these for sun protection if they are applied liberally and evenly all over the face. If you prefer to wear a sheer, thin layer of foundation or don't want to wear foundation all over your face, then a moisturizer with sunscreen must be worn underneath. To ensure your foundation with sunscreen is protecting you all day, consider setting your makeup or touching up your makeup during the day with a pressed powder that contains sunscreen.

<u>**Oil-free and matte liquid foundations:**</u> Most of these contain oils (even though the names don't sound as though they do) or ingredients that act or feel like oils, such as silicones. These oils and oil-like ingredients are not necessarily bad for any skin type, but their presence demonstrates that the term "oil-free" is another cosmetics industry contrivance that won't necessarily help you find the best product for your skin type. Keep in mind that what most of these foundations have in common when they are well formulated is that they dry to a matte finish, with no shine or dewy appearance whatsoever. On the skin, "oil-free", matte foundations look like a traditional liquid foundation, although they are often thicker in appearance and have no shine.

**Examples:** Clinique Stay-True Makeup Oil-Free Formula *($16.50)*, Almay Wake Up Call! Energizing Makeup SPF 15 *($9.99)*.

**Application:** See the section "Blending Foundation" that follows.

**Pros:** These foundations are the best choice for women who want balanced coverage with no shine at all, and who like a smooth, matte look. They last much longer on oily skin or oily areas than most other foundations (except for the ultra-matte foundations), which for some women is a very desirable, if not essential, effect.

**Cons:** There aren't many disadvantages to using this kind of foundation. Some of them can make the skin look or feel dry and flaky, but this is usually true only for those that contain talc or other absorbent ingredients.

**Ultra-matte foundations:** These are an amazing group of products that truly stay put. Most have a very liquid consistency and are blended on like any other foundation, though precision blending is key. You have to be very careful about using a moisturizer under ultra-matte foundations. If you use too much, if it's too greasy, or if you don't allow it to be adequately absorbed, it can make the foundation gunk up or streak.

The major drawback with foundations like these used to be the lightning-quick dry time, as that meant blending had to be absolutely perfect from the start or you would end up with a streaky, uneven application. Today's ultra-matte foundations are less tenacious than earlier ones, but they are also noticeably easier to blend and more forgiving of mistakes. The trade-off for this added convenience is that these do not wear as long as they used to, but most women will appreciate the extra "play" today's ultra-matte formulas have.

**Examples:** Maybelline Non-Stop Makeup *($8.75)*, Estee Lauder Double Wear Stay in Place Makeup SPF 10 *($28.50)*, Revlon ColorStay Lite SPF 15 *($12.95)*.

**Application:** See the section "Blending Foundation" that follows.

**Pros:** These foundations are a superior option if you have seriously oily skin, have trouble with makeup slipping or disappearing as the day goes by, live in a humid climate, exercise but still like your makeup to stay put, or like a completely matte finish. Ultra-matte foundations will outlast any other foundation, with no slippage or movement. If you have very oily skin, these are an absolute must to try.

**Cons:** Regrettably there are many disadvantages to using oil-free, matte foundations. Primarily the problem is that most of them go on rather heavy and look masklike, leaving the skin feeling very dry and taut. To get this makeup on evenly, you must blend quickly or it will dry in place before you know it, and then it can be difficult to blend further. This foundation type can also be hard to work over when applying cream eyeshadows and blush. Ultra-matte foundations have less movement than more emollient foundations, which means eyeshadow and blush have a tendency to stick to them; that can make blending and correcting mistakes a bit irksome, but not impossible.

Women of color should be careful when choosing ultra-matte foundation. Even if it is the right color, these foundations can tend to look gray and ashen after being applied to darker skin tones. Skin that shows no shine or reflection in general tends to look dull gray with this kind of foundation, and that effect is even more pronounced for women of color.

Ultra-matte foundations like this are also the most difficult to remove. The number of options for ultra-matte foundations is dwindling, as women have undoubtedly had problems with them. This is unfortunate because these ingenious formulations can work so well for truly oily skins.

**Water-based and standard liquid foundations:** Water-based does not mean oil-free, even if the label says so; what it does generally mean is that the first ingredient is water and the second or third ingredient is some kind of oil or emollient slip agent. These foundations look like a somewhat thick liquid and pour slowly but easily out of the bottle. They are perfect for women with normal to dry skin, and the number of foundations fitting this description and performance abound.

**Examples:** Laura Mercier Moisturizing Foundation *($38)*, L'Oreal Visible Lift Line-Minimizing Makeup SPF 12 *($9.99)*.

**Application:** See the section "Blending Foundation" that follows.

**Pros:** Most water-based foundations are best for those with normal to dry skin. They are perfect for these skin types to wear without a moisturizer, or they can be worn with a moisturizer or a moisturizer that contains an SPF. The oil or emollient part of these foundations gives them good movement, which makes blending a pleasure and allows blushes and eyeshadows to blend on effortlessly and evenly over the face. Mistakes are easily buffed away with the sponge.

**Cons:** If you have oily or combination skin, this is not the foundation type for you. Even the little bit of oil or emollients in a water-based foundation show shine almost immediately if you have oily skin. Those who do not have oily skin but have a paranoia about any shine on the face will not like the effects of a water-based foundation either; and for those with breakout-prone skin, the small amount of oil or emollients in this cosmetic may make you nervous. For the most part, I personally don't believe there are any disadvantages to using water-based foundations and I recommend them wholeheartedly. Water-based foundation is also a great option for women of color. The slight amount of emollient these contain helps create a nice glow on the skin, preventing darker skin tones from appearing dull or ashen. That same glow is also most attractive for women with dry skin.

If you are concerned about the small amount of shine that water-based foundations leave behind on the skin, try adding a light dusting of loose powder. After you've blended the foundation in place, you can apply the powder all over the face to reduce the shine.

**Oil-based foundations:** Oil-based foundations list oil as their first ingredient and water usually as their second or third ingredient. Oil-based foundations feel greasy and thick, look greasy and thick, and go on greasy, yet can blend out quite sheerly and softly. You can blend an oil-based foundation to a very thin, subtle layer of makeup.

**Examples:** Alexandra de Markoff Countess Isserlyn Cream Makeup *($47.50)*, NARS Balanced Foundation *($38)*.

**Application:** See the section "Blending Foundation" that follows.

**Pros:** Oil-based foundations can be very good for women with extremely dry or wrinkled skin. The emollient ingredients help the skin look very dewy and moist, which can minimize the appearance of wrinkles.

**Cons:** Oil-based foundations tend to be very greasy and thick and can look that way on the skin unless you are very adept at blending. They also have a tendency to turn orange on the skin because the extra oil in them affects the pigments in the foundation. This can be true for women of color, too, and it explains why oil-based foundations can look orange after they are worn for awhile. The typical recommendation for applying an oil-based foundation is to add water to your sponge so that it goes on thinner, and more like a water-based foundation. But that can be tricky to gauge and can cause the makeup to streak. Why not just use a water-based foundation in the first place and skip the negatives of the oil-based foundation? That would be my recommendation. Additionally, if you wear face powder over this type of foundation, the oil grabs the talc and the face can appear coated and heavily made up even if you blend it on thinly. The same is true for blushes and eyeshadows— they will go on more heavily because of the increased oil on the skin, and they will also become darker once applied. Traditional cream blushes tend to work best over this type of foundation.

**Pressed powder–based foundations:** These foundations come in a compact and appear and perform much like any pressed powder, which is what they really are, only with a bit more coverage and ability to stay put. Almost all of them have a superior creamy, silky feel, but when applied to the skin they blend on as easily and lightly as any pressed powder.

**Examples:** Laura Mercier Foundation Powder *($38)*, Chanel Double Perfection Makeup SPF 8 *($45)*, M.A.C. Studiofix Powder Plus Foundation *($22)*.

**Application:** You can apply these foundations with either a sponge or a brush all over the face, including the eyelids. This is the easiest way to get a smooth, light, and fast application. You might have to worry about a smooth application if you have dry skin, but these powder-based foundations go on evenly for other skin types, providing extremely sheer to medium coverage. For more specifics about blending techniques, see the section "Blending Foundation" that follows.

**Pros:** Powder-based foundations are great for women with normal to oily or combination skin. They blend on easily and quickly, last all day, generally don't change color, and feel exceptionally light on the skin. They are best for those who want a minimal feel and appearance from their foundation. They also work very well over sunscreens, and can help reduce the shine some sunscreen ingredients (even those in a matte base) leave on the skin.

**Cons:** Women who have dry skin should not wear powder-based foundation. This is also not a good option if you have flaky skin, regardless of your skin type. The powder content makes this type of foundation too drying for someone with dry skin, and the way it goes on can make the skin look more dry and flaky. Also, women with very oily skin might want to be cautious, because powder-based foundations can get a thickened, pooled appearance as oil resurfaces on the face during the day.

**Cream-to-powder foundations:** These foundations are an interesting cross between a pressed powder and a creamy liquid foundation. They come in a compact and have a very creamy, almost greasy appearance. When you blend them on, the creamy part disappears and you are left with a slightly matte, powdery finish. Cream-to-powder foundations provide much better coverage than pressed powder–based foundations.

**Examples:** Clinique City Base Compact Foundation SPF 15 *($21)*, Maybelline True Illusion Liquid to Powder Makeup SPF 10 (despite the name this is definitely a cream-to-powder makeup) *($6.99).*

**Application:** Cream-to-powder foundations are best applied with a sponge. Some women have success using a brush, but I think this is a difficult, messy technique. See the section "Blending Foundation" that follows.

**Pros:** Cream-to-powder foundations blend on quickly and easily and provide a semi-matte, soft, medium coverage. They work great for someone with normal to slightly dry or slightly combination skin. The consistency doesn't require powdering after you apply it. If you wish to use powder, make sure you apply it as lightly as possible to avoid a caked, heavy look.

**Cons:** Cream-to-powder foundations can blend on slightly thickly, providing a made-up look rather than a sheer, natural appearance. They don't work well for someone with oily skin because the cream components can be too creamy, making skin look more oily, and they don't work well for dry skin because the powder part can be too powdery looking and cause more dryness. Essentially, they are best for normal skin types.

**Liquid-to-powder foundations:** These liquidy powders with a gel-like wet feel apply easily and dry to a satiny-smooth, sheer, slightly matte finish. They typically contain water as the first ingredient, along with a slip agent such as glycerin. In contrast to cream-to-powder foundations, liquid-to-powder foundations feel significantly lighter on the skin. They also tend to last longer over combination or oily skins because the creamy, waxy ingredients are either decreased or altogether absent.

**Examples:** Vincent Longo Water Canvas *($45)*, Aveda Cooling Calming Cover Sheer Face Tint *($18)*, Cover Girl Aqua Smooth Makeup SPF 15 *($8.50)*.

**Application:** Liquid-to-powder foundations are best applied with a sponge. Some women have success using a brush, but I think this is a difficult, messy technique. See the section "Blending Foundation" that follows.

**Pros:** Liquid-to-powder foundations blend on quickly and relatively easily and provide a semi-matte to matte finish with sheer to medium coverage. They work great for someone with normal to oily or slightly combination skin. The consistency means that it doesn't require powdering after you apply it. If you wish to use powder, make sure you apply it as lightly as possible to avoid a caked, heavy look.

**Cons:** Liquid-to-powder foundations dry quickly and can, therefore, blend on choppy, making application tricky. This type of foundation does not work very well over dry skin because the water portion tends to cling to dry areas, leaving a powder finish that is not easily moved. If you have dry skin and want to try this type of foundation, use an emollient moisturizer or sunscreen beforehand. The product itself must be kept tightly closed between uses because the water component will evaporate if left exposed to air for long periods. Some of the compact liquid-to-powder makeups can chip or break apart if you are not careful while swiping your sponge over the makeup.

**Stick foundations:** These foundations are essentially cream-to-powder foundations in stick form, and the application, pros, and cons mentioned in that section are the same. The main difference between stick and cream-to-powder foundations is the variety of coverage available from sticks. Whereas cream-to-powder makeups typically provide medium coverage, stick foundations come in formulas that range from full to sheer coverage with either matte to creamy texture. Many stick foundations also feature effective sunscreens, making them a great all-in-one option. In addition, they can do double duty as a concealer, and most product lines offer a wide selection of shades.

**Application:** These can be swiped onto the skin right from the stick and then blended with a sponge, fingers, or—if you're up for the challenge—a foundation brush.

**Examples:** Elizabeth Arden Flawless Finish Stick Makeup SPF 15 *($18)*, Trish McEvoy Foundation Stick *($38)*, Almay One Coat Light & Easy Liquid Stick Makeup SPF 15 *($12.49)*.

**Pros and Cons:** Refer to the section for cream-to-powder foundations.

**Foundations with shine:** A definite trend in the world of makeup is having your entire face shine, either with a makeup primer that shines, a foundation that has shine, or a powder that shines. Shimmering shine (as opposed to naturally pro-duced shine) seems to be "in" and I have to admit that it does look great in pictures. In real life (and especially in daylight) it tends to look sparkly or extremely artificial, and if you have normal to oily skin, it looks like the very oil you were trying to do away with. Try this one and check it out in daylight before you splurge. It works better as an evening look than for a classic daytime look.

**Examples:** Revlon Skinlights Diffusing Tint SPF 15 *($11.99)*, Prescriptives Luxe Soft Glow Moisture Makeup SPF 15 *($30)*.

**Application:** The method of application varies, depending on if it comes in a stick or has a cream-to-powder, liquid, cream, or powder base (refer to those sections for more information on performance and texture). Generally, a sponge can be used for all of these. A brush can be used if the intent is to highlight spe-cific areas.

**Pros:** For dull, lifeless skin, the best of the foundations with shine can indeed add a subtle glow to the face, but the more product applied, the more the glow turns into obvious, sparkly shine or looks somewhat greasy.

**Cons:** In a word, shine. There's a lot of variation when it comes to how much visible shine you'll get from these products, so pick and choose based on whether you want a subtle glow or high-wattage shimmer.

**Self-adjusting foundations:** These foundations supposedly can absorb oil, stop oil production, and also prevent moisture loss. I've yet to see one perform as prom-ised, though it would be great if someone came up with one that could!

**Custom-blended foundations:** If a foundation is blended for you and you only, will that get you the best shade? This style of selling makeup is very enticing. The customer-service interaction is impressive. Your foundation is supposedly mixed and matched for your exact skin color and needs. The premise is that there are only so many ready-made shades and you might be better off having one custom-blended. Unfortunately, the idea sounds better than the reality. The major problem with custom-blended cosmetics is that the success of the match depends on the expertise of the salesperson—and there are huge variations in skill.

As nice as custom-blended foundations sound, the formulations are not neces-sarily superior to (or sometimes even as good as) standard products. The founda-tion may be too greasy or too dry and it might turn to rose or peach as you wear it. With so many off-the-shelf foundation products available, in many excellent colors, custom blending turns out to be more an expensive gimmick than any-thing else.

When should you try a custom-blended product, particularly foundation? When you have tested many standard foundations and are still frustrated with the color of your foundation.

## BLENDING FOUNDATION

**When it comes to blending foundation over your face, keep one mantra in your head: Blend, blend, and blend again, and then, just to be sure, blend one more time.** All the other details are, well, just details, and not anywhere near as important as buffing off the excess foundation and smoothing out the edges to be sure you have the thinnest possible layer of foundation over the skin (see photograph on page 461).

**Exception to the rule: If you are using a foundation that contains an effective sunscreen, a thin or sheer application will not provide adequate protection from the sun. To ensure you will be getting the stated SPF, it is essential to apply the foundation liberally and in an even layer all over the face. If you prefer a sheer or spot-application, then you will need to wear a separate sunscreen underneath your foundation or consider a tinted moisturizer with sunscreen or a pressed powder that contains sunscreen.**

Keep in mind that the goal of wearing foundation is to create the illusion of smoother-looking skin, not a noticeable mask of color. Of course, the best place to check your blending technique is in broad daylight. Unfortunately, most of us apply foundation in bathroom light, with only minimal exposure to sunlight. Once you get into daylight, even on a cloudy day, the areas you missed, particularly next to the ears, mouth, jawiine, sides of the nose, and temples, often look streaked, show a line of demarcation (even when the color matches perfectly), or appear blotchy or smudged. This is not the effect you are trying to achieve! Smoother-looking skin takes diligence and daylight, or the very best lighting you can create in your home, where you apply your makeup. But whenever possible always check your foundation in daylight before showing your made-up face to the world!

I never recommend blending foundation with fingers. Instead, use a sponge. **Painting a wall with your fingers would leave streaks and lines, and the same is true for applying foundation to your skin. Using the flat, smooth surface of a sponge is the best way to get a smooth application.** The best tool is a flat, square, or round one-quarter-inch-thick sponge that doesn't have holes and is not made of synthetic foam rubber. Together, the shape and density of this kind of sponge provide the smoothest application possible. I know that many makeup artists, from Kevyn Aucoin to Bobbi Brown, advocate finger application of foundation. The rationale is that the warmth of your fingers will help the foundation mesh with the skin and provide a more natural look. If you feel more comfortable finger-painting than using a sponge, go for it. But humor me and make sure you always smooth out the edges of your finger-applied foundation with a sponge. I think you will find the results will be well worth the effort!

Be good about cleaning or changing your sponges frequently, particularly if you tend to break out or have rosacea, psoriasis, seborrhea, or eczema. While sponges are great blending tools, they love holding on to bacteria, fungi, and yeast that can aggravate those conditions.

The sponges frequently found for sale or in use at most cosmetics counters are the thick, wedge-shaped, foam-rubber ones. These sponges are compact, but they drag over the skin, and that makes blending difficult. Also, because they're so thick, most of the foundation is absorbed into the sponge, where you can't get to it, which can waste a lot of product. Wedge sponges are used for traditional theatrical makeup. They are great for applying grease stick or pancake foundations, which require more "pull" across the face to apply them evenly, but that is the last thing you need when you're wearing a lightweight foundation. Shiseido, Sephora Collection, and Paula's Select make some excellent makeup sponges—and these can be washed repeatedly without falling apart.

To achieve an even application with your nice, thin, flat, square or round sponge, shake some of the foundation from the bottle onto the sponge, then transfer the foundation to the face and over the eyes by dabbing the sponge over the skin. You can also use your fingers to transfer the foundation in dots from the bottle to the face and then use the sponge to blend the dots. Start by placing the foundation generously over the central area of the face, including the eyes but avoiding the sides of the face near the hairline, jaw, and chin. The foundation can go on in large patches or small dots all over the nose, eyelids, cheeks, and forehead, but only in this central area. Avoid placing the foundation all over the face unless you want a full makeup application or are using a foundation that contains sunscreen as your only source of sun protection. By concentrating the foundation over the central part of the face, as you blend down and out from the center there will be less foundation at the jaw and hairline. When applying a foundation with sunscreen, apply an even layer all over the face, and use the clean side of your sponge to softly feather the edges of the makeup at the jaw and hairline. The objective is to soften, but not wipe off, the foundation.

Once the foundation is on your face, begin using your sponge to blend the foundation evenly. **Holding the sponge between your fingers and thumb, spread the foundation down and out over the entire face with a stroking, buffing motion, going in the direction of the hair growth.** (Going against the direction of the hair growth on your face coats the hair with too much foundation.) The idea is to blend the foundation color out from the center of the face, where you initially placed it, to the perimeter of the face, leaving no line of demarcation at the jaw or hairline. Use the edge of the sponge *without* foundation (or turn the sponge over to the clean side) to dab or buff away any of the excess that tends to collect under the eye or around the nose. You can also use the sponge to wipe away any of the excess that gathers at the jaw or hairline. When blending the foundation, do not try to force it into the skin. There is a fine line between blending something on and wiping something off. Instead, blend a thin layer over the face, smoothing it with your sponge as you go. Using this technique, you can build coverage as desired. At this point your sponge should not be full of foundation; if it is, you've used too much.

If you did not apply a concealer before the foundation, you can apply it now and blend that into place. Apply the concealer, which is a shade or two lighter than the foundation, over the under-eye area and other areas you want to highlight, then dab it into place with your finger or sponge.

Watch out for the jaw and neck. This is very important. **Never, ever put makeup of any kind on the neck; you do not want your makeup to end up on your collar.** Always double-check your blending. Places on the face that you are likely to miss with foundation include the corners of the nose, the tip of the nose, the corners of the eyes (especially over the concealer), and the edge along the lower eyelashes. Also, some places are likely to end up wearing foundation that shouldn't, including the ears, the jawline, and the hairline—especially blonde hairlines. Be careful to remove this foundation if you've gone past your mark. Both situations can make your makeup appear sloppy.

**Your sponge is an exceptional blending tool that you should keep near you at all times. When the edges of your blush or eyeshadow need softening, you can blend out the hard edges with the side of the sponge that was used to spread the foundation over the face.** Using the side of the sponge that has foundation on it as opposed to the dry edge allows the sponge to glide over the blush or eyeshadow without streaking or rubbing it off.

## APPLYING A MINI-APPLICATION OF FOUNDATION

If you dislike the feel of foundation or if you want to wear the least amount of foundation possible, yet you still want the benefits that wearing a foundation provides (mainly helping blush and eyeshadows go on more evenly) there is an alternative. The thing most women don't like about foundation is how it feels when it's applied all over the face. One way to solve that problem is to not apply foundation all over, basically because it isn't necessary. (Of course, if your foundation contains your sunscreen, that does require applying it evenly all over the face.) The key points to remember, aside from the question of sunscreen protection, are that foundation is needed primarily to give the blush and eyeshadows something to adhere to, and to even out skin tone. This means that if your foundation color matches the face exactly—and after you finish this section, it will—you can apply a mini-application of foundation just over the areas where you will place the blush and eyeshadows. This way you won't feel heavily made up and the blush and eyeshadows will still go on evenly.

For a mini-application, place the foundation only over a mask-shaped area between the eyes and mouth, including the nose and cheeks. Coverage is not needed on the chin, forehead, or jaw area. Be sure to blend the edges carefully with your sponge. Apply the concealer the same way you would for a full makeup application. You may also want to consider a tinted moisturizer if you want a touch of color and minimal coverage. Lancome, Aveda, Neutrogena, and Bobbi Brown all have excellent options for tinted moisturizers.

## BLENDING OVER THOSE FINE LITTLE WRINKLES

If you've started to notice that foundation or concealer is sinking into some of those little wrinkles on your face, especially the laugh lines, lines under the eyes, or near the crow's feet (I have no regard for the person who came up with the term "crow's feet" to describe the lines extending from the back corner of the eyes!), you have to be even more meticulous about how you blend your foundation into place. In this regard, less is best. Blend, blend, and blend again, being sure to remove the excess in those areas with the clean side of the sponge. Continue blending intermittently while you apply your lipstick, blush, and/or eyeshadow to ensure that you have removed the excess.

Minimize your use of moisturizers over the areas where you have lines, and use a foundation or concealer that's neither greasy nor too emollient. Anything with movement and slip gives the foundation a free ride into the lines.

As for those concealers and foundations that claim to deflect, reflect, or somehow improve the appearance of wrinkles: They don't. And the cosmetics lines that sell foundation primers, which are usually just moisturizers with extra film-forming agents (hairstyling-type ingredients), don't work all that well either, plus they just add another layer of product to the face, which increases the likelihood of clogging pores, exacerbating breakouts, or creating dull-looking skin. **The truth is, a face without foundation always looks less wrinkled. I'm not sure why this has to be so, but it is. You can test this for yourself.** Go to the cosmetics counter, find the most expensive foundation with the most elaborate claims about making the skin look less wrinkled, apply a sample to one side of your face, and leave the other side naked with just a dab of moisturizer over dry areas. Then check out your face in the daylight. You will be amazed how much more noticeable the lines on the foundation side of the face are. Of course, the foundation side will look smoother and will have a more even tone, the redness and blotchiness will be gone, and the pores will have virtually disappeared. But the wrinkles will be more noticeable than on the side without foundation. That's the agony and ecstasy of foundation!

## FOUNDATION MISTAKES TO AVOID

1.  **Do not buy a foundation before trying it on and checking it in the daylight.**

2.  **Do not wear foundation unless it matches your skin color.**

3.  **Do not wear a foundation that is lighter than your skin, or you will end up looking chalky or pale.**

4.  **Do not wear pink, peach, rose, orange, or ash-colored foundation.**

5.  **Do not wear oil-based foundations unless you have very, very dry skin. Oil-based foundations can look greasy and appear more orange and pink than other types of foundation.**

6.  **Do not wear oil-free or ultra-matte foundations unless you have very oily skin. Oil-free and ultra-matte foundations can look quite thick and matte and make lines on the face more evident.**

7.  **Cream-to-powder foundations work best for normal skin. The cream part can be too greasy for oily skin and the powder can be too dry for dry skin.**

8.  **Use foundations that have shine for a special evening look.**

9.  **Do not apply a thick layer of foundation; thin and sheer are the operative words when it comes to applying foundation unless you are wearing a foundation with sunscreen, in which case liberal, even application is essential.**

10. **Do not use your fingers to blend your foundation over the face unless you're willing to go over your handiwork with a sponge.**

# BRUSHES

Before we go on to powders, eyeshadows, and blushes, it is crucial to discuss the most important blending tools you can use (besides the sponge for blending on foundation)—brushes. Brushes are simply the best way to apply almost all types of makeup, and you'd be hard put to find a makeup artist anywhere who disagrees. Moreover, after years of struggling with those tiny, pre-packaged sponge eyeshadow applicators and doll-sized blush brushes, we now have a profusion of brushes to choose among. Whether they're from M.A.C., Prescriptives, Bobbi Brown, Trish McEvoy, Stila, Maybelline, Aveda, Lorac, BeneFit, Paula's Select, or other lines, good brushes are available in an impressive array of sizes, shapes, and sensual textures that facilitate makeup application in ways that feel artistic and effortless. As with anything related to cosmetics, though, a high price does not always mean superior performance. And having more brushes does not mean you will be able to apply your makeup better.

The personal set of brushes you choose is determined strictly by how you prefer to apply your makeup. If your makeup application is elaborate and nuanced, involving several eyeshadows, contour, and highlighting, you need a variety of brushes. If your makeup application is uncomplicated and basic, you need fewer brushes. It's that simple. (The reason makeup artists carry an arsenal of brushes is because they see a vast assortment of eye and face sizes.) All you need is a group of brushes that match the areas of your face and the kinds and colors of makeup you apply. A good, basic collection of the brushes I recommend is shown in the photographs on pages 428 and 429.

**As a general guideline, it is best to not purchase a pre-packaged set of brushes unless you know you will use all of them and the particular shapes and sizes will meet your needs.**

The general rule to follow when considering what size brush to purchase is: **Does the size of the brush match the size of the area you are working on?** Too small and it will take longer to apply your makeup and it can end up looking striped. Too large and you can end up with a messy application. If you are lining the eye, a tiny thin brush with few hairs and that doesn't scratch or feel stiff is best. If you are filling in the brow, a small angle brush with a slight amount of stiffness to control the color is best. (It should be small and stiff enough to fit through the spaces in the hair and follow the edge of the brow with pencil-like control.) For the eyelid, choose a brush size that fits the curve of your lid, and the same reasoning applies for the crease area. Both should be determined by the size of your eye, and there are countless eyeshadow brush sizes to choose from. To highlight along the brow, a soft, small wedge brush (less stiff than the brow brush), fitting just that area, is best. Try not to use the same brush for both lighter and darker shades of eyeshadow.

**How many and which brushes do you need?** A full makeup application can require three basic eyeshadow brushes, an eyeliner brush (for liner and brows), a blush brush, contour brush, large powder brush, a lash brush (an old clean mascara wand will do), a brow brush (here a toothbrush will do nicely), and a lip brush.

Here is a good basic group to consider. I recommend **two or three eyeshadow brushes**, including one for the lighter eyeshadow colors and one for the crease. If you want to save time and money, you can use the edge (side) of the eyeshadow brush you use for the lid to place a light color under the brow. If you want the perfect tool, a small, soft **wedge brush** for that area is best. If you are shading the back (outside) corner of the eye with a dark eyeshadow, you may want to select a **smaller eyeshadow brush** than the one you use for the lid or crease. Again, the shape of your eye determines the size of the brush you choose.

If you don't use a pencil, a **tiny, thin eyeliner brush** is best for building either a thick or thin line along the upper and lower lashes. While some makeup artists use thicker brushes that are more square or wedge-shaped for this purpose, I think they are harder to control (they can make a thick line, but it's hard to get them to create a thin line, while a tiny thin brush can do either). If you're unsure, experiment with both styles and see which you prefer. A **wedge-shaped brow brush** can be used just for the brow to apply eyeshadow powder or to smooth out the line of an eyebrow pencil. Personally, I use a tiny eyeliner brush to fill in the brows to keep the shading soft by creating hair-thin strokes. An old **toothbrush** is still the best tool for combing through the brows. For combing through the lashes, I strongly recommend a good, densely packed **used mascara wand** that you wash clean, like the ones in L'Oreal Voluminous, Maybelline Illegal Lengths, and Lancome Definicils mascara. Most lash brushes that are sold separately have bristles that are too far apart to be helpful for easy unclumping and separating. Avoid metal eyelash combs—these can be incredibly painful and damaging if you accidentally poke yourself in the eye.

Both the **blush brush** and **powder brush** should have a soft, firm texture and not splay out when placed on the skin or into the color (no brush should be so loose as to splay when used either on the face or in the product). They should also feel soft and silky, yet hold their shape. If a brush is too wobbly, it will be hard to control the color. I often recommend getting two good blush brushes in the same size and using one for powder and one for blush (you don't want to dust color over the face). Many powder brushes, though they may feel incredibly soft and luxurious, are too large, cumbersome, and hard to control. It's nearly impossible to maneuver some of these behemoth brushes under the eye, along the corner of the nose, or along the cheek without hitting other areas of the face that may not need powder, and using too much powder is extremely likely.

If you are looking for a **contour brush** to shade along the temple, jaw, or cheekbone, a smaller blush brush is a great choice. Brushes specially designed for this area come in a variety of sizes, but the flat edge of these specially designed brushes, though impressive in appearance, can create just that, a hard edge, which takes more blending to soften than necessary. Simply use a small, half-inch-wide version of your blush brush; the idea is that this contour/blush brush should fit the hollow of the cheekbone.

I'm not among those who diligently apply lipstick with a **lipstick brush**. I just don't have the time. Generally, I save this precision for special occasions or when I want to use up every last drop in the tube. But if you like this option, look for a

Now This Is A
# GREAT BRUSH COLLECTION

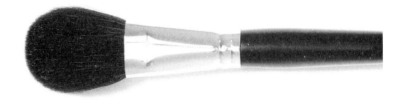

**1 POWDER BRUSH:** Don't get one that's too big or you will end up spreading too much powder over your face or powdering areas you don't want powdered.

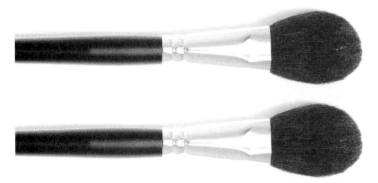

**2 BLUSH BRUSHES:** One for blush and one for contouring.

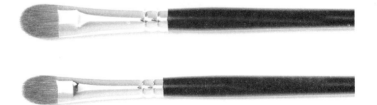

**2 EYESHADOW BRUSHES:** One small rounded brush for the crease and back corner of the eye and one large rounded brush for the lid and under-brow area.

1 ANGLE BRUSH: For shaping eyebrows.

1 EYELINER BRUSH: For lining eyes or for shaping eyebrows.

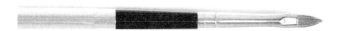

1 TOOTHBRUSH: For combing through eyebrows and eyelashes.

1 CLEAN MASCARA WAND: For combing through eyebrows and eyelashes.

1 RETRACTABLE LIP BRUSH, OR LIP BRUSH WITH CAP

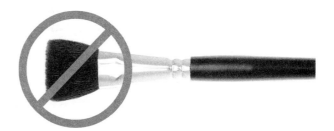

AVOID SHARPLY ANGLED CONTOUR BRUSHES—They can leave streaks.

brush with bristles that are strong and slightly stiff. Tug hard on the brush and make sure it doesn't move in the least. Look for a brush the size of your lips. Too small and it can take forever; too big and you'll be applying lipstick to your face. You know those retractable metal brushes you see almost everywhere and in every price range? They are all the same, and they are excellent! Retracting the bristles neatly back into place beats trying to keep the little plastic protective sheath on a wood-handled brush. (They never stay on and lipstick ends up getting all over your purse and makeup bag!)

You may notice that some brush collections sport a white, thin, slightly stiff brush sold as a **concealer** or **highlighter brush**. If you use a lighter shade of concealer for smile lines, under the eyes, on the corners of the nose, in the center of the chin, a dab in the middle of your lips over lipstick, or to spot-cover a blemish, this brush is a consideration. Many makeup artists use this type of brush to do things that most people (including me) do with their finger or their foundation sponge. Supposedly it allows better blending with less drag. It definitely helps you use less product, and also let you more easily reach tight spaces, such as along the lower lash line, the corner of the nose, and the edge of your lips. One thing it does not help in the least is keeping the concealer or highlighter from creasing into lines, despite what the salesperson will probably tell you.

I am not an advocate of foundation brushes, despite the fact that many lines now offer these as part of their brush collections. Quite simply, using foundation brushes takes longer than using a sponge (or fingers if you're so inclined) and they require more maintenance between uses. Depending on the type of foundation being used, these brushes can create a striped or streaked appearance. If you are tempted to try them, experiment with them before making a purchase so you can be sure you like the final result with whatever foundation you use.

## BRUSH QUALITY AND CARE

As you check out the different lines of brushes, the first thing you will hear about is the so-called quality of the bristles, and the salespeople will use this to justify the cost. Depending on the line, you will hear pretentious claims about squirrel, sable, pony, goat, and several other animals that did not give up their coats voluntarily. Synthetic brush hair is an option for those who are 100% vegetarian. However, synthetic brush hair is not preferred for most makeup application other than foundations and concealers. The most reliable synthetic brushes are from Origins, Paula Dorf, and Shu Uemura.

Although natural bristles are definitely softer (and often more expensive) than synthetic, it does not take sable to make the perfect brush, and mixed-hair bristles can make for a stronger, more pliable brush that doesn't lose its shape. Natural hairs tend to get softer over time, which means a firm, well-controlled brush can eventually become floppy and too soft. Salespeople who encourage you to buy the expensive brushes will claim that synthetic hairs get coarser and stiffer, or fall out after a year or two of usage, but that is not true. Synthetic hair brushes hold up as well if not better than natural hair brushes.

Ignore the claims about hair quality and trust your own **touch and feel tests.** Brush the bristles along the nape of your neck and ask yourself, "Is it smooth? Do the bristles hold their shape? Does it feel too loose, too stiff, or too soft? Does the brush feel densely packed, meaning lots of hairs, or flimsy?" Once you decide which feel you prefer, you can determine which brushes you want to work with.

Now that you have a sense of the feel part of the test, use the touch test to ascertain how the brush will hold up. Simply tug at the bristles, pulling away from the handle end, to see if there is any give. Do any hairs fall out? If you feel any release whatsoever, this is not a well-constructed brush. Some brushes are not well anchored and bound into the base of the brush. For example, Maybelline's incredibly inexpensive brushes beautifully pass the feel test (they are wonderfully soft and firm), but fail the touch test (the bristles tend to pull out). In the short term they are a superior bargain, but they won't hold up over the long haul.

Some cosmetics lines still sell the bamboo-handled brushes with white bristles. These are often the sparsest of brushes and are not constructed very well. They are a great example of the type of quality to avoid. Yes, they are attractive, but they are a waste of money. Along a related line, the more elaborately adorned a brush is, the more likely it is to fall apart. Look for simple, solid, streamlined construction.

When it comes to the **shape of the brush**, generally it is best to avoid blunt brushes and brushes with the bristles lined up flat with a severe edge. For most brushes—eyeliner, lip, eyeshadow, blush, and powder—look for ends that are more dome-shaped. Not only do these have a softer feel, but they also allow for a softer, less hard-edged application, which is almost always the goal. The only exception is the wedge brush for the brows or under the eyebrow.

When I'm doing my own makeup for media appearances or doing someone else's makeup, I personally favor brushes with long, elegantly tapered wood handles. But when I try to squeeze these long-stemmed beauties into the small makeup bag I travel with or keep in my briefcase, I realize how cumbersome they can be. For women who want to invest in only one set of brushes, short handles are not only more convenient, they are essential.

When it comes to **caring for your brushes**, some people claim you must wash them frequently. If you are a makeup artist working on lots of people, you should be washing your brushes every day. But for those of us who are working on ourselves only and not changing colors on a daily basis, once a month is just fine (and I won't tell anyone if you don't do it that often). Especially for natural-hair brushes, frequent washing breaks down the hair shaft and that breaks down the brush hairs. Also, washing too often can loosen the glue in the handle that holds the bristles together and keeps them in place. When you clean the brushes, concentrate your effort on the bristles, not the handle.

It is best to use a regular shampoo instead of a special brush-cleaning solution (which is just shampoo anyway). The shampoo shouldn't contain any conditioning agents, which can build up on the brush just like they do on the hair. L'Oreal Colorvive Gentle Shampoo and Paula's Choice All Over Hair and Body Shampoo are great inexpensive options. A conditioner is not necessary when caring for your brushes. Brush hair is extremely healthy. It isn't damaged from dyeing, perming, styling, brushing, and the other things people do to their own hair, which requires the use of conditioners. When washing your brushes, carefully follow these steps:

- Gently but thoroughly wash the brush in tepid water.
- Meticulously rinse the brush.
- Carefully press out the excess water and dab the brush dry.
- Arrange the bristles back into their original shape.
- Let the brush air dry flat on a towel without the help of a blow dryer, which can damage bristles.

## BRUSH TECHNIQUES

Brushes can be foolproof tools for applying makeup, yet it is definitely possible to use brushes incorrectly. I've seen enough women use their brushes in a rubbing or wiping motion on the face to know how often it can happen. Many women beat at their faces with a wild brushing motion as they attempt to apply their blush and eyeshadows. There truly is an easier and more effective method. When you wipe, beat, or heavily rub the brush against the face, it may be removing what you just put on, not to mention wiping off the foundation underneath, which can result in a streaky uneven appearance. The best technique is to brush in short, light, purposeful motions that glide over the skin.

If there is a distinct line where the brushstroke was placed or if you feel an urge to use your finger to blend what you've just applied, most likely you are not using the brush properly or your brush is too stiff for a soft application. (You may also have applied your foundation too thickly or used a foundation that is too greasy, or the blush color you've chosen is too strongly pigmented for your skin color.) You should avoid blending anything with your fingers—use your brush or the flat, square, thin sponge you use to apply your foundation. Remember, use your sponge for applying foundation and softening edges of your blush, contour, and eyeshadows.

Something else that is critical to using brushes effectively—even though it may seem insignificant at first—is the way you pick up the powder on your brush before you apply it. **Never smash or rub your brush into the powder. Rather, gently place your brush into the powder without moving the bristles.** You don't want to see the brush hair bend or splay. Always stroke through the powder evenly and always knock the excess powder off the brush before you apply it to the face. This prevents applying too much color to the first place your brush touches. When it comes to makeup, it is always easier to add than subtract!

## Brush Mistakes to Avoid

1. **Do not use hard or stiff brushes.**

2. **Do not use a brush that is too big or too small for the area of the face you are working on.**

3. **Do not use brushes that are too soft or ones with bristles that are too sparse, they won't hold up over time.**

4. **Do not forget to knock the excess powder off the brush before you apply the color to your face.**

5. **Do not wipe or rub the brush across the face; instead, gently brush on the color with short even strokes.**

6. **Do not forget to use your sponge to blend out hard edges and soften your color application.**

7. **Do not forget to gently wash your brushes every month or so, unless you are using them on a variety of people, in which case you should be washing or disinfecting them every day.**

# POWDER

Classic makeup application requires powdering after you've applied your foundation, but powdering doesn't work for all types of foundation. Powdering works best after applying a water-based, oil-based, or matte foundation that isn't all that matte. It is either unnecessary or problematic to apply powder over most oil-free or matte foundations, all of the ultra-matte foundations, or any of the pressed powder, cream-to-powder, or liquid-to-powder foundations. Some stick foundations that dry to a powder finish do not need extra powder, but those that remain creamy do.

If you are using a water-based or oil-based foundation, you may indeed want to apply powder to absorb any excess moisturizer or emollients that may make the face look too moist or too dewy. However, the less powder you build up on your face, the less made-up you will appear. Overpowdering also makes the face look dull and dry, especially if you have dry skin or darker skin tones. Some amount of natural, dewy shine to the face is very attractive. **I think it is a 1950s' notion that the face should not shine at all and that a woman must constantly wipe powder over her face to reduce the shine (and then apply shiny eyeshadows, blush, lipstick, or powder so the skin shines, but artificially).** After a foundation is applied, the slight shine that is left behind (except with oil-free, matte, ultra-matte, and pressed-powder foundations) gives the face a radiant glow. Powder is great for touch-ups as the day goes by to dust down excessive shine (see the photograph on page 461), just avoid overpowdering.

## TYPES OF POWDER

**Loose powder and pressed powder:** Loose powder is exactly what the name suggests. It tends to provide a more sheer, light application and can be best for someone with normal to oily skin. Pressed powder is merely loose powder with added waxes or emollients to keep the powder in a solid form. While pressed powder is heavier than loose powder, it is more convenient and a lot less messy. Both loose and pressed powders are perfectly fine options and it is a matter of personal preference which you use. What is essential, though, is to choose a powder that is the same color as your foundation. If your powder is lighter than your foundation, you can end up looking pasty and pale; if your powder is darker, you will look like you're wearing a mask.

**Pressed powder with sunscreen:** A few cosmetics lines, including Paula's Select, Jane Iredale, and Neutrogena, offer pressed powders that contain effective sunscreens. These powders are nearly identical to regular pressed powders except that they have a slightly thicker texture and provide more substantial coverage, along with an SPF 15 or greater including UVA-protecting ingredients avobenzone, titanium dioxide, or zinc oxide. Because sunscreens must be applied liberally to ensure sun protection, I generally do not recommend relying on pressed powders with sunscreen as your sole source of UV protection. Most women simply would not use enough of the powder to get the designated SPF number, and overpowdering is not an attractive option. Therefore, pressed powders with effective sunscreens are an excellent way to add to the UV protection you get from your sunscreen or foundation with sunscreen, particularly for those with oily skin. For longer days in the sun or times when it is not feasible to redo your makeup to maintain sun protection, pressed powders with sunscreen can be very convenient and extremely practical.

Talc is the basic element in almost all loose and pressed powders, but some companies opt to use mica (which lends a shiny finish), cornstarch, or rice starch (both starches have a light but very dry feel). Keep in mind that using powders made from corn or rice is not the best option if you're prone to breakouts. The bacteria that cause acne thrive on food ingredients like this, so why would you give something you don't want (blemish-causing bacteria) what it needs to grow?

**Application:** Apply the powder with a large (but not too large), full, round brush. Avoid using a sponge or powder puff, which can put too much powder onto the face. Pick up some of the powder on the full end of the brush, knock off the excess, and brush it on using the same motion and direction as you did for the foundation. Apply everything in the same direction to help retain a smooth appearance.

If you are touching up your makeup later in the day, before powdering, use your sponge, a facial tissue, or special oil-absorbing paper to dab away excess oil from the face. Then apply the powder.

Some makeup artists use a powder puff to press the powder into the skin for a very flat, matte finish. As professional a touch as this may be, it is best only for photographs. A powder puff places too much powder on the skin and can look thick and heavy in real life. Powdering with a makeup sponge has the same effect as using a powder puff, although the "pores" of the sponge do allow for a slightly less matte look. However, this can still lay too much powder on the skin.

**Pros:** If you want to reduce shine or moisture on the face, powdering is the fastest, easiest way to get the job done. Sans foundation, powder can lend a polished, sophisticated look to the skin.

**Cons:** There are really no drawbacks to wearing powder, except overdoing it, using the wrong color, or building up too much powder on the skin. There are also some powders that have sparkles or shine added to them. I have even seen some matte or oil-free powders that contain shine. If powdering is meant to reduce the shine produced from your oil glands or from your foundation or moisturizer, it is a huge mistake to do that with a shiny powder. Clearly, that would defeat the entire purpose. If you do want to use powder to add shine, see the next entry, "Powder that shines." Other than that, powdering is a basic step for almost all skin types to help keep makeup looking fresh during the day.

**Powder that shines:** If you want to use something to make the skin look luminescent and shiny, one of the best ways to do that is with powder that has shine. Apply this after your foundation and regular powder, and only dust it over the areas you want to glow, such as the cheeks, chin, center of the forehead, shoulders, neck, and décolletage. Most makeup lines offer at least one shiny powder, and some lines offer several. If you want to try a shiny powder, be sure to check the finish in daylight so you can really see how shiny it is and decide if this is the look you had in mind.

## TALC IN FACE POWDERS: FRIEND OR FOE?

Talc is often maligned as an awful cosmetic ingredient that should be avoided, but I do not agree in the least with that assessment when it comes to makeup products. The concern about talc is not about how it is used in makeup, but, rather, when it is used in pure, large concentrations in the form of talcum powder. Part of the story here dates back to several studies published in the 90s that found a significant increase in the risk of ovarian cancer from vaginal (perineal) application of talcum powder (Sources: *American Journal of Epidemiology*, March 1997, pages 459–465; *International Journal of Cancer*, May 1999, pages 351–356; *Seminars in Oncology*, June 1998, pages 255–264; *Cancer*, June 1997, pages 2396–2401.)

However, subsequent and concurring studies have cast doubt on the way these studies were conducted or the conclusions they reached (Sources: *Journal of the National Cancer Institute*, February 2000, pages 249–252; *American Journal of Obstetrics and Gynecology*, March 2000, pages 720–724; *Obstetrics and Gynecology*, March 1999, pages 372–376).

While more research in this area is being carried out to clear up the confusion, none of the research about the use of talc is related to the way women use makeup. There is no indication anywhere that there is any risk for the face when using products that contain talc. That means you need not avoid using eyeshadows, blushes, or face powders that contain talc. But it absolutely means you should consider never using talcum powder on your children or on yourself vaginally. If you still wish to avoid talc in makeup, it is easy enough to do so simply by checking the ingredient list.

## POWDERING MISTAKES TO AVOID

1. **Never buy powder without testing it over your foundation first. Even if the powder is translucent, it always has some amount of color to it, and that color and its extra texture over the skin can greatly affect the appearance of your foundation. Powder should match the color of your skin (and foundation) and not change the color of either. Never powder with a color that is lighter or darker than your foundation.**

2. **Never powder with a white, orange, pink, or coral shade of powder; it will make you look either pale or overly made-up.**

3. **To help prevent a caked appearance don't forget to dab off excess oil from the face before you apply your powder during the day to touch up your makeup.**

4. **Do not apply more than the sheerest layer necessary to take away excess shine; the face can handle only so much powder before it starts looking thick and heavy.**

5. **Do not powder more than necessary during the day. Powder only once or twice a day to prevent buildup, even if you are using a pressed powder with sunscreen.**

# EYESHADOW

I've been watching and evaluating other makeup artists and their eyeshadow techniques for years. Though there are myriad alternatives, eyeshadow design is usually built on an application sequence that allows you to create a flow of colors in either one, two, three, or four steps. The four steps involve applying a succession of colors that can be anything you want them to be, but if the goal is a classic makeup application, the colors proceed gradually from light to darker. The basic technique is to apply the lightest shade either just on the eyelid or all over the entire eye area (including the crease and up under the eyebrow) and then to place each progressively darker shade in a more specific section of the eye area, such as the crease and/or the back corner of the eye (see the photographs on page 462).

## TYPES OF EYESHADOW

**Aside from powder eyeshadows, other types available include liquids, pencils, cream-to-powder, and creams. Though these can be fun and easy to use, they are hard to blend and control.** Makeup artists rarely, if ever, use the liquids or pencils, but some opt for creams as a change of pace from powder eyeshadows. Overall, I don't recommend them. I admit they're fun, but I just wish they worked better to create a more sophisticated blend of colors. Almost without exception, cream eyeshadows crease and fade, and they're not the type to choose if you have trouble making mascara or eyeliner last because their emollient consistency can cause smearing and smudging of these other products.

## USING BRUSHES TO APPLY EYESHADOW

Eyeshadow should be applied exclusively with brushes, and it's best to use brushes that are designed specifically for eyeshadow. Never use sponge-tip applicators—they drag across the eye and tend to blend colors in streaks. Once you get used to good brushes, you will never go back to the sponge-tip applicators again.

When applying eyeshadow, use the flat side of the brush against the eye. Gently wipe the brush across the eyeshadow, knock the excess off the brush, and apply it with long, stroking motions across the eyelid, crease, or under the eyebrow area. This motion of laying strips of color that overlap and blend together over the eye as opposed to beating the brush back and forth across the eye is the way to achieve an even, well-blended design.

Remember that the size of the brush should match the size of the eye area you are working on. If you have a large eyelid area, use a brush that is wide and full. If your eyelid is small, use a smaller brush that's the same width as the lid. The same rule is true for the crease area (if a specific color is being placed just there) and the under-eyebrow area. Using brushes that match the job is essential to putting makeup on effectively and efficiently. Do not purchase or use brushes that have hard, coarse bristles or you will end up with hard edges where the eyeshadow couldn't be blended, not to mention irritated skin.

## DESIGNING THE EYE MAKEUP

Makeup books and cosmetics salespeople describe and demonstrate all kinds of eye-makeup designs—say, a dab of pastel yellow in the center of the lid, teal across the crease, taupe above the teal, pink above the teal, and gray in the back corner of the lid. Not only do I think those designs are too complicated, I've never, at least not that I can recall, seen a model on the cover of any fashion magazine wearing a multicolor pastel eye design.

**The most beautiful makeup applications, the ones you see and admire the most on models and actresses, are neutral, not colorful.** Look at any fashion magazine. You're not going to see pastel or vivid eyeshadows on many faces, unless it's a purposely eccentric or bizarre montage. Too many competing pastel or vividly colored shadows make the eye design distracting. Pastel and primary colors (green, blue, red) are hard to blend together, so they stand out. Besides, the general purpose of eyeshadows is to shape and shade the eye, not color it. **The only way to shape the eye is by shading it with neutral shades such as taupe, brown, gray, ash, beige, tan, mahogany, redwood, caramel, sable, charcoal, and black.** Eyeshadows are called *shadows* for a reason—they build shape, movement, and interest via shading, not with color.

The list of appropriately neutral colors and tones available is actually quite extensive. Yet color on the eyelid is best kept as subtle as possible, or you will end up creating an eye makeup design that is more noticeable than your eye. **As a general rule, for a classically applied makeup, the lips and cheeks provide color on the face. More color standing out around the eyes can be overkill.**

Be cautious about thinking you need to choose a design based on the need to correct a perceived facial problem, such as your eyes being too close together, too far apart, too round, or not round enough. There are no standard facial dimensions that define how attractive you or your eyes are. You can end up with a contrived look that allows the makeup to be more noticeable than your eyes.

The best way to choose which design to wear is to decide what image you want to project. The more shading you use, the more dramatic and formal the eye makeup design; the less shading, the more subtle and casual the design. Other considerations when choosing one eye-makeup design over another involve your skill at applying makeup, your personal preference, and the amount of time you want (or have) to spend. For example, if you are new or unaccustomed to wearing makeup, keep your entire makeup look simple until you become adept at the different application techniques. The same thing goes if you have only a few minutes in the morning to put your makeup on—it is best to keep your routine simple. Trying to apply full makeup very quickly can result in mistakes or a sloppy application.

## APPLYING AN EYE-MAKEUP DESIGN

Options for building an eye design are almost too numerous to list. The basic concept is to shade the eye to accent its shape, or to change its shape by using a progression of light to dark colors across the eye, blending one over the other so that you can't see where one stops and another starts. Here I will explain, step by step, how you can use one eyeshadow or several different eyeshadows to create a well-blended, classic eye-makeup design. Even for the most formal eye-makeup design, four different colors should be plenty. Whether you use one, two, three, or four different eyeshadows, they become a full design when worn with eyeliner, temple contour (see the "Contouring" section later in this chapter), and mascara.

**One-color eye-makeup design:** This design blends one soft, subtle color all over the eye area, from the lashes to just under the eyebrow, with no patches of skin showing through. You should not wear only a splash of color over the eyelid and ignore the rest of the eye area.

**Application:** When applying a single color, first place it from the lashes to the crease, making sure that you do not extend the color into the inside corner of the eye (off the lid area) or out beyond the lid onto the temple. Also be certain there are no patches of skin showing through on the lid next to the eyelashes. The entire lid at this point is one solid color.

Next, place the color from the crease up to the brow, following the entire length of the eyebrow from the nose out to the temple area. Avoid leaving a hard edge at the back (outside) corner of the eye where the eyeshadow stops. If desired, fade the eyeshadow as you blend up and out from the crease. This will create subtlety and a soft highlight under the eyebrow. Because the eyeshadow for the one-color eye-makeup design is so soft and subtle, blending and application is quite easy. The best colors for this design include light tan, neutral taupe, beige, pale mauve brown, pale gray, light golden brown, camel, and light auburn. Whatever the color, it should definitely not be obvious.

**Two-color eye-makeup design:** This is one of the most common, practical eye designs for many women. You can approach this design by applying the lighter color to the eyelid and the deeper color from the crease up to the brow, or you can apply the deeper color to the lid and the lighter color from the crease to the brow. Generally speaking, the under-eyebrow color should be a shade or two darker than the lid color. You do not want it to be a distinctly different color, just a different shade. The lid can be taupe, beige, tan, camel, gray, light auburn, golden brown, or any light neutral shade, and the under-eyebrow color would be a deeper shade of the same color. Women with darker skin tones can wear muted rose, mauve, or peach as long as it doesn't make their eyes look irritated or isn't too obvious. Bright, shiny, or whitish shadows can look dated and make the brow bone look more prominent and heavy.

Which color and what shades go where? **The general rule is that the larger or more prominent the eyelid area is compared with the under-brow area, the darker or deeper the eyelid color can be; the smaller the eyelid area is compared with the under-brow area, the brighter or lighter the eyelid color can be.** The notion is that if the eyelid area is already prominent or large, it isn't necessary to make it appear any bigger by applying a light color to it. If the eyelid area is small, it is appropriate to make it more prominent by wearing a lighter color.

**Application:** Whichever way you choose to apply this design, the lid and under-brow shades should meet—but not overlap—at the crease. As an option for the two-color eye-makeup design, you can apply the light shade to the lid and the darker shade from the crease up to the brow. Then, using a small wedge brush, you can use the light color again as a highlight just along the lower edge of the eyebrow. This can bring dramatic, but subtle, attention to the shape of the brow and the eye without the need for another eyeshadow color. You can also apply the lighter color from the lid to the under-brow area and use the darker color in and slightly above the crease. Then take the brush and use the darker color to softly shade the back corner of the eye, being sure this shading is an extension of the crease color. For more dramatic variations on this theme, see the descriptions below.

**Three-color eye-makeup design:** Start by applying either of the basic one- or two-color eye-makeup designs mentioned above. Once you have done that, the third shade, an even deeper color than the two previous colors, is added to the back (outside) corner of the lid or in the crease, or over both the crease and the back corner of the lid.

In this design, the lid and under-brow colors are softer and less intense than the color at the back corner of the lid or in the crease. Regardless of where you place this third, darker color, it can be a beautiful deep shade of brown, charcoal, cedar, mahogany, sable, red-brown, slate, chocolate brown, camel, deep taupe, or even black.

**Application:** If you apply the third eyeshadow in the crease, the trick is to not get the crease color on the lid, but rather to blend it slightly up into the under-eyebrow area and out onto the temple. Be sure, when sweeping the crease color across the eye, not to follow the down-curving movement of the shape of the eye. The best look is achieved if you blend the crease color out and up into the full back (outer) corner of the eye, and up onto the back of the brow bone.

When you apply the crease color, be sure to watch the angle of your brush as you blend the color from the crease out and up toward the under-brow area. If you place your color with the brush straight up at a 90-degree angle, you will look like you drew on wings. The softer the angle and the fuller the sweep, the softer the appearance, so be certain you blend *out* and slightly *up* from the lid area toward the under-brow area.

If you apply the third color at the back corner of the eye, the color hugs a small section of the lid, blending out and up into the crease and temple area. I explain this step in more detail for the four-color eye-makeup design.

**Four-color eye-makeup design:** In this design, you again start with the one- or two-color eye-makeup design, then add a darker color to the crease and an even darker color such as black or deepest gray to the back corner of the eye. Shading the back corner of the eyelid involves the arts of placement and blending. Because this area almost always requires a dark color, blending is essential to make it look soft, with no hard edges.

Why bother with a crease color and more shading at the back corner of the eye? The best part of this full eye-makeup design is that it shades, defines, and creates movement by adding a shadow in a curved flowing motion that follows the natural shape of the eye. The difficult part of this design is blending the crease color across the entire length of the eye without making it look obvious, choppy, or smeared. The goal is to tuck the color just in the crease at the fold nearest the nose and have it hug the crease until you get to the back corner of the eye, where you start the movement of the eyeshadow up and out onto the brow bone. Again, this sweep of color should not look like a stripe across the eye.

**Application: Be sure to knock the excess eyeshadow off your brush, and apply the color with very small strokes over the back corner of the lid only.** The problem here is keeping the color on the back of the lid only. If you don't know how to handle the brush, the back wedge can take up more than half of the eyelid (looking more like a mistake rather than carefully blended shading) or look like a stripe across the temple.

As mentioned above, when you apply the crease color, be sure to watch the angle of your brush as you blend the color from the crease out and up toward the under-brow area. If you place your color with the brush straight up at a 90-degree angle, you will look like you drew on wings. The softer the angle and the fuller the sweep, the softer the appearance, so be certain you blend out and slightly up from the lid area toward the under-brow area.

Remember, the center or fold of the crease area is always the darkest, so start your brush there and blend out in each direction. Concentrate your efforts on how much of the crease area you want to shade. You can start all the way at the front part of the eye area under the front third of the brow, then follow the crease through the center, blending slightly up toward the brow. As you approach the back corner of the eye, begin your movement up and out toward the temple, aiming toward the eyebrow.

## EYESHADOW TIPS

1. Matte powder eyeshadows in an array of neutral tones from light to dark are your best bets for a classic, sophisticated eye design that accents the shape and color of your eyes.

2. Unless you're using just one eyeshadow color, use at least two eyeshadow brushes for application.

3. Prime the eyelid and under-brow area with a matte-finish concealer, foundation, and/or powder before you apply eyeshadow. This helps to ensure a smooth, even application and (if you have fair to medium skin) will also neutralize the red and blue coloration of the eyelid.

4. Tap off any excess eyeshadow from your brush before applying—this will prevent overapplication as well as flaking eyeshadow.

5. If you really want to make the color of your eyes pop, choose a contrasting color in a soft tone and apply this to the lids. Blue eyes come alive with pale peach or cantaloupe hues, green eyes seem richer with light bronze or caramel tones, hazel eyes become more alluring with chestnut and golden brown shades, and brown eyes are nicely accented by almost all neutral tones.

## EYE-DESIGN MISTAKES TO AVOID

1. **Do not overcolor the eyes; too many bright colors can be distracting, not attractive.**

2. **Do not create hard edges; you should not be able to see where one color stops and another starts. Practice your application and blend well!**

3. **Do not wear bright pink or iridescent pink eyeshadows; they make eyes look irritated and tired. Muted or pale pink is an option, but be very, very careful. If it makes the eye look irritated or "red," it isn't the color for you.**

4. Do not wear shiny eyeshadows of any kind if you are concerned about making the skin look more wrinkled because they exaggerate the appearance of lines. If you have smooth, unlined eyelids and prefer a touch of shine, apply it sparingly and look for a low-wattage glow instead of distracting glitter.

5. Do not apply lipstick or blush over the eye area; it might sound like a time-saver, but if you have a lighter skin tone, it can make you look like you've been up all night crying. However, most bronzing powders can work as eyeshadows.

6. Do not match your eyeshadow to your clothing or your eye color. If you have blue eyes, blue eyeshadow would make the blue of your eyes look duller. And complementing your clothing is at best dated; besides, what do you do if you're wearing red or black?

7. Unless your goal is short-lived, messy eye makeup, avoid eye glosses and other greasy colors at all costs. These may look intriguing in photographs, but are more annoying than alluring in real life because they smear and smudge all over the place in a very short period of time.

# EYELINER

Do you need to wear eyeliner? As with any makeup step, eyeliner is completely optional. From an artistic perspective, if you are wearing eyeshadow, I almost always recommend wearing eyeliner, unless your eyelids and eyelashes are obscured by the eyebrow area. Eyeliner is a basic part of an eye-makeup design because it shapes and defines the eyes and makes the eyelashes look thicker. If you are wearing only mascara and not eyeshadow, or if you want an extremely soft look, eyeliner is not necessary. If you do decide to wear eyeliner when you are wearing mascara and no eyeshadow, be sure to line the eyes with only a very soft, well-blended eyeshadow color.

As with most aspects of makeup, eyeliner presents a host of options. There are eye pencils (both traditional and chunky), liquid liners, gel eyeliners, cake eyeliners, and powder eyeliners. When it comes to colors, what used to be a simple choice of black or brown has morphed into a range of hues that can be overwhelming. Depending on the look you're after and your personal taste, the color of your eyeliner can be anything from crimson to silver to gold, bronze, or even olive green. Although I strongly suggest staying with tried-and-true colors like black, brown, and gray, the final decision is yours.

## TYPES OF EYELINER

Since you can choose from among several styles of eyeliner, it is more important than ever to be aware of which ones have the best staying power, and which ones it's best to avoid. What kind of eyeliner should you use? Eye pencils are a quick, convenient option, but they do have problems; they tend to smear and unless you are using a twist-up pencil they are tricky to keep sharpened.

My favorite option over the years for applying a line is to use a tiny eyeliner brush with an appropriate color of traditional eyeshadow powder. I recommend using a dark-toned, matte eyeshadow color (almost any medium to deep eyeshadow color can work) and a tiny brush. I often apply the eyeshadow by wetting the brush and using it as "liquid" liner. The application is more controlled, but once it dries you have the soft look and the staying power of a powder without the hard edge that liquid eyeliners can create. A tiny, thin eyeliner brush allows absolute control over the thickness of the line around the eye. Another benefit to using powder and a brush is that you can use the powder as an eyeshadow just by selecting a different brush size.

**Pencil eyeliners** can often work well if you follow these basic rules:

- Self-sharpening pencils are by far the product of choice. Sharpening regular eye pencils is difficult, and keeping the point sharp without chewing up the pencil can be tricky.

- Remember that not all automatic pencils have a wind-down feature. That means if you wind up the tip of the pencil too high, it cannot be retracted and will likely break off.

- It is easier to apply pencil along the lower lashes than along the upper lid because the eyeshadows on the lid are harder for the pencil to stick to. You may want to consider using a greasy pencil for the lid and a firmer, less greasy pencil for the lower lashes. (If a pencil flattens when you press it, it will blend on more easily—but also will tend to smear more easily.)

- Warm the pencil between your fingers to apply a softer line of color; just remember this is not a surefire way to get a smooth application.

- To get a more precise line, if you have the time, leave the pencil in the freezer for a minute or two.

- Apply matching or similar powder eyeshadow over pencil to get the best of both worlds.

**Liquid eyeliner**, in general, is the most dramatic option, and when applied correctly (meaning a well-controlled, even line with no patches of skin showing through) it can definitely have an impact! However, getting the application right is more than half the battle with liquid liners. Even those that have well-tapered and firm but flexible brushes can be difficult to control and apply evenly to both eyes. Yet if you're intent on trying a liquid liner, the easiest (and I use this term loosely) way to apply it is after your eyeshadow design is done and before mascara. Do not blink excessively or touch your eye until you're sure the liner has dried. If you wish to apply liquid liner to the lower lash line (which almost always looks overdone), get the tip of the brush underneath the lashes and draw a thin line using light but steady pressure. For best results, liquid liner should be used only on the upper lash-line. Powder eyeliner is a softer choice for the lower lash-line, and you will lose none of the oomph that comes with well-applied liquid liner. Make sure the liners meet at the outer corner of the eye.

**Powder eyeliner** can be applied with almost any eyeshadow you have, but by far the best products for this are Bobbi Brown, L'Oreal, M.A.C., Trish McEvoy, and Paula's Select eyeshadows. Choose a dark shade of eyeshadow. Always line the eyes last—after all the other eyeshadows have been applied. Use a tiny, thin, slightly stiff brush. Whether you use your powder wet or dry (both are fine, but dry is softer and wet can be more dramatic), stroke the brush through the color, keeping the bristles together. Do not dab or rub the brush into the color. Move the brush across the eyeshadow in the direction of the bristles, making sure the form of the brush is not destroyed. Knock the excess color from the brush, then apply the color to the eyelid next to the lashes and under the eye near the lower lashes.

**Gel eyeliner** is similar to liquid liners in almost every respect, except the gels tend to go on sheer and need to be layered to achieve the same depth of color you get instantly from a liquid liner. Some gel eyeliners come in small jars and are painted on with the brush of your choice. These tend to go on like a true liquid liner and often have incredible staying power. Bobbi Brown's Long Wear Gel Eyeliner *($18)* is a good example of this type of eyeliner.

**Cake eyeliner** has been around for years and most of us have either seen or tried it at some point. Compared to a well-pigmented powder eyeshadow or even a standard liquid liner, cake eyeliner is more of an antiquated choice that has no distinct advantages over other types of eyeliners. If you're a devoted user of cake liner and like the results, stick with it. Otherwise, I encourage you to try other types of liner before considering this one to achieve a softer look with more options for neutral color choices.

## APPLYING EYELINER

Assuming you have a steady hand (if not, try this sitting down so you can steady your arm by placing your elbow on a table), position the brush, pencil, or applicator so it is as close to the lash-line along the eyelid as possible. Then draw a line from the inner to outer corner using one fluid stroke, following the curvature of the eyelid. Do not extend the line past the outer corner of the eye or hug the tear-drop area of the eye. To start, keep the line as thin as possible, and if a thicker line is desired, repeat the process either across the entire lash-line or simply on the outer third of the lid along the lashes. Making the line along the eyelid a solid, even one, starting thin at the front third of the lid and becoming slightly thicker at the back third of the lid can be an attractive classic look.

You can line all the way across the eyelid if you like, from the inside corner to the outer edge, or you can stop the line where the lashes stop and start. Along the lower lashes, line only the outer two-thirds of the eye. **Be sure the lower liner is a less-intense color than the upper liner. Also make sure that the two lines meet at the back corner of the eye.** As a general rule, avoid lining all the way across the lower eyelashes. Leaving some space on the inside corner of the eye where the lashes end near the tear ducts gives a softer less severe look. Plus, wrapping a complete circle of eyeliner around the eye tends to create an eyeglasses look and can make the eyeliner a stronger statement than the eye itself.

Makeup artists sometimes recommend that women over 40 not line the inner corner of the eye either on top or on the bottom. I think that's a fine suggestion. Instead, highlighting this area with a light shade of matte eyeshadow can be a very attractive alternative.

**How thickly can you line the eye?** As a general rule, for a classic look, the thickness and intensity of the eyeliner is determined by the size of the lid—the larger the eyelid area, the thicker and softer the eyeliner should be. The smaller the eyelid area, the thinner and more intense the liner should be. If your lid doesn't show at all, forget lining altogether.

You may have seen or heard a dozen other ideas as to how to apply eyeliner. Half-way across the lid, or one-third, or one-fourth, and three-fourths of the way under the lower eyelashes, or one-third, or one-fourth, and on and on. You are more than welcome to experiment with all these placements, but I encourage you to try the classic way first and see how you like it. Because the major reason to wear eyeliner is to shape the eye and make the eyelashes look thicker and deeper, I believe it is important to line where the lashes are and not just arbitrary sections of the lid. You can always line with a very soft color if you are concerned about overdefining the eyes, but I am not convinced that these "adjusted" lengths of placement look very natural.

**Should you apply 1960s-style liquid eyeliner?** Overexaggerated eyeliner with wings beyond the corner of the eyes is not a good idea. Depending on the effect you are trying to create, you can use a more definite eyeliner look most anytime of day. But for a more classic look, it is best to keep eyeliner soft by using powder or (if you prefer) by using a pencil and then applying powder over it.

**What about applying eyeliner in the rim of the eye?** There are many reasons why this is not a good idea. The first is that this kind of application smears in a very short period of time and creates goopy dark specks in the eye. Applying any makeup that is destined to smear in less than an hour or two is not a good idea. Pencil applied along the rim of the eye usually causes the area to become irritated; after all you are putting a foreign substance next to the mucous membrane of your eye. I am equally concerned about the health of the eye area when this technique is used. While there are no studies indictating there are any risks associated with pencil being applied to the rim of the eye, it seems problematic to put cosmetic ingredients (that include coloring agents and preservatives) that close to the eye.

**Which eyeliner color should you use?** For a classic eyeliner application, choose shades of dark brown, gray, or black eyeshadow for the upper lid and a softer shade of those—tan, taupe, chestnut, soft brown, soft gray, or soft black—along the lower lashes. Eyeliner is meant to give depth to the lashes and make them appear thicker. If the liner is a bright color or a true pastel, attention will be focused past the lashes to the colored line, as opposed to the more subtle flow of color from dark lashes to dark liner. Test it on yourself. Line one eye with a vibrant color, the other eye with brown or black, and see which one looks like it has thicker lashes. Then, if all my attempts to convince you have failed, and you still prefer to use bright or pastel liners, go for it.

## CHECKING FOR MISTAKES

After using powder eyeshadow as eyeliner, check for drippies under the eye and on the cheek. Drippies are those little powder flakes that fly off the brush and land on the cheek. Knocking off the excess from the brush every time helps prevent drippies, but there will always be flakes that end up where they don't belong. The best way to go after drippies is to use your sponge and simply wipe them away. If you do this, your next step is to touch up your foundation if that has gotten smeared.

Some makeup artists recommend applying a thicker layer of loose powder under the eyes and onto the upper cheekbone to catch the inevitable drippies, allowing them to be whisked off with a powder brush. If you have relatively smooth, unlined skin in this area you may want to try this. Otherwise, it can make the under-eye area look dry and enhance lines and wrinkles.

Always double-check the intensity of your eyeliner application and blend away any thickness or color that is more dramatic than you intended. It is not possible to blend or correct mistakes with liquid liners, which is one of the reasons I generally don't recommend them.

If you do choose to wear pencil eyeliner, check for smears under the eye as the day goes by. This is annoying, but letting it go without blending away the smears can make any well-applied eye-makeup design look like a mess.

## EYELINER MISTAKES TO AVOID

1. **Do not use greasy or slick pencils to line the lower lashes; they smear and smudge.**

2. **Do not use brightly colored pencils or eyeshadows to line the eye; they are distracting and automatically look like too much makeup. All you'll see is the color and not your eye.**

3. **Do not extend the eyeliner beyond the corner of the eye (no wings).**

4. **Do not make the eyeliner the most obvious part of the eye-makeup design.**

5. **Do not line the inside rim of the lids, between the lash and the eye itself; it is messy and can be unhealthy for the cornea.**

6. **If you do use pencil to line the eye, apply a small amount of eyeshadow over your pencil eyeliner to help set it and keep it from smearing.**

7. **Do not apply thick eyeliner to small or close-set eyes.**

8. **Do not use eyeshadow as eyeliner unless you use the proper brush.**

9. **Do not line the eye with a circle of dark or bright color. Both are too obvious and create an eyeglass-style circle around the eye.**

10. **Do not overblend, spilling your eyeliner onto the skin under the lower lashes; that makes dark circles look worse.**

# MASCARA

Mascara is an amazing invention and is considered basic to any kind of makeup application. Many makeup artists, including myself, say that if you're not wearing any other makeup but still want to wear something, wear mascara. On the other hand, many of us—and I'm guilty of this, too—get carried away and wear way too much mascara.

Women overdo mascara in part because the cosmetics industry tells us loudly and clearly that long, thick lashes are to be coveted, but even unadvised we covet someone else's long, beautiful lashes. When we apply mascara, visions of longer, thicker lashes sometimes come into view and then we get carried away and decide to apply more and more. Unfortunately, applying too much mascara increases the chances that the mascara will flake, chip, or smear, and that the lashes will appear hard and spiked. Also, the eyelashes can take only so much weight, and excess weight can break them. Lashes gunked-up with tons of mascara do not resemble long, thick lashes—they resemble gunked-up lashes!

The desire for longer, more noticeable lashes brings up the image of that ever-popular device that curls the lashes by squeezing them into a bent-upward shape. The problem with curling lashes is that it can bend the lashes into a severe angle that can look unnatural; and, although it can make them more noticeable (sometimes in an odd sort of way), it can also end up breaking them and pulling them out. Doesn't that defeat the purpose of making your lashes look longer? If you're still gung-ho on doing this, curl lashes only before you apply mascara, never after, or you will end up with broken, strangely bent lashes. The best lash-curlers are the ones with a sponge-tip section where the eyelashes are squeezed for protection. Squeeze gently with even pressure. Hold for a few seconds as you "walk" the curler along the length of the eyelashes, and release slowly. Some fashion magazines recommend heating the rubber pad of the eyelash curler by running your blow dryer over it for a few seconds. This may be worth trying, but be extremely cautious that the pad does not get too hot (touch it with your finger to be sure) because you don't want to fry fragile lashes or burn the eyelid skin.

## Types of Mascara

Mascara comes in two basic types: waterproof and water-soluble. Mascaras should not smudge, flake, or clump, and it is not your fault if they do. As is true for any aspect of the cosmetics industry, price does not tell you anything about how well a mascara performs. Drugstore mascaras can be as good as more expensive department store brands, and sometimes even better. **Regardless of where you buy your mascara, you might find that upon opening it, it already seems dried up. This is a recurring problem in the cosmetics world. Take it back immediately and get a refund or another tube.**

Can you extend the longevity of your mascara? If you want to, there are a few possibilities. First, do not overpump the wand into the tube in an attempt to build up mascara on the brush. All that really accomplishes is pumping more air into the tube, which makes the mascara dry up faster. Another solution is to avoid mascaras with a wide-bristled brush. To accommodate the wider brush, the tube opening needs to be larger, and this allows more air inside, again causing the mascara to dry out faster. Don't be fooled by the promise that wider bristles will make lashes longer. If anything, big brushes are clumsy to use, and they make it harder to get to the lashes at the corners without making mistakes. One last thing you may want to try is rotating the mascara wand around the inside of the tube. This will ensure you get any mascara that has been clinging to the sides of the tube and can help stretch mascara a bit further.

**Water-soluble mascaras:** The problem with some water-soluble mascaras is that they don't come off all that easily with water, even though they should. However, a great water-soluble mascara can go on beautifully and wash away easily. Again, there are many superior mascaras at the drugstore—this is not an area where you need to splurge!

**Waterproof mascaras:** These cause problems because to remove them you usually need to pull and wipe at the eyes, which can pull out lashes. I understand the desire to go swimming while wearing your makeup or to cry at weddings and not have mascara streaming down your cheeks, especially if you're the bride! Waterproof mascara is fine for occasional use, but wearing it every day can cause more headaches in the long run. Another drawback is that although most waterproof mascaras hold up well under water, they can still break down and smear when they meet the oil from your skin or emollients from your moisturizer or foundation. Do not make the mistake of thinking that waterproof means smearproof.

For those times when you do need waterproof mascara, the most effective way to remove it is with a silicone-based makeup remover that won't leave a greasy film on the skin. To be as gentle as possible, soak a cotton pad with the remover and lightly press and hold this against your lashes (make sure the eye is closed) for a few seconds. This helps loosen the mascara from lashes. Using very light pressure, move the pad down over the lashes and then back and forth, paying close attention not to pull or tug the skin. You can perform this step before or after cleansing.

## APPLYING MASCARA

The traditional upper-lash application of rotating the mascara wand by round-brushing from the base of the lashes up to cover all the lashes around the entire eye is the most efficient, expedient method. **Keep an old, cleaned-up mascara wand in your makeup bag to use for removing occasional mascara clumps (it can happen with the best mascaras) and separating lashes.**

Apply mascara to the lower lashes by holding the wand perpendicular to the eye and parallel to the lashes (using the tip of the wand). This prevents you from getting mascara on the cheek. It also makes it easier to reach the lashes at both ends of the eye. If you want a softer application on the lower lashes, wipe the wand down with a tissue and then apply lightly.

Have you ever had mascara end up on the eyelid or under the eye while you're applying it? Wait until it dries completely and then chip it away with a cotton swab or your sponge. Most of it will just flake off, with very little repair work needed. Always check for mascara smudges; they can look very sloppy and distracting.

## FALSE EYELASHES

Although I am not a fan of false eyelashes (primarily because you can almost always tell that they're fake), I realize that many makeup artists love to use them, and because they do, women wonder if they should try them, either to be doing the "proper thing" or for fun. Basically, false lashes are available in full sets or as individual lashes. Application always involves the use of an adhesive gel (such as Duo) and must be precise if you want the effect to look convincing. Removing false eyelashes can also be tricky, not to mention hazardous to your real lashes. Remember, there are lots of mascaras available that can come pretty close to giving a false-eyelash effect—you may want to experiment with these before ever considering falsies.

## MASCARA MISTAKES TO AVOID

1. **Do not wear colored mascara such as blue, purple, or green if you're going for a classic daytime look.**

2. **Do not wear mascara that smears or flakes; don't put up with those that do, because there are lots that don't.**

3. **Do not use waterproof mascaras on a daily basis; they can be difficult to remove and hard on fragile eyelashes.**

4. **Do not forget to apply mascara evenly to lower lashes.**

5. **Do not overapply mascara; your lashes will look clumpy or like thick-barred windows.**

# EYE MAKEUP—IS IT SAFE?

Mascara, eyeshadow, and eyeliner are intended to make women more attractive. One thing they shouldn't do is harm the eyes! Yet each year, many women suffer eye infections from cosmetics. At the time of purchase, most eye cosmetics are free from bacteria that could cause eye infections. Problems happen when they aren't adequately preserved against microorganisms or if they are misused by the consumer after being opened. Poor preservation or misuse of an eye cosmetic can allow dangerous bacteria to enter and grow in the product. Then, when the cosmetic is applied to the area around the eye, it can cause an infection.

The Food and Drug Administration has taken numerous steps to make sure that eye cosmetics are free from contamination when they reach you and that they contain preservatives to inhibit the growth of bacteria. The cosmetics industry generally makes products that will not harm you. Nevertheless, the FDA urges you to follow these 11 tips on the use of eye cosmetics.

1. **Discontinue immediately the use of any eye product that causes irritation. If irritation persists, see a doctor.**

2. **Recognize that bacteria on your hands could, if placed in the eye, cause infections. Wash your hands before applying cosmetics to your eyes.**

3. **Make sure that any instrument you place in the eye area is clean.**

4. **Do not allow cosmetics to become covered with dust or contaminated with dirt or soil. Wipe off the container with a damp cloth if dust or dirt is visible.**

5. **Do not use old containers of eye cosmetics. If you haven't used the product for several months, it's better to discard it and purchase a new one.**

6. **Do not spit into eye cosmetics. The bacteria in your mouth may grow in the cosmetic, and subsequent application to the eye could cause infection.**

7. **Do not share your cosmetics. Another person's bacteria in your cosmetics can be hazardous to you.**

8. **Do not store cosmetics at temperatures above 85 degrees Fahrenheit. Cosmetics held for long periods in hot cars, for example, are more susceptible to deterioration of the preservative.**

9. **Avoid using eye cosmetics if you have an eye infection or if the skin around the eye is inflamed. Wait until the area is healed.**

10. **Take particular care in using eye cosmetics if you have any allergies.**

11. **When applying or removing eye cosmetics, be careful not to scratch the eyeball or other sensitive areas.**

## EYEBROW SHAPING AND SHADING

No aspect of makeup seems to go through such dramatic fashion changes as eyebrow styles. Eyebrows are as representative of each fashion decade as clothes are. We've gone from overtweezed, pencil-thin, tortured brows to overdrawn, thickly penciled brows, to a full, bushy natural look, and now we've settled on very soft, natural, but definitely shaped brows. The best idea is for the eyebrows to be natural in appearance but not bushy or thick, with an expertly defined, but not pointed, arch.

## SHAPING THE EYEBROWS

Full, softly shaped eyebrows are easier to keep up but there is a balance between overtweezing and no tweezing. We are talking about natural, not Neanderthal. There is a middle ground between Groucho Marx and Greta Garbo when it comes to the appearance of your brows!

Discovering the best shape for your eyebrows without sacrificing a natural appearance is what you want to accomplish. The eye is framed by the arch, length, and thickness of the eyebrow. Just as the shape of a mustache can change the appearance of a man's face, the shape of the eyebrows can affect the appearance of the eyes. For example, if you tweeze too much off the front part of the eyebrows (near the nose), the eyes will appear smaller. If you tweeze too much from under the eyebrows, increasing the distance between the eye and the eyebrow, you can look permanently surprised.

Which hairs you leave and which ones you remove makes all the difference between attractively shaped brows and misshapen ones. And go slowly—because for some reason, over time, eyebrow hair does not always grow back after it is tweezed (there is no known physiological reason for this, but that is what many women experience). You can use an eyebrow pencil and a diagram to help you line up the following parameters for shaping your eyebrow.

The beginning of the brow should align with the center of the nostril, the arch should fall at the back third of the eye, and, although the eyebrow should be as long as possible, it still shouldn't extend into the temple area (see the diagram on page 457). **The basic rule is that the front part of the brow should never drop below the back part of the brow.** Allowing this to happen, either with the way you tweeze your eyebrows or the way you draw them on, makes you look like you're frowning and overemphasizes the downward movement of the back part of the eye.

What are the best tools? The best tweezers are the ones from Revlon or Tweezerman with tips that are slightly rounded to a soft point. Tweezers that are too pointy can stab the skin; if they're too flat across the top they can grab skin along with the hair. There are lots of other tweezers around in all kinds of shapes or with handles that snap together, but these all pose problems when it comes to reliability and ease of use.

## STEPS TO SHAPING A PERFECT BROW

1. **Before you start tweezing, use a lip or brow pencil to heavily draw on the shape you want; you can adjust it as you decide on the look you want.**

2. **Once the shape is drawn on, tweeze any hairs that fall outside the line of the brow.**

# EYEBROWS 101

Tweezing a soft natural shape is the goal; eyebrows that are too thick or too thin can take attention away from the rest of your face. Follow these steps to create beautiful eyebrows.

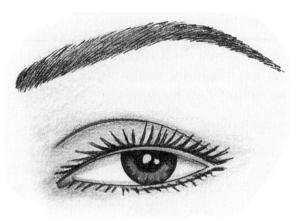

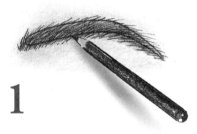

## 1

Draw on the shape you want with an eyebrow or lip pencil, following the natural growth as much as possible. Take your time with this step, repeating it until you get the look you want.

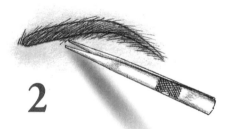

## 2

Tweeze hairs that fall outside the brow you penciled on. Use rounded or needle-nose tweezers for accurate removal.

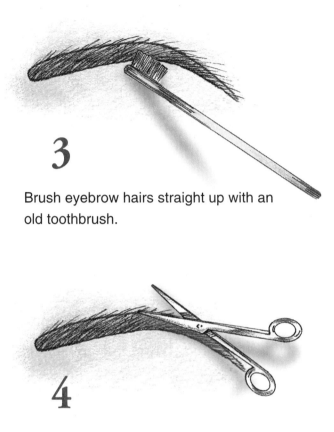

## 3

Brush eyebrow hairs straight up with an old toothbrush.

## 4

Trim hairs that are too long with a small pair of scissors.

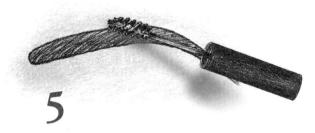

## 5

To keep brows in place, smooth the hairs with an old mascara wand and then apply brow gel or clear mascara, or spray the mascara wand with hair spray and then comb it through the brows.

3. Next, brush the brows straight up with an old toothbrush. Any hairs that are too long and floppy should be trimmed with small scissors. Tweezing long brow hairs rather than trimming them can result in gaps in the eye brow or a patchy look.

## TYPES OF EYEBROW PRODUCTS AND APPLICATION

**Powder eyebrow colors or eyeshadows used to fill in the brow** should be applied using a soft-textured powder (either an eyeshadow or a powder designed for the brow; both work great) that matches the brow color exactly and a soft wedge brush or a tiny eyeliner brush (I prefer the control of a small eyeliner brush). Follow the basic shape of the brow, using the same guidelines as for tweezing. Fill in only at the front or underneath the brow, or through the brow itself. Avoid drawing on color above the brow. For a softer look, brush through the eyebrows using a clean, old toothbrush.

**Eyebrow pencils:** These are a perennial option but be careful when deciding which one to use. Eyebrow pencils can can produce a greasy, hard look and mat the eyebrow hair, and too often you end up looking like you live in another decade. If you are presently penciling your eyebrows, seriously consider changing to powder. If penciling doesn't look absolutely natural, don't do it. Better to go without any eyebrow makeup at all than to be adorned with a line of pencil above your eye.

Many makeup artists use both pencil and powder to create natural-looking brows for women with little or no eyebrow hair, and this can be a great alternative. This way you can get the control and delineation of a pencil, and then soften and shade the effect with a powder. If you decide to try this, look for brow pencils that have a firm but smooth texture and slightly powdery finish. Avoid using any brow pencil that is painful or that applies color too dramatically or thickly.

**Application:** To apply the powdered brow color or brow pencil, brush the brow up with an old toothbrush and then apply the color with an angled wedge brush, filling in the shape of the brow between the hairs where needed. If your eyebrows are set high, away from the eye area, and you want to reshape them, place the color directly under the eyebrow. The closer the brow is to the eye area (meaning the height from the brow to the lid or eyelashes is small), the more you should fill in the color in the existing brow itself rather than shading just below the brow. As much as possible, work only with the hair that is there. The idea is to shade rather than draw on eyebrows. Do not place your brow color, whether it is pencil or powder, more than one-quarter inch away from where the natural hair growth stops. It simply looks fake and accentuates the fact that there is no brow there in the first place! What you want is the suggestion, the shadow of a brow—not a line and not an obvious application of color (see the photograph on page 463).

# BEAUTIFUL
# EYEBROW SOLUTIONS

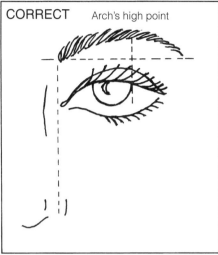

CORRECT — Arch's high point

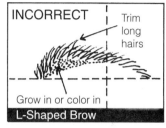

INCORRECT — Trim long hairs
Grow in or color in
**L-Shaped Brow**

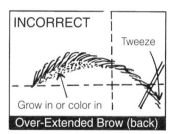

INCORRECT
Grow in or color in
**U-Shaped Brow**

**Perfectly Shaped Eyebrows:** The shape of the eyebrow is correct when the beginning of the brow is aligned with the center of the nostril and the arch falls over the back third of the eye.

**L-Shaped Brow**
**Problem:** The arch is over the front third of the eye.
**Solution:** Grow in or color in the indicated area.

**U-Shaped Brow**
**Problem:** The eyebrow has no arch.
**Solution:** Grow in or color in the indicated area.

**Over-Extended Brow (back)**
**Problem:** The back third of the brow is lower than the front third of the brow.
**Solution:** Grow in or color in the indicated area and tweeze the end of the brow to align it with the front of the brow.

**Over-Extended Brow (front)**
**Problem:** The front third of the brow is lower than the back third of the brow.
**Solution:** Tweeze the front of the brow to align it with the back of the brow.

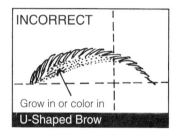

INCORRECT — Tweeze
Grow in or color in
**Over-Extended Brow (back)**

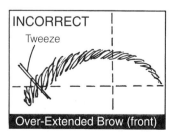

INCORRECT
Tweeze
**Over-Extended Brow (front)**

**Colored eyebrow gels:** These are a fairly recent development and a good option for making the most of sparse, light-colored eyebrows or for giving a thicker look to most other eyebrows. These products look like mascara but they have a much lighter consistency. Examples are Paula's Select Brow/Hair Tint *($8.95)*, Origins Just Browsing *($12)*, and Bobbi Brown Natural Brow Shaper *($16.50)*.

**Application:** Apply the color through the brow in much the same fashion as you apply mascara to the eyelashes. Brush the wand through your brows, being careful not to get the product on the forehead or other areas of the skin and not to leave the brows standing straight up. It will probably take you a few times to get the hang of it. You also might have trouble at first controlling the amount of gel from the tube to the brow. But if you want your brows to look fuller, give this one a try—it really works. The products mentioned above all have dual-bristled brushes, which can be used for a soft, full look or for more definition. Be wary of brow gels and tints with single- or small-bristled brushes because these can make application trickier (they often produce a lined or spotted effect).

## WHAT EYEBROW COLOR SHOULD YOU USE?

Generally, you should match the exact color of the brows rather than your hair color or a color you think would look better than what already exists. You don't want to see a difference between the eyebrow hairs and the shadow or gel used to fill them in. However, if you have pale eyebrows and want to darken the brow color, use a soft shade of brown that is as close to your brows' natural color as possible. If you have red hair and brown eyebrows, using a red pencil or red-brown powder will look unnatural; just stick with brown. If you have blonde eyebrows, you could use a slightly darker blonde or taupe color on your brows to make them visible. For those with well-shaped, naturally full brows, a clear brow gel (Cover Girl and Max Factor have good ones) is a great option for lightly grooming the brows without adding any color. You can also spritz some hair spray on an old toothbrush and comb through your brows, or add a dab of non-sticky styling gel to keep unruly brow hairs in place.

**What if you don't have any hair at all where the eyebrows are supposed to be?** This is the only circumstance that requires applying a brow color that matches the hair on your head. It will look the most natural. Use the wedge brush and powder to follow the bone above the eye, applying to whatever hair is there. Usually there's enough shape to create a natural, shaded impression of a brow. Use a light touch, with short, quick motions, and avoid the temptation to exaggerate the shape by arching it severely or extending it into the temple area. Downplay the fact that there is no hair; it's better not to overexaggerate the area with a strong, eye-catching line. Also, don't place a highlighter or light-colored eyeshadow under the brow to further emphasize the brow. Putting something dark next to something light makes it look even more prominent. Use what you have as the basis for any makeup application, and avoid making any obvious, theatrical changes. Once the brows are softly accented (or left alone), play up your lips or cheeks instead so that these will become the focus rather than your absent or too-sparse eyebrows.

## EYEBROW MISTAKES TO AVOID

1. **Do not overtweeze, and never tweeze above the brow, only underneath. Tweezing above the brow can ruin its natural shape.**

2. **Do not overstate the shape of the brow; minimal brow alteration is best.**

3. **Do not pluck brows into a thin line thinking it will make your eyes look larger. It will only look strange, contrived, even sinister. It can also give the face a surprised look, and none of this is attractive or natural—or easy to correct once the damage is done.**

4. **Do not use eyebrow pencil or eyeliner pencil to fill in your eyebrows unless you are adept at making it look very soft and shaded.**

5. **Do not apply eyebrow powders that are a different color than your own eyebrows; it is best to always match your existing brow color.**

6. **Do not apply brow color that is obvious or has a drawn-on look.**

7. **Do not forget that eyebrow color should look shaded and soft, not like a straight, hard line.**

8. **Be careful of brow colors that look red on the skin, which can make the eyebrow look fake and the skin look irritated. If you're in doubt when choosing between brow shades, go with the more muted option.**

# CONTOURING

Contouring is the art of creating or increasing shadows in certain areas so the face appears to have more structure and definition. It involves using brown tones of blush or pressed powder to contour along the sides of the nose, at the sides of the forehead, under the cheekbones, and in the center of the chin to add color, definition, and shape to the face. Although contouring is an optional step for most daytime makeup applications, it is still rather intriguing and is worthwhile for some women.

For the most part, the popularity of using contouring to reshape the face has subsided somewhat. The likely reason for its demise is that believable-looking contouring is difficult to master (even more difficult than believable-looking blush). Contouring takes skill and patience, and very few women have the time to deal with it every morning. Women who do decide to take the time often end up with a brown stripe under their blush, and that is not the way contouring is supposed to look! Think twice before incorporating this step into your daily makeup routine until you've practiced and developed the skill to apply this look softly. Without careful application and conscientious blending, what looks sculptural from the front may look odd from other angles.

Contouring is always done as a separate step, using a completely different brush and shade of powder than for the blush application. Shades of pink, red, and orange are used as blushes; only shades of brown are used in contouring. The safest contour shade to use if you have fair to medium-dark skin tones is one that looks like your skin color when it is tanned. A soft or rich golden shade of brown is generally the perfect color to use when trying to produce realistic shadows on the face. Shades of gray-brown can look dirty, and shades of red-brown and mauve-brown can look like bruising on women with fair to medium-dark skin tones. For women of color, particularly African-American women, either an extremely dark shade of golden brown or a deep chocolate brown color can work exceptionally well.

## Types of Contour

Contour is essentially blush in a golden brown or reddish-brown color. For the varying types of contour, take a look at the "Types of Blush" section below. The easiest type of contour to work with is applied with powder-based color. Cream and cream-to-powder contour colors can be extremely difficult to control and blend, which can interfere with proper placement—a major no-no when it comes to natural-looking contour color.

## Applying Contour

Instead of using a brush designed for contouring, use a brush designed for blush or rouge. (But avoid traditional blush brushes that often come packaged with the blush; they are too small for most cheeks, and so are a poor choice for blush or contour application.) Surprisingly, traditional contouring brushes are also a poor choice for applying contour because they are usually too stiff, have a flat edge, and can leave visible edges when you apply your color. Instead, use the full end of the blush brush when contouring. Knocking off the excess powder before applying, and brushing on the color in short, quick motions going back to the ear will net the best results. Here are some rules of placement to help you most effectively contour your face.

# MAKEUP APPLICATION
# STEP BY STEP

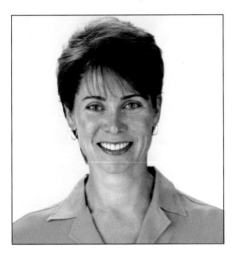

Jonette
Entrepreneur & Model

"Before"

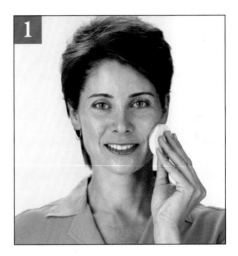

Foundation
Evenly blended application
using a thin sponge
(See page 421)

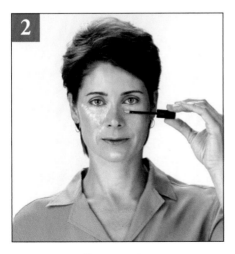

Concealer
Applied to dark circles and
areas to be highlighted
(see page 403)

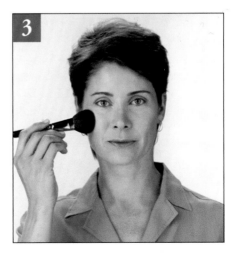

Powder
An even, light dusting "sets" makeup
and creates a perfect palette
(see page 434)

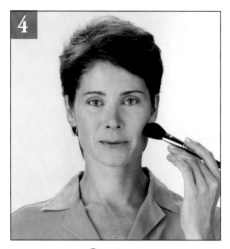

### Contour
Adds definition and some color
(see page 466)

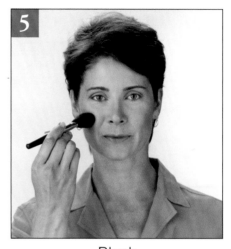

### Blush
Lightly applied along the entire
cheek area, from the "apple" to the
back of the ear (see page 467)

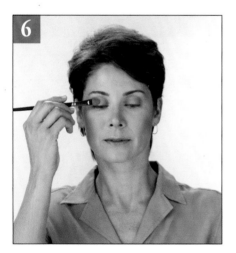

### Eyeshadow
Use an appropriately-sized brush
for the lid (see page 437)

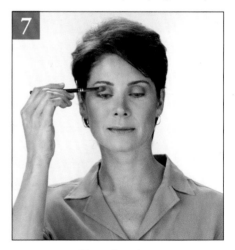

### Eyeshadow
... and a smaller brush for the
crease (see page 437)

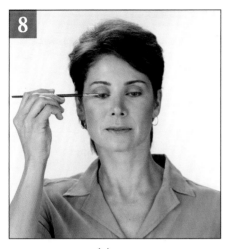

### Liner
Here, a slender brush is used wet
with powder (see page 445)

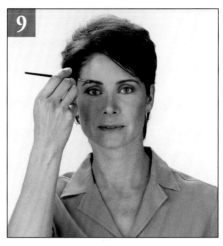

### Eyebrow
Defined brows help frame the face
(see page 456)

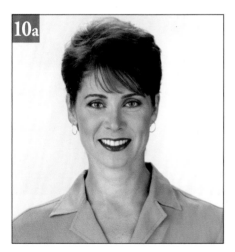

### Lipliner, Lipstick & Mascara
### Finished Daytime Look

The face is softly accented in neutral earth
tones on the eyes and light rosy-brown
tones on cheeks and lips. Each feature is
played up, but no single feature is more
prominent than another. The goal is a
flawless gradation of color with no hard,
abrupt edges.

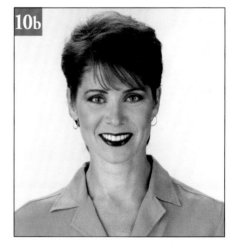

### Modified Eyes & Lips
### Finished Evening Look

Her daytime makeup was made more
dramatic by intensifying the eyeshadow
using a darker brown in the crease and
back corner of the lid. The eyeliner was
deepened with soft black powder
eyeshadow. Blush was left alone, and the
lips were played up with liner and a classic
red lipstick topped with a dab of gloss.

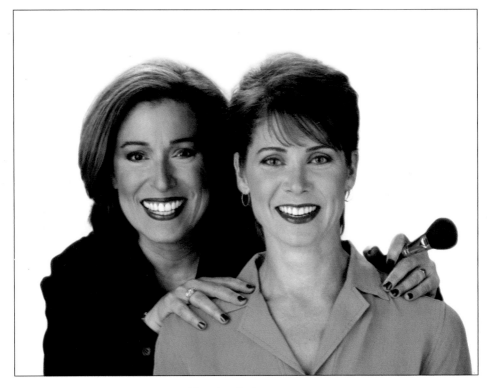

Paula & Jonette

**Contouring under or along the jawline:** Avoid contouring or shading along any portion of the jawline for daytime. Though this technique can make you look like you've lost a few pounds, you can end up with a line of demarcation around the jaw, negating the trouble you went through to find a foundation that leaves no such line. That means it will not look like natural shading. Nevertheless, shading the jawline or just under the chin can be passable for pictures or possibly for evening, but it must be applied very carefully. Shading under the jawline can also result in shading your collar at the same time. Be careful! Be sure to blend well and soften any noticeable edges or concentrations of color.

**Contouring under the cheekbone:** Place the center of your brush about one-quarter to one-half inch behind the laugh line, and stroke the color straight back, aiming toward the middle of the ear. The area of application should be approximately a half inch in width, with no definite edges visible. Use your sponge to soften hard edges. The starting point for under-cheekbone contouring is almost always the same regardless of the face shape, because the cheekbone corresponds nicely to the laugh line and middle ear area for most women. You can adjust the angle depending on your preferences. The steeper the angle going toward the top of the ear, the longer the face will appear. If you have a square or round face, you might want to try contouring at a steeper angle. The longer the face (as an oblong or triangular face might be), the more horizontal (straight back toward the middle of the ear) the line can be. This, in effect, de-emphasizes the length of the face. All this takes experimentation, so be patient until you achieve the look you want. Be sure to blend well and soften any noticeable edges or concentrations of color.

**Caution:** When applying the under-cheekbone contour, be sure never to blend or place the contour color below the mouth area, below the middle of the ear, or onto the cheekbone itself. There is also no need to suck in your mouth to help find your cheekbones—that will only help you find the sides of the mouth, not the cheekbone.

**Contouring the sides of the nose:** Although most women think that contouring the nose is strictly to make it look smaller or narrower or longer, there is actually a more artistic reason for using this shading technique. If you're applying a full makeup, particularly for evening, and you ignore the nose, you will have color everywhere on your face except for a blank spot in the center of the face. Contouring the nose helps to achieve color balance for the whole face when you choose to wear a formal, full makeup application. It isn't essential, but it's a great trick—and one that can be seen on models gracing the covers of almost every fashion magazine out there.

The goal is to make the contour color look absolutely as soft as possible. The challenge is to restrict the color to the sides of the nose. You never want to accidentally blend the color of the nose contour onto the area under your eyes or onto your cheeks. Take extra care to blend only a small amount of contour color on such an obvious focal point.

The best technique for applying the nose contour is to place the brush itself between your fingers and thumb, so the brush tip becomes somewhat flattened. This way the brush tip can more easily follow along the sides of your nose. (You can use the same brush you use for contouring or a very large, flat eyeshadow brush.) Now, take the index finger of your other hand, place it flat down the center of the nose, and apply the contour color along the side of your finger. Where the brush falls against your finger is the area to be contoured. Once you've done this, remove your finger and softly apply the contour fully around the tip of the nose and on the flare of the nostrils. Continue the contour in a narrow, soft line up under the eyebrow, avoiding the corner of the eye and the area between the eyebrows. Be sure to blend well and soften any noticeable edges or concentrations of color. Blend using very soft, short strokes and pay careful attention so that you do not spread the contour color onto the cheeks (see photograph number four on page 462).

**Contouring the temple area:** Temple contour is a traditional step that is as basic as applying blush. The difference is that most women don't know about it. Take a look at the cover of any fashion magazine or ad for designer clothes, and you will notice this contouring on most of the models. When temple contour is neatly applied, the eyeshadows at the back of the eye can be blended into it so they don't end abruptly with a harsh edge of color. Without temple contour, the forehead becomes a great bare wall against the colored background of the cheeks and eyes.

The temple contour is placed next to the back third of the eye near the brow bone, directly out and up onto the forehead like a pie wedge, but without the edges. Temple contour can be applied either before or after the eye-makeup design is in place. If you apply the contour after the eye-makeup design, it is important to place the brush directly over the eyeshadows at the back third of the eye and then brush the contour all the way back to the hairline. If you do the contour first, apply it in the exact same place and in the same way, but when you apply the eyeshadows, blend them directly over and onto the temple contour. Either way, the contour softens the back edge of the eyeshadows.

When temple contour looks wrong or unnatural, it's usually for one of three reasons:

1. Forgetting that this step begins at the back third of the under-eyebrow area, right on top of and over the back third of the entire eye area. It does not float on the forehead unconnected to the back corner of the eye.

2. Not brushing the contour directly over the eyebrow itself, which can make the application look choppy instead of smooth and even (you should apply the eyebrow color after the temple contour).

3. Applying the color in a straight one-inch strip next to the eye instead of in a softly blended two-inch pie wedge that is partially blended onto the forehead. Temple contour is a shaded area, like the blush area, and it should never look like a stripe. Be sure to blend well and soften any noticeable edges or concentrations of color.

## CONTOUR MISTAKES TO AVOID

1. **Do not use a blush color to contour any part of your face. Contour only with golden brown, chocolate brown, or dark brown shades.**

2. **Do not use contour under the jaw or at the chin area during the day; it can look too obvious and possibly get on clothing.**

3. **Do not apply contour as part of your regular makeup routine until you get used to blending it on softly; it should never look like stripes or brown lines on the face.**

4. **Do not forget to blend hard edges; contour should always look soft and as natural as possible on the face.**

# BLUSH

Knowing how to choose a great blush color and apply it correctly is essential to successful makeup application. Blush adds life and a hint of healthy color to the face and its importance should not be overlooked when you're deciding how to go about doing your makeup.

Blush is one part of makeup application many women take for granted. The comment I hear most often is, "I've been doing that for years. I know how to put on blush." Yet it is so easy to make mistakes, and I see them all the time. Blush is one of the more prominent parts of any makeup routine, so if you do make a mistake—such as applying it too close to the lines around the eye, applying it like a stripe of color across the cheek, applying the wrong color, or applying it underneath the cheekbones as if it were contour—it is very noticeable. I urge you to take time to learn how to apply blush properly.

I can't say that everyone agrees exactly where you are supposed to place blush! There are many opinions on where it should start, where it should end, and how high or low to place it along the cheekbone. My strong preference—one that is shared by many, as is evident in fashion magazines—is to keep the blush on the cheekbones and away from the eye area, blending the color just on the cheekbones and starting it about one-half inch behind the laugh lines. Some women start the blush no farther into the center of the face than the center of the eye. That can make the blush look very strange. The idea is to blush the entire cheekbone, and that means full across the cheek.

## TYPES OF BLUSH

**Powder blushes:** Powder blushes are an excellent choice for all skin types. They go on easily, blend beautifully, and come in great colors. A brush is essential for applying these smoothly, softly, and evenly.

**Application:** To find the area to be blushed, place the full end of your brush about one-quarter to one-half inch behind the laugh line. Starting here, brush downward and back toward the center of your ear, being careful not to place any color below the level of the mouth. Applying your blush by brushing down as opposed to back and forth eliminates a stripe effect. The blush area should be about two inches across, with no hard edges. Always use your sponge to soften edges.

**Pros:** There are only pros to this type; it works for just about everyone! The only possible negative for powder blushes is due to powder's naturally drier texture that can sometimes appear to sit on top of the surface of the skin, although this effect is usually short-lived. It can be eliminated altogether by choosing a silky-smooth, perfectly soft powder blush.

**Liquid, gel, cream, and cream-to-powder or stick blushes:** These are not my favorites and I recommend considering these carefully. The only real advantage they have over powder blushes is that they tend to mesh better with the skin, which on some women can look more natural—as if it were a "glow from within." Yet in spite of this minor positive point, liquid, gel, and cream-type blushes don't perform reliably for most skin types. They can be very awkward to blend evenly, and they tend to streak whether you use your fingers or a sponge. They can also stain the pores, making the face look dotted with color, and they don't work well over foundation—the foundation gets wiped off as you apply the blush. Still, if you have near flawless, smooth skin (no dryness and not oily), no visible pores, and have a deft touch at blending, you are a candidate for liquid, gel, or cream blush. It does help that many of today's cream blushes are silicone-based, which allows a clean, smooth application and a soft powder finish. Just don't buy anything until you check it out in the daylight and see how it wears during the day.

**Application:** There isn't one best way to apply these types of blushes. A sponge is my first choice, but some women do fine using their fingers or even a synthetic brush. Use whatever works best for you and always double-check to make sure there are no hard edges to soften. Gel blushes can be the hardest to blend evenly, so you may want to start with cream or cream-to-powder formulas.

## APPLYING BLUSH AND CONTOURING

If you are applying both blush and under-cheekbone contour, apply the contour color first and then blend the blush on top of and gradually down into the contour color. Then, using your sponge, blend until you meld the colors together into an attractive design. The hallmark of an attractive design is not being able to see where one color stops and the other starts. When done properly, blush and contour add color, depth, and dimension to a face—and that's always attractive.

## CHOOSING A BLUSH COLOR

How much color and which color should you use? That is not an easy question to answer. When it comes to a fashion statement the trends seem to change on a monthly basis. One month sheer, almost no blush color is the rage and the next mauve is the style. But by the time the next issue of your favorite fashion magazine is launched, peach, rose, pale red, and apricot blushes may be the style. What to do? Let go of the trends, they are exhausting, and what is trendy may not look good on you. Pale blush can look ghostly on many women, peach can look too sallow for some skin tones, and mauve can look ashen on olive tone skin. In the long run the color that looks best and most natural to your skin tone is the best place to start.

An option to consider when choosing blush color is to go neutral; a soft golden brown, tannish-looking color is a great foolproof choice for many skin tones. I personally use this look for the summer. For darker skin colors, a deeper golden brown works perfectly. Whatever option you choose be sure your lipstick colors match the underlying tone of your blush. In other words, if you are wearing a blush with a blue undertone, the lipstick should be in that same color family; rose blush means rose lipstick; coral blush coordinates with coral or coral/tan lipstick; though a soft tan-looking blush works with almost any color of lipstick. You absolutely do not want to wear pink blush and coral lipstick or mauve blush with orange lipstick. The point is for lipstick and blush colors to work together and not look like opposite, clashing ends of a rainbow.

Your blush color does not need to match your clothing, shoes, or any other accessories, although if you wear vivid clothing colors (fuchsia, turquoise, royal blue) your blush should ideally be in the same tonal family as your clothing to prevent an overly contrasted look.

## BLUSH MISTAKES TO AVOID

**1. Blush and lipstick colors should never clash; they should either complement each other or be in the same color family.**

2. **Never put blush close to or on the lines around the eye; it makes them look more evident, and if you are using a pink, peach, or coral shade of blush, the eye area can also look red and irritated.**

3. **Do not apply blush below the mouth or the laugh lines; blush is for the cheekbones only.**

4. **Do not blush your nose, forehead, hairline, or chin; it can make the face look overly pink or red or made-up. It may look great in professional photographs, but can look blotchy and uneven in daylight.**

5. **Do not forget to use your sponge to blend out hard edges or smudges of blush. Blush should always be well blended, with no visible edges where the blush starts and stops.**

# LIPSTICK AND LIP PENCIL

I'd hardly lose the bet if I said most of you already know about lipstick, but I've talked to enough women to know that my next sentence needs to be said. Luckily, it's not complicated: If you're wearing makeup, your lips need lipstick—not lip gloss, but lipstick. Lip gloss doesn't last, but lipstick does. Lip gloss provides a sheer, temporary look that can be great but doesn't go with a full or classic makeup look. Lipstick (cream, matte, or semi-matte lipstick, not overly iridescent) provides a polished and put-together look that can last at least until your second cup of coffee. If your lips are naked while your eyes and cheeks are made up, you will look like you forgot you had a mouth when applying your makeup. For the sake of balance, remember lipstick.

## TYPES OF LIPSTICK

Are there differences among lipsticks? Well, yes! In fact, there are vast differences. As you probably already know from experience, lipstick colors and textures can vary even within the same cosmetics line. Some are creamy; others are dry, greasy, shiny, or flat. Some melt easily; others go on stickily, smearily, evenly, thickly, thinly, and all combinations thereof. I recommend lipsticks that go on creamily, in an even layer that doesn't smear or look thick or greasy. Whether or not to go with a matte or creamy finish is your own personal preference. True matte-finish lipsticks do last noticeably longer than creamy (and especially sheer) lipsticks. The only way to find out which ones you prefer is to be patient and try on various formulas in the colors you like and see how they feel and look. But whatever you do, avoid wearing overly shiny or glittery lipsticks, particularly if you are an adult with a serious career. Glaring iridescence is best reserved for evening, not for daytime.

**Note:** If your lipstick has a tendency to cake or to dry out as the day goes by, avoid reapplying more lipstick over semi-worn-off lipstick. Wipe off all your lipstick first and then reapply. You may also want to apply a bit of lip balm under your lipstick if the problem of caking persists.

**What about lipsticks with sunscreen?** When it comes to sun protection, ignoring the lips is problematic. Not only is the skin on the lips very thin, it does not contain any melanin—essentially the rest of the skin's built-in defense against UV radiation. Although conventional, opaque lipsticks do provide a barrier (which is one of the reasons skin cancer on the lips is markedly higher in men than in women) for true sun protection, a lip balm with sunscreen applied underneath lipstick, or better yet a lipstick with built-in sunscreen is a must. A few cosmetic companies offer wonderful lipsticks with effective UVA/UVB sunscreens. The ones to look for are: Revlon Absolutely Fabulous Lip Cream SPF 15 *($8.99)*, Almay Protective Lip Tints SPF 25 *($4.99)*, and Cover Girl Triple Lipstick SPF 15 *($5.89)*. When checking an SPF-labeled lipstick, make sure the UVA-protecting elements of avobenzone, titanium dioxide, or zinc oxide are listed as one of the active ingredients. If they don't appear, or if they are listed anyplace other than the active ingredient list, you can't count on getting reliable sun protection.

**What about ultra-matte lipsticks?** Ultra-matte lipsticks are all essentially identical. They all go on moist and wet, then dry within a few seconds to form a dry, matte layer with no movement or creaminess. The dry texture does prevent transference to coffee cups, glasses, the food you eat, and the significant other you kiss. But it isn't indelible; this stuff does eventually rub off. Actually, it tends to chip or peel off. **Ultra-matte lipsticks are not for everyone, particularly not for those with a tendency toward chapped lips, because they will make the lips even drier.** Ultra-matte lipsticks can feel very uncomfortable during cold, dry winters or in hot, arid climates. Also, while ultra-matte lipsticks tend not to bleed, if you have wrinkles on or near your lips, these lipsticks will accentuate them. Due to trade-offs like this, which are inherent with ultra-matte lipsticks, many cosmetics companies have either reduced the number of or entirely discontinued these products. It seems that most women were not keen on putting up with the drawbacks in exchange for longer wear, and I understand the logic. However, if you have not done so already, you may want to consider the latest ultra-matte hybrids—the ones that use PermaTone technology to create truly long-lasting, comfortable color.

**Permanent Lipcolor:** The world of lipstick changed considerably when Max Factor launched Lipfinity in early 2001. Shortly thereafter, Cover Girl (a sister company to Max Factor, as both are owned by Procter & Gamble) launched the identical (and less-expensive) Outlast lipstick. What makes both of these products unique is that they use something called PermaTone technology to enhance application, wear, and—most significantly—comfort. PermaTone is a silicone-based ingredient complex that provides semipermanent color by gently attaching color pigments to the lips in a flexible mesh effect. The PermaTone "sets" (after approximately 60 seconds), yet the flexible mesh means the color is able to move and breathe, so that it doesn't dry or cake. Once the color has set, you apply a special top coat, an emollient, clear lip balm that does not disturb the color and provides a soft, glossy finish and comfortable wear. This top coat does not contain ingredients like mineral oil or petrolatum that could break down the color, which is good. But you may definitely need such ingredients to provide some extra help to remove it at the end of the day!

As great as this all sounds, there are some drawbacks to be aware of. First, these formulas offer opaque coverage and are not forgiving of application mistakes. That means you need to get the color on evenly and correctly the first time, or it's back to square one. If your lips are at all chapped, Lipfinity and Outlast will look terribly uneven, so be sure your lips are perfectly smooth and dry—no lip prepping with lip balms or Chap Stick because this will prevent the color from adhering to and setting on the lips. Once you have mastered the color application, you may find you need to reapply the moisturizing top coat frequently, which means you'll be using up more top coat than color (a common complaint from Lipfinity aficionados). Thankfully, you can purchase the special top coat separately. If you're willing to practice with this new breed of semipermanent lipsticks, you will find that unless you're eating very oily foods (such as salad with oil and vinegar dressing), they really do last all day (and often all night or into the next morning!) if properly applied. There is much less chance of cracking or peeling color with these when compared to traditional ultra-matte lipsticks, thanks mostly to the ingenious top coat. Lipfinity and Outlast come in a broad range of shades, and can be removed with plain mineral oil, Vaseline, or most other nonvolatile oils. If long-lasting lip color is important to you, these are a must-try.

## CHOOSING LIP COLORS

When choosing lipstick colors, there are three basic rules. (1) Thinner or smaller lips look best with brighter, more vivid colors. Brighter colors may take a bit of getting used to, but they truly make a smaller mouth more noticeable. Occasionally I read about or hear makeup advisors suggesting that women should wear a neutral color on small lips and instead play up the eyes (as if the notion is ever to play down the eyes or ignore the mouth!). Test this technique for yourself before you give in to this nonsense. (2) Avoid darker colors on thin lips; they make the mouth look severe and harsh. (3) Larger lips can wear just about any color, but softer shades look better because darker or vivid colors can make large lips look too prominent.

## APPLYING LIP COLOR

A lip brush or lip pencil is an optional accessory. You can use a lip pencil to draw a definitive edge around the mouth to follow when applying lipstick, and a lip brush to control your application. A tube of lipstick makes too wide a mark for some lips and too narrow a mark for others. If your lips are small, it is best to use a lip brush; if your lips are large, the only reason to use a lip brush is to improve your accuracy.

If you do choose to work with a lip pencil, always place the color on the actual outline of your mouth. Do not use corrective techniques that make the mouth look larger or longer, especially for daytime makeup. **If you try to change the outline of your mouth with a lip pencil by drawing outside the lips, some time later when your lipstick wears off, the lipliner, which almost always lasts longer than the lipstick, will still be in place and it will look like you missed your lips.** Always line the lips following their actual shape, then fill in the lipstick color, using either the tube or a lip brush.

**What about the center outline of the mouth? Do you round the point of the lips or make the point more obvious?** As a general rule, a softer appearance is better than a hard one. Leave the points neither rounded nor pyramid-like—someplace in between with a soft arch is best.

To prevent lipstick from gunking up in the corners of the mouth, don't place lipliner or pencil in that area. Stop before you get to the very corners of the mouth. If you feel doing this makes you look as if you have missed a spot, carefully fill in this area with color using a lip brush, but only the smallest amount.

Lip pencils should never create an obvious dark, brown, or clearly visible line around the mouth. Delineations like this keep showing up as if they were the latest thing, and women hold on to the look for some unknown reason, but I've yet to see a professional makeup artist choose this design. **Your lip pencil should not make an obvious line that shows up as a colored border around the lipstick. The goal is to have the lipstick and lip pencil meld so that you can't see where one starts and the other stops.**

If you wear lipliner and you want to help your lipstick last longer, apply the lip pencil all over the lip area, including the outline of the lips, and then apply your lipstick over it. This extra step puts a more permanent color on the lips, so the lipstick won't wear off as quickly as it normally does. **With the exception of Lipfinity and Outlast, there is no such thing as an all-day lipstick.** Even Lipfinity can present some reapplication issues if you eat oily foods, and there is still the issue of touching up with the moisturizing top coat. For years the cosmetics industry has been proclaiming new "all-day" or "long-wearing" lipsticks, yet women continually need to reapply their lipstick. To date it remains impossible for 99.9% of all lipsticks to make it past lunch, or even past midmorning, still looking the same as when you first put them on.

**How can you stop lipstick from traveling into the lines around your mouth?** The first step is to stop wearing greasy lipsticks and lip glosses. **The greasier the lipstick or lip pencil, the faster the color will slip into the lines around your mouth.** The drier-feeling lipsticks are best for conquering this problem. Powdering the mouth with loose powder before applying the lipstick also helps, but can be a bit messy. Lip pencil will not stop greasy lipsticks from traveling, but can slow them down.

Several years ago, some cosmetics companies came out with new products that were supposed to prevent lipstick from bleeding. I tried a lot of them and many never worked, but I finally found three that changed the way I wear lipstick. Regrettably, all of the options I used to love are no longer made. Refusing to be dismayed by this, I simply found out which company produced the formula (there are only a handful worldwide that make almost all cosmetic pencils) and added the formula I loved to my own line. If you were a fan of products like Coty's Stop It, Revlon ColorLock, or The Body Shop's No Wander, you should consider trying my Long-Lasting Anti-Feather Lipliner in Clear.

**Does using a lipstick brush help keep lipstick on longer?** Why using a brush would have this effect has never been explained to me in a manner that makes any logical sense, and it simply doesn't work. What does make lipstick stay on longer? When you wear strong, vivid colors that are not greasy, avoid wearing lip glosses, and put on a lot of lipstick!

## LIPSTICK AND LIP PENCIL MISTAKES TO AVOID

1. **Do not use a lip pencil that contrasts with your lipstick; it has been unfashionable since the '80s and it almost always looks severe and gives a contrived appearance to the mouth area.**

2. **Do not wear lipstick that is a different color tone from the rest of your makeup. For example, if you are wearing a rose-toned blush, wear a rose toned lipstick.**

3. **Do not use lip gloss in place of lipstick during the day; it can bleed and won't last as long as lipstick.**

4. **Do not wear noticeably iridescent lipstick; when it wears off, it can look dry, white, and caked; it also looks too distracting for daytime.**

5. **Do not exaggerate or change the shape of your mouth with your lip pencil or lipstick; it will look like you missed your mouth.**

**6. If you want your lipstick to last, wear more of it and don't blot; blotting takes off several layers before you've even left the house.**

# TOUCHING UP

As the day goes by, even the best-applied makeup can slip, fade, and get phone- or finger-printed. Lipstick can become thick and clumped, too. Long days call for a few quick touch-ups to revive beautifully applied makeup. Following the steps below, in order, will revive the look you started with.

- If you have oily skin, blot away the excess oil by laying either a tissue or one of the face-blotting papers sold by some cosmetics companies over the face and blotting. Perm endpapers also work well. Do this before you do anything else.

- Remove all of your lipstick so you can start over after you have touched up your face makeup. Apply a light layer of lip balm if your lips feel dry.

- Once the excess oil on your skin has been absorbed, take a fresh sponge and smooth out the foundation, blush, and contour (women with dry and normal skin should also follow this step). Use a gentle buffing motion, making sure to smooth things as you go.

- Apply a little extra concealer under the eyes if that area looks a bit dark.

- If you need a little more foundation over blemishes or discolorations, blend it on now, avoiding the blush and contour area.

- Dust a light layer of pressed powder over the face. A pressed powder with an SPF 15 including UVA-protecting ingredients of avobenzone, titanium dioxide, or zinc oxide is an excellent option to ensure all-day sun protection.

- Apply more blush or contour if needed, but *only* if needed, and be careful color "grabs" more over makeup that has been on the face awhile.

- If you want to touch up your eyeliner, particularly under the eyes where it might have smeared, use a powder shadow instead of a pencil. Use the corner or side of your makeup sponge to remove any smeared eyeliner.

- If your eyeshadows have creased, blot the area gently with a tissue or blotting paper and then use a brush to smooth out the color. Apply a powder over the area to even out the shadows and add whatever color is needed to make the eye makeup look balanced.

- Finally, reapply your lipstick and lipliner.

**Note:** If you are wearing an ultra-matte foundation, you may find that touch-ups are tricky because ultra-matte makeup doesn't move and reblending is almost impossible. In that case, you may very well be stuck with starting over. But it's worth a shot to see if you can blend things smoothly and do a simple touch-up. For me, ultra-matte foundations stay so well that my makeup never slips in the least once it's in place.

## TURNING DAYTIME MAKEUP INTO NIGHT

All right, you've touched up your makeup, but suppose you now want to change it from your office or daytime look to a knockout evening visage? Here are some ideas to consider:

- Add a dark or black shade of eyeshadow to the back corner of the lid or in the crease.
- Use the same shade of dark or black eyeshadow to create a more dramatic line around the eye.
- Use a wedge or angle brush to add extra definition to the arch of your eyebrows, or add a bit more brow powder to the ends of your brows (but don't overdo it).
- Use a powder that has shine to add some shimmering highlights to the cheekbones, center of the forehead, chin, neck, shoulders, or décolletage.
- A vivid red lipstick always makes a dramatic evening look, especially if you are wearing black.
- Avoid overdoing your blush. Making the cheeks look overly colorful doesn't improve an evening look.
- Avoid applying more mascara, unless you're adept at doing so without creating a clumpy, spiky mess.

## BALANCE, PROPORTION, AND DETAIL

Have you ever wondered exactly what it is you admire when you see a well-made-up woman? You may not be able to pinpoint what it is you find appealing, but you probably envy her skill and wish you could figure out how she did it. At the airport a few years ago, I noticed such a woman and watched other women (and a few men) turn their heads and take notice. It wasn't just that she was attractive and her clothes were stylish, but her makeup in particular was impeccable. Her face looked smooth and was accented with rich, though subtle, blush and contour tones. All the colors, from her lipstick to her eyeshadows, softly mingled into a harmonious sweep of light to dark, with just the right amount of shading—not too much and not too little.

That's when it occurred to me that any woman can revitalize her makeup by going over a list of everyday makeup guidelines and just omitting the mistakes that detract from, rather than enhance, her appearance. Recognizing the nuances of a well-done makeup application versus one that is not so good can make all the difference in helping a woman look great all day long. Considering all the time most women spend buying makeup and wearing it, putting it on wrong just doesn't make sense.

Besides the essential rules regarding application and blending techniques, there are only three basic concepts you need to keep in mind to achieve a flattering look: balance, proportion, and detail. **Balance** is about making sure the different elements of your makeup go together and that no one aspect is more prominent than any other. In other words, if you are wearing a dark, rich, brownish red lipstick, you must choose blush in a harmonious color (shiny pink blush is not going to work with a lipstick in that color range). Meanwhile, make sure your eyeshadows accent the eyes so they don't get lost because too much attention is directed toward the lips. When colors and tones are in balance and no one aspect of the makeup shouts over another, you don't notice the makeup as much as you notice the woman. Don't forget little things, like lining the upper lashes if you line the lower lashes (otherwise the line underneath will look too heavy and obvious all by itself). If you choose to wear blush, blend the color well so it doesn't stand out as a visible swipe of color across your cheek.

**Proportion** is about the total package of selecting what to wear. It's about paying attention to symmetry, to how your makeup colors, wardrobe, and hairstyle work together. If you are wearing a classic, tailored business suit and the eyeshadows you have on range from tan to black, with a wine-colored lipstick and blush, that may indeed be a stunning combination, but a bit too dramatic and overpowering with what you're wearing. The same is true for someone with very light hair and fair skin: the color combination may be dramatic and beautiful, but it will look out of place in sunlight or office light. Proportion is making sure that everything works together, with nothing looking out of synch, so your makeup doesn't upstage you.

**Detail** is the most essential and perhaps the most difficult area because it takes so much effort and concentration. Pay attention to every nuance of your makeup. If necessary, apply your makeup using a magnifying mirror so you don't leave the house with eyeshadow sprinkles on your cheek or mascara smudges at the back corner of your eyelid. Do not be satisfied with doing a ten-minute makeup application in only five minutes when you're in a hurry. **If you don't have enough time to do your normal makeup routine, be ready to change your look; do only what you have time to apply well.**

I can't tell you how often women have asked me what they can do differently with their makeup, and my responses were that they needed to blend their foundation better because it looked patchy and uneven, or the eyeshadow area looked uncertain or too obvious. Often these women reply, "Things were just frantic this morning, and this was the best I could do." I then say, "I notice you have your blouse buttoned and your skirt zipped up." Typically their answer is, "Of course!" I in turn comment, "Well, even though you didn't have much time, you didn't leave the house undressed. You should apply the same rule to your face." It doesn't mean being late because of your makeup; it means doing less so it goes faster. But whatever you do, take the time to do it right. Because when makeup is sloppy, it just looks wrong.

As I mentioned above, I use several levels of makeup application, depending on the time I have and what the makeup is for. For me, and I've done this a lot, full makeup for a television appearance takes 20 to 25 minutes. Makeup for a business meeting or a formal event takes 15 minutes. Makeup for casual daily business or informal get-togethers takes 5 to 10 minutes. Makeup for running to the gym to work out takes a minute and a half (lipstick and mascara only).

## GETTING YOUR MAKEUP TO LOOK THE WAY YOU WANT IT TO

- Foundation color should always match the skin exactly—no exceptions. Watch out for lines of demarcation in any light, but most of all in daylight.

- Be sure your foundation is best for your skin type. If you have oily skin, do not use a foundation for dry skin, and if you have dry skin do not use a foundation for oily skin.

- Concealer and foundation should blend together seamlessly. Be sure your concealer is not too light or white and is not a noticeably different texture than your foundation.

- Colors on the face should blend softly and without stop-and-start lines; that is, no stripes of blush or eyeshadow.

- Go light with the powder. After you find a foundation that matches your skin exactly and blend it on smoothly and sheerly, loading your face with powder would negate all your previous efforts. As a rule of thumb, the more wrinkles you have on your face, the less powder you should wear. Shiny powders (even the subtle ones) can magnify large pores as well as wrinkles and lines on the face.

- Powder should either match the color of your foundation or should be transparent and sheer enough to have no color effect on the foundation at all.

- Powder without any added oil is best for oily skin; powder with some amount of oil is best for dry skin.

- Blend, blend, and blend again.

- I know you have been staying away from shiny eyeshadows if you have wrinkles on your eyelids (right?), but many cosmetics lines are busily adding them to their collections and calling them matte, even though they have some shine. I highly recommend staying away from them. No matter how minimally shiny they may appear in the container, once they are on your eyelid, the shine will make the skin look wrinkly, plus they don't wear as well as matte eyeshadows during the day. Unless that's the look you want (and you can always check this out in daylight) don't wear them.

- Always check for eyeshadow that may have flaked onto your cheek while you were applying it.

- If your eyebrow and eyeliner pencils are smearing during the day, try using powder instead. Why continue using products of any kind that don't hold up during the day?

- Thickly clumped-on mascara does not look like defined, long eyelashes. A neat, clean application will look far more appealing.

- Consider avoiding heavy, greasy lip glosses. Even if you're young, these can look sloppy and messy.

- Greasy lipstick or gloss can look wet and slippery as opposed to creamy and smooth. Be certain your lipstick looks soft, not damp. Also, the greasier the lipstick, the more quickly it will come off.

- Lipliner is a nice touch, and using a lip brush can provide a great professional flair. If you don't have time, you can apply lipstick evenly from the tube and still look terrific.

- Dark lipsticks can be quite attractive, but if they are too dark they can make you look cadaverous unless you are going "Gothic" on purpose. Also, wearing dark lipliner with a lighter shade of lipstick hasn't been in fashion since 1980, and even then it looked peculiar. It is too obvious and makes your mouth look hard and severe.

- When you apply makeup, take into consideration how it will look by midday and at the end of the day. Don't buy products that look great for an hour or two but by lunchtime make you look like you forgot to wash your face the night before. If you have a problem with eyeliner or mascara that smears, reconsider the products you use or the look you are trying to achieve.

- Don't trust the color if it doesn't make sense on your skin. If you buy a gray eyeshadow and it goes on blue, even though it looks gray in the container, it isn't gray, it is blue. Likewise with a foundation that is the right color in the bottle but looks peach, ash, or rose on your skin. Believe what you see on your face, not what you see in the container. If it is not right for you, take it back for a refund or exchange. And always check how the color looks on your skin in daylight—it's the least forgiving, but most realistic, way to gauge if the color you've chosen is a keeper.

## CHOOSING COLOR

Finally, we come to the most difficult subject of all to discuss, at least on paper. I would love to have the time to sit down and create a makeup look that works for everyone. That isn't humanly possible, but I do have some rules that can help you create the makeup look you want.

- Foundation matches the skin exactly so there are no lines of demarcation. (I know this is getting repetitive, but I can't emphasize this point enough.)

- Concealer is only a shade or two lighter than the foundation.

- Powder should match the foundation exactly or go on transparent so it does not affect the color of foundation in the least.

- Eyeshadow colors should be neutral shades ranging from pale beige to tan, brown, dark brown, and black (and the thousands of shades in between).

- Eyebrow color should match the exact shade of the existing brow hair, unless your brows are naturally blonde, in which case the brow color should be slightly darker.

- Eyeliner on the upper lid should be a darker color (all the way to black, depending on the look you want) than the line along the lower lashes, which should be a softer shade of brown or gray.

- Blush can be almost any color as long as it coordinates in some logical fashion with the lipstick color, but it must be blended on softly, without any noticeable edges whatsoever.

- Lipstick can be bold to neutral—there is a fantastic range of great colors. When you're choosing, remember that smaller lips should wear brighter shades than larger lips.

- Less is best.

- To create a tanned appearance, use golden brown and chestnut shades for your blush, eyeshadows, contour, and lipstick. Never apply a foundation or bronzer all over the face if that means you'll end up with a line of demarcation at the jaw or hairline.

- It is best not to clash color tones. For example, if the outfit you are wearing is peach or coral, your blush and lipstick should have that same underlying color tone or be neutral enough not to clash.

## COLOR MISTAKES TO AVOID

- **Don't wear white or very pale lipstick with a white cast to it. This can look ghostly and ghastly.**

- **Don't wear blue, green, or overly pastel anything, including eyeliner, eyeshadow, and mascara.**

- **Avoid navy blue eyeshadow. (Stick with black—it looks smoky, while navy just tends to look "ashen.")**

- **Don't wear dark brown or black lipstick. (On Dracula it's great; on women it may suggest a cartoonish appearance.)**

- **Don't wear shiny eyeshadows (they exaggerate any wrinkles around the eye); they may be fun occasionally, but only if you have smooth, unlined eyelids.**

- **Don't wear rainbow-style eyeshadow designs.**

- **Don't wear eyeshadow applied as a smudge of black around the eye (unless the members of your rock band insist on it).**

- **Don't wear blush and lipstick colors that clash; they should be in the same color family, not glaring opposites.**

# CORRECTING SOME POPULAR MAKEUP MYTHS

- Some makeup artists declare that you shouldn't be afraid to touch your makeup. The truth is, you should be very careful about touching it. After you've taken time to apply your foundation smoothly with a sponge and your eyeshadows evenly with brushes, there's no reason to use your fingers unless it's absolutely necessary, and only lightly at that. Touching your face during the day will rub off all your nicely applied makeup. In a pinch, clean fingers can be used to soften color or smooth out mistakes, but use a light touch.

- Don't spray water or toner on makeup to set it or freshen things up. It doesn't work. A mist of water can streak foundation, powder, and mascara. How this makeup myth got circulated is anyone's guess!

- Don't change every part of your makeup with every season. If you want to go softer during the spring and summer, that's fine, but it isn't an absolute must. Makeup should reflect how you want to be seen by the world and what makes you feel good—not a seasonal dictate.

- Don't use makeup to correct the shape of anything on your face, especially the lips. Close up and in person you can absolutely tell when lipstick has been applied beyond or inside the natural lip line. If you overcontour, you will look like you have brown stripes all over your face.

- Don't use foundation or color correctors to change the color of your skin. Foundation must match the underlying skin tone exactly. That will soften any skin discoloration or redness. If you have yellow or olive skin there's nothing you can or should do to change it. It's best to accept it and work with it for your own look. Even if you succeeded in changing the color of your face, it would look strange next to your neck and along the hairline.

- To keep pencil eyeliner in place, many makeup artists recommend going over it with a matching powder eyeshadow. That works, but why do two steps when only one is needed? Forget the pencil and just use dark eyeshadow to begin with.

- Glowing skin does look nice, but mostly just in pictures. In real life, the same skin looks like it is covered with glitter. That isn't bad, but it isn't as appealing as the pictures make it seem, and any wrinkles will be illuminated, too. It is an option for an evening out, but that's about it.

- No single set of colors is absolutely right for any skin color. The days of being typed into one color grouping are long gone. Just because you have red hair doesn't mean you *have* to wear corals and avoid blue-red lipstick. It's all up to experimentation and finding what looks best. Quite honestly, most women can wear just about any color they want to, as long as they pay attention to color intensity and application and adjust the details accordingly.

## GROWING UP IN THE MILLENNIUM

In our society, for young girls on the perilous journey from preadolescence and adolescence to young adult status, one of the emotional pitfalls is the social pressure and self-awareness that precipitates wearing makeup. Putting on blush, lipstick, mascara, and eyeshadow has become one of the primary rites of passage that marks the moment when changing hormones begin to influence both mind and body. As this new style of expression is developing, teenage anxiety begins to take on a whole new depth (witness a teen's explosive desperation at a single perceived insult or problem). What do you do when the little girl in your life (who is looking less and less like a little girl) wants to start wearing makeup? Particularly when her sensitivities are overflowing but her sophistication is lagging? And it isn't just that she *wants* to wear makeup—she *has* to. To make things even more confusing, teenagers continually demonstrate an inexplicable duality of independence and fierce individualism, while at the same time buying only what everyone else is wearing. How many times have you heard the teen in your life proclaim loudly that she doesn't care what anyone else thinks, while at the same time she refuses to wear anything else but the same style of makeup, shoes, skirts, blouses, sweaters, and dresses her friends or latest rock-star idol is wearing? Too many to count!

Feeling attractive is an overwhelmingly important aspect of life for many teenage girls. It is often complicated by well-meaning adults who don't quite know what to do or say. "You look beautiful, you don't need to wear makeup" is just as irksome as "A little pink blush, rose lipstick, and brown mascara will make you look beautiful." The first statement, "You look beautiful just the way you are," comes off as a thunderous lie. It discounts what the teenager sees all around her on television and in magazines—that women can look more exciting and glamorous with makeup on (or why else would Mom and the rest of the world be wearing it?). The other comment about adding just a little color here and there suggests that the girl is unattractive and would be better off hiding her face behind a layer of cosmetics (albeit a small one). Then there's the ever-popular, "You can start wearing makeup when you're 16 and that's that." At best, an arbitrary date like this ignores the specific needs and development of each teen.

What to do? I wouldn't recommend any of the above approaches, that's for sure. Instead, I suggest incorporating all three positions into a compassionate compromise. The goal is to acknowledge the teenager's needs, letting her know they are valid and important. Tell her something along the lines of "I know wearing makeup is important to you and it could look lovely on you. But at the same time I want you to know that I think you are beautiful just the way you are." Then the two of you can decide together what is appropriate, giving in a little as you go. Remember, what you think is important may not be what the teen thinks is important. Gloss yes, lipstick no; blush yes, but only a little; mascara yes, but only brown; concealer yes, but foundation no; and so on. Mostly this process is about being gentle and respectful of the teen's feelings as they arise (and not about trying to control or contradict).

Another option is going together to a professional makeup artist or makeup demonstration. This can be a positive experience as long as you are careful to ward off any attempt on the part of the salesperson to foster insecurity and vulnerability via sales techniques. Let the salesperson know ahead of time, in no uncertain terms, that you don't want her to use any language that suggests something is unattractive or wrong with any aspect of your teen's appearance. If the salesperson wants to introduce something different she can easily say, "I think a softer blush can be an attractive look," instead of "The blush you have on is all wrong for you." Don't let the counterperson get away with "You have small lids and a bright color will make them look larger," when a simple statement such as "A pale brown eyeshadow on the lid is a good color choice for you" can go a long way to build self-esteem instead of makeup addiction and insecurity.

If the age of your teen is of great importance to you in making your decision about when to allow makeup, you can put off the inevitable by intervening with an emphasis on skin care (which is a good starting point in general). Encouraging the everyday use of UVA-protective sunscreen, regular cleansing with a water-soluble cleanser, exfoliating gently with baking soda or an AHA or BHA product, and using 2.5% benzoyl peroxide over blemishes is a great way to start paying attention to beauty issues without getting into makeup, except maybe for mascara or lip gloss. At the same time, it is essential that you take the time to share information about how the cosmetics industry can take advantage of women and stress why it is a waste of money to buy expensive products. That combination is an excellent and beautiful introduction to the world of cosmetics.

You and your teen can even read one of my books or visit my Web site together, marking areas to discuss. If you reach a crossroads and cannot agree, seek out an impartial third party to mediate (preferably not male unless you're looking for a "Who cares?" response!).

Most of us grown-ups started off on the wrong foot with makeup and skin care, somehow learning incorrectly from the outset that it would make us perfect and correct all our flaws (of which there were always too many—eyes too close together or too far apart, nose too broad or too narrow, face too square or too round, skin too yellow or too pink, and on and on). We are now in a good position to hand the next generation a new measure of self-worth and to tell them the truth about cosmetics and what they can and cannot do. That's something the cosmetics industry probably isn't expecting.

# CHAPTER 19

## PROBLEMS? SOLUTIONS!

## WHEN SHOULD I THROW OUT A PRODUCT?

**Problem:** I've heard a lot of different information regarding when I should throw away a cosmetic. Is there a time limit when products should be thrown away?

**Solution:** There isn't an easy answer to this question because there are no regulations or agreed-upon guidelines on the expiration times for skin-care or makeup products, and the FDA has no rules on the issue whatsoever. Cosmetics companies generally test their products for stability, but some do one-year assays while others do three-year assays. Clouding the stability testing issue even more is that the cosmetics companies typically look only at temperature variables (freezing or overheating, for instance). The testing doesn't take into account how consumers use the products. Cosmetics that have been improperly stored—for example, exposed to sunlight, left open, or become contaminated (any product packaged in a jar has almost a 100% risk of being contaminated)—may deteriorate substantially before a year is up. On the other hand, products stored under ideal conditions may be acceptable long after the suggested "use by" dates. An additional stability issue, which is not related to stability testing, is that there is no way to tell how long a product has been sitting on a shelf before you buy it.

So what should you do? In general, it's best to toss out cosmetics that you place near the eye (mascara, for example) after four to six months, and to dispose of face products (moisturizers, foundations) after one to two years. The toss time for eye-area cosmetics is more limited than for other products because of repeated microbial exposure during use by the consumer and the risk of eye infections. Some industry experts even recommend replacing mascara after only three months from the date of purchase. Another thing, if mascara becomes dry, discard it. Don't add water or, even worse, saliva to moisten it, because that will introduce bacteria into the product. And if you have an eye infection, consult a physician immediately, stop using all eye-area cosmetics, and discard those you were using when the infection occurred.

Among other cosmetics that are likely to have an unusually short shelf-life are certain "all-natural" products that contain plant-derived substances conducive to microbial growth. It's also important, for both consumers and manufacturers, to consider the increased risk of contamination in some "natural" products that contain nontraditional preservatives or no preservatives at all.

Sharing makeup also increases the risk of contamination, and the testers commonly found at department store cosmetics counters are even more likely to become contaminated than the same products in your home. If you must test a cosmetic before purchasing it, apply it with a new, unused applicator, such as a fresh cotton swab. But remember, these are merely suggestions; they are not based on any established research or guidelines (Source: FDA *Office of Cosmetics Facts Sheet*, March 9, 2000, "Shelf Life-Expiration Date").

# DARK CIRCLES

**Problem:** I have dark circles that seem to get worse as the day goes by! What can I do to make my concealer last?

**Solution:** Dark circles can be caused by several factors, and each needs to be dealt with in a different way. Dark circles can be caused by sun damage, veins and capillaries that show through skin, irritation, the natural dark pigment that can occur in this area, and by dry skin that just makes the area look dull and tired. Dark circles can also be the result of natural shadows that fall within the eye area due to the fact that the eye is set back and the brow bone can cast a shadow, making that area appear darker.

Be sure you are using a lightweight moisturizer (gel or silicone-based moisturizers are best) under the eye area; too much moisturizer or too heavy a moisturizer can make your concealer slide off. And always use a sunscreen over this area during the day, or wear sunglasses, to prevent the sun from stimulating melanin (dark pigmentation) production.

Matte-style (rather than creamy or greasy) concealers are best to cover natural shadows or natural dark pigmentation, and concealers such as Revlon ColorStay Concealer *($9.49)*, Maybelline Great Wear Concealer *($4.69)*, and Elizabeth Arden Flawless Finish Concealer *($14)* work particularly well. The color of the concealer must be light enough to cover the dark circles, but not so light that it gives the appearance of a white mask around the eyes. Avoid using greasy pencils along the lower lashes, and stay away from mascara that smears; these can both slide during the day, making the under-eye area even darker. Use only a powder to line the lower lashes, and then the thinnest line possible, or wear no lower liner at all. City pollution can get to your eyes by day's end, too, so you may want to consider using an air filter in your home or office (talk to the building or office managers to see if they are willing to accommodate this request).

If you have allergies that get worse as the day goes on, you may want to consider taking an antihistamine. Although uncommon, food allergies may also be to blame, but this would need to be confirmed by an allergist.

If all else fails, you may want to consider laser treatments for lightening (and in some cases eliminating) dark circles. Traditional skin-lightening products used for sun or hormone-induced skin discoloration do not have any effect on dark circles. For more information on lasers, refer to Chapter 14, *Cosmetic Surgery*.

# LASHES FALLING OUT

**Problem:** My lashes are falling out! Is there anything I can do to stop this from happening?

**Solution:** It is natural for lashes to shed and then regrow, but if you are noticing bald spots along your lash line, you may need to change some habits that might be making the condition worse. For example, don't wipe off eye makeup (or any makeup, for that matter) because wiping and pulling at the eyes can pull out lashes. Don't rub your eyes, even if they itch, especially when you are wearing mascara. Also, do not overuse mascara. I know it's tempting to have long, dramatically thick lashes, but the weight of the mascara (and what it takes to remove it later) can be too much for delicate lashes. Waterproof mascaras are the most difficult to remove and often take many lashes with them, so you might want to consider changing mascaras. It is unlikely that you are allergic to your mascara, but on the remote possibility that it may be the cause of the fallout, switch brands and see how that works.

By the way, you aren't using an eyelash curler are you? Over time, that consistent tugging can certainly pull out lashes. Another possibility is that noncosmetic allergies could be playing a part in your eyelash dilemma. Your only recourse, if that turns out to be the cause, is to use antihistamines or eliminate from your environment the allergens causing the problem. For example, if you are allergic to the down in your pillows, use pillows with a synthetic fill. Hay fever can also cause the eye area to swell severely, damaging eyelashes, a problem that could be alleviated by using over-the-counter or prescription antihistamines.

Medically speaking, doctors refer to the loss of eyelashes as *madarosis*. According to ophthalmologist Dr. William Trattler, "While it may seem like mainly a cosmetic problem, the condition can be an indicator of something more serious, such as eye trauma, eyelid infections and even cancer of the eyelid. In addition, metabolic conditions such as hypothyroidism and pituitary insufficiency can cause madarosis" (Source: http://ivillagehealth.com).

It is also possible that the eyelash loss can be attributed to the presence of a mite called *Demodex folliculorum*. When it is active in small hair follicles and eyelash hair follicles it can consume epithelial cells, causing the hair follicle to become swollen, inflamed, and plugged. All of this can cause the eyelashes to fall out. Fortunately, this problem is easily treated once correctly diagnosed (Source: *eMedicine Journal*, May 11, 2001, volume 2, number 5).

If your loss of eyelash hair is chronic, you should see an eyelid specialist (called an oculoplastic surgeon) and have him carefully examine your eyelid to determine the cause of the madarosis.

# SELF-TANNERS

**Problem:** I tried an expensive new self-tanner from a line called Decleor at Neiman Marcus. It just smelled so much better than the one I was using from Coppertone. Now my palms are striped, one leg is darker than the other, and my knees and elbows look mottled!

**Solution:** Believe it or not, the Decleor product, though absurdly expensive, is not at fault for your chameleon-like dilemma; rather, it is most likely due to uneven application. First, all self-tanners, regardless of price, use the same ingredient, dihydroxyacetone, to create the color change in your skin. The scent that attracted you to the Decleor product (some women tell me the Clarins, Origins, and Bain de Soleil self-tanners smell great, too) helps mask the naturally sweet smell of this ingredient. However, the fragrance is temporary and fades in a brief period of time. The color, on the other hand, affects the skin cells, and it takes time to get your skin back to its normal color. The cell itself changes color. Sloughing can remove altered skin cells, but at this point you can't quickly slough off all the layers of skin that have been affected. That takes time. Well-formulated AHA or BHA products can make mistakes fade faster and sometimes even remove them entirely. To a lesser extent, you can try baking soda mixed with Cetaphil Cleanser, sea-salt scrubs, and even a washcloth massaged over the problem areas twice a day—but, in most cases, time is the only real cure.

Once your skin is back to normal, you can try again. Remember that when it comes to self-tanners, application is everything! Be patient. Apply the self-tanner only over a clean, dry, exfoliated body, giving special attention to the knees, elbows, and heels. Do not apply self-tanner in a steamy, hot room where perspiration or condensation may make it run. Do one area of your body at a time. Watch what you are doing, and apply the self-tanner thoroughly and evenly. If you miss an area, you are going to look noticeably streaked or blotchy. Wash the palms of your hands as soon as you are done applying the self-tanner, and then stand still until it is completely absorbed, with no after-feel. Some women think that using a fast-darkening self-tanner is best because it changes the skin's color immediately and you can more easily see your mistakes and correct them. Others prefer a self-tanner that changes color slowly, so you can build a tan slowly and evenly. The choice is yours.

## SERIOUSLY OILY SKIN

**Problem:** I have seriously oily skin in the T-zone (forehead, nose, and chin), and it is driving me crazy. I've tried matte foundations, even Lancome MaquiControle, all kinds of oil-control gels and powders, and my face still feels like an oil slick by midday. Surely there must be something I can do?

**Solution:** Aside from doing all the right things (see Chapter 4, *Skin Care Basics for Everyone*), it is essential to be sure you aren't doing anything to your face to make matters worse. For example, if you are using a moisturizer, even an oil-free moisturizer, stop immediately. Your oil glands are already working overtime as a result of hormonal activity, and this oil is also your own built-in moisturizer. There is no reason to add more. If your oily skin is still driving you nuts, my favorite trick is to take milk of magnesia (the one I recommend as a facial mask for oily skin) and apply an extremely thin layer of it over the most oily areas. Let it dry, and then apply your foundation over that. It works great! When it comes to powdering, try loose powder instead of pressed powder in a compact. Even when a pressed powder is oil-free, the waxlike ingredients that keep it in a pressed form can add to a slick feeling on the face. As a last resort, ask your dermatologist about medical options for taming oily skin, which range from birth control pills to hormone blockers and, in extreme cases, even Accutane.

## SMALL LIPS

**Problem:** I have small lips. Any lipstick color I put on seems to make this more noticeable. What should I do?

**Solution:** The best way to deal with small lips, is to not overline them to make them look larger. That technique of creating a new lipline works great in photographs, but in real life it looks like you missed your mouth. Also, to maintain the look, you have to diligently touch up your lipstick and use your pencil the moment any wears off. What works best is lining just to the outside or edge of your true lipline with a natural-colored lipliner. Do not wear dark lipstick, because dark colors applied to any surface make it look smaller. A true red or any vivid color will make your lips look bigger. Of course you can always consider cosmetic surgical procedures that enlarge lips, but that should be a last resort after experimenting with lipstick options.

## FLAKING EYESHADOW

**Problem:** Whenever I apply eyeshadow, I always find eyeshadow sprinkles on my cheeks and under-eye area. What am I doing wrong?

**Solution:** Sprinkles are almost inevitable, but knocking the excess powder off the brush before you apply your eye makeup will help a lot. Some eyeshadows are more powdery than others and cause more sprinkles. Eyeshadows made by M.A.C., Physicians Formula, Shu Uemura, Bobbi Brown, Jane, Iman, and Paula's Select are more reliable in this respect. Another technique that some makeup artists use is to apply foundation and concealer to the eye area first; then the eyeshadow, liner, and mascara; after that, apply foundation to the rest of the face, touching up the concealer if "drippies" have made a mess of things. Although I find that approach time-consuming, it does help eliminate any trace of stray eyeshadow.

## BLEEDING LIPSTICK

**Problem:** I like a sheer lipstick look, but every one I've tried (and I've tried them all) just feathers into the lines around my mouth and looks like a mess! I've tried several of the ultra-matte lipsticks, but they look so hard and dry, and pencils are useless. I'm too young to have this problem. Is there something out there I've missed?

**Solution:** No, you haven't missed anything; sheer lipsticks (which are just glosses in a stick form), both the expensive and inexpensive ones, are slippery by nature and don't stay put. Pencils are helpful, but they can't block a creamy, glossy lipstick all day. If you have any lines around your mouth—and that's not necessarily related to age—sheer, creamy lipsticks and lip glosses in general will follow those pathways. Your only option is to give up the notion of a completely sheer look. Try a semi-matte lipstick such as Elizabeth Arden Semi-Matte, Clinique Long Lasting Soft Matte, M.A.C. Matte, or Revlon Absolutely Fabulous LipCream. Once you apply it, blot with a tissue until it looks more or less sheer. I know it won't have the sheen you're looking for, but it also won't travel into the lines around your mouth. Don't try to put a gloss over it; that will only encourage the lipstick to bleed. Matte lipstick isn't a shield that's impervious to the effect of the gloss. Gloss creates movement no matter what it goes over. Perhaps the best option is Cover Girl's Outlast or Max Factor's LipFinity. These are semi-permanent lip stains that don't move and really do stay on, and on, and on. These are discussed more fully in Chapter 18, *Makeup Application Step By Step* in the section "Lipstick and Lip Pencil."

## BLOODSHOT EYES

**Problem:** I have red, bloodshot eyes that just look awful. It seems to have nothing to do with sleep and I don't drink alcohol, so what am I doing wrong, or, better yet, what should I be doing right?

**Solution:** Many things can cause the blood vessels in the eye to swell and look more obvious. Lack of sleep and alcohol consumption are only two possibilities; there are lots more. For example, contact lenses, exposure to smoke, rubbing the eyes, allergies, dry air (from heat or air-conditioning), makeup particles getting in the eye and causing irritation, bad pollution days, staring at a project or computer monitor all day without giving your eyes a break, and overusing eyedrops can all make the tiny blood vessels in the eye look like roadmaps.

A humidifier in your home or office can help, and so can remembering to blink regularly during the day, especially when working at the computer. Not wearing contact lenses all day, using antihistamines for allergies, keeping your hands away from your eyes, and zealously keeping makeup out of your eyes are all exceptionally helpful. To reduce dryness, the "natural" tear products and eyewashes found at the drugstore are a great option (but use only disposable eyecups; repeatedly using the same eyecup can cause or aggravate problems such as eye infections or irritation). Eyedrops such as Visine used repeatedly can actually aggravate the problem by causing a rebound effect, making the blood vessels swell even more (Sources: Visine product warning label; *Ophthalmology*, November 1991, pages 1364–1367). You would want to use Visine-type products only occasionally, not as a regular routine.

## PUFFY EYES

**Problem:** I have puffy eyes every morning that sometimes don't go away until midday. They look awful and I've tried lots of eye products that don't change a thing.

**Solution:** There are no cosmetics or miracle eye moisturizers that can alter puffy eyes, but lots of things, including water retention, can cause the skin around the eye area to swell. Lack of sleep is probably not as big a factor for puffy eyes as it is for bloodshot eyes. If anything, sitting up instead of lying down would prevent fluids from collecting in the tissues around the eye. Of course, no one should sit up day and night! Sleeping with your head slightly elevated, and making sure you give your neck the support it needs, can help prevent fluid retention. Alcohol consumption and a diet high in salt also can cause water retention and increase the puffiness around the eyes.

Another factor to consider is contact lenses, which can cause irritation and swelling of the eye, so be sure you are wearing the most comfortable type available for your vision correction. As with bloodshot eyes, exposure to smoke, rubbing the eyes, allergies, dry air (from heat or air-conditioning), makeup particles getting in the eyes, allergic reactions to skin-care or makeup products, bad pollution days, leaving makeup on overnight (which can cause inflammation), and using irritating skin-care products around the eyes can all make the eye area swollen.

Be sure to take your makeup off meticulously at night, don't rub your eyes during the day, and take an antihistamine if you have allergies. If you are allergic or sensitive to certain skin-care or makeup products, avoid them.

Preventing dryness around the eyes can also help reduce irritation and swelling that can cause a puffy appearance. If that's your problem, a lightweight, fragrance-free moisturizer will help a lot. Be certain the moisturizer does not contain any irritating ingredients that could make matters worse, such as witch hazel, volatile plant oils, and sensitizing plant extracts like lemon oil or menthol. If you have time in the morning, place cool compresses on the eyes (low temperatures can make the skin contract); if you don't have time for that, leave your moisturizer in the refrigerator so it's cool when you apply it in the morning.

If none of these things help alleviate the problem, it may be that your eyes are just naturally puffy. Most typically this results from overly large fat pads around the eye (everyone has fat pads around the eye) creating a puffy-looking bulge. If that's the case, the only way to get rid of the problem is with cosmetic surgery, which in most cases is incredibly effective at eliminating the problem.

## CHAPPED LIPS

**Problem:** What should I do about my eternally chapped lips? No matter what I use, the chapping never goes away.

**Solution:** Whether they are responding to cold weather, an arid climate, or are just naturally dry, chapped lips are a pain. Cracking, flaking, and chapping are not only uncomfortable but also unsightly, and lipstick only seems to make the situation worse. You can solve those dry-lips blues with consistency and patience. Chapped lips are not going to disappear in a day, and missing even one day of treatment can drive lips back to dryness.

Lips are more vulnerable to the environment than any other part of the face. This means that keeping your lips moist and sealed against the weather is essential. There are lots of emollient lip products that do just that, and the more emollient they are, the better. Ingredients like lanolin, oils of any kind (including castor oil, lanolin oil, safflower oil, almond oil, and vegetable oil), and shea and cocoa butter are all excellent, especially if they are listed at the beginning of the ingredient list. However, many lip products are little more than waxy coatings that make lips feel thick and protected when they are applied (Chap Stick is a great example), but they don't really moisturize or provide adequate protection from the weather or from the dry heat and air-conditioning you find indoors.

Lots of lip products also claim to be medicated. "Medicated," however, is a dubious term at best, and it has no regulated meaning. These "medicated" products usually contain camphor, menthol, peppermint oil, eucalyptus, but these are not medicines for dry lips! They mostly irritate and can actually make lips burn, which is neither disinfecting nor helpful for lips that are already dry and chapped. Products like Blistex, which includes 0.5% phenol, are the exception, because they truly are medicated; phenol kills anything that gets in its way. However, phenol is strong stuff and actually can trigger serious irritation and dryness all by itself. It is not something I would recommend for anything but extremely limited use.

You may have heard a rumor that lips can adapt to or become addicted to lip balm. It isn't possible. But if the lip balm you are using contains irritating ingredients (and lots of them do), your lips will stay dried up. When a lip product contains irritating, drying ingredients, there is no way the other, more emollient ingredients can help. Likewise, if you are using a lip product that is just waxy, with no emollients or water-binding agents, it can only plaster down the dry skin; it doesn't reduce the dryness.

I am quite fond of BeautiControl's LipApeel. This two-step product exfoliates the chapped skin with a waxy cream you rub over the lips; then, after that's rubbed off, you apply a very emollient balm. It is one of the only really gentle and effective exfoliating products I've ever seen for lips. It's a bit pricey, but it can last for years. BeautiControl's ordering number is (800) BEAUTI-1. I also developed two products for my Paula's Choice skin-care line that work similarly, Protective Lip Balm SPF 15 (with titanium dioxide) and Exfoliating Treatment.

At night you can apply almost any lip balm that contains some of the emollients I mentioned above, but no irritants. **For daytime care, it is best to use an SPF 15 lip balm that contains avobenzone, titanium dioxide, or zinc oxide.** However, if you wear an opaque lipstick, it may not be essential to have that kind of SPF protection. Research has shown that women who apply lipstick more than once a day are at a much lower risk of getting lip cancer than women who apply lipstick only once a day (Source: *Cancer Causes and Control*, July 1996, pages 458–463). Theoretically, opaque lipsticks have enough sun-blocking protection to enable them to screen out the sun's skin cancer–causing rays. Still, you may as well play it safe and use a lip balm or lipstick with sunscreen daily, especially if you are outside for long periods of time in the sun or if you live in a sunny climate.

# DRY SKIN AROUND THE LIPS

**Problem:** For some time now I have had a strange red, dry irritation, just along the skin around my mouth. Moisturizers don't seem to help.

**Solutions:** One of the first things you can do is determine whether you've developed an allergic reaction to fluoride toothpaste. Fluoride can cause irritation around the mouth. Try a fluoride-free toothpaste for a while and see what happens. If that seems to be the solution, check with your dentist to see how this will affect your dental health.

The dryness and irritation around your mouth could also be caused by a significant other who happens to have a rough beard. There isn't much you can do about that, but occasionally using a little cortisone cream around the area can help minimize the irritation from almost any source. Another possibility is frequent, unconscious licking of the lips. Saliva can be an irritant for the lips, causing flaking and dryness. Lip balm won't be able to keep up with this bad habit.

If the area around the mouth is dry and irritated, that can also affect the lips. What's important here is to treat the root of the problem, which in this situation may require using an emollient moisturizer around the edge of the mouth as well as a lip exfoliant and lip balm for the lip area.

# PERIORAL DERMATITIS— RED BUMPS AROUND THE MOUTH

**Problem:** I can't seem to get rid of these red, swollen, sometimes crusty bumps around my lips and at the sides of my nose. Nothing seems to help, including over-the-counter acne products and cortisone creams. What can I do?

**Solutions:** What you describe sounds like an almost classic case of perioral dermatitis. According to the American Academy of Dermatology (http://www.aad.org) "Perioral dermatitis [POD] is a common skin problem that mostly affects young women [20 to 45 years of age]. Occasionally men or children are affected. Perioral refers to the area around the mouth, and dermatitis indicates redness of the skin. In addition to redness, there are usually small red bumps or even pus bumps and mild peeling. Sometimes the bumps are the most obvious feature, and the disease can look a lot like acne. The areas most affected are within the borders of the lines from the nose to the sides of the lips, and the chin…. Sometimes there is mild itching and/or burning."

POD is actually quite common and, according to most dermatologists, is increasing in incidence (Source: *Australasian Journal of Dermatology*, February 2000, pages 34–38). While little is known about what causes this disorder, there are theories that overuse or chronic use of topical cortisone creams, fluoridated toothpaste, or heavy or occlusive skin-care ointments and creams (especially those with a petrolatum or thick wax base) and foundations may be responsible. Exposure to sunlight, heat, and wind can also make matters worse (Source: *eMedicine Journal*, August 1, 2001, volume 2, number 8).

You can experiment by stopping the use of any of the potentially problematic products mentioned above. It would be a great idea to stop using topical cortisone creams, but be advised that this step can initially make matters worse before any improvement takes place. That can feel self-defeating, but be patient, at least for a few weeks, to see if the condition finally improves.

It would also be helpful to find out if fluoridated toothpaste is the source of the problem. You can try brushing with fluoride-free toothpaste such as Tom's of Maine Natural Fluoride-Free Toothpaste (*$2.99 for 4 ounces*) and see if that makes a significant difference. If fluoride-free toothpaste turns out to be the solution, check with your dentist to see how this will affect your dental health.

If these experiments lead you to suspect POD is indeed the cause of the bumps around your mouth and nose, it is best to see a dermatologist because there are no cosmetics or over-the-counter medications that can treat the condition. A dermatologist can prescribe topical metronidazole (MetroGel, MetroLotion, or MetroCream), alone or in combination with either oral tetracycline or erythromycin. Even though topical cortisone creams may be the cause of POD, you may be prescribed a low-potency cortisone cream to reduce the inflammation and to help you wean off the stronger topical cortisone cream you may have been using (Source: *Seminars in Cutaneous Medical Surgery*, September 1999, pages 206–209). For more information on POD, visit http://www.aad.org/pamphlets/Perioral.html (this URL is case-sensitive).

# EXPENSIVE VERSUS INEXPENSIVE

**Problem:** I'm not one to fall for a company's enthusiasm for its products, but surely some companies can have secret or special ingredients and formulas, or use more expensive, superior ingredients. A friend mentioned that her chocolate chip cookies contain flour, sugar, shortening, eggs, vanilla, chocolate chips, and nuts, but they still don't taste like Mrs. Fields'. I have used your inexpensive recommendations and they have worked great, but I am so tempted to buy the more expensive stuff!

**Solution:** I understand the concept your friend is suggesting when it comes to her cookies. However, some people may prefer Mrs. Fields cookies while others would prefer your friend's. If she does have a secret ingredient, that may taste great to you but not to someone else. When it comes to shopping for makeup and skin-care products, there are unquestionably great formulas out there that work better for different skin types and different needs, in all price ranges, but the notion that expensive is better isn't supported by any of the research I've seen or done. We know this is true, because we've all bought expensive products we didn't like. After interviewing dozens of cosmetics chemists and cosmetic ingredient manufacturers, I have yet to find any that agree with this theory that secret ingredients provide superior benefits for the skin. There are ingredients that can make a difference, but almost without exception they are accessible to every cosmetics manufacturer. Further, even if there were "secret ingredients," keeping them secret wouldn't be legal. According to the FDA, *every* ingredient except fragrance must be included on the ingredient list or the product would be subject to seizure.

I rate lots of expensive and inexpensive products as both excellent to poor, so I've come to know that judging by price alone can hurt your skin and waste your money.

## USING DIFFERENT PRODUCTS FROM DIFFERENT LINES

**Problem:** I've been following your advice and am using products from several different lines. My skin is doing great, but all the cosmetics salespeople say it is a mistake to mix and match. They say products are designed to work together, and that is what helps the skin best.

**Solution:** Stop listening to the cosmetics salespeople; they are wrong. If every line had SPF 15 sunscreens with the requisite UVA protection, gentle cleansers with nonirritating ingredients, foundations that aren't peach-colored, and on and on, I would agree that you don't need to mix and match. But I have found good and bad products in every line (and I've reviewed hundreds of cosmetics lines and thousands of products). Many lines don't have adequate sunscreens, have products that contain irritating ingredients, or offer rose, peach, and ashen foundation colors, though they may have superior mascara and blushes. Staying with the same line for all your skin-care or makeup needs almost always ensures that you end up with some bad products! Mixing and matching is the only way to go. You don't wear clothes from one designer, buy furniture from one manufacturer, take medicine from one pharmaceutical company, or eat food from just one company. The only way to develop a successful skin-care or makeup routine is to select what works best for your skin type and needs, not what one line happens to be selling.

## FEELING BEAUTIFUL DURING THE TRAUMA OF CANCER

**Problem:** I have a dear friend who has just been diagnosed with breast cancer. I want to be a support for her. I know how important feeling beautiful is for her. Any suggestions from you would be truly appreciated.

**Solution:** I've spoken with many women who have lived through the ordeal of radiation and chemotherapy, and they all agreed that paying attention to how they looked helped their emotional well-being a lot during the trauma of diagnosis and treatment. Having gone through this life-threatening event with my older sister, I had a reason to look further into these issues, and now I have the opportunity to share some solutions and possibilities with you and your friend. Given the number of women who have breast cancer or other cancers, surely most all of us know someone who can benefit from this information. One thing my sister found immensely helpful was talking openly about her cancer experience without embarrassment or reservation. Perhaps your friend or someone else in your life would appreciate that kind of support and openness.

**Body care:** Because chemotherapy and radiation make the skin ultra-sensitive and even sunburned, as a general rule it is best not to use any types of adhesives, tints, bleaches, waxes, harsh or irritating chemicals, or to take hot baths or showers. Even deodorants and shaving can be problems. Saunas, Jacuzzis, loofahs, strong soaps, and washcloths can also exacerbate irritation. Anything you can do to reduce the hypersensitivity will go a long way to making the skin feel soothed and less irritated.

Instead of bar soap, which can be extremely drying and harsh on sensitive skin, try a gentle liquid body cleanser such as Nivea Moisturizing Shower Gel, Dove Nutrium Body Wash, or Olay Daily Renewal Body Wash. Keep the skin moist with lightweight gels that don't trap heat, such as pure aloe vera (found at most health food stores). If the skin becomes dry, use a nonfragranced, nonirritating moisturizer (the fewer plants it contains, the better) such as Lubriderm Seriously Sensitive Moisturizing Lotion. Take tepid or slightly warm showers and baths, and try to enjoy cool baths whenever possible, adding a little bit of light oil, such as safflower or sunflower oil, to the water. Avoid heavy oils such as vitamin E. Despite the fact that vitamin E has a reputation for healing the skin and can help the skin after the radiation and chemotherapy are over (as can other antioxidants), in the midst of treatment keep in mind that vitamin E is a potential allergen, and that its occlusive attributes can trap heat in the skin when it needs to dissipate heat instead.

Many women worry that even washing the skin may increase irritation. It turns out that gentle washing is better for skin than just leaving it alone. According to an article in *Radiotherapy & Oncology* (March 2001, pages 333–339), "Washing the irradiated skin during the course of radiotherapy for breast cancer is not associated with increased skin toxicity [or irritation] and should not be discouraged."

To keep her skin feeling soft and light, one of the first things my sister and I did before she went in for her radiation was to buy silk underwear, including T-shirts, underpants, teddies, and pajamas. She had to give up wearing a bra because the irritation from the straps and the tightness around the breast was just too uncomfortable. The silk was not only soothing, it also helped her feel more feminine and attractive.

**Hair care:** Some women feel compelled to shave their head in anticipation of losing their hair. That can be the worst possible solution for dealing with the inevitable. Shaving your head may look exotic, but unless you plan to shave every day, it can itch like crazy when it starts to grow back between treatments. It's best to cut your hair very short and consider wearing designer baseball caps or wigs. Scarves always make it look like something is wrong, while baseball caps and wigs are quite normal nowadays.

By the way, the American Cancer Society can provide you with a free wig; call (800) 227-2345. The wigs have been donated and are clean, but use them as a springboard for finding one that is perfect for you. You can buy a wig at a specialty salon or wig shop, but the trick is to find a good one and go to someone who knows how to style it. Wigs almost always need to be cut and styled to match your face. If you live in or near a large metropolitan area, your absolute best option is to find out who styles wigs for the women in the Orthodox Jewish community. For religious reasons, many Orthodox Jewish women cover their own hair with a wig. The shatelmacher (wig maker) is a mainstay of the Orthodox community and knows better than anyone how to make a wig look natural and attractive. Just call the Orthodox synagogue in your area and ask for the number of the woman who styles wigs for the community. The larger the metropolitan area, the more choices there will be.

One woman told me that after she purchased her first quality wig (around $100 to $500), she was a changed woman. "Not only did it fit great, but it looked so real that no one could believe it was a wig. I still wear it now and then, and get the biggest kick out of telling people it's a wig."

When your hair starts growing back, you may find that it grows back in thicker and straighter or curlier than it was. As tempting as it will be to dye your hair or perm it, be patient. Wait for the hair to go through a few normal cycles of growth before using chemicals on it. The skin and hair may still be sensitive or altered by the radiation and chemotherapy, and could react in a way that can cause problems.

**Skin care:** All of my recommendations for gentle skin care are doubly true during radiation and chemotherapy. And it is even more imperative than usual to avoid the sun, because the skin can become photosensitive. Sunscreen is essential, and the less the body and face are exposed to the sun, the better. That means wearing hats, light, tightly woven cotton pants, and light, long-sleeved blouses whenever possible. Because the skin can become dry, it is important to follow my recommendations for dry-skin care, which include using a gentle cleanser, a skin-softening toner, an emollient moisturizer, and plant oils such as safflower, olive, or sunflower oil over dry patches.

**Eyebrows and eyelashes:** Accompanying the loss of hair on your head is the probable loss of eyebrows and eyelashes. Avoid the natural tendency to pencil in new brows, which look fake and dated. Instead, try powder shadows to draw on a soft arch of a brow. If you have any eyebrow hair left, consider using the colored brow gels from Bobbi Brown, Origins, or Paula's Select; these can add definition and shape to whatever hair you have left. Another option is to use a waterproof mascara or a waterproof eye pencil that matches your brow color. Although waterproof mascara and waterproof eye pencils can look slightly more artificial, they are worth trying because chemotherapy or other drugs can bring on menopause or menopausal symptoms, and the accompanying hot flashes, followed by profuse sweating, will wash the others away. This one takes some experimenting, so be patient until you find what works for you.

If you do lose your eyelashes, it's best to not use any mascara, even if you have a few lashes left, because gaps in your application will be quite noticeable and mascara can shorten the life of the lashes you still have. Instead, consider lining the eyes with a dark brown shade of powder that you draw on more as shading than as a line. Lining with a pencil or liquid liner and no mascara can look odd, but shading the eye with a dark powder can look smoky and defining without making the lack of lashes more obvious.

Remember that brows and lashes grow back quickly, so that part is the most temporary!

**Makeup:** When it comes to concealer, foundation, blush, lipstick, and the rest, do whatever you are used to doing. Not only will it make you feel good, it will also normalize much of the process.

One woman wrote me a wonderful e-mail about this issue: "I cannot stress enough the concept that *look good and feel better* really works. I thought I was doing OK and I was, until I found out what it felt like to go out in public with hair and makeup (eyebrows) that looked real. I never lost my sense of humor or my positive outlook; but when I got a great wig and wore makeup (and eyebrows), I felt fantastic."

One of the most powerful things you can do for yourself is to pay attention to your physical appearance and experiment to find what works. Don't try to pretend that feeling and looking beautiful doesn't matter during this time or that it is a waste of your energy. It may provide some of your most pleasant and uplifting moments until you are on the other side of your treatment.

# DOES HAIR DYE CAUSE CANCER?

**Problem:** I had a nurse tell me not to use any dark brown or black hair coloring because it might cause cancer. I read your book on hair care about this particular subject explaining there is nothing to worry about, but it seems to still be an issue in the medical world. Is *dark* hair color safe, or isn't it?

**Solution:** I would suggest that few, if any, of the 75 million women who color their hair on a regular basis even know that there is an issue about hair dye and its association with certain types of cancers. However, although the issue is real, what it means isn't settled or conclusive in any regard. The best I can do is to provide you with the information and research available that may help you make a final determination for yourself.

Much of this controversy began when a study conducted by the American Cancer Society found that women who used black hair dye for more than 20 years had a slightly increased risk of dying from non-Hodgkin's lymphoma and multiple myeloma (a bone-marrow tumor that is usually malignant). Researchers surveyed 573,369 women who completed questionnaires about their use of permanent hair dye. However, this same study concluded that women who dyed their hair showed a slightly *reduced* risk overall of dying of cancer than women who never used dyes (Sources: *Journal of the National Cancer Institute*, February 2, 1994, pages 210–215; *Environmental Health Perspectives*, June-July 1994, volume 102, number 6–7).

Subsequent studies looking at hair dyes in general found no correlation and did not support any risk of any kind. An article in *FDA Consumer* magazine (January-February 2001) explained that in a "...study, published in the October 5, 1994, issue of the *Journal of the National Cancer Institute*, researchers from Brigham and Women's Hospital in Boston followed 99,000 women and found no greater risk of cancers of the blood or lymph systems among women who had ever used permanent hair dyes. Then in 1998, scientists at the University of California at San Francisco questioned 2,544 people about their use of hair-color products. After integrating the results of this study with those of animal and other epidemiological studies, they concluded that there was little convincing evidence linking non-Hodgkin's lymphoma with normal use of hair-color products in humans. The study was published in the December 1998 issue of the *American Journal of Public Health*."

There have also been other subsequent studies showing hair dye to have no association with cancer or other diseases. One noted that: "The lack of an association between exclusive use of a single type of hair coloring application and breast cancer risk argues that hair coloring application does not influence breast cancer risk among reproductive-age women. Thus, the results of the present study, as well as negative ones from most (but not all) prior studies, are most consistent with the conclusion that neither hair coloring application nor hair spray application influences breast cancer risk" (Source: *Cancer Causes and Control*, December 1999, pages 551–559). Another stated: "We found no evidence that permanent hair dye use, age at first use, frequency of use, or duration of use is associated with the development of systemic lupus" (Source: *Arthritis and Rheumatism*, April 1996, pages 657–662).

This issue was given new life in February 2001 when researchers from the University of Southern California (USC) reported a link between the use of permanent hair coloring and bladder cancer. "They analyzed questionnaires from 897 patients with bladder cancer and compared them to questionnaires from 897 similar individuals without bladder cancer. They found that individuals with bladder cancer were three times as likely to have used permanent hair dyes at least once a month for 15 years or more. In addition, subjects who worked for 10 or more years as hairdressers or barbers were five times more likely to have bladder cancer than people who were not exposed to permanent hair dye" (Source: http://www.sciencedaily.com).

It is important to point out that this study was an epidemiological investigation looking at behavior and the possible relationships between products and their effect on health. Epidemiological studies are not definitive in any way. For example, it isn't clear from this study what percentage of this group smoked, what kind of diet they had, or whether or not they had other mitigating illnesses. It also doesn't say that hair dye causes cancer, just that it has a casual relationship (meaning there is no definite or conclusive evidence).

As you can tell the jury is still out on this issue. There truly is not enough information or research to assert with any confidence that you should avoid dark-colored hair dyes.

If you want to be extra cautious you can avoid dark permanent or intermediate hair dyes. In view of the USC study showing that women who dye their hair 12 times or more each year for a period of 15 years were at a higher risk, you may want to consider dying your hair less frequently, no more than say 6 or 8 times a year. It is also important to keep in mind that although hair dyes may increase the risk of getting bladder cancer, such a risk would represent a relatively small number of cases, since women account for only about 15,000 of the 40,000 new cases of bladder cancer diagnosed each year (Source: http://www.webmd.com).

## FOUNDATION SETTLING INTO PORES AND LINES

**Problem:** What causes foundation to settle into the pores and leave tiny little spots, or settle into laugh lines? I do not know whether my moisturizer is too heavy or not heavy enough, whether the foundation is too heavy or too light, or whether I have not waited long enough for the moisturizer to be absorbed.

**Solution:** Most foundations contain ingredients that allow some amount of movement. If they didn't, they wouldn't blend easily and would feel dry and matte on the skin, making wrinkles look worse. But that also means that those foundations can easily slip into pores, making the skin look mottled. Moisturizing when you don't need it creates even more slippage. Unless you have dry skin, there is no reason to wear a moisturizer under foundation. Most foundations for normal to dry skin have enough emollient ingredients to make an extra moisturizer unnecessary. Too much moisturizer (not too little) or too much foundation can absolutely cause slippage into lines and pores. Once you've blended on a foundation, apply a light dusting of powder to set your makeup. Also, try blending on your foundation with a sponge, not with your fingers. A flat sponge can pick up excess foundation from the skin and blend it on in an even layer. Most important, if you have normal to dry skin, you may want to consider changing to a more matte foundation to avoid slippage. If you have oily skin then you may want to consider an ultra-matte foundation, which won't move throughout the day.

# EYELASH DYES

**Problem:** A friend of mine gets her eyelashes and eyebrows dyed at the hair salon. The effect is really rather impressive and I'm tempted to try this myself. Her blonde lashes look dark and long, even without mascara. What do you think?

**Solution:** Unfortunately, my solution isn't much of a solution, because all I can do is strongly say, "Don't do it!" The only safe solution for making lashes and brows more visible is to use mascara on the eyelashes and shade your eyebrows, either with an eyeshadow that matches your hair color, an eyebrow pencil, or a brow mascara like Bobbi Brown's Natural Brow Shaper. But first let me give you a little history on why my answer to your question is such an emphatic "no." Back in 1933, a congressional controversy was brewing over the need for new and stronger food, cosmetic, and drug laws. At the time, the FDA had no authority to move against a cosmetic product called Lash Lure that was causing allergic reactions in many women. Two women, in fact, suffered severe reactions to the product; one woman became blind and the other woman died. When the new Food, Drug, and Cosmetic Act was passed in 1938, Lash Lure was the first product seized under its authority. A lot of time has passed since then, but although hair dyes (and that includes lash dyes) have changed a great deal, they are still formulated with peroxide and ammonia or ammonia-like ingredients. If a hair dye doesn't contain those ingredients, it can't affect hair color.

No one should ever dye her eyelashes or eyebrows. An allergic reaction to the dye formulation could prompt swelling, inflammation, and susceptibility to infection in the eye area. These reactions can severely harm the eye and even cause blindness. The FDA absolutely prohibits the use of hair dyes for eyebrow and eyelash tinting or dyeing, even in beauty salons and other establishments. The FDA has also continually warned the public about the use of coal-tar dyes on the eyebrows and eyelashes, stating that such use could cause permanent injury to the eyes, including blindness.

(Using eyelash and eyebrow dyes or hair dyes for the eyes or brows should not be confused with using mascaras, eyeshadows, eyebrow pencils, and eyeliners, which contain ingredients that have been approved by the FDA for use in the eye area.)

Be aware that there are no natural or synthetic color additives (or coloring agents) approved by the FDA for dyeing or tinting eyelashes and eyebrows—either in beauty salons or in the home. In fact, the law requires all hair-dye products to include instructions for performing patch tests before use, to identify possible allergic reactions, and to carry warnings about the dangers of applying these products to eyebrows and eyelashes. The health hazards of permanent eyelash and eyebrow dyes have been known for more than 60 years. These dyes have repeatedly been cited in scientific literature as capable of causing serious reactions when placed in direct contact with the eye.

## SEASONAL CHANGES

**Problem:** During the winter I use an emollient moisturizer you recommend and it works great, but during the summer it seems a bit much. Should I change what I do with the seasons?

**Solution:** Summer can absolutely require a change in skin-care products, particularly moisturizers. Instead of the richer or more emollient moisturizers you were wearing at night to combat the dry heat indoors and the dry cold outdoors, consider using lighter moisturizers that come in gel or gel/lotion consistencies. Keep in mind that the major concept here is to cut back on the amount of moisturizer you use. Moisturizer is for dry skin, so if you don't have dry skin, you really don't need moisturizer. Also, remember that no matter how much moisturizer you wear, and no matter how many antioxidants it contains, it won't change or stop one wrinkle on your face. What a lightweight moisturizer can do is soothe spot dryness and make fine lines less noticeable. Nothing is erased or changed, but wrinkles do look better, and that's great. And this is at night, right? Because during the day you should be using a sunscreen with UVA-protecting ingredients for your face and exposed parts or your body.

Please ignore the fact that many of the products recommended below are labeled "oil-free." This is a meaningless term. What makes these products good for those with minimally dry skin is they contain fewer thickening agents and emollients. Also ignore words and phrases such as "oil-control," "lift," and "firming." None of these products can control oil, lift the skin anywhere, or firm it even a little. These are all good, very lightweight moisturizers, and that's enough.

Here's a list of some of the better lightweight gel moisturizers, regardless of price (remember, price often has no relation to quality): BioMedic High Density Gel;

Chanel Hydramax Balanced Hydrating Gel; Clinique Moisture Surge Treatment Formula; Estee Lauder Future Perfect Skin Gel and Clear Difference Oil-Control Hydrator; Lancome Oligo Major Mineral Serum, Vinefit Cool Gel, and Hydra Controle Oil-Free Fresh Gel; L'Oreal Revitalift Night; and Prescriptives Super Line Preventor.

## MAKEUP COLOR SELECTIONS FOR REDHEADS

**Problem:** I am a natural redhead and have problems finding makeup professionals who are trained to advise someone with my coloring (I have bright red hair, pale skin, and freckles). I've had lots of makeovers at department store makeup counters and always walk out looking either overly made up or wearing colors that clash with my hair! What colors do you suggest?

**Solution:** The answer to your question seems rather simple to me, so I'm not sure what's going wrong when you get your makeup done professionally. For you, the sheerest foundation is best. If a makeup artist is trying to cover up your freckles, he or she should be reprimanded. Neutral golden tan as well as shades of camel and chestnut brown for eyeshadows, blush, and lipsticks are made for your coloring. You can try a golden coral-brown for lipstick or blush if you want a dash more color. Although those colors are considered tried and true for redheads, there really is no color barrier these days when choosing colors. A vibrant red with a soft reddish-brown blush can look wonderful and quite dramatic on someone with your coloring. In the long run, experimenting until you find colors you're comfortable with is the best way to go.

When it comes to mascara, stay with brown and avoid black, which can be too hard a look on fair, freckled skin. Also keep in mind that makeup is not supposed to match hair color. A woman with gray hair doesn't need to wear gray colors, and you have alternatives, too.

## WHITER TEETH

**Problem:** I would so love to have a perfect white smile. I hate my yellowing, stained teeth. What should I do?

**Solution:** There are many reasons why someone may have yellow or stained teeth. Silver fillings might have grayed the surrounding tooth enamel, so replacing those fillings with the new tooth-colored material dentists use can make a world of difference. Lots of foods such as coffee, tea, and berries can cause stains. You can cut back on the foods causing the problem, but who's going to give up their coffee in the morning, much less fresh berries? Smoking is also a major cause of yellow and brown staining on teeth. And, unfortunately, some people just have natural yellow-colored teeth. Serious staining and discoloration (natural or otherwise) cannot be corrected with toothpaste, but some minimal improvement can be achieved with this kind of product. Colgate Total Plus Whitening Toothpaste is as good a place to start as any (Source: *Journal of Clinical Dentistry*, 2002, volume 13, pages 91–94).

Abrasive toothpaste can be a problem because over time the abrasives erode the surface of the tooth, and that can further complicate yellowing. The external part of the tooth is white, but underneath the white enamel is a yellow dentin core. The white part erodes naturally as part of aging, but it's speeded up by using hard toothbrushes or abrasive toothpaste.

For startling results that can make teeth whiter than you ever thought possible, one remarkable solution is to ask your dentist to bleach your teeth. Teeth-bleaching treatments used by dentists come in two forms, one you use at home and the other is done at the dentist's office. The whitening process done at the dentist's office can take several weeks, at about a half-hour per visit, for a cost of $300 to $800. The kit you buy from a dentist and take home uses a similar carbamide peroxide–based bleaching gel. Your dentist will fit a mouth guard to your mouth, and it must be left on for several hours over several days or nights. These at-home kits can cost between $300 and $400. The whitening effect can last up to 47 months in 82% of the patients who use it with no adverse side effects (Source: *Journal of Esthetic and Restorative Dentistry*, 2001, volume 13, number 6, pages 357–369). One major drawback of this process is increasing and even painful gum sensitivity.

The teeth-whitening kits with mouthguards that you buy at the drugstore ($15 to $25) use a substantially weaker hydrogen peroxide-based bleach and the mouth guard is not specially fitted to your mouth. If your teeth are even, that's fine, but if they aren't, the mouth guard will not fit correctly and you can get uneven results. The mouth guard the dentist makes for you is created from an impression taken from your mouth and has individual spaces for each tooth. If the teeth do not lighten evenly you can do extra treatments for only the teeth that didn't become light enough.

Bleaching or whitening strips were created to eliminate the problems associated with having to use mouth guards and a bleaching solution (not everyone is comfortable wearing a mouth guard). Whitening strips are available either over-the-counter or from your dentist. Both types of whitening strips use hydrogen peroxide to whiten teeth. The strips that are available from your dentist use a stronger concentration of hydrogen peroxide than those available at the drugstore. Both types of whitening strips can be very effective when applied twice daily for 14 days, yielding a highly significant improvement in tooth color versus baseline (Source: *Compendium of Continuing Education in Dentistry*, June 2000, Supplement, pages S22–S28). Drugstore versions will require more applications to net the same results as those from the dentist. Regardless of your choice there are definite drawbacks to these strips. They can leave a yellow area on the teeth near the gumline. Whitening strips also are limited because they can only cover the front teeth, which means only those will be lightened, leaving all the other teeth unaffected. Perhaps most discouraging is that whitening strips have a short shelf-life. This is because whitening strips use hydrogen peroxide as the active agent, and it is an exceptionally unstable ingredient. It can happen that by the time you find, buy, and start using your whitening strips the hydrogen peroxide may have become inactive. The teeth-whitening kits available through dentists have mouth guards that use carbamide peroxide, which is far more stable than hydrogen peroxide and has a very long shelflife.

It is important to keep in mind that none of these treatments is very effective if your teeth are grayed rather than yellowed, or if they are completely yellowed or have brown in color. Teeth-bleaching systems work best for partially yellow or food-stained teeth.

Other than bleaching, if the yellow or dull color of your teeth is from tartar buildup, get your teeth cleaned, and have them cleaned regularly. If you can, avoid foods that can grab onto teeth and make them look darker, such as chocolate, dark-colored berries, red wine, and coffee. Milk and rice can also bond to front teeth and cause a buildup of yellow tartar. Clearly, it is best to brush immediately after eating these foods, but if that isn't possible, rinse your mouth well with water and then chew sugarless gum. Many dentists recommend using the Sonicare electronic toothbrush as a way to prevent tartar or plaque buildup. You definitely cannot manually brush your teeth as well as the Sonicare can, and it is a worthwhile option to check out. And, above all else, don't smoke!

# CHAPTER 20

## ANIMAL RIGHTS

### BEAUTY VERSUS ANIMAL RIGHTS

Politically, I'm a moderate. I haven't always been. I grew up in the 1960s, and my politics have ranged from idealistic liberal to confused bipartisan. Now, as I stand loosely planted in the new millennium, I can earnestly say I am convinced that few, if any, issues in life are black and white, or all or nothing. I find more and more often that there is truth on both sides of the issues and the middle ground is often the only reasonable position. At least the middle ground is the only position that acknowledges the whole picture and not just one side.

This middle position also reflects my perspective on animal testing as it pertains to cosmetics products and the health-care industry. While I unquestionably advocate the humane and ethical treatment of all life, especially unprotected and dependent life, I am not in favor of eliminating all forms of animal testing when it comes to health-care issues or human safety issues.

I feel terrible pain and anguish when I think of animals suffering in any way so that I can put on mascara or clean my face. Many animal tests that are used to ascertain whether a cosmetic will hurt people are cruel and gratuitous. No one is ever going to eat 50 pounds of mascara. Forcing animals to do so in order to demonstrate how much mascara people can eat before they die makes me want to resign from the human race. How can anyone put an animal through such torture?

On the other hand, my older sister who had breast cancer, my father who had prostate cancer, my friends whose parents have suffered through Alzheimer's, my friends who have multiple sclerosis, and my brother-in-law who has diabetes all take or have at some point taken medication or undergone medical procedures that improved their quality of life or facilitated recovery. All of these medications and procedures had been proven effective and safe as a result of animal testing. I absolutely do not want to see even one animal die by being force-fed foundation or eyeshadow to prove a favorable formulation. Yet, if sacrificing an animal's life can help find the cure for Alzheimer's, prevent more cancers, or reduce the risks of high blood pressure and a host of other illnesses, I would and do support that research.

Most of us are aware of the dramatic pictures distributed by animal-rights groups showing the terrible torment of animals in research laboratories. They have exposed conditions that are indeed grotesque and painful and that all of us should be sickened by and do our best to change. But this narrow, shocking display does not address the positive results of animal research (the creation of safe products and medical treatments), nor does it represent the labs that treat animals humanely by caring for them and anesthetizing them.

Children who survive leukemia owe their lives to animal testing. Arthritis patients who can walk again owe their agility to animal testing. Successful excisions of brain tumors are due to animal testing, and on and on. Human health-care advancement and the use of animals to test various protocols and risks are inextricably linked and cannot be separated. This is the dilemma of animal testing.

There are many arguments surrounding this issue from both points of view. On one side are the animal-rights activists who claim there is no need or reason to ever use animal testing (or eat meat, use leather goods, or use animals for any purpose other than as pets). When it comes to animal testing, they point to alternative methods of research assessment that can be used. Spokespeople for People for the Ethical Treatment of Animals (PETA) and the National Anti-Vivisection Society (NAVS) claim that a preponderance of research proves that all animal testing is inconclusive and has no relation to what takes place in humans. Animal activists insist that all animal testing is motivated by financial profit and stubborn old-fashioned doctors or "good old boys" who refuse to change. Their reasoning is that animal testing is big business, and no one wants to alter what they are doing and potentially lose money.

On the other side are the vast majority of physicians, medical research groups from most major universities, national medical organizations representing everything from cancer to heart disease, and pharmaceutical companies, all of which believe the use of animal models for research is essential to evaluating new and old medical treatments and procedures. These physicians and organizations often agree that in vitro (test tube–oriented) tests and computer model studies can replace some animal testing, but definitely not all of it.

No one among these countless medical professionals would concede that all or even most animal testing is futile and immaterial. They can point to thousands of chemical substances and operations that were first determined to be safe and effective or dangerous and deleterious because of animal testing. Suggesting that these be stopped would halt most medical research, from AIDS to Alzheimer's, and the development of any new drug. Even physicians deeply involved in finding alternative research methods to replace animal testing would not agree that we should close the door to that ultimate and desirable goal.

The truth probably lies somewhere in the middle. Medical, pharmaceutical, and cosmetics industry experts freely admit that in the past, they were doing far more animal experiments than were needed to prove safety. Animal-rights activist campaigns inspired a vocal consumer base to force a major change in the number and type of animal tests being done. Many companies responded by reducing animal testing, changing to alternative methods whenever possible, and instituting humane treatment of their animals. Yet all or nothing is the goal of animal activists, and it may not be the goal of all consumers buying makeup, taking medicines, or considering medical procedures. Consumers should look at the whole issue, not just at shocking pictures.

For example, according to an article in the January 1997 issue of *Drug and Cosmetics Industry* magazine (*Drug and Cosmetics Industry* magazine's name has been changed to *Global Cosmetic Industry*), Gillette has been a boycott target of PETA since 1986. What PETA does not acknowledge is that, since its boycott, Gillette has reduced tests on animals by over 90%, has contributed millions of dollars to alternative research, and has donated over $100,000 to the Humane Society. You would think PETA would ease up on Gillette, but that isn't the case. It still lists Gillette among its companies to boycott. As long as a company does any animal testing, humane or otherwise, it is a target for PETA's condemnation. That is regrettable, because as a consumer you get only a limited perspective.

As a result of PETA's and NAVS's black-or-white position, you may be led to believe that The Body Shop is the greatest ally of animal rights since the inception of the concept. Yet, when faced with the publication of an article exposing The Body Shop's ambiguous animal-testing policy, owner Anita Roddick had her cabal of attorneys suppress the story from running in *Vanity Fair*. That only fueled the ire of reporter Jon Entine, who was then able to get his story published in *Business Ethics* and *Drug and Cosmetics Industry* magazines. It seems The Body Shop didn't want people to know its product development included use of ingredients that had been tested on animals; in fact, The Body Shop was banned from using the term "not tested on animals" on their products by West German courts in 1989. (The company subsequently began using the term "against animal testing.") According to a January 1997 article in *Drug and Cosmetics Industry* magazine, a research executive at The Body Shop in 1993 was quoted as saying that "the technology of alternative testing for raw materials has not yet sufficiently advanced to guarantee product safety." This story about The Body Shop was overlooked or completely ignored by both PETA and NAVS.

Most of us are against animal testing, but we also have the right to safe products and straight information about how that can best be accomplished. It would be wonderful if alternative, computer-based, and test-tube models were sufficient to establish a cosmetic, drug, or medical procedure's safety, but that doesn't seem to be true, at least not now or in the near future. If alternatives do become common practice, that will probably happen in the world of cosmetics first, mainly because cosmetics are not ingested and alternative research methods for irritation studies are showing promise.

Frank Fairweather, head of clinical and pathological programs at the British Industrial Biological Research Association, is a frequent spokesperson in Europe on alternatives to animal testing of cosmetics. In a presentation he made in 1996 at the Second World Congress on Alternatives to Animal Use in the Life Sciences, he said that "none of the alternative techniques could yet be reliably substantiated." He is hoping that research protocols can be quantified and then mimicked via in vitro methodology. At this point, procedures like this don't exist; however, he is optimistic that in the next several years tests will be developed that finally do away with the need for testing cosmetics on animals. I hope so, too.

I will continue to earnestly support the humane and ethical treatment of animals, but I do not at this time support a complete ban on animal testing. I personally do not use animal testing for any of my Paula's Choice skin-care products, either directly or indirectly (meaning I don't hire third-party testing facilities to do my testing for me). I use only proven, long-established formulations and ingredients, as do many other companies that make claims about no animal testing. But because all of the cosmetics ingredients currently in use have at some point been tested on animals, including everything from vitamin C to sunscreen ingredients, no one can claim that the ingredients in their products involved no animal testing.

By creating products that are not tested on animals and by my supporting through financial contributions such organizations as animal welfare groups and legal groups that fight for animal causes, I feel I am doing my part to help create a world where fewer and fewer animals will be used for testing, and those that are will be treated humanely and ethically every step of the way.

I want my readers to know that I believe their decisions and consumer activism in this area have been and continue to be vital. Cosmetics companies only started changing and looking for alternative methods because you, the consumer, brought pressure to bear and forced them to change. It is important to keep up this pressure. However, I feel it would be foolish to follow organizations like PETA and NAVS blindly unless you truly agree completely with their goal of abolishing all animal testing and creating a completely vegetarian or vegan society. **Instead, I encourage you to support organizations fighting for the welfare and safety of all animals, limited and humane animal testing, and continued research to find alternatives to animal testing in hopes that eventually someday no animals will have to be used in any research experiments.** This is completely in your power, because you, the consumer, have everything to say about what you buy and whom you buy it from, and your actions speak loudly and clearly to all kinds of corporations and enterprises the world over.